Changing
Perspectives
in Mental Illness

Changing Perspectives in Mental Illness

Edited by

STANLEY C. PLOG   *and*   ROBERT B. EDGERTON
Behavior Science Corporation   *Center for the Health Sciences*
Panorama City, California   *University of California, Los Angeles*

Holt, Rinehart and Winston, Inc.

NEW YORK · CHICAGO · SAN FRANCISCO · ATLANTA
DALLAS · MONTREAL · TORONTO · LONDON · SYDNEY

Copyright © 1969 by Holt, Rinehart and Winston, Inc.
All rights reserved
Library of Congress Catalog Card Number: 69–13563
SBN:03-074680-9
Printed in the United States of America
1 2 3 4 5 6 7 8 9

Contributors

Herbert Barry, III—UNIVERSITY OF PITTSBURGH
Ernest Beaglehole (deceased)—VICTORIA UNIVERSITY OF WELLINGTON
James H. Bryan—NORTHWESTERN UNIVERSITY
Fred R. Crawford—EMORY UNIVERSITY
H. Warren Dunham—WAYNE STATE UNIVERSITY
Troy Duster—UNIVERSITY OF CALIFORNIA, BERKELEY
Robert B. Edgerton—U.C.L.A. CENTER FOR THE HEALTH SCIENCES
Jerry Hirsch—UNIVERSITY OF ILLINOIS
Mildred B. Kantor—ST. LOUIS COUNTY HEALTH DEPARTMENT, MISSOURI
Ari Kiev—CORNELL MEDICAL CENTER
Harry H. L. Kitano—UNIVERSITY OF CALIFORNIA, LOS ANGELES
Robert J. Kleiner—TEMPLE UNIVERSITY
Thomas S. Langner—NEW YORK UNIVERSITY SCHOOL OF MEDICINE
Alexander H. Leighton—HARVARD SCHOOL OF PUBLIC HEALTH
Perry London—UNIVERSITY OF SOUTHERN CALIFORNIA, LOS ANGELES
Craig MacAndrew—U.C.L.A. CENTER FOR THE HEALTH SCIENCES
William Madsen—UNIVERSITY OF CALIFORNIA, SANTA BARBARA
Benjamin Malzberg—RESEARCH FOUNDATION FOR MENTAL HYGIENE, ALBANY,
        NEW YORK
Peter McHugh—YALE UNIVERSITY; HUNTER COLLEGE
Ivan N. Mensh—U.C.L.A. CENTER FOR THE HEALTH SCIENCES
Raymond J. Murphy—UNIVERSITY OF ROCHESTER
Harry G. Murray—UNIVERSITY OF ILLINOIS
Raoul Naroll—STATE UNIVERSITY OF NEW YORK AT BUFFALO
Marvin K. Opler—STATE UNIVERSITY OF NEW YORK AT BUFFALO
Seymour Parker—MICHIGAN STATE UNIVERSITY
Stanley C. Plog—BEHAVIOR SCIENCE CORPORATION, PANORAMA CITY (LOS ANGELES),
        CALIFORNIA
Bernard Rimland—INSTITUTE FOR CHILD BEHAVIOR RESEARCH, SAN DIEGO, CALIFORNIA
Alexander C. Rosen—U.C.L.A. CENTER FOR THE HEALTH SCIENCES
Theodore R. Sarbin—UNIVERSITY OF CALIFORNIA, BERKELEY
Edwin Schur—HARVARD LAW SCHOOL
L. Douglas Smith—VETERANS ADMINISTRATION HOSPITAL, PALO ALTO, CALIFORNIA
Leo Srole—COLLEGE OF PHYSICIANS AND SURGEONS OF COLUMBIA UNIVERSITY
A. F. C. Wallace—UNIVERSITY OF PENNSYLVANIA
John H. Weakland—MENTAL RESEARCH INSTITUTE, PALO ALTO, CALIFORNIA
Richard E. Whalen—UNIVERSITY OF CALIFORNIA, IRVINE

Preface

We became aware of the need for a volume of edited papers approaching concepts of mental illness from different perspectives through our involvement as instructors in the Training Program in Social Psychiatry at U.C.L.A. One of us was Associate Director of the program and the other was Research Social Scientist. Most of the trainees had strong backgrounds in mental health fields, but their concentration had been in the clinical practice of psychiatry and psychology. To introduce them to basic concepts of epidemiology and the multiple determinants of community pathology, it was necessary to assemble a large bibliography of references that often were difficult to locate and, when only a single copy could be found, impossible to use as basic source materials for an entire class. Many such works were not even appropriate because they dealt with esoteric problems or did not provide adequate summaries of the current status of research in the field.

Our search for suitable materials led to discussions with academicians and researchers in various mental health specialties who quickly revealed that they too felt a need for a reference work that would summarize much of current thought about the determinants of mental illness. The need was apparent to professors responsible for courses dealing with pathology and to investigators who wanted a reference work that quickly brings them up to date in specialized fields related to their own research interests.

Through these discussions we developed the outline of contributions included in this volume. At first we believed the volume should be updated every five years, but since the gestation process from inception to final production for the first edition has consumed more than six years, we doubt that any editor, new or old, will want to face the task so frequently.

The undertaking was far larger than either of us realized at first, and it would not have been possible without the help of many people. William C. Beckwith provided many useful ideas on the organization of the materials and the need for the inclusion of particular contributors. Theodore R. Sarbin reviewed the original outline submitted to the publishers and offered helpful suggestions on content, style, and format. Sascha Kaufman diligently uncovered new source materials on the history of epidemiologic research. Mildred Burkhalter guided the crucial work of reviewing galley and page proofs. And not to be forgotten are the patience and understanding of the individual contributors that have helped to sustain us through long delays.

In spite of this considerable amount of help, we alone assume responsibility for any shortcomings apparent to the casual or the involved reader. We have found, as we have explored these new fields of inquiry, that our old concepts and beliefs about mental health and illness have changed and that old certainties and convictions have disappeared. We can only plead with Goethe, "We know accurately only when we know little; with knowledge doubt increases."

Robert B. Edgerton
Stanley C. Plog

LOS ANGELES, CALIFORNIA
FEBRUARY 1969

Contents

PREFACE   *vii*

Introduction   *1*

chapter one
Theoretical Perspectives

1.1   Introduction   8

1.2   Orientation   *9*

1.2   The Scientific Status of the Mental Illness
      Metaphor · THEODORE R. SARBIN   *9*

1.3   Orientation   *31*

1.3   Morals and Mental Health · PERRY LONDON   *32*

1.4   Orientation   *48*

1.4   On the "Recognition" of Mental Illness ·
      ROBERT B. EDGERTON   *49*

chapter two
Does Culture Make a Difference?

2.1   Introduction   *71*

2.2   Orientation   *74*

2.2   Cultural Change and Mental Illness ·
      A. F. C. WALLACE   *75*

ix

2.3   *Orientation*   *87*

2.3   Anthropological Contributions to Psychiatry and
      Social Psychiatry · MARVIN K. OPLER   *88*

2.4   *Orientation*   *105*

2.4   Transcultural Psychiatry: Research Problems and
      Perspectives · ARI KIEV   *106*

2.5   *Orientation*   *127*

2.5   Cultural Determinants and the Concept of the Sick
      Society · RAOUL NAROLL   *128*

2.6   *Orientation*   *155*

2.6   Cultural Variations in the Development of Mental
      Illness · HERBERT BARRY, III   *155*

2.7   *Orientation*   *179*

2.7   A Comparative Study of Psychiatric Disorder in
      Nigeria and Rural North America ·
      ALEXANDER H. LEIGHTON   *179*

2.8   *Orientation*   *199*

2.8   Pathology among Peoples of the Pacific ·
      ERNEST BEAGLEHOLE   *200*

2.9   *Orientation*   *217*

2.9   Mexican-Americans and Anglo-Americans: A
      Comparative Study of Mental Health in Texas ·
      WILLIAM MADSEN   *217*

2.10   *Orientation*   *241*

2.10   Variations between Negroes and Whites in Concepts
       of Mental Illness, Its Treatment and Prevalence ·
       FRED R. CRAWFORD   *242*

2.11   *Orientation*   *256*

2.11   Japanese-American Mental Illness ·
       HARRY H. L. KITANO   *257*

chapter three
Social Complexity

3.1   Introduction   *285*

3.2   *Orientation*   *287*

3.2 Urbanization, Psychological Disorders, and the Heritage of Social Psychiatry · STANLEY C. PLOG 288

3.3 *Orientation* 312

3.3 Stratification and Mental Illness: Issues and Strategies for Research · RAYMOND J. MURPHY 313

3.4 *Orientation* 336

3.4 City Core and Suburban Fringe: Distribution Pattern of Mental Illness · H. WARREN DUNHAM 337

3.5 *Orientation* 364

3.5 Internal Migration and Mental Illness · MILDRED B. KANTOR 364

3.6 *Orientation* 394

3.6 Are Immigrants Psychologically Disturbed? · BENJAMIN MALZBERG 395

3.7 *Orientation* 422

3.7 Protestant, Catholic, and Jew: Comparative Psychopathology · LEO SROLE · THOMAS S. LANGNER 423

3.8 *Orientation* 440

3.8 The Aging Population and Mental Health · IVAN N. MENSH 441

3.9 *Orientation* 457

3.9 Social Mobility, Anomie, and Mental Disorder · ROBERT J. KLEINER · SEYMOUR PARKER 457

chapter four
Social Deviance and Mental Illness

4.1 Introduction 480

4.2 *Orientation* 482

4.2 On the Notion that Certain Persons Who Are Given to Frequent Drunkenness Suffer from a Disease Called Alcoholism · CRAIG MAC ANDREW 483

4.3 *Orientation* 501

4.3 The Addict and Social Problems · EDWIN SCHUR 501

4.4 *Orientation* 522

4.4   Mental Illness and Criminal Intent · TROY DUSTER   *523*

4.5   Orientation   *538*

4.5   Structured Uncertainty and Its Resolution: The
      Case of the Professional Actor · PETER MC HUGH   *539*

4.6   Orientation   *556*

4.6   Occupational Socialization and Interpersonal
      Attitudes: A Partial Failure in the Acculturation
      of High-Class Prostitutes · JAMES H. BRYAN   *556*

4.7   Orientation   *577*

4.7   The "Beats" and Bohemia: Positive Social Deviance
      or a Problem in Collective Disturbance? ·
      L. DOUGLAS SMITH   *578*

chapter five

Nature-Nurture and Perspectives on Pathology

5.1   Introduction   *594*

5.2   Orientation   *596*

5.2   Heredity, Individual Differences, and
      Psychopathology · HARRY G. MURRAY · JERRY HIRSCH   *596*

5.3   Orientation   *627*

5.3   The Determinants of Sexuality in Animals ·
      RICHARD E. WHALEN   *627*

5.4   Orientation   *653*

5.4   The Inter-Sex: Gender Identity, Genetics, and
      Mental Health · ALEXANDER C. ROSEN   *654*

5.5   Orientation   *672*

5.5   Schizophrenia: Basic Problems in Sociocultural
      Investigation · JOHN H. WEAKLAND   *672*

5.6   Orientation   *701*

5.6   Psychogenesis versus Biogenesis: The Issues and the
      Evidence · BERNARD RIMLAND   *702*

      NAME INDEX   *737*

      SUBJECT INDEX   *743*

Changing
Perspectives
in Mental Illness

Introduction

If we may harken back to the world of earliest man—perhaps to those curious small manlike creatures who lived in Olduvai Gorge more than a million years before our time—it is not at all far-fetched to imagine that some among them were as strange, as troubled, as troublesome, and as incomprehensible as some persons are in all human societies about which we have knowledge. So, too, we can readily imagine that these first men were concerned with taking action to reduce the strangeness, troublesomeness, and incomprehensibility of their fellows. We cannot know what words were used to describe these troubled folk, or what actions were undertaken in their behalf—or against them—but we can be certain that these men had words for troubled and troublesome people and that they took some actions toward them. So it is with modern man, and so, we suppose, it must always have been.

The history of man's concern with what we have come to know as mental illness is, like the history of most things, vast and largely unwritten. However important this history may be, our interest here is not with the history of man's understandings regarding mental illness, but rather with the prevailing state of knowledge among those men of today who have become involved in the study of mental illness. We have chosen this interest at this time because traditional understandings of mental illness are now being challenged, cherished beliefs have been assailed, and many established truths are being trampled in the relentless march and countermarch of competing ideas and evidence. It is commonplace to note that many fields in the sciences, or in the humanities, are in flux, for indeed many are undergoing change. The study of mental illness, however, is not experiencing any commonplace change—it is in the ferment of fundamental and far-reaching reassessment.

In the wake of this change, we begin to recognize the passing of those halcyon days when medical men had successfully arrogated to themselves the study of mental illness and had exclusively allocated the treatment of persons designated as mentally ill to a properly ordained medical specialty, psychiatry. To be sure, these days of medical monopoly over mental illness were not always completely tranquil, for there were problems which led to no little acrimony. However, these problems were usually confined to the sancta of medicine, where they were discussed, and sometimes settled, safely out of the scrutiny of nonmedical scientists and scholars. Occasionally, internecine problems became public, as those who have followed neo-Freudiana will recall, but the domain within which answers to such problems were properly to be found remained the domain of medicine. Outsiders sometimes railed against this medical monopoly—"intellectuals" assailed the theories upon which medical psychiatry was founded, the public complained about the care offered in mental hospitals, erstwhile patients likened psychoanalysis to alchemy, and jurists warned that psychiatry was poaching upon the realm of law —but their voices remained those of outsiders. If there were to be changes in the study of mental illness or the treatment of the mentally ill, these changes would take place within an appropriately enlightened psychiatry. Or, so it seemed. Thus, while psychiatry expanded greatly, it did so largely by annexing satellite fields such as clinical psychology, social welfare, nursing, and education, with the sometimes tacit, but usually explicit, understanding that both in development of theory and in treatment of patients medical suzerainty would prevail.

It may be stretching a point to argue, as several authors have done recently, that there is a revolution within psychiatry, but there may well be a revolution against psychiatry. Psychiatric dominion over the study and treatment of mental illness is being challenged as never before. Outsiders are now insisting that their right to explore man's mental condition is as legitimate as psychiatry's. As a result, the walls of the psychiatric citadel are being shouted down by an astonishing multitude of voices. Some of the most penetrating come from within, as from Thomas Szasz or the many others who have argued that psychiatric theory rests upon a quicksand of unproven assumption, and that psychiatric treatment works, when it works, largely through the operation of suggestion. But nonpsychiatric voices are creating an equal clangor. The credentials for psychiatric treatment are being claimed not only by clinical psychologists, psychiatric social workers, and others trained in approved procedures, but also by existentialists and religionists of every stamp. Those who now demand equal entitlement to study mental illness, or to discuss it, represent a bewildering variety of fields and professions.

The social sciences are particularly active, but so too are the more physical and natural sciences, among them ethology, zoology, and biochemistry. But not only the so-called sciences are involved. Philosophers, historians, lawyers, and humanists of many orientations have joined the chorus that is demanding a more comprehensive view of man's mental health and illness than traditional psychiatry has offered.

The outcome of this invasion of the province of psychiatry by so many nonpsychiatric disciplines is impossible to anticipate. There may be a détente that will permit a concerted attack upon the problem. And a problem it is, for even if we agree that mental illness is a misnomer, a myth, and a metaphor, it remains as a hard fact that our hospital beds are filled by patients whose infirmities are mental or social, not organic. But perhaps the babble of voices now heard will not coalesce into a stronger and clearer voice, perhaps the contesting views will separate into competing camps where differing orthodoxies will become established. We can offer no auguries here. We cannot even provide a comprehensive view of the present ferment, for it is too diverse and too complex to be reviewed in any single volume.

What we hope to accomplish is less ambitious but no less important. We hope to offer a glimpse into some of the changing perspectives in the study of mental illness by addressing ourselves to basic questions in the field of contemporary social psychiatry—questions that are of utmost import to all who are concerned by or who must contend with disordered behavior in a population of people, questions that demand answers before social psychiatry can demonstrate that it is a field of study deserving the attention of professionals and concerned laymen. Thus, this is not a book of case histories written by men whose clinical views of the world are often as confining as the four walls that serve as the habitat for their private practice in psychoanalysis or psychotherapy. This is a book by researchers impatient with the fact that so many men of today do not grasp the fact that man can only be fully comprehended by studying his intricate relationships to other men within a social or cultural context. Mental illness is a social problem, and it has social origins. This we cannot lose sight of.

Except for two chapters (modified for current publication), this is a book of original contributions. Our original letter to contributors stated what we continue to see as the central purpose guiding our efforts:

> The book to which you have been invited to contribute is intended to be a basic inquiry into the social psychiatry of mental illness. We hope to accomplish this inquiry by organizing a number of original writings around a set of basic questions and problem areas. We believe that the field called 'social psychiatry' is particularly beset by problems of inadequacy in conceptualization, theory,

method, and comparative substantive data. As a consequence, what is taken for granted in one discipline is challenged in another; what is accepted by some is rejected by others; and, what is accepted by *all* is by no means demonstrably true.

We believe that these problems are exacerbated by an insufficient exchange of information among interested disciplines. Thus, we hope that this book will provide a forum within which essential questions in social psychiatry can be exemplified, discussed, and debated. We expect that some postulates now taken for granted will be shown to be highly problematic and some apparently insoluble problems to be less refractory than had been thought; at the very least, we hope that a wide readership will be made aware of the basic questions that must be answered before social psychiatry can improve understanding of mental disorder. The purpose of the book is to present a stock-taking of current social psychiatric thought about mental illness. It would be useful if such an inventory could be taken each year, but we shall feel fortunate if someone performs this task every five years. Social psychiatry, as we think of it, is not exclusively a *medical* or a *psychiatric* discipline. To us, the term connotes a concern with those social forces that can contribute to the development of disordered or pathological behavior. There are other terms in common usage, but each has its self-limiting features. "Community psychiatry" more commonly refers to the *practice* of social psychiatry in community settings, and it specifically focuses on the amount and kinds of psychiatric services needed for the care of substantial populations of people. "Community psychology" is a vague reference to the fact that psychology is a Johnny-come-lately in the area of concern about community-based treatment for specific psychological disorders. The term is even more limiting in scope than "Community Psychiatry." Were it not for the fact that "social psychology" is the term applied to an established discipline with a history of concern about particular kinds of problems, that term might have served our purposes well. Beyond this, there are no other descriptive competitors. "Social psychiatry" at least has the virtue of implying that many social factors contribute to patterns of mental illness.

In organizing this book, we were forced to examine our own basic beliefs and biases before we could develop a final conception of the kinds of contributors and papers we wanted to include. Our primary questions are few, and they are reflected in the titles of each chapter. The first necessity was to ask some of the theoretical questions that continue to plague most investigators concerned with pathological behavior. Of primary concern is whether or not the term "mental illness" accurately reflects the phenomenon under study. The paper by Theodore R. Sarbin is addressed to this problem; not only is Sarbin's incisive analysis convincing in its logic and presentation of evidence, but it confronts us with a dilemma which pervades the entire book. Probably none of the thirty-five contributors is entirely satisfied with the connotations of "mental illness." Yet most authors, in this book and in others, continue to use the term, however hesitatingly, and we have used it in the title of this book. Our reason, developed after considerable debate and soul-searching, is that no other term in common usage conveys a similar meaning to most readers. "Mental illness" at least implies a prescribed field for legitimate study, with recognized professional disciplines in attendance, and it holds a widely understood meaning for the general public.

Following Sarbin's paper, we direct our attention to two related theoretical problems. Once having decided to live with the phrase "mental illness," we examine its *moral* implications and consequences in contemporary Western civilization (Perry London). Then we ask: Are there behaviors in primitive cultures that also are identified as mental illness, and what is the process through which such identification takes place (Robert B. Edgerton)?

Next, we turn our attention to one of the basic questions of this book: Does culture make a difference? We are concerned here with whether or not cultural differences are related to the amount or kind of mental disorders produced in a population, and in what way they are related to these disorders. The presentations are not meant to exhaust the world's cultural groups; rather, we have sought authors who have been deeply involved with this question, and whose views are based on years of research. A related subtopic is whether or not membership in an ethnic subgroup within a dominant population has important consequences for the production of mental illness in its members. Since the number of societies with their corresponding subgroups throughout the world is so vast as to preclude any thorough overview, we have limited ourselves to considering theoretically relevant questions about some of the major ethnic groups within the United States.

Our next major question area looks at "Social Complexity and Contemporary Life." Our previous concern with "culture" carries with it an underlying assumption about the relative stability of the various cultures compared. However, contemporary life is characterized by rapid technological and social change and the concomitant need for personal and social reorganization. Our questions are about the effect of such changes, and about whether or not man has the capacity to adapt to a world that offers relatively little stability, as compared with the world of his grandfathers.

Next, we turn our attention to the potential relationship between "Social Deviance and Mental Illness." Our reasons for treating this question as a major section heading in the book center around the fact that it is widely assumed that social deviance is rapidly increasing on a worldwide basis, and that this is a reflection of the increasing personal and social "stress" of living in complex societies. The crux of the discussion generated by such observations is whether deviant members represent a measure of the amount and kind of "pathology" of a society or subcultural group, or whether their deviance is an expression of "health" in breaking away from restrictive norms and social conventions. The latter assumption suggests that deviance may be a positive self-corrective mechanism for a society.

Our final major section, "Nature-Nurture and Perspectives on Pathology," reminds us that all behavior, however much it may be influenced by its social or cultural environment, still has a hereditary base. Thus, we need to understand the interactions of nature *and* nurture for an adequate understanding of the epidemiology of mental illness. Does one predominate over the other, or are there interactive effects? What is the status of current research and thought in the field? We believe that "social" psychiatry too often ignores this problem. Consequently, the discussions that we have included in this final section will be of value to a wide range of workers, researchers, and students concerned with mental health and illness.

In selecting the contributors for this book and in asking them to address certain general questions, we have had to omit much that is important. We have not, for example, dealt with the treatment of mental illness, except in passing. Neither have we examined the many public and polemic questions about mental illness that are now current. Furthermore, we have not even attempted to give all sides of the story that we have told. We have not, for example, made an extensive inquiry into the modern existentialist and philosophical contributions, nor have we attempted to represent the changing perspectives within psychiatry itself. We have not done so because we believe that existing books do so adequately.

Instead, we have concentrated upon the perspectives offered by the social and psychological or, if you prefer, the behavioral sciences. These perspectives are themselves immensely varied, and even within our prescribed area of concentration we have omitted much. We have not systematically covered research into early experience or socialization, again because existing books do so with more thoroughness than we could hope to match; and we have, this time unintentionally, scanted the work of psychiatrists. That so few of our contributors are psychiatrists is in part a reflection of our social orientation, but it is far more an accidental result of the relative availability of contributors to a book of this sort.

By including so few psychiatrists here, we do not mean to imply that they cannot escape a narrow medical perspective or that they have contributed little to a broadly social or behavioral perspective on mental illness. As this book amply attests, they have contributed much that is fundamental.

In what we present here there is no nostrum for the cure of all the ills of society, not even for the cure of those maladies that are mental. At best, we offer improved understanding of the social ambiance within which mental maladies arise and become problems.

chapter one

Theoretical Perspectives

1.1 Introduction

Many of us refer to *mental illness* with such sublime disregard for our own confusion regarding the meaning of the term that we violate the teachings of Ludwig Wittgenstein and confirm the wildest fantasies of Lewis Carroll. We display an inconsistency comparable to Polonius', when he so willingly saw in the same cloud anything that Hamlet suggested might be there. In like manner, we have come to see in mental illness as much or as little as fad, theory, or doctrinal zeal would dictate. We have been guilty not only of reifying a metaphor, but also of losing sight of the explanatory purpose the metaphor was intended to serve. Instead of explaining an otherwise disparate set of phenomena as "diseases of the mind," we have, like Procrustes, more often merely attempted to coerce an ever less similar set of phenomena under the authority of this label. As a result, there is a growing realization that the term *mental illness* is both more and less than we would have it be, and the concept has come under increasingly critical scrutiny.

It is only proper that a book purporting to examine mental illness begin with an examination of the term itself. This examination is no idle exercise in epistemology, for the term has come to have an enormous social reality with important moral and legal implications. The three papers of this section are concerned with metaphors and reality. The consistent threads are the authors' attempts to raise very basic, theoretical questions about what mental illness is and the fact that each author recognizes that metaphors become realities in the minds of the beholders, whether they are "mental health" professionals or members at large of a society. The ideas of Theodore Sarbin, Perry London, and Robert Edgerton are clear and logical statements of their positions on the issues, backed up by years of personal thought and research. Perhaps some of the most challenging conclusions of the entire book are contained in these early pages.

1.2 Orientation

Theodore R. Sarbin is not the first professional researcher to attack the mental illness model, or "metaphor" to use his term, of pathological behavior, nor will he be the last. In fact, he quickly recognizes some of the other professionals who have concerns similar to his. However, he has the capacity to provide persuasive arguments based on solid information, which is lacking in the presentations of most other critics.

Sarbin's basic thesis is that "mental illness" was first used to describe behavioral disorders for persons whose symptoms made them appear "as if sick," but that over a period of time the "as if" disappeared in usage and the metaphor seems to have become "real." He provides evidence for his position, dating back to the fifteenth century, and he traces the implications that such a metaphor holds for contemporary thought. Unlike most critics, he provides us with an alternative to the mental illness metaphor and spells out its social implications.

The concepts presented by Sarbin are central to nearly all theoretical considerations in a book of this type. For this reason, we have selected his paper as our first contributed chapter. We wholeheartedly agree with his criticism of the mental illness metaphor, but it remains to be seen whether or not his alternative will become part of the everyday vocabulary of the professionals who work with disordered personalities.

1.2 The Scientific Status of the Mental Illness Metaphor

Theodore R. Sarbin

INTRODUCTION

One of the most perplexing problems in contemporary behavior science is that of defining instances of conduct that are not easily assimilated to concurrent norms. The persons who exhibit such misconduct are frequently labeled disordered, insane, psychotic, mentally ill, crazy, lunatic, aberrant, deranged, and so on. The problem may be stated simply: Under what conditions should certain acts be defined as a basis for applying a label to a person, the result of which may have far-reaching consequences?

Our problem is not unique. In every age and in every culture, acts that violate certain (but not all) normative prescriptions pose a problem to the immediate or remote observers of such acts. The need to locate such misconduct on meaningful dimensions is as urgent for the illiterate Chukchee as it is for the modern behavior scientist. Perplexing conduct that cannot readily be accounted for by rule-following models—based on the concept that man's conduct is rational, purposive, and intelligible —invokes a *causal* explanation. When the observed conduct is an exception to a rule, and when the conduct under consideration is not inconsequential, a causal explanation *must* be invoked, and the posture of the observer reflects a *why?* or *what for?* question. Entrenched cultural thought models provide the starting point for such causal explanations.

We have fallen heir to a deeply entrenched thought model that is symbolized by the term "mental illness." Although the model is part of Everyman's stock of conceptual equipment, certain specialized agencies and professions employ it to form and to justify decisions about persons who fail to enact certain expected and required roles. More specifically, the person whose conduct is designated, through a series of inferential steps, as "symptoms" of "mental illness" is subject to isolation, segregation, degradation, incarceration, surgery, chemical and/or psychological treatment, and so on. The assignment of a person to the class "mentally ill" is its own warrant for decisions related to management and treatment. Historians of science have concluded that entrenched thought models of the type that includes "mental illness" are particularly resistant to change or abandonment. They become convenient myths that are unbending against the flow of rational argument or empirical nonconfirmation. It is not until a new metaphor is introduced and accepted because of its kinship to other tolerated or acceptable thought models that the old myth is exposed and exploded.

The mental illness model has been attacked from a number of quarters. Szasz (1963), Goffman (1961), Scheff (1966), and Sarbin (1964, 1967, 1968), among others, have argued that mental illness is best regarded as a myth; a myth that, among other things, supports the status quo in the medical profession, giving to physicians the power (and obligation) to pass judgment on the acts of others.

This chapter is intended

1. to uncover the metaphoric roots of the concept "mental illness" and to show, from our present perspective, how the metaphors were illicitly transformed and combined into a myth;

2. to review the social implications of maintaining the mental illness concept;

3. to propose a new metaphor for labeling persons whose actions embarrass, annoy, perturb, or endanger others; and

4. to sketch some of the heuristic and pragmatic implications of the new metaphor.

HISTORY OF THE MENTAL ILLNESS CONCEPT

The answer to our first question requires a brief excursion into historical linguistics. Where and when did the expression "mental illness" arise? We may stipulate at the outset that from the dawn of civilization individuals have performed acts that were judged by their contemporaries to be extraordinary, bizarre, inexplicable, and perturbing. Our concern is not with the truth of the statement that an individual's performances may set the stage for his being declared possessed, psychotic, or mentally ill. Our concern is with the cultural conditions that led our predecessors to regard the inexplicable event (1) as an illness or sickness and (2) as being located "in the mind."

Lest the impatient reader offer the criticism that semantic analyses fail to illuminate problems, let me declare that the choice of metaphor to denote a set of observations is not merely a rhetorical exercise. Every metaphor is potentially rich in connotations; each connotation is potentially rich in implications; each implication is a directive to action. Appropriate here is Szasz's argument (1961) that we regard deviant conduct as "problems in living." The connotations (and concurrent implications for action) of the predicate in the statement "He is mentally ill" are dramatically different from the connotations of the predicate in "He has problems in living."

It is important to note that the label "mental illness" represents a combining of two unrelated concepts, the mind and illness. Our first focus is on the illness concept; the mind will be discussed later. The basic referents for illness, and for synonyms such as sickness and disease, have not changed in any substantial way over the centuries. To medieval man, no less than to contemporary man, the referent for the symbol "illness" or for its cognate "disease" was discomfort of some kind, such as fevers, chills, aches, pain, cramps, shaking, and so on. Parenthetically, the word disease was originally equivalent to discomfort, or "not at ease" (dis + ease). Some of the meaning has been retained in "malaise"

(aise = ease). In both cases, the referent is a self-assessment through attention to compelling stimuli located "inside" the organism. These internal
(proximal) stimuli, when they occur simultaneously with dysfunction or
incapacity of bodily organs, are the so-called symptoms or signs of illness.
A diagnosis of illness or disease meant not only that a person complained
of discomfort but that the associated somatic dysfunction rendered him
incapable of performing some of his customary and expected roles. This
general paradigm of sickness, illness, and disease is widespread and may
be noted in ancient writings as well as in the observations by anthropologists of esoteric societies.

How did the class name "illness" come to include misconduct, a term
relating to behavior, rather than somatic symptoms and complaints, the
defining criteria of pre-Renaissance medicine? What other criteria were
employed to increase the breadth of the concept "illness" in the absence of
self-observations described as aches, pains, chills, fevers, or other dis-
comforts?

A search into historical sources suggests that the inclusion of conduct
disorders in the concept "illness" did not come about suddenly or accidentally. Rather, the label illness was at first used as a metaphor. As is
the case with metaphors, they are frequently transformed into reified
entities, thus setting the stage for myth-making. The history of the employment of the concept "illness" seems to fit this sequence.

The beginning of this metaphor-to-myth transformation appears to
have been an achievement of the sixteenth century. The demoniacal
model of conduct disorders, so thoroughly exploited in the fifteenth-
century *Malleus mallificarum,* had embraced all deviant or perplexing
conduct. The most significant outgrowth of this model was the Inquisition, a social movement that reached into every nook and corner of
Western civilization, including the diagnosis and treatment of perplexing
behavior, unusual imaginings, esoteric beliefs, and so on. Such diagnosis
(nearly always witchcraft) and treatment (invariably burning) was the
special province of the priestly hierarchy.

The sixteenth century witnessed a number of reactions against the
excesses of the Inquisition. The discovery and serious study of Galen and
other classical writers, the beginnings of humanistic philosophy, in fact,
the whole thrust of the Renaissance was opposite to that of the Inquisition.

One of the outstanding figures of this period was Teresa of Avila. Her
efforts to save a group of nuns from the Inquisition contributed to the
shift from demons to "illness" as the cause of conduct disturbances. The
nuns exhibited conduct that at a later date would have been called mass
hysteria, a condition arising from cloister life. By declaring these women

to be infirm or ill, Teresa could fend off the impending Inquisition. That illness is something that happens *to* a person, rather than something over which one has control, was (and is) the traditional and thoroughly accepted viewpoint. However, the appeal that a diagnosis should be changed from witchcraft to illness did not result from a direct straight-forward fiat. Rather, Teresa asked whether the observed behavior could be explained by *natural* causes. Among the natural causes that she sug-gested were (1) melancholy (Galenic humoral pathology) (2) weak imagi-nation, or (3) drowsiness. Persons whose conduct could be accounted for by such natural causes were to be regarded not as evil, but *comas enfermas* —"as if sick." By employing the metaphor "as if sick," she implied that physicians rather than priests should be the social specialists responsible for dealing with the problem (Sarbin and Juhasz, 1967).

When employing metaphorical expressions, there is a common human tendency to drop the qualifying "as if." That is to say, the metaphor is used without the label that designates it as figurative rather than literal. In the case of illness as a metaphor for conditions not meeting the usual criteria of illness, the dropping of the "as if" was facilitated by the practitioners of "physik" (predecessors to medical practitioners). It was awkward for them to talk about two kinds of illnesses, "real" illness and "as if" illness. The "as if" was dropped, especially when Galenic classifications were reintroduced. Thus, Renaissance and post-Renaissance practitioners could concern themselves with illness as traditionally under-stood and *also* with misconduct as illness. A review of the sixteenth- and seventeenth-century treatises on "physik" reveals clearly that Galen's humoral theory was widely accepted. In many cases, writers copied verbatim the declarations of Galen and of others of the Greco-Roman period. Hunter and McAlpine (1963), historians of psychiatry, in repro-ducing some excerpts from Barough (1583), explain that the treatise

shows the main divisions of mental and neurological disease based on Galen's classification which remained in use into the nineteenth century. Equipped with only the crudest notions of pathology, the presence or absence of fever measured by the pulse was the main diagnostic guide. In consequence there was much con-fusion between organic and nonorganic conditions; that is, between neurological and psychological disorders [p. 24].

That Barrough (and nearly every other writer on "physik") was influenced by Galen's humoral theory is readily documented. The point is clearly illustrated in the following description of "madness," one of a dozen disorders differentiated according to the then-current beliefs about the conditions, amount, and location of actual or imaginary humors within the body.

Mania in Greeke is a disease which the Latines do call *Insania* and *furor*. That is madnes and furiousnes. They that have this disease be wood and unruly like wild beastes. It differeth from the frenesie, because in that there is a fever. But *Mania* commeth without a feaver. It is caused of much bloud, flowing up to the braine, sometime the bloud is temperate, and sometime only the aboundance of it doth hurt, sometime of sharpe and hote cholericke humours, or of a hote distempure of the braine. There goeth before madnes debility of the head, tinckling of the eares, and shinings come before there eies, great watchings, thoughtes, and straunge thinges approach his mind, and heavines with trembling of the head. If time proceed, ther is raised in them a ravenous appetite, and a readines to bodily lust, the eyes waxe hollow, and he do nether wincke nor becken. But madness caused of bloud only, there followeth continuall laughing, there commeth before the sight (as the sicke thinketh) things to laugh at. But when choler is mixed with bloud, then the pricking and fervent moving in the braine maketh them irefull, moving, angry and bold. But if the choler do waxe grosse and doth pricke and pull the brain and his other members, it make them wood, wild, and furious, and therefore they are worst to cure.

Greco-Roman medicine provided Renaissance scholars with the basic model of illness, a model that continues into the present. The patient's complaints of pains, aches, fevers, and so on, are integrated with observations of skin color, pulse, respiration, and so on, and an inference is constructed as to the probable humoral imbalance. Similarities among persons in complaints and observed signs were taken to indicate similarities or identities in the underlying etiological agent—the presence or absence of humors in certain parts of the body.

The decline of the importance of the Church in matters of unusual imaginings and conduct was parallel to the rise of science. The prestige of the scientist and his utility in filling the gap left by the withdrawal of the temporal priesthood helped in establishing the model of Galen for all kinds of illnesses—those with somatic complaints and observable somatic symptoms *and* those without somatic complaints but with conduct disorders substituted for somatic symptoms.

Whereas the concept of illness had been satisfied by the exclusive use of conjunctive criteria (complaints *and* observable somatic symptoms), now it was satisfied by the use of disjunctive criteria (complaints and somatic symptoms *or* complaints by others of perplexing, embarrassing, or mystifying conduct). As a result of the uncritical acceptance of the humoral pathology of Galen as the overriding explanation for both somatic and conduct disorders, the latter became assimilated to the former. That is to say, to meet the requirements of the basic Galenic model, symptoms of disease had to be observed. So the form of the conduct disorder was regarded as if it were the observable symptom. Thus, the verbal report of strange imaginings, on the one hand, and fever on the other, were both treated as equivalents. As a result of shifting from a metaphorical to a literal interpretation of conduct as *symptom,* Galenic medicine embraced not only everything somatic but also all conduct. Now, any bit of behavior—laughing, crying, spitting, silence, imagining, lying, and believing—could be called a symptom of underlying, internal pathology.

Such a state of affairs held until the nineteenth century, when neurology, influenced by the development of the telephone, precipitated the distinction of organic and functional disorders. The former, of course, had demonstrable pathology, but the latter had no demonstrable organic signs. Organic medicine continued to use the conjunctive criteria of Galen: self-report of discomfort and observed symptoms leading to a search for neoplasms, germs, toxins, and so on. Probably because of the intrinsic dissimilarity of the "functional" disorders, psychiatry arose as a medical special that concerned itself exclusively with conduct perturbations as symptoms of underlying disorder. However, nineteenth-century replacements for humors, specific microbes, localizable neoplasms, and specific toxins, were inadequate to account for the behavioral symptoms of misconduct, particularly those bits of misconduct called hallucinations, delusions, phobias, and compulsions. In this connection, it is important to note that patients with somatic complaints in general seek out physicians for help. Patients whose conduct is not assimilable into current norms are usually referred to psychiatrists by relatives or law-enforcement agencies.

The basic Galenic model was not rejected by psychiatry and its immediate antecedents. Microbes, toxins, and growths, which were material and operated according to mechanical principles, were appropriate "causes" of diseases of the body. They were *inside* the body. The appropriate causes for abnormal *behavior* had to be sought along different lines. Since the dualistic mind-body concept was everyone's heritage, the hypothesis could be entertained that the causes of abnormal conduct, conduct already considered as nonsomatic disease, were *in the mind.* If this were so, then the most appropriate label for such nonsomatic diseases would be *mental illness.*

Before considering the meaning of "mental" in the phrase "mental illness," let me recapitulate. I have tried to show that "illness," as in "mental illness," was an illicit transformation of a metaphorical to a literal concept. To save unfortunate people from being labeled witches, it was useful to regard persons who exhibited misconduct of certain kinds as if they were ill. The Galenic model facilitated the eliding of the hypothetical phrase, the "as if," and the concept of illness was thus stretched to include events that did not meet the original conjunctive criteria for illness. A second transformation assured the validity of the Galenic model. The disturbing modes of behavior could be treated as if they were symptoms equivalent to somatic symptoms. By dropping the "as if" modifier, observed behavior was taken to be symptomatic of underlying internal pathology.

Our question has now become this: How did the notion of illnesses "of the mind" become so widely accepted that it served as the groundwork for a medical specialty? A searching analysis of the history of the concept makes clear that "mind" was originally employed as a metaphor to denote such events as remembering and thinking. (Colloquial English still uses mind as equivalent to remember, as in "mind your manners.") The shift of meaning to that of a substantive and an agency can best be understood as another instance of metaphor-to-myth transformation (Ryle, 1949).

The modern practitioner of Galenic psychiatry operates from the principle that the illness about which he is concerned is *in the mind* (or psyche, or psychic apparatus). Further, just as special techniques may be employed to examine the body, so are there special techniques for examining the mind. But the mind, even for Galenic practitioners, was too abstract and undifferentiated a concept. It had to have certain properties, just as the body had specific properties.

Since visual, palpable organs were obviously assigned to the material body, the differentiating characteristics of the invisible, impalpable mental entity were expressed as states. States of love, fear, anxiety, apathy, and so on were invented to account for differences in observed conduct. Since the mind was invisible and immaterial, it could not have the same properties as the body—properties that could be denoted by physicalistic terms. A new metaphor was required—the metaphor of states of mind. The practitioner now had the job of discovering through chains of inferences which mental states were responsible for normal and abnormal conduct.

For our purposes we can begin our linguistic analysis of mental states with the language of the Middle Ages. The natural history of word formation seems to be, first, the forming of words to denote objects and events in the distal environment, such as sun, fire, water, people, clouds, and so on. These distal objects are primarily mediated by the receptors of vision and audition. Later, terms are invented for denoting proximal events, such as pains, itches, pressures, soreness, and so on. Words already in existence to denote distal objects are borrowed through metaphor to denote proximal events. Just as distal events are mediated by visual and auditory receptors, proximal occurrences (and not mental states) are mediated by somasthetic receptors. The construction of a language to denote distal and proximal events was no mean achievement. Such a language served the purposes of men who had to communicate about things of importance to their survival.

The achievement of a language to denote mental states—the purported object of study by mentalistic specialists—required a tour de force, a special set of circumstances. What were these special circumstances? In short, how did the concept of mental states, whose relation to empirical events was unknown or presumed to be inconsequential, derive from the distal-proximal language?

Before the great religious and scientific transformations of the Renaissance, the language of conduct was essentially a distal-proximal language. The available stock of words denoted objects and events in the distal and proximal ecologies that had concrete reference. This is not to say that terms were not at hand for denoting imaginary things such as angels, leprechauns, and demons. However, these imaginary objects were regarded as if they belonged to the distal world, not to a shadowy inner world. A review of early writers, such as Chaucer, reveals almost no reference to internal mental states. The motivation to go on pilgrimages, for example, is in the world of nature and in the changing seasons—it is not a result of the activation of a special mental state.

Three developments contributed to the postulation of a mind as the repository of mental states—a postulation that made possible the further invention of illnesses of the mind: (1) a linguistic factor—the availability of dispositional terms, (2) the introduction of new terms of faith and religion that located religious experience "inside" the person, and (3) the development of scientific lexicon that tried to break away from theology.

(1) Dispositional terms are shorthand expressions for combinations or orderings of distal and/or proximal events—in principle a dispositional term may be reduced to a series of observable occurrences. For example, "courage" implies a set of concrete behaviors under certain conditions. There is no necessary implication that the referent is an internal mental state. The development of dispositional terms, however, appears to be a necessary (although insufficient) prerequisite for the postulation of mental states. In time, the detailed, concrete occurrences (for which the dispositional term is a sort of shorthand) became elided and remote from the original metaphoric beginnings. It is as if some dispositional terms were free-floating and distant from their empirical moorings.

(2) Terms of our second class were conveniently borrowed when religious conceptions shifted from emphasis on ritual and ceremony to "inward," personal aspects of faith. Theologians and preachers gave a new

set of referents to these dispositional terms, referents that changed dispositional terms from shorthand descriptions of conduct to descriptions of states of mind.

The context in which mental states are employed is best expressed by the polarity *inside-outside*. The problem for the medieval thinker was to find a model for locating events on the inside. Such a model could have been constructed from the following observations and inferences: Two classes of proximal inputs may be identified. The first occurs in a context of external events. For example, pain in the ankle occurs in a context of tripping over a curb; discomfort in the head occurs in the context of a blow from a baseball bat; a burning irritation in the fingers occurs in the context of accidentally leaning on a hot stove. The second class of proximal inputs occurs *in the absence* of recognizable distal events, such as toothache, headache, gastritis, neuritis, and so on. Since the antecedents of the latter inputs could not be located in the outside world by medieval man, the locus of the somatic perception was taken as the causal locus— inside the body. Medieval man had little reliable knowledge of anatomy save that there were bones, sinews, tubes, and fluids, and there were also empty spaces. Under the authority of the priests, he acquired the belief that an immaterial and invisible soul resided in these otherwise empty spaces. Within this system of beliefs, events for which there were no observed distal contexts could be attributed to the workings of this inner entity or soul. Proximal events that could not be related to occurrences in the distal environment were related to the spiritual happenings inside the person.

Such an analysis probably prepared the way for locating dispositions inside the person and calling them states of mind. If the cause of an event had no obvious external locus, then it must have had an internal locus. Dispositions, when they are codified as substantives, tend to be treated in the same way as other nouns, as possessing "thingness." Thus, courage, lust, conscience, purity, devotion, all dispositional terms originally tied to orderings of behavior were framed as nouns. If some nouns are names of things—and things are frequently located on spatial dimensions—then dispositional terms may refer to things that have location. But how to locate the disposition? In the same manner as locating the cause of pain in the absence of external occurrences—*inside* the person. Thus, anger, joy, courage, happiness, and so on came to be located in the soul.

(3) The displacement of theologians by scientists in the sixteenth and seventeenth centuries in matters pertaining to strange and mysterious conduct made necessary a shift from theological to scientific metaphors.

The soul had too much surplus meaning to be useful to materialist scientists. However, they could not break completely with the entrenched dualistic philosophy so well enunciated by Descartes. Renaissance scientists took as their point of departure the facts of thinking and knowing, and, as a substitute for the soul, employed mind as the organ for such activities. With the development of classical scholarship, Greek terms were substituted for the vernacular, the most popular being "psyche" (Boring, 1966). The efforts of the post-Renaissance Galenic practitioners, then, were directed toward analyzing states of mind and psychic processes. Those sequences of perplexing conduct that could not be related to external occurrences were declared to be outcomes of internal mental or psychic processes.

In the preceding paragraphs I have tried to show that mental states— the objects of interest and study for the diagnostician of "mental illness" —were postulated to fill gaps in early knowledge. Through historical and linguistic processes, the postulation was reified. Contemporary users of the mental illness concept are guilty of illicitly shifting from metaphor to myth. Instead of maintaining the metaphorical rhetoric "it is as if there were states of mind" and "it is as if some states of mind could be characterized as sickness," the contemporary mentalist conducts much of his work as if he believes that minds are "real" entities and that, like bodies, they can be sick or healthy.

IMPLICATIONS OF "MENTAL ILLNESS" CONCEPTION

Having sketched the metaphoric history of the phrase "mental illness," we now address ourselves to its implications. As was suggested earlier, the choice of metaphors is not inconsequential. The concepts embraced by a particular term contain their own implications; and implications are directives to action.

The most potent implication of the metaphor is that persons labeled mentally ill are categorized as significantly discontinuous from persons labeled with the unmodified term "ill." Of course, referring to persons as simply ill or sick suggests that they belong to a class different from the mutually exclusive class "not ill" or "healthy." Assigning persons to the class "ill" carries the meaning of objective signs and symptoms of a recognized or named disease in addition to subjectively experienced discomfort. In most societies, persons so classified are temporarily excused from the performance of selected role obligations. The label carries no hint of negative valuation. Sickness, in general, is something for which one is not responsible.

However, when the modifier "mental" is prefixed, a whole new set of implications follows. Contrary to the humane intent of those who resisted the diagnosis of witchcraft by employing the nonpejorative diagnostic label of illness, present usage is transparently pejorative.

In adding the word "mental" to "illness," the whole meaning-structure changes. In the first place, the necessity for adding a modifier to "illness" imposes a special constraint on the interpreter—he asks, "What is it about this person or his behavior that calls for a special designation?" Since it is a special kind of illness, does the same expectation hold that he is to be temporarily excused from the enactment of his roles?

The answers to these questions may be found in a number of studies (J. Cumming & E. Cumming, 1962; Nunnally, 1961; Goffman, 1961; Phillips, 1963). Persons who are labeled mentally ill are not regarded as merely sick, but are regarded as a special class of beings, to be feared or scorned, sometimes to be pitied, but nearly always to be degraded. Coincident with such negative valuations are the beliefs that such "mentally ill" persons discharge obligations of only the most simple kinds. Elsewhere I have argued that the process whereby a person is converted into a mental patient carries with it the potential for self-devaluation. The stigmatization, then, may work in the nature of a self-fulfilling prophecy (Sarbin, 1968).

Further, because of the inherent vagueness in the concept of mind, its purported independence from the body, and its permanence (derived from the immortal soul), there is a readiness to regard this special kind of sickness as permanent. Thus, a person who has a broken leg or suffers from barber's itch, that is, a sick person, may take up his customary roles upon being restored to health. A person diagnosed as mentally ill, however, is stigmatized. Although "cured" of the behavior that initiated the sequence of social and political acts that resulted in his being classified as mentally ill, his public will not usually accept such "cures" as permanent. It is as if the mental states were capable of disguising the person as healthy, although the underlying mental illness remained in a dormant or latent state.

Another implication of the mental illness concept, stemming from the demonstrated utility of germ theory for nonmental illness, is the internal causal locus of mental illness. The interior of the mind, rather than the interior of the body, is the object of study and inference. But that shadowy interior is not easily entered. The experts must depend on chains of inference forged out of the patient's verbal and nonverbal communications. From such communications, the experts draw conclusions about the mental structures, their dynamic properties, and their relation to observed behavior. One outcome of the exclusive verbal preoccupation with the interior of the mind is the neglect and avoidance of events in the exterior world that might be antecedent to instances of misconduct arbitrarily called symptoms.

The heuristic implications of the mental illness metaphor are no less important than the practical implications. Scientists of many kinds have discovered the causes for many (nonmental) illnesses by looking inside the body. By adding a postulate that all mental states are caused by organic conditions (the somatopsychic hypothesis) and also accepting disordered conduct as symptomatic of underlying disease entities, one is then forced to consider the corollary that the ultimate causal agents will be discovered through biochemical, toxicological, and bacteriological investigations. Again, such search methods deploy attention and effort away from the distal ecology as the source of possible antecedent conditions of misconduct.

A further implication of the illness metaphor is that physicians should be assigned the task of diagnosing and treating mental (along with nonmental) illness. But those persons assigned the mental patient role, characteristically allowed to meet only minimal social demands, required special kinds of medical treatment. Since the middle of the nineteenth century in the United States, such treatment has been carried on in asylums and hospitals where policies and practices were within the province of physicians. Szasz (1961) has convincingly discussed the biases introduced into legal procedures as a result of labeling a person "mentally ill."

It is interesting to note that a euphemism is only effective for a short time. "Asylums," at first a term used to suggest a haven of safety and security, deteriorated in meaning along with the degrading practices of the keepers and inmates. Its pejorative character made it inappropriate for the new humanism of such forceful figures as Dorothea Lynde Dix. "Hospitals" became the new euphemism. However, when "hospital" is now employed as in State Hospital or Mental Hospital, the image of bedlam is reconstructed, including locked wards, barred windows, keepers and wardens, and so on. The degraded status of the inmates has generalized to their institutional residences.

In the interest of brevity, we must eschew further discussion of the implications of the mental illness myth. To recapitulate, the choice of "mental illness" to denote conduct that violates certain cultural norms carries with it some definite implications for practice and theory. Among these implications are the following:

1. The diagnosis "mentally ill" is a pejorative; its use has the effect of publicly degrading a person and also of providing the basis for self-devaluation.

2. The belief in the "reality" of mind and mental states has directed the attention of scientists to the interior shadowy mind. The effect of this concern for the "inner life" has been a systematic rejection of possible causal factors in the exterior world.

3. The force of the illness metaphor is that physicians should be the specialists of choice. Along with this implication is the continued search for internal mental state causality on the model of germ theory.

4. Special kinds of illness require special treatment centers. Euphemistically called mental hospitals, such centers are managed by physicians and in the main serve merely to segregate the diagnosed mentally ill from the community.

A NEW MODEL: THE TRANSFORMATION OF SOCIAL IDENTITY

In the natural history of science, a myth is exploded when evidence of its inutility accumulates concurrently with the exposition of a new metaphor that better captures the essence of the events under examination. The remarks in the preceding pages were aimed at "undressing" the metaphor (Turbayne, 1960) of mental illness. The purpose of this undressing was to show that "mental illness," originally a pair of metaphors introduced to facilitate communication about certain kinds of conduct, has been transformed to the status of a myth.

Metaphors have great utility in opening new frontiers for exploration and in suggesting new directions for research and practice, as well as in modifying the connotations of a concept. The time has come for replacing the old myth with a new metaphor. The assertion can be readily supported that the mental illness model of dysfunctional conduct is no longer helping us to understand, predict, or control disordered behavior. The current trend for dealing with deviant and disordered persons is away from the tradition of the physician's being sought out by the patient or by his relatives. The efforts of professionals are no longer exclusively directed toward the more dramatic instances of disordered conduct for which our predecessors coined sesquipedalian Greco-Latin terms such as agoraphobia, pyromania, catatonic schizophrenia, and psychasthenia. Modern efforts are directed toward controlling the mystifying conduct denoted by such opaque metaphors, as well as the garden varieties of disordered behavior. The grand strategy is to reach out into the community and help those people who lead lives of quiet desperation, some of whom occasionally break out of their social entrapment with bizarre conduct or violence. To be effective, this new strategy must take into account two postulates: (1) that man as a social creature must confront and solve certain ongoing problems, and (2) that man as a social creature acquires modes of solving problems that may be successful under some conditions and not successful under others. These postulates are irrelevant to practitioners and theorists of Galenic medicine, whether ancient or contemporary.

As a replacement for the older concept, I propose that disordered conduct follows from, or is concurrent with, attempts to solve certain problems generated in social systems. The metaphor of choice is "the transformation of social identity." The conception flows from a dramaturgical stream of ideas. The establishment of a social identity occurs in a context of enacting roles in such a manner as to make good one's granted and attained roles. The dimensions of social identity are formed out of the components of the role system in which the person operates.

Borrowed from the theater, role is a metaphor to suggest that public conduct is associated with certain "parts" or statuses rather than with the players who recite their "parts." The guiding motive to the writing and later acting of such parts was the conduct of representatives of mankind struggling to make their way in imperfectly organized social systems. Thus, there is a continuity in the role metaphor: from problem-solving in social life to the drama, and from the drama to a theory about persons enacting real life drama (Sarbin & Allen, 1968).

A basic postulate in the proposed model is that human beings act to locate themselves accurately in their environments. In order to make efficient choices from among behavior alternatives, a person must locate himself with regard to the world of occurrences. This world may be differentiated into a number of ecologies, among them the social ecology or role-system. Constantly faced with the necessity of locating himself in the role system, any misplacement of self may lead to embarrassing, perilous, or even fatal consequences.

Locating oneself in the social system follows from an inferential process: on the basis of clues available and of his knowledge of the role system, the individual infers the role of other and concurrently of self. The essence of the process of locating oneself in the social system is caught in the efforts of a person to find answers to the question "Who am I?" The answer is achieved in locating answers to the reflexive question "Who are you?" Finding one's place in the social system is a reciprocal event—the answers to the question "Who am I?" are determined by the answers to the question "Who are you?" and vice versa. *It is the totality of such answers that defines a person's social identity.*

Answers to "Who am I?" questions are drawn from the categories of the role system, such as name, age, sex, occupation, memberships, religious affiliation, marital status, and political party affiliation. It is important to note that all role categories imply relationships—there can be no role of teacher without the complementary role of student, no role of mother without the role of child, and so on. Further, such relationships are imbedded in the social systems in which the person operates.

Role-relationships being the definers of one's social identity, planned or unplanned changes in role-relationships will alter the answers to the "Who are you?" questions and the simultaneous inferences about social identity. Changes in social identity are the rule, occurring with changes in the roles of complementary others, for example, one's location in social space is different when one interacts with an adult and with a child. Such ordinary shifting of perspectives do not lead to dysfunctional conduct. To understand disordered conduct with the aid of social identity concepts requires that we construct a set of dimensions that make it possible to determine the relative contribution of *particular roles* to one's social identity; further, these dimensions should facilitate recognition of the effects of shifting one's placement in the role system. For this purpose, we have constructed a three-dimensional model that provides the means for assessing the total value of a person's social identity at any point in time (Sarbin, Scheibe, & Kroger, 1965; Sarbin, 1968). The three dimensions are (1) the status dimension, (2) the value dimension, and (3) the involvement dimension. The appropriateness of this model to displace the mental illness model will become apparent in the following paragraphs.

The term status is used in the sociological sense as being equivalent to position in a social structure. The relationship between role and status is governed by the conventional definitions: A status or position is an abstraction or set of beliefs defined by the expectations held by members of the relevant society; role is a set of public modes of behavior enacted by an individual in order to make good his occupancy of a particular status or position. Another way of differentiating among these related concepts is to regard position or status as a cognitive notion, a set of expectations that is carried around in one's head; and to regard role as a unit of conduct, characterized by overt actions. The point of departure is Linton's classification of statuses (and their corresponding roles) as *ascribed* or *achieved*. For conceptual analysis Linton separated statuses that are defined by biological characteristics, such as age, sex, and kinship, which he called *ascribed,* from those statuses characterized by attainment or option, which he called *achieved*. Examples of ascribed statuses are mother, son, adult, child, uncle, male, and female; of achieved statuses, physician, high school student, and voter (Linton, 1936). This two-valued dimension is too limiting, primarily because of instances that show the contribution of both ascriptive and achievement factors. Rather than being two-valued, the dimension is a continuum. The underlying conception is the degree of choice prior to entry into any particular status. At one end point of the dimension are statuses *granted* an individual simply by virtue of his membership in a society, that is, *cultural man,* or *person,* sex roles, age roles, and kinship roles are in the same region. The other end point is defined by statuses that involve high degrees of choice, such as member of the Book of the Month Club. Several paths lead to adopting a role at the choice end, among them, election, nomination, training, revelation, and achievement.

At the granted end, statuses may be further defined as less differentiated. These statuses apply to large numbers of participants in a culture. Thus, every adult member of a culture is, in principle, granted the minimal status of cultural participant or person; that is, he is expected to perform according to certain propriety norms that take priority over specific expectations attached to any attained or choice status. By the same token, the occupant of this granted status of person may lay claim to certain minimal rights.

At the achieved end of the continuum, statuses may be additionally defined as optional and highly differentiated, their requirements applying to a very small number of potential candidates. Examples would be Pulitzer Prize winner, a skating champion, and Prime Minister of Great Britain. The dimension is highly correlated with legitimate power and social esteem. In addition to the bare minima of rights granted by virtue of an individual's holding the granted status of person, he acquires grants of legitimate power and esteem according to the location of his statuses toward the achievement or choice end of the dimension. Thus, the social identity we assign an individual will in general include several roles located at different points on the status dimension, some carrying explicit grants of power and esteem, others little or none.

The model becomes more useful when we add the second component: the value dimension. At the same time that role-enactments provide the basis for locating an individual's identity on the status dimension, they provide the basis for declarations of value. The value continuum is constructed at right angles to the status continuum. It has a neutral point and positive and negative end points. The range of potential value, in this model, is different for the *performance* of roles and for the *nonperformance* of roles at different points of the status dimension.

First, consider the range of potential value to be applied to the occupancy of statuses at the achievement end: The valuations declared on nonperformance or poor performance tend to be neutral. In general, negative valuations are not applied to persons whose enactments do not validate statuses heavily weighted with choice, such as occupational and recreational statuses. Being laid off from a job, dropped from a team, or dismissed from school does not enrage or perturb a community. The responses to such outcomes of nonperformance may be formalized as failure, underachievement, poor judgment, or misfortune. On the other hand, the *proper* performance of role behaviors at the choice end earns high positive valuations, such as Nobel prizes, public recognition, and monetary rewards. For role-enactments that validate achieved statuses, then, the range of potential value is from neutral to positive.

Now consider role-enactments aimed at validating statuses that are primarily ascribed or granted. Little or no positive value is declared for the enactment of granted roles. An individual is not praised for participation in a culture as a male, an adult, a father, a person. One is expected to enact such roles without positive public valuations. The *nonperformance* of such roles, however, calls out strong negative valuations. Common examples are the male who fails to perform according to the expectations for masculine sexuality, the mother who fails to be interested in the care and welfare of her children, persons who fail to act according to age standards or to kinship norms. The status of *person*—the very end point of the first dimension—carries with it expectations that the status occupant will engage in role behavior to meet minimal expectations. These expectations may be listed as *propriety norms* dealing with age-sex graded behavior, with kinship, and with reciprocal social interaction (communication), modesty, property, and ingroup aggression. When these role-requirements are perceived as being violated, the individual holding the minimal granted position is negatively valued and marked with a pejorative label. There are many forms of the label and they all denote the social identity of a nonperson. That is to say, if the pejorative label is applied by a person who is granted the power to apply such labels, then the society goes to work to treat the individual as if he were a nonperson. The term most widely used to represent nonperson is brute, sometimes rendered as beast, animal, or low-grade human (Platt & Diamond, 1965). The reason that such labels are not a part of our scientific and professional lexicon is that we have coined special euphemisms that for a short time attenuate the strong negative valuational component— for example, patients, wards, lunatics, slum-dwellers, inmates, schizophrenic, psychotic, rabble, charity cases, paupers, mentally ill, welfare recipients, and so on. These labels carry much of the meaning of nonperson—the labeled individual is likely to be handled as if he were without grade on the first dimension and with negative value on the second. The pejorative labels provide a means of codifying answers to the "Who are you?" question *and to designate a degraded social identity*.

Parenthetically, it is interesting to speculate about the motivational theories brought forward to account for the nonperformance of granted roles, on the one hand, and for the nonperformance of chosen roles, on the other. The latter case is seldom taken as a starting point for elaborating a causal theory. When a champion loses his title, an industrial executive is demoted, or a politician defeated, explanations are drawn from rule-following models. Failure is attributed to lack of practice, aging, superior competition, economic considerations, and so on. The nonperformance of granted roles, however, calls out explanations of a causal kind, such as heredity, humoral displacements, somatotypes, unconscious conflicts, toxins, psychic forces, psychosexual complexes, and so on (Peters, 1958). From Galen to Freud, causal explanations have been proferred for nonperformance of granted roles.

Involvement, the third component, may be recognized in two ways: (1) the amount of *time* a person devotes to certain role-enactments, and (2) the degree of *organismic energy* expended. An individual whose identity includes a status at the achievement end of the continuum may sometimes be highly involved in the role-enactment and not involved at other times. In short, the possibility exists for variation in time and energy expended in enacting attained roles. A teacher may be highly involved in his role when in the classroom, in the library, or when grading term papers. He may be relatively uninvolved in the teacher role when listening to music, when selecting a wardrobe, or when visiting friends. At the ascribed or granted end, involvement is typically high. To be cast in the role of adult male, for example, means being in the role nearly all the time. To be cast in the role of "old maid," similarly demands high involvement. To be cast in the extreme granted role of person, or its negatively valued counterpart, nonperson, similarly means being in role all the time. Examples of roles that are highly involving and without choice are prisoners in maximum security institutions, committed inmates of state mental hospitals, inmates of concentration camps, and unemployed workers in urban ghettos. The social identity of a member of these classes of persons includes few, if any, achieved roles, the enactment of which is cyclical. Legitimate opportunities for obtaining role-distance, in Goffman's (1961) terms, are absent when one's identity is composed exclusively of granted roles.

People with degraded social identities are the potential, if not the actual, candidates for the diagnosing, judging, helping, and treatment facilities usually called "mental health services." From the preceding remarks, it follows that to degrade an individual's social identity, one need only remove from him the opportunity to enact roles that have elements of choice. The more one's identity is made up of granted roles, the fewer opportunities he has of engaging in role behavior that may be positively valued. The best he can hope for is to be neutrally valued through the proper, appropriate, and convincing enactment of his granted roles, all of which are highly involving. Such a state of affairs is achieved, if at all, only at the cost of high degrees of strain, a neutrally valued social identity being the maximum possible reward. At what point does the individual raise the question of whether the payoff is commensurate with the high degree of strain? Indexes of social pathology are highest among populations that exhibit these characteristics. If a man's job and other vehicles of his achieved identity are removed, he has few chances of displaying conduct that may be positively valued by self or relevant others. The difference is only one of degree between the unemployed urban ghetto dweller and the more commonly used examples of degraded identities, inmates in a maximum security prison, patients in back wards of mental institutions, and prisoners of war in thought-control camps. Totalistic social organization and control of achieved statuses leads to extreme degradation, to the identity of a nonperson.

The differences in degree between these totalistic settings and the settings that induce norm violations in persons often labeled "mentally ill" are reflected in the fact that the relevant societies are not completely totalistic. During their early socialization experiences, these potential norm-violators acquire beliefs that they may someday perform roles-by-choice and thus attain a valued social identity. First, in the bosom of the family, then in the early years of street and community play, then through the mass media, the child is led to believe that he has a chance to occupy statuses that have achieved as well as granted components. Such a system of beliefs might be compressed into the following premise: *In addition to being a person, a male, a son, and so on, I am a worthy and valued member of society.* Relevant others in the social ecology, however, withhold confirming positive valuations because the individual does not in fact occupy achieved statuses. A contrary premise is thus formed: *I am not a worthy and valued member of society.* Such paired contrary premises are the conditions of cognitive strain (Sarbin, 1964)—a state of affairs for which the common word *problem* is a more felicitous expression than *sickness.*

Parallel to the restrictions in the range of values assignable to occupants of granted statuses are restrictions imposed on the form and content of problem-solving. The social networks of individuals valued for their performances of roles-by-choice provide large numbers of avenues for reducing strain and reconciling contrary premises. The social networks of degraded individuals are limited—usually to individuals whose identities are made up exclusively of granted roles.

In addition, the social conditions that promote degradation also retard development of differentiated concepts and modulated action (Bruner,

1961; Bernstein, 1960; John & Goldstein, 1964). For this reason, the employment of universal adaptive techniques to reduce strain, to find solutions to problems, tends to be more extreme among degraded people. Their use of instrumental acts, for example, tends to be unmodulated by verbal controls. Thus, they are described as assaultive and violent. Their use of attention-deployment is more likely to be focused on syncretic imaginal products: traditional diagnosticians call them hallucinators or schizophrenics. Their use of the releasing powers of unregulated motoric activity (as in spontaneous dancing) is characteristically without well-defined social or verbal controls; they are called "acter-outers." Their use of the tranquilizing features of sleep, sex, and drugs tends toward the extreme: they are diagnosed as escapists. Their use of superordinate belief systems to reconcile contrary premises tend to be messianic, fundamentalistic, and highly personalized: they are labeled superstitious or delusional.

The implications of this model—designed to displace the entrenched mental illness model—are transparent. In the first place, our technique for case-finding is to be guided by a theory of social identity and the socially dysfunctional outcomes of degradation. That is to say, we would try to locate those individuals and groups whose efforts to establish acceptable social identities have been unsuccessful. These persons would show the characteristics of degraded identities, as indicated before. In the second place, the theory makes possible the construction of a set of propositions to be tested empirically. These propositions include hypotheses about the behavioral effects of prolonged degradation, the outcomes of upgrading social identities through commendation, promotion, and so on. Further, the heuristic implications are not to be minimized. The search for "causes" will be in social systems, not in mythic internal entities.

The process of reorganizing conduct takes on a new set of characteristics. In the place of "psychotherapy"—a derivative of Galenic medicine—opportunities arise for the use of a social systems approach. Rather than direct the efforts of the helping professions to the "insides" of the individual, the focus is the role-set, the constellation of persons in complementary and reciprocal relations one to the other (Kahn, Wolfe, Quinn, Snoek, & Rosenthal, 1964). Further, the degradation and upgrading metaphors suggest an entirely new approach to behavior change or conduct reorganization. From an analysis of systems of behavior change that have been successfully employed in religious, military, and other non-medical settings, we have been able to isolate components that bear a striking resemblance to the components of the model presented here under the heading: the transformation of social identity (Sarbin & Adler, 1967).

SUMMARY

Traditional metaphors for conceptualizing socially dysfunctional conduct are unsatisfactory. The illness and mind metaphors have led us astray. We suggest a fresh perspective—that we follow the implications of social role theory and concern ourselves with the shaping and transforming of social identities. To approach the etiology of dysfunctional conduct, we must take into account the effects of the degradation of social identities. The new metaphors must flow from a comprehensive social theory; they must replace "mental illness"—the older metaphor-turned-myth, the heritage of Galenic medicine.

REFERENCES

Bernstein, B. Language and social class. *British Journal of Sociology,* 1960, **11,** 271–276.

Boring, E. G. A note on the origin of the word psychology. *Journal of the History of the Behavioral Sciences,* 1966, **2,** 145–147.

Bruner, J. S. The cognitive consequences of early sensory deprivation. In P. Solomon (Ed.), *Sensory deprivation.* Cambridge, Mass.: Harvard University Press, 1961. Pp. 195–207.

Cumming, J., & Cumming, E. *Ego and milieu.* New York: Atherton Press, 1962.

Goffman, E. *Asylums.* Chicago: Aldine, 1961.

Hunter, R. A., & MacAlpine, J. *Three hundred years of psychiatry.* New York: Oxford University Press, 1963.

John, V. P., & Goldstein, L. S. The social context of language acquisition. *Merrill Palmer Quarterly,* 1964, **10,** 265–276.

Kahn, R. L., Wolfe, D. M., Quinn, R. P., Snoek, J. D., & Rosenthal, R. A. *Organizational stress: Studies in role conflict and ambiguity.* New York: Wiley, 1964.

Linton, R. *A study of man.* New York: Appleton-Century, 1936.

Nunnally, J. C. *Popular conceptions of mental health.* New York: Holt, Rinehart & Winston, 1961.

Peters, R. S. *The concept of motivation.* London: Routledge & Kegan Paul, 1958.

Phillips, D. L. Rejection as a consequence of seeking help for mental disorders. *American Sociological Review,* 1963, **28,** 963–972.

Platt, A. M., & Diamond, B. L. The origins and development of the "wild beast" concept of mental illness and its relation to theories of criminal responsibility. *Journal of the History of the Behavioral Sciences,* 1965, **1,** 355–367.

Sarbin, T. R. Anxiety: the reification of a metaphor. *Archives of General Psychiatry,* 1964, **10,** 630–638.

Sarbin, T. R. The concept of hallucination. *Journal of Personality,* 1967, **35,** 359–380.

Sarbin, T. R. Notes on the transformation of social identity. In L. M. Roberts, N. S. Greenfield, and M. H. Miller (Eds.), *Comprehensive mental health: The challenge of evaluation,* Madison: University of Wisconsin Press, 1968.

Sarbin, T. R. Role-theoretical analysis of schizophrenia. *Journal of Personality,* in press.

Sarbin, T. R., & Adler, N. Communalities in systems of conduct reorganization. Paper read at the meeting of California State Psychological Association, Jan., 1967.

Sarbin, T. R., & Allen, V. L. Role theory. In G. Lindzey & E. Aronson (Eds.), *Handbook of social psychology,* Vol. I. Cambridge: Addison-Wesley, 1968, pp. 488–567.

Sarbin, T. R., & Juhasz, J. B. The historical background of the concept of hallucination. *Journal of the History of the Behavioral Sciences,* 1967, **3,** 339–358.

Sarbin, T. R., Scheibe, K. E., & Kroger, R. O. The transvaluation of social identity. Ms., 1965.

Scheff, T. J. *Being mentally ill: A sociological theory.* Chicago: Aldine, 1966.

Szasz, T. S. *The myth of mental illness.* New York: Hoeber, 1961.

1.3   Orientation

It is only in recent years that social scientists have recognized that the existence of the mental health movement presents special moral and ethical questions. Critics of current practices for the care, treatment, and diagnosis of the mentally ill no longer are a small minority of the disgruntled or malcontent. Rather, thoughtful and concerned citizens from all walks of life and professions are raising serious questions about the direction of the mental health movement in America, and its potential influence on our basic social fabric.

Perry London, who has written extensively in the area of the moral problems confronting professionals in the mental health fields, points out some of the important questions that all practitioners must face. How much destructive deviance can any society tolerate? Is good mental health merely good citizenship? Where does the ultimate responsibility of a psychotherapist lie, to the individual or to the larger social group, when the values or behaviors of his patient run counter to the best interests of society? When is "social engineering" justified? Are there important differences in the ways that mental health experts respond to their patients on the basis of their personal value systems or kind of professional training.

London presents a lucid conceptual analysis of these and other problems. The important ethical, political, and social issues are raised and examined in light of contemporary practicing psychiatry and psychology, and a conceptual framework is provided for interpreting the trends and counter-trends in the mental health movement.

1.3   Morals and Mental Health[1]

Perry London

Almost any human problem with many different and difficult possible solutions has some moral implications, because morals are the main systems by which people evaluate what they ought and ought not to do. This essay concerns some of the moral issues raised by problems of mental health and illness and the things that are done about them in America.

Mental illness is as much a social as a personal problem, partly because it is epidemic, and therefore costly to society, but also because its symptoms are not disorders of body but of behavior, as likely to make their victim offend society as withdraw from it. It is here, in the ambiguous encounter between individuals and institutions, that the moral issues of mental illness are mostly joined. Professional healers, with their investments in preventing, treating, and profiting from mental illness, must confront this ambiguity when the needs of their patients are incongruent with the demands of society. Society's agents, chiefly its police and welfare workers (and ultimately its lawyers), routinely must present ad hoc solutions to the threat of destructive deviance implicit in the forms of aberration they most often see—and must do so without knowing whether to loathe or pity the strange, suffering people they inevitably fear. Meanwhile too, special auxiliary groups of public spirited laymen play an enthusiastic but ill-defined role in the widespread but ill-defined struggle against these maladies.

Each of these perspectives—the social, the professional, and the aux-

[1] The preparation of this material was supported by a Public Health Service Research Scientist Development Award No. K3-MH-31, 209, from the National Institute of Health.

iliary—lends itself to somewhat different ambiguities, crises, and resolutions, to different tensions and equilibriums, and thus to different focuses of moral concern. Their examination forms the body of this work.

THE SOCIAL PROBLEM

The attitude of an organized society toward mental illness is a special case of its general moral outlook on the relation of the individual to the group. Societies are naturally conservative; their functions cannot be organized and regulated unless people can be depended on to adopt common public practices and to avoid deviating from them unexpectedly. For the group establishment to serve the interests of its individual members, they must share enough common causes to permit an establishment to work.

But even the best social organization, it seems, is purchased only at the cost of the ease with which individuals could once dissent or withdraw from the group. Eventually, customs become laws, plausible conveniences turn into moral proprieties, and trivial habits into public manners—until any irregular and deviant public behavior by individuals may seem to threaten the organization of society and create suspicion and alarm. Such is the case with the mentally ill.

Mental illness threatens society in two general ways. One is economic: it is the threat to productivity that exists when large numbers of people in the labor force are disabled. The economic loss from mental illness in America is great, but certainly not crippling and probably not widely recognized. The second source of threat is psychological: it is the socially deviant, nonconforming, unpredictable nature of mental illness which, translated politically, ultimately threatens the power structure of society. Operationally, these both reduce to the fact that mentally ill people do not behave in ways expected of regular citizens; it is the fact of *deviance,* not of *disability,* that finally makes them the objects of tense public concern.

A society's potential sufferance of individual dissent depends partly on its population density and technological development. A small, technically primitive social organization cannot function very well if any of its members fail to do their assigned jobs, regardless of the reasons for their failure. If the food-getting member of a three-man society goes on strike, for example, the consequences for the others may be disastrous, and their demands that he resume work will not be stilled by his insistence on his individual moral prerogatives. In a technically advanced society like ours, however, a given person's refusal to join the Army, pay income taxes, or even work for a living, has so little effect on the conduct of the nation's business that any decision to indulge or punish him can rest more on

the abstract rights and wrongs of the case than on the assessment of any
material damage he inflicts on society. In general, a primitive society *must*
treat individual deviance as a functional problem while an advanced one
can treat it as a moral problem.

The economic and political history of the United States makes it inevitable for social deviance in general and mental illness in particular to
be moral rather than functional problems in this country, despite any
damage they do to our gross national product. A political ideology of
individualism that officially authorizes the pursuit of happiness, exon-
erates the entrepreneurial spirit and, by implication, invites people to be
as free of society as they wish, is ideally suited to social deviants. The
viability of such a society depends on its wealth, on there being few
enough deviants so that they can be supported, on a relative dearth of
external enemies, and on a lot of good luck. The United States has had
all these in abundance, and the favorable combination of technology and
ideology has brought us to a position where we can "afford" mental illness
economically but may be endangered morally by the very freedom from
social responsibility that is implicit in our political ideals.

As our growing wealth has gradually lightened the conventional burden of work on the shoulders of individual Americans, the conventional
prerequisites for freedom from such responsibility have become less
stringent. Extreme youth and old age are valid exemptions from gainful
labor; delaying work to get more education has increasingly become the
right rather than privilege of all classes and strata of our society. Illness,
which has always been good and sufficient reason for withdrawal from
ordinary society, has become a broader and more inclusive concept in
our day than ever before. The more common and extreme mental disorders like psychoses and neuroses have long been considered illnesses
for this purpose, but in this century there has been a reduction in the
opprobrium and scandal (if not the fear) connected with them. Wealth
makes compassion easier, and as our society has grown richer, it has
become more liberal too. The individualistic disposition has become more
tolerable in socially deviant forms than was ever previously true, the more
so when it can be rationalized. And the mentally ill, like everybody else,
have benefited from it. Our moral tolerance for deviations has grown to
the extent that automated production has increased our economic capacity for such tolerance.

Mental illness, perhaps always the vaguest of ailment classifications, has
now become the broadest as well, gradually incorporating virtually any
kind of personal ineffectiveness or disorder of character. Deviations once
dismissed as criminal are now redefined as pathological. This is easy to
rationalize for things like sexual deviance, which are defined as crimes

because of religious traditions even if they do not directly affect the productive capacities of society or hurt people. Such redefinitions are sometimes extended still further, however, to the point where theft caused by a personality disorder can be judged in terms of the disorder's need for treatment rather than out of concern for anybody's loss of property.

As might be expected, the terminology of crime, mental illness, and other kinds of social deviance has shifted to accompany the shifting contemporary view of these events. Conditions for which the appropriate epithets were once *evaluative* have become *scientific,* that is, factual or technical or merely descriptive. Where it was once implied, if not stipulated, that deviance is bad (as when Kraft-Ebbing described sexual disorders as the result of "hereditary taint"), deviance is now treated in purely descriptive, even sympathetic ways which say nothing worse than that it is unhealthy.

Regardless of the language used to discuss it, the fact is clear that, from the social point of view, *healing* mental illness means *dealing* with social deviance—and the moral problems engendered by the social perspective all reduce to questions of how society ought best to deal with people who are misfits in it.

The most useful analogy to *mental illness,* from this point of view, is *crime,* not because the two are often confused (as they are), but because when they are kept quite clearly separated in mind, there are still important parallels between them. Both involve nonconformist behavior, both are socially unacceptable, both are commonly seen as attributes of adults (judging from the extant social machinery for handling them), even though widely observed in children too and, in more or less enlightened societies, both are handled in ways that are in constant transition and result in constant tension between punishment and rehabilitation. A naïve observer of our social organization might think that the differences between them rest entirely on one assumption, from which all else follows: The criminal, it seems, *chooses* to violate the rules of society; the mentally ill *cannot choose* to observe them.[2] This belief contributes to some unfortunate practices from which one might well conclude that, if a person is going to be socially deviant, it is wiser to commit crimes than follies. Since an accused criminal presumably is capable of rational

[2] The belief that criminals are themselves mentally ill is growing; some of them certainly are, which is an important reason for handling their treatment by rehabilitation rather than punishment. The distinction is still valid, however, for the mentally ill often commit no crimes, criminals often show no demonstrable mental disorders—and the argument for rehabilitation instead of vengeful punishment is quite plausible without any assumption that criminals are deranged.

encounter with the social system on the same terms as any citizen, he is granted all the civil rights that anybody else would require for his defense; but since mentally ill people, by definition, are believed incapable of such encounters, they are more liable to legal restraint than criminals and, once subjected to such restraints as commitment proceedings, are generally denied ordinary civil rights. Imprisonment denies a convicted criminal his civil rights also, but the sentence imposed on him is finite, subject to mandatory and periodic review and, presumably, to termination.

The imprisonment of the mentally ill, however, is often interminable and, should he lack interested champions outside the asylum walls, is not necessarily subject to anybody's scrutiny. The deviance of the mentally ill seems less intelligible, hence less predictable than that of criminals, and in this sense is less tolerable to society. The fact that the reason for their incarceration may be their own good, in effect, simply gives their keepers more authority over them than over criminals.

Stated another way, a benevolent society serves the mentally ill *in loco parentis,* where it would not choose to do so for criminals. The same assumptions that prevail about children are made about the mentally ill, namely that they are presently incapable of making defensible choices about allegiance to social conventions, and it is therefore the duty of society both to protect them from harm and to educate them to a modicum of productive conformity.

There are a number of circumstances, and a number of mental illnesses, where hardly anyone would take exception to these principles. In particular, these are (1) organically based mental illness, such as traumatic brain damage or paresis, a deteriorative neurological and behavioral condition which stems from untreated syphilis, (2) criminal mental illness, such as homicidal tendencies or unchecked impulses toward sexual violence, and (3) what might be called "word salad" or "drifter" styles of functional disorders, that is, disabilities where there is no sign of physiological damage nor any known propensity to commit crimes, but where the victim's functioning is simply so impaired that he can neither shift for himself in the world nor communicate to others what deliberate goals he might pursue. Such conditions are popularly thought of as simplemindedness or feeble-mindedness, but technically they are as often found among schizophrenics as among the mentally retarded.

In all such cases, the congruence of *restrictive social control* with *mental healing* goes morally unchallenged, sometimes because the misbehavior in question is demonstrably *not* the fault of the disordered individual, as in (1), where mental illness really does mean disease; or because continuing his behavior presents a clear and present danger to other people, as in (2), so he may therefore be restrained as a criminal would be; or because there is nothing in the person's behavior to indicate that he is making deliberate choices for the conduct of his own life, and there is some evidence that he cannot make such deliberate choices, as in (3).

The moral issue that appears when mental illness is viewed from a social perspective assumes the obverse of the conditions where social control and mental healing go hand in hand. It assumes first that the individual is capable of expressing his desires, second that no external agent, such as organic illness, is responsible for his condition, and third that the need or title of society to protection against his expressed desires is doubtful. The two common conditions that probably address this problem most clearly are *suicide* and *sexual deviation*.

There are any number of suicides and deviate sexual acts committed or attempted by people who are blatantly psychotic or otherwise fall within the three criteria of true irresponsibility discussed above. The problem does not arise in connection with them, however, but only with those people for whom the very definition of disorder is implicit in the behavior in question. If an otherwise sane person, for example, attempts suicide or is discovered in some homosexual act, is he properly considered a criminal, mentally ill, or neither one? The fact that the act is illegal and the man evidently responsible and communicative might lead us simply to call him a criminal, but most sophisticated people in our society would not accept this idea. But it is difficult to say that the act shows he is mentally ill because that would rest the definition of mental illness on the person's willingness to conform to some modal and therefore normative social standards. In that event, the meaning of mental health converges on good citizenship, the "whole" man becomes political man, and the only moral question then at issue is the implied contract that exists between the individual and the social order in which he lives.

This position has some puzzling effects, not the least of which is that it obscures or destroys the meaning of *crime* to say that a person who knows what he is about and feels responsible for his actions too can still be mentally ill with respect to them. But whatever logical problems are thus created, this idea is nevertheless widely accepted among enlightened people.

The treatment of extremely disturbed persons under an implicit contract between the individual and society is easy to understand on both technical and moral grounds. Since the patient cannot assume responsibility for his behavior, he cannot be blamed for performing harmful acts or for failing to contribute productively to society. A benevolent social organization is morally obligated to protect and nurture him if it must and rehabilitate and restore him to itself if it can. It thus reciprocates in an implicit bargain where he has agreed to avoid harming others in his social system and to conduct his own life in a way that adds to the total output of goods, services, and pleasures available within society's domain.

Sexual deviates may be violating the prohibition on harming others (whether physically or in their sensibilities), while suicides, all else aside, violate the agreement to contribute by removing their own productive capacity from society. (Historically, neither harm to others nor the good of society were the explicit reasons for which laws banning suicide and sexual deviations were passed—but reasons like these are used to argue for their retention today, and it is only their ominous legal status that makes them subject to debate with respect to mental illness in the first place.)

If the issue of harm to others, like the seduction of children, is removed from consideration, then such deviates as adult homosexuals can claim the right to maintain whatever private relationships they can negotiate with others of their kind and that society has no right to interfere with them merely because some people's sensibilities are injured by homosexuality. Potential suicides can make a similar case proposing that as long as their demise does not actively harm other people, society has no right to prevent it on the highly abstract grounds that suicide destroys their productive contribution. Certainly American society makes no explicit demands on people for productive work in order to survive or even to be taken care of. And if people who kill themselves do not work, they also do not eat, thus removing their consumptive potential along with their productive one.

In both cases, society's right to intervene on grounds of mental illness is plainly doubtful unless this claim is justified to some extent by a definition that includes social conformity, good citizenship, or the like. Such a definition would make crime a subtopic of mental illness distinguished only by the fact that people are intentionally harmed by the antisocial behavior. But it might make Bohemianism, fanatical bird watching, writing novels, or almost any other unconventional behavior subject to the same definition, which seems senseless.

THE PROFESSIONAL PROBLEM

As difficult as it may seem to find a reasonable social definition of mental illness, the task is only abstract and parlor-gamish compared to that which faces the mental health professional in the routine management of his practice. His job is to serve the needs of individuals, but his sanctions come from a society that usually assumes that the disordered individual is out of phase with it and that the mental health expert will restore the person to it. The problem of defining mental illness does not confront the professional worker *because* his role is socially sanctioned, and the moral issues he faces are not only the results of such sanctions, but the sanction of society does make a difference to his functioning.

First, it gives him a form of economic protection that ordinary trades-men do not get. The laws that license and certify mental health experts are meant to protect the public against harmful treatment by charlatans or well-meaning but poorly trained pretenders to expertise—but they inevitably restrict the practice of mental treatment to a relatively small group of people drawn mostly from three professions, psychiatry, clinical psychology, and social work. Since there are terrible personnel shortages in all three professions, and since nobody, least of all the professionals, has tried much to solve the manpower shortage by mass training of sub-professional groups or the like, they have a virtual monopoly on treat-ment of the mentally ill both inside and outside the mental hospitals of the nation.

Second, because of its sanction, society continually imposes on the mental health professions, especially psychiatry, the hopeless responsibil-ity of helping to apply its own peculiar legal definitions of mental illness in individual cases, especially criminal cases involving questions of in-tent and responsibility.

The legislators of our social system are sensitive to the need to have some social agents transcend some of the ordinary strictures of the law, and it is for this reason that privileged communications are permitted between individuals and their priests, lawyers, and doctors. Privileged communication is designed only to enable someone who has committed a crime to reveal himself without peril of retaliation and to let the person who hears his secrets listen without fear that he will then be compelled to betray the trust of his confidant. These sanctions are not meant to authorize priests, doctors, or lawyers to counsel clients on whether or how to break the law efficiently, so as not to be arrested in due course.

But that is exactly the problem that perenially confronts the mental health expert who works face to face with clients. The gambler whose game is off, the anxious homosexual, the compulsive thief, and a host of others with a host of other problems, all want to commit the expert to helping them—and doing so requires that the expert juggle his obli-gations to the individual and to society as best he can.

The moral problems of the mental health expert begin with the fact that he is socially sanctioned to serve persons whose best interests, he may judge, run counter to the needs of society. As long as the behavior he treats is not glaringly criminal in the narrowest sense (like threaten-ing violence to others would be), he need not be obsessively concerned with the social sanctions on his practice. Even so, the professional perspective on mental illness brings some important moral problems into focus, especially those of (1) criteria of disorder, (2) the morals of social engineering, and (3) the social biases of the mental health industry.

The Criterion Problem

There are some elementary and fairly good criteria for most conditions that most people call illness. For one thing, the person who has it usually hurts; for another, it is generally difficult for him to work or otherwise function while he is ill; for a third, he is likely either to recover from it or get worse in reasonably short order. If he recovers, either there will be no trace of his having ever been ill or he will retain some visible stigma, defect, or disability that rather clearly shows that he was sick. If he does not recover, he will probably die of the malady, again clearly suggesting that he had been ill.

In the case of mental illness (and now from the professional rather than the social view), nothing could be less clear more often than what defines the condition. Toward the end of the nineteenth century, most psychiatrists were convinced that the basis of virtually all mental disorder was physiological. This opinion was reflected not only in the learned texts of the day, but also in the extreme decline in discharges from mental hospitals resulting from the learned incompetence or total lack of treatment which the "organic" or "disease" approach to mental conditions brought about.

At the present time, it is generally conceded that, whatever anatomical or physiological basis may exist for psychological disorders, the disorders themselves are mostly reflections of troublesome learning patterns, usually acquired in childhood, which tend to be sustained by the exigencies of the person's contemporary life. (The *educational* perspective thus lent to mental illness presents the professional with another moral conundrum, for it suggests that his function is often to restore the patient's functions whether or not he approves of them.) But the learning approach to disorders leaves the healer, now perhaps educator, in the same position the legislator finds himself with regard to mental illness and crime. Restated for therapists, the question becomes: If the troubled individual is not "ill" but has only learned some behavior pattern that is unacceptable to most other people, if not to him, who is to be responsible for dealing with it? If the patient does not think he is sick, then why should the doctor be obliged to make him well? It is true that doctors often function as public health officers and authorize quarantine and other restrictive procedures—but they do so only where there is clear and present danger to everyone if the sick person walks around untreated. Contagion is not a common problem with psychiatric disabilities.

The Morals of Social Engineering

The mental health expert faces the criterion problem most dramatically where the patient is not hurting because of his condition but some social convention is. A related difficulty occurs when the patient is suffering also, but suffering more from the social stigma attached to his condition than from the condition itself. Homosexuality is a good example; many homosexuals are less disturbed by their sexual behavior than by the social scorn they feel because of it. In such cases, discretion about what treatment should accomplish often rests with the psychotherapist. He may find it easier to free the homosexual of anxiety about social disapproval than to change his sexual style, and such a course is easy to justify if the therapist himself does not truly regard homosexuality as immoral or injurious. At the same time, however, the operations he then attempts make him a social engineer, and it may give him legitimate pause to think that he is thereby deliberately working to reconstruct the sexual mores of society.

The potential of mental health experts for social engineering is quite large, although relatively few of them are publicly concerned about it. Homosexuality is itself a statistically common problem for American men, and other problems of sexual conduct and morals have also been increasingly confronting psychotherapists in their routine dealings with patients. With the exception of those therapeutic personnel whose religious or institutional affiliations make it easy to recognize the conservative bias of their outlook, it is clear that most practitioners in most private offices and outpatient clinics are liberal in their own moral judgments of sexual freedom, if not in their own private activities. At the least, this means they support a changing sexual morality that is permissive of extensive sexual activity prior to marriage, frowns on sexual deviancy mostly because of its social stigma alone and would not have it outlawed, and even judges hitherto more or less inviolate social norms of sexual restriction with major concern for the psychological rather than other consequences of their breaching. At least one formal study has shown that psychotherapists tend to fall ideologically among the most Bohemian groups in American society.

For their own part, most practitioners would probably say that the positions they take on any kind of problem depend on the unique attributes of the situation and the patient being served. Their work is done if they are able to change the person's life in some beneficial way, which usually means in a way that makes it more pleasant. Of course, many people suffer in the same way and can be changed in the same way by treatment, but this does not usually make the therapist feel that he has become a social engineer as long as he has not gone into collusion with his colleagues to produce the changes for which he is individually responsible.

The argument has some value in that there must be some limit on the responsibility an individual must bear for the consequences of his activity; otherwise, responsibility would be a meaningless idea. But the position may not be entirely valid in the case of psychotherapists because, in the first place, changing behavior is precisely their business and, in the second, they do not really need to operate in genuine isolation from their colleagues. Being in the behavior changing business to begin with, commits them to some engineering of people's lives, and the only possible defenses against being called social engineers are then either *incompetence* or *individualism;* that is, either they are ineffective or that they do not change people in standard ways. The first position cannot be justified; the second is the argument of noncollusion mentioned above.

It is true that individual therapists generally do not know just what is going on behind their colleagues' doors, and in that sense there is no agreement on what to do to people. On the other hand, there is a great deal of discussion among therapists about behavior disorders and about what should be done to treat them, and these ideas are incorporated into training procedures and supervision, into books, journals, lectures, and seminars, and into the standards of ethics and of practice of virtually all the professional organizations from which psychotherapists seek credentials. In this connection, the main difference between mental health experts and other social engineers, like educators and legislators, is that the former are able to operate in relative secrecy and to disclaim responsibility, while the latter must work their changes under public scrutiny and only after publicly defending their goals. The relative privacy in which the mental health expert can work out his social goals permits him to think them through more carefully perhaps than some other professionals do and to be more selfconscious and ingenuous in discovering their eventual possibilities. But it also permits him to be irresponsible, even incompetent—and if he insists on totally denying responsibility for the social changes he fosters, then his role becomes insidious and potentially destructive.

The Social Biases of the Mental Health Industry

The moral issues of social engineering are derivatives of the conflict between those therapists who feel that they serve on their patients' own behalf and those who feel an ultimate responsibility to the social order that appoints and sanctions them. But the morals of mental health experts are also products of their own social and political biases or the biases forced upon them by the projections of political and social extremists. The ferocious attacks on psychological testing, psychiatric treatment, and the mental health movement leveled by right wing political extremists have tended to produce a sort of shotgun wedding between mental health and political liberalism, enough so that even within the professions some people who oppose many current programs of psychological testing or practices of commitment to mental hospitals become identified with political positions. The psychoanalyst Thomas Szasz, for example, was recently excoriated (and redeemed) politically by a colleague for having written an article in the very conservative *National Review* (Leslie Farber in *Commentary*, November 1965). By the same token, the radical political left, especially its younger advocates, sometimes equates the extreme social changes it promotes, especially in standards of sexual morality, with political objectives and assumes, without evidence, that the liberal opinions of many mental health experts on sex imply corresponding political biases. This may, in fact, be true, but it has only been argued, not substantiated.

It is difficult to know, and perhaps irrelevant to care, about the actual political ideas of mental health experts, but it does seem that the views therapists have of their goals with patients parallel conventional kinds of political and social views in Western countries. Mental health, like government, has Conservative, Liberal, and more or less Radical exponents. The Liberal bias is not a firm one in its own right and effectively reduces to the Radical one.

The socially conservative bias of psychiatry sees individual *adjustment* as the aim of treatment. The object of this adjustment may be called "reality," "adulthood," or "socialization," but its meaning, regardless of label, is that the individual must learn to conform to the modal public behavior of others who occupy the same social station. Some advocates of adjustment also imply their approval of conformist private behavior as well, although it is always harder to be sure of what a man is thinking than of how he acts. The conservative position can be said to serve the best interests of the individual by making him more socially acceptable, and by that means more happy, but it argues, in any case, that the individual should not prick the fabric of social norms.

The historical roots of the conservative bias in psychiatry lie in the idea that mental illness is a straightforward variation of organic illness. This view became popular in the United States in the middle of the nineteenth century, and, according to statistics compiled by Bockoven, we have been paying for it ever since in excessively low discharge rates from our mental hospitals. It is easy to see how such a perspective on mental illness supports a socially conservative approach to it. After all, if the trouble with a mental patient is that he has some kind of infection, and it is only this that damages his relationship to society, then it is his malady alone that needs repair and not the social conditions in which it originated. This argument is specious even with respect to organic illness (as any intelligent garbageman or sanitary engineer can testify), but it is easily come upon and has some heuristic appeal, just as it is easy to think of syphilis as a strictly organic disease until one remembers that you must be in the right social situation to catch it. At all events, what Redlich and Hollingshead call the "organic" approach to psychiatry has dominated mental health in this country for many decades and is still associated with a conservative view of prevention and treatment.

The psychological approach to the conservative bias has only recently found a very capable spokesman in William Glasser, whose *Reality Therapy* is a practical and cogent argument that restoring the mentally ill to health means restoring them to modal social functions. Disordered behavior, it says, is irresponsible, and responsibility, by implication, means the assumption of congenial social roles. Whether social acceptability is worth striving for or makes life worth living in either a moral sense or a physically gratifying one is not the immediate problem of this position. Its first concern is that a person must recognize the limits imposed on him by these realities if he wishes to occupy even a nondescript, let alone honored position in society. On the other hand, merely to recommend that anybody get along in society is to endorse it in some measure, and if the point at issue is some sort of responsible deviance to begin with, then prescribing adjustment amounts to an endorsement either of the social norms or of their subversion, but not of defiance. Since subversion smacks of dishonorable conduct, and since psychiatrists are about as well bred as anybody, they are understandably loathe to promote it, which propels conservative doctors toward supporting social norms, adherence to which will secure their parents' places in society. But if this commitment conflicts with the doctor's simultaneous commitment to the patient's individual benefit, then he must rationalize his position to the patient. He often does so with the notion that social deviance is "unhealthy," and then often proceeds, instead of explicating this opinion, to analyze the patient's deviant action. The therapist's proposal to analyze something is often a substitute for openly disapproving it, which is then the doctor's own form of subversion.

The conservative doctor has an especially hard time being honest and helpful because he upholds social norms that his client may not. The liberal position has no such strictures. It gives the client latitude to settle with society whatever way best suits him, assuming generally that a viable social order can stand a good deal of deviance and that it is not, in any case, the business of mental doctors to negotiate with individuals on society's behalf. Neither is it the business of the liberal therapist to challenge social norms, and he can therefore take or leave them as suits his client without compromising himself. His object too is the adjustment of his client, but more to the client's own needs than to society's demands.

The socially radical bias of psychiatry views *self-fulfillment* as the goal of treatment. This may sound like the same thing as adjustment, but it is far from it. Adjustment implies that the object of treatment is the *comfort* and well-being of the patient, whether conservatively achieved by conformity to society or liberally left to him to decide. The idea of fulfillment, however, means that the patient needs to become either a different kind of person than he is or a lot more of it; that is, he needs to achieve the maximum personal maturity of which he is capable. For many people, that means discovering their niche in life and adjusting to it—they can be comfortable and fulfilled. But for most, as the radical position would have it, self-fulfillment involves no surcease of struggle and inner turmoil, but the direction of them toward personally productive ends which will make life most meaningful. For such cases, the probability is high that successful treatment will, if anything, foster rather than inhibit social deviance, though perhaps an ultimately more useful deviance than that with which the patient entered treatment. Should his personal development make him more acceptable to society, so much the better, but it is not likely that a more "individuated" person, as some radical positions would label him, would become a very conforming member of a very imperfect and homogenized society.

The conceptual roots of the radical position are to be found in a strictly psychological view of mental illness, but, as we have seen, a psychological view can be used to support a conservative position as well. Whatever the historical origins of this position, its individualistic orientation is clearly most congenial to a democratic and rich society, capable at once of sustaining an ideology that fosters the utmost personal liberty and surviving the people who make the most of it.

Subversion holds the same ethical dangers for the radical therapist as for the conservative one, but rather than subverting libertarian impulses, he would be more likely to subvert the patient's feelings of guilt and moral anxiety, if not all social responsibility. Only the liberal position escapes this conundrum, and it does so at the sacrifice of firm commitments in either direction. If the liberal doctor has nothing much to hide, he also has nothing much to promote—and while that may do well enough for him when the patient's needs are themselves clear-cut, it may not be worth much otherwise. In an age of anxiety, where what Wheelis calls *the quest for identity* is the core problem of those who seek therapeutic advice, there is little of comfort or fulfillment in the counsel that says it is all right to be fish or fowl or stew. This fact and their intuitive sensibility to it makes most liberal psychiatrists into de facto radicals; the liberal message that "it is permissible to get what you want" gives way to the radical message that "it is mandatory to discover what you must have."

Despite all this, most mental health people would claim the liberal position as their own, and it is indeed this position that expresses the dilemma of any conscientious mental health expert, right or left, who thinks about the relationship of individuals to society. *His object, if he were left alone, would be to create a conformist deviant who can contribute to society without being enslaved to it, who can gratify himself without violating it, and whose most profound and fulfilling experiences of self would ultimately make society change, so that his very individuation would enrich and bless the rest of us.* But the needs of single men are not so neatly scaled to the demands of men in multitude contesting with and ruling over each other. So the dilemma remains just that.

THE WILLING HANDS

The legislators and executives of the social order face moral dilemmas over mental health, as we have seen, because they must be concerned with crime as well as health and with social regulations and restraints as well as illness. The merchants of the health industry too face moral dilemmas created by the difficulty of defining mental illness precisely, the challenges and dangers of social engineering, and the influence of their personal biases on the lives of their clients. There is but one body of concerned people who can hurl themselves into the breach without anxiety or hesitation and with no need to scruple about the outcome of their work. These are the laymen who have organized and operate the Mental Health Associations of America.

On the face of it, the Mental Health Associations are probably indistinguishable from any other of the layman's auxiliary groups that help combat major menaces to the nation's health. Its membership is drawn chiefly from the upper middle socio-economic strata of the population, undoubtedly consists largely of women, and reflects political biases ranging from mildly conservative to mildly liberal views. On the face of it too the goals of these organizations are like those of the other health auxiliaries—to stamp out mental illness just as we stamped out polio. The difference, as we have seen, is that polio can be treated this way and mental illness cannot, for not only is it more than one thing, but most of the things it is are not even illnesses.

Such niceties have not retarded the Mental Health Associations at all, though plenty of other things have, including the ambivalence of psychiatrists about whether they really want laymen getting into the mental health act. This has been analyzed at length by the Joint Commission on Mental Illness and Health, in *Action for Mental Health* (Basic Books).

To say that the goals of the Mental Health movement are to stamp out mental illness says also in effect that its goals are vague and uncertain and suggests that they fluctuate with style changes in mental health, especially as these vary among psychiatrists. It is a benevolent uncertainty, however; the associations are *for* everybody concerned, the patients, the doctors, and society, and their activities reflect none of the moral dilemmas that are intrinsic to the mental health business.

Theirs is a naïve position indeed, if one wishes to examine the movement from the point of view of its moral implications or of the moral awareness of its members and advocates. It is, however, a very useful one, and perhaps a necessary one if the movement is to do much toward solving the nation's problems of mental health and illness. There are at least two vital functions this movement can fulfill without any pretense of concern over lofty moral dilemmas. It can marshall the force of public opinion to assure that humane treatment is given the hospitalized mentally ill. And it can finance and sustain community mental health enterprises, the most important of which are undoubtedly clinics and other facilities devoted mostly to service for children. Perhaps it will not be long until these associations also assume some role in the provision of community facilities for the aged and indigent. The only moral presupposition involved in serving all these groups is opposition to a kind of individual suffering usually unrelated to the conflicts of individual and society. If such commitments fail to tax the moral fiber of mental health movement members or to build their characters, they nevertheless permit them to perform a human kindness the importance of which is not diminished by its philosophic flaws.

When all is said and done, perhaps the chief moral significance of the Mental Health Associations lies in just this fact, that they represent the main moral stance of the American people, not just toward mental illness and health, but toward the very character of the rights and needs of individuals from life and from society. Above all else, it is an unreflective position which, by its nature, grants individuals the right to be left alone by others, to live their lives as they choose and, within some limits of respect for the similar individualism of others, commends them to whatever success they can have from exploiting the world around them.

The auxiliary health associations have always reflected this position, and perhaps even arose as an extension of the mixed tradition of self help and community cooperation that marked the pioneering and land conquest of America until the frontier expired in 1890. Certainly this attitude was integral to the mental health movement since its very beginning less than twenty years later. The very name that Clifford Beers, the movement's founder, gave his book, *A Mind That Found Itself,* is true to the American approval and admiration for self help.

But underlying even this entrepreneurial morality is another characteristic, perhaps uniquely American, morality of faith in the benevolent solubility of all human problems, however difficult they seem or hopelessly warped by inherent contradictions. It is a part of what is too contemptuously called "the American Dream" to believe in the essential intelligibility of the universe and sufficiency of its resources so that some combination of energy, pluck, ingenuity, good will, and fortune must make it ultimately possible to elaborate some kindly scheme by which all men will be able to live individually happy and free lives.

The naïveté of this argument goes without saying, and it is easy to see how it can be understood historically as a result of the good fortune that has characterized so much of the American experience for so long. But at the same time that this position leaves its advocate disarmed against hypothetical dilemmas like the moral problems of mental health, it also leaves him motivated, hopefully and perhaps industriously, to discover the practical resolutions of the suffering and disability of mentally disordered persons. Perhaps kindness is thus purchased at the cost of wisdom. If so, here is another moral dilemma for the philosophically minded—but not for the American mental health industry, whose commitment, like the humane commitment of the populace it serves, is to allay suffering, not to reflect upon it.

1.4   Orientation

The process through which persons come to be recognized, or diagnosed, as mentally ill has been little studied. This chapter, by an anthropologist, attempts to examine this process. Mental illness is viewed as a social status that is probably present in all societies. The process by which persons become recognized as mentally ill, and hence as entitled to this status, is described in four East African societies. In these societies, a few persons seem to be accorded this status because they are chronically unable to account for their behavior. Others—by far the majority—become labeled as mentally ill only after a complex social process which can profitably be thought of as a negotiation. Since the status of mental illness has both moral and jural involvements, the negotiations that surround the recognition of mental illness are played for high stakes. This article explores the nature and importance of these negotiations.

1.4   On the "Recognition" of Mental Illness

Robert B. Edgerton

THE PROBLEM

The problem that I wish to explore here can be introduced by this deceptively simple question: How is it that some people come to be recognized as being mentally ill? To come to terms with this question requires that the process whereby "recognition" takes place be examined, carefully and without presuppositions. To open this complex and little-studied process to preliminary scrutiny may improve our understanding of mental illness, but it will certainly call forth an entire galaxy of equally complex new problems. Even though this is a chastening prospect, the task of beginning to outline the process through which mental illness becomes recognized should be undertaken, because an understanding of this process is of fundamental importance for any fully adequate view of mental illness itself.

In beginning this preliminary task, I shall first provide illustrations from the non-Western world; next, I shall turn to the possible relevance of these illustrations for our own society.

Some Definitions: "The Recognition Process"
and "Mental Illness"

Some initial definitions are required, not because the issues can be resolved through sheer skill of definition, but because working definitions are necessary in order to provide a basis for subsequent discussion.

As conceived here, the "recognition" process has three aspects: perception, labeling, and action. *Perception* refers to an observer's initial subjective realization that something is "wrong"—that someone is behaving in a "crazy" (irrational, unreasonable, inexplicable) way. This may be a private realization, known but not expressed to others. It is cognitive, but it need not be verbalized, or even verbalizable. *Labeling* refers to the verbal expression of such a perception; for example, the person who is perceived as behaving in a "crazy" way is now designated a "crazy" person. The label "crazy" is now applied to him by one or more members of his society. *Action* is likely to follow once such a label is applied. Action tends to result because the label always confers a status, and this status will require that other persons adopt new modes of interaction with the "crazy" person, modes such as avoidance, assistance, ridicule, punishment, or protection.

To be sure, these three aspects of the recognition process, perception, labeling, and action, are not merely related—they tend to be causally connected. For example, perception tends to lead to labeling, and the label in turn may require certain action. Indeed, it can be argued that the three are inseparable aspects of a single process, and that to speak of recognition is necessarily to speak of all three. However, this unity is not always present. For one thing, perception and action not only stand at opposing poles of a process, they can also be quite different phenomena, with perception being a problem in psychophysics and action a problem in the management of a deviant person. Thus, the three aspects of recognition are not separated simply for convenience of analysis. In the world of social reality, perception, labeling, and action can be separated, and they often are.

The second matter for definition is the term "mental illness." To deal properly with the problems of such a definition would require another essay at least as long as this one. And under any conditions, defining mental illness can be a morass from which there is no exit, as witness the murky metaphysics that so often appear in answer to the question of how best to define "mental illness." By way of example, it has sometimes been argued that while "mental illness" is many things, it is neither mental nor an illness.

For the purposes of this discussion we need only agree that there are certain terms (labels) that are everywhere applied to persons who are thought to be conducting themselves in a manner that is inappropriate, abnormal, or unreasonable for persons in that culture who occupy a similar social position; that is, to persons who can provide no otherwise acceptable explanation for their conduct. Such labels in English would include, "craziness," "madness," "insanity," "nervous breakdown," "psychosis," "schizophrenia," and the like. Of course, the repertoire of labels differs somewhat from one culture to another, but every culture has labels that imply some version of "mental illness." The point is that we are dealing with labels, and these labels have their own reality, as even that most extreme doubter, Thomas Szasz, insists (1963): "While I argue that mental illnesses do not exist, obviously I do not wish to imply that the social and psychological occurrences *so labeled* do not exist [p. 16]."

The central concern of this discussion is with *how* these labels come to be applied.

The Thesis

The thesis that I offer here contains these three postulates:

1. The recognition of persons as mentally ill who are both severely *and* chronically psychotic usually proceeds with relative ease and consensus, because persons such as these are typically so dramatically, and enduringly, far beyond the pale of everyday rationality.

2. However, most persons who behave strangely, even "crazily," are not both extremely and chronically outside of their culture's view of rational conduct. Where such persons are concerned, the recognition process is infinitely more complex. In fact, it is a social transaction that often involves extensive negotiation.

3. Negotiations concerning the appropriate application of labels signifying mental illness inevitably have both moral and jural implications. Because of these moral and jural involvements, the negotiation that surrounds labeling comes to influence both the action that flows from the labeling, and the original perception itself. Thus, the crucial dimension of the recognition process is *negotiation*.

It should be noted that I have referred only to "mental illness" and "psychosis," not to finer diagnostic categories. For the purposes of this general discussion the important question is not the nature of the mental disorder, but its severity and chronicity. As employed here, psychosis refers to a severe degree of mental illness, and chronic means either perpetually present, or regularly recurring. It must also be made clear that I refer only to recognition of one person by others, not to self-recognition.[1]

[1] The analysis of self-recognition of mental illness can be extremely revealing, whether it be based upon the words of a famous European psychotic, as in Perceval's "Narrative" (Bateson, 1963), or discussed by a formerly psychotic Hehe tribesman who said, "I knew I was mad because my head felt so strange, and I was afraid that if I bent over, my head would fall off." Regrettably, I was unable to collect any adequate amount of material on self-recognition in East Africa. For some interesting examples from other areas, see Devereux (1963) and Bowers (1965).

The Cross-Cultural Evidence

Turning to non-Western societies for answers to psychiatry's perennial questions, although still very much in its groping stages as a technique, has nevertheless shown promise, both because of the comparative perspective it affords, and because of the less obstructed analytic view one can sometimes find in these relatively small and less complex societies. Unfortunately, while the volume of psychiatrically relevant research in these non-Western societies is increasing, where recognition is concerned, the currently available information remains very sketchy.

There is some evidence to suggest that certain mental illness labels are easily and consensually applied. Some reports imply that this is the case with certain of the exotic psychotic states apparently not known in the West: for example, the *koro* psychosis of Southeast Asia, *windigo* among some North American Indian tribes, *imu* among the Ainu, *latah* in Central Asia, *pibloqtoc* among the Eskimo, and so on.[2] There is also some evidence from various mental hospitals in non-Western countries,[3] from a few epidemiologically oriented studies, and from studies of native conceptions of mental illness,[4] to suggest that some psychotics can be easily recognized as such. An excellent example of the extent to which patterns (and labels) of psychotic conduct are recognized (and known) in non-Western societies is provided by Devereux (1963) in his discussion of "malingering." Devereux contends that there are shared "thought models" or "templates" that permit a malingerer effectively to simulate psychosis. These same "thought models" also guide an "actual" psychotic in the appropriate display of his "symptoms."

There is also some evidence, frequently from the same sources, to suggest that many cases of presumed mental illness are less easily recognized.[5] Here we receive the impression that the routine of recognition is complex, and that labels are often applied with difficulty, and without consensus.

However, even when all available sources on mental illness in non-Western societies are considered together, the *process* by which recognition takes place remains essentially undescribed. As Devereux (1963) has written, what we find in the existing literature is the finished product of the recognition process, not an understanding of the process itself.

---

[2] See Teicher (1960), Aberle (1952), Wallace (1962), Yap (1952), Linton (1956), and Kiev (1964).

[3] Leighton (1963), Opler (1959), Linton (1956), Rogler & Hollingshead (1965).

[4] See Brelsford (1950), Lee (1950), Edgerton (1966), and Kiev (1964).

[5] For an example of contrastive views on similar societies in Highland New Guinea, compare Newman (1964) and Langness (1965).

Devereux himself (1961, 1963) has come closest to providing a beginning toward an understanding of this process, but despite Devereux's own worthwhile analysis, much remains to be understood.

SOME EAST AFRICAN ILLUSTRATIONS

The following material from four East African tribal societies will illustrate some aspects of the recognition process. The observations recorded here were collected in 1961–1962 during participation in the "Culture and Ecology in East Africa" project, directed by Walter Goldschmidt. In the course of this project, I spent fifteen months in East Africa doing research in these four tribal societies: the Hehe in Tanzania, the Kamba and Pokot in Kenya, and the Sebei in Uganda. In addition, research was conducted in three East African mental hospitals.[6]

Recognition of "Chronic Psychotics"

As reported elsewhere (Edgerton 1966), most persons in all four East African tribes were able to describe the behaviors said to characterize a psychotic person, and this catalogue of psychotic behavior was widely known within each society even by people who had never seen a psychotic themselves. In effect, there was a known pattern of expectations for psychotic behavior. The following four cases, one from each of the tribes, illustrate the degree of agreement present in these societies concerning the recognition (perception, labeling, and action) of a chronically psychotic person.

Case 1.   Nzomo: A Kamba chronic psychotic   Among the six or seven chronic psychotics I saw during my research with the Kamba, one particularly stood out. Perhaps because he was so regularly in evidence, this man, whose name was Nzomo, was known to many Kamba in the area, and I often saw him as I drove along the road. Nzomo was a man of about 35, who dressed in rags. He came to be known as the "bus driver" because he was usually to be seen "driving" an imaginary bus along the main road between the administrative center of Machakos and the more remote mountain farming areas. Nzomo "drove" his bus by trotting along this road, making loud, humming engine noises, and dramatically shifting gears with his hands as he changed the speed of his "bus." When he encountered someone along the road, he would bring his bus elaborately to a stop, beckon the person aboard, and then hold out his hand for the

[6] This research was supported by a research grant from the National Science Foundation, and Public Health Service Research Grant M-4097 from the National Institute of Mental Health.

fare. When approached by Nzomo, people usually laughed or merely
ignored him. They did not abuse him or attack him, but they did not give
him any money, either. Children sometimes mocked him by giving him
a twig or stone or leaf as the fare and then lining up behind him single-
file. As he drove off, they would run along behind him until they tired of
the game and then they would fall behind, sending along their laughter
and mocking cries. Nzomo ran along this road almost every day, often
covering over 30 miles in a day. He was said to live alone in a tiny hut
in the low brush country on the far side of the mountains, and it was
also said that he lived by stealing maize at night. But no one really
knew anything about Nzomo, and I was never able to find out where
he actually spent the night because he would never respond to any
question or greeting, and if approached too closely, he would run away.
No one could be found who had seen him at any activity during the day
other than his "bus driving." I asked over forty Kamba men and women,
and some dozen children, about him, and every single person agreed that
Nzomo was psychotic; and they agreed in labeling him *kichaa*. Furthermore, all said that he was harmless.[7] Some complained mildly about his
alleged stealing, but no one felt that anything should be done about him.
Most added, "He harms no one, let him live."

Case 2. Daudi: A Hehe chronic psychotic   During my stay among the
Hehe, I saw only two persons whom I thought to be chronic psychotics.
One of these was a very agitated young woman who constantly ran about
aimlessly and frantically. The other was Daudi. Daudi was seemingly
everywhere—in the villages, on the road, and in the nearby European
town. He was a large man of about 45, who even on the very hottest of
days was swathed in no fewer than three ragged British Army greatcoats.
His feet were wrapped in yards of rags, while on his head and in every
pocket were masses of leaves, twigs and grass. Daudi was always on the
move, singing as he trotted here and there between the town and the
surrounding farming areas. He often trotted down the center of the
road, nimbly dodging the cars that he encountered. Sometimes he would
stop to importune some passerby with a spate of incoherent speech, but
except for these excursions into the world of ordinary man, he seemed
to have little use for people. Nor did people have much desire to be
near him, for he was incredibly dirty and foul smelling. Daudi's passion
was automobiles. In the town or wherever else he saw a car, he fondly
rubbed and polished it with rags or leaves that he always had with him. I

[7] The term *kichaa* and other equivalent terms for psychosis are discussed in
Edgerton (1966).

often found him polishing my own car this way, humming and laughing to himself, but when I approached him, he backed off scowling, and refused to answer any of my greetings. Once as I stopped at a station to fill the car with petrol, I saw Daudi standing nearby, watching. He watched as the station attendant filled the tank, then as the attendant left the car to go to the cash register, Daudi rushed up to the car and filled the tank himself—by urinating into it. Eventually, the attendants chased him away, but Daudi refused to be hurried, and when he finally desisted he seemed to be immensely pleased with himself.

I asked twenty-six Hehe men and fourteen women about Daudi. All firmly declared that he was psychotic (*lisaliko*) and, as far as they knew, always had been; but they unanimously added that he was completely harmless. None felt that anything should be done about him. One added grimly: "Why bother? A motorcar will run over him someday."

Case 3.   Cheposerra: A Pokot chronic psychotic   Although I was told about many chronic psychotics among the Pokot, I saw only one— Cheposerra, a widow of about 50. Cheposerra lived alone in a small house that was hidden away from people in a wooded area some distance from any other house. It was said that she had been psychotic for many years; it is surely true that during the six weeks that I knew of her, she was acutely psychotic. She constantly laughed to herself, sang, and, especially at night, she screamed and howled like a dog or hyena. She was often seen walking about the populated areas. She usually did so nude except for the leaves she draped over her head and the feces that she smeared on her forehead and stuffed into her ears. As she walked about, she laughed or moaned, and sometimes she chased small children or goats, but she apparently never caught them or hurt them. Her most notorious —and spectacular—behavior earned her the nickname of "the grabber." She quite often sneaked up upon a group of unsuspecting men who were sitting together talking. Although Pokot women (save for psychotics such as Cheposerra) are never nude, Pokot men usually are. Cheposerra would rush out of her hiding place, grab the penis of one of the men and pull it vigorously, despite his howls of painful and embarrassed protest. As she did so she would call loudly, "You are my son. Come and have sexual relations with me!" Cheposerra always seemed to manage her assault before a good-sized audience, which, except for her unfortunate victim, enjoyed itself hugely.

Every one of the seventeen men and twenty-two women whom I asked about Cheposerra said that she was psychotic (*kipoiyi*). All but a few volunteered the opinion that she was harmless and, indeed, sometimes amusing. None suggested that anything should be done to restrain her.

Case 4. Andyema: A Sebei chronic psychotic I saw three chronic psychotics among the Sebei: a young man, a young woman, and an old man. The old man was at least 65. He still lived where he had been living for a great many years, near the Greek River in the low plains country close to the northern perimeter of Sebeiland. He lived with his two wives and several grandchildren in what appeared to be a normal homestead, and his early life appears to have been nonpsychotic. However, for at least the four years prior to my visit, and perhaps for longer, he had been acutely psychotic. He talked only nonsense, indeed gibberish, except for an occasional phrase that he repeated, such as "I have a chicken in my head," or "I have countless wives." He ate cow dung, the walls of his mud house, the roots of trees, and his own feces. He sometimes wandered naked and made loud noises at night, but most characteristically he hung from the limb of a tree or from a rafter in his house. Each morning he would climb to his perch and hang all day by his knees. A grandchild or his eldest wife cared for him, even feeding him as he hung upside down. He was a reasonably well-to-do man, and his relatives tried all the available native treatments, but nothing improved his condition. He continued to hang upside down all day.

I asked twenty-one adults and several children about Andyema. With one exception, they said that he was psychotic (*punmit*). The one exception was a grandson who argued that Andyema could not be psychotic because he had managed to marry a young wife. However, that marriage was contracted more than four years earlier, and the grandson was probably concerned lest the psychosis of his grandfather implicate him, for the Sebei believe that madness can be inherited and that it can skip generations.

To summarize these examples, it is apparent that at least some chronic psychotics are recognized with ease. Such persons are totally unable to provide good reasons to account for their actions, nor are they able to conduct themselves so that others impute good reasons for their actions to them. They remain outside all acceptable rationality. Those chronic psychotics who represent an obvious threat to life or property are kept in restraint, are killed, or in some instances, are sent away to the authorities. Those who are not dangerous are usually permitted to live on the fringes of the society, where they remain outside the ordinary network of cultural understandings and human relationships, without responsibilities (except for staying out of trouble) and without rights (except for the right to go on living).[8]

[8] Compare Spiro (1950).

In occupying the permanent status of "psychotic," such persons come to most members of the society pre-labeled as persons who are already known by all to be "crazy." Thus, there need not be a continuing process of recognition. Neither is there typically a problem of negotiation, because in most instances the chronic psychotic has so completely lost his social value (his rights and responsibilities) that there is no longer any socially viable basis for negotiation.

Recognition of Cases
That Are Not Both Severe and Chronic

A great many, indeed most, of the cases of "mental illness" that occur in any society, are not both severe and chronic. Some cases are severe but by no means chronic, and others are chronic but not severe. Still others are neither severe nor chronic. With all such cases, the process of "recognition" becomes much more complex, and the degree of agreement among observers concerning the labeling diminishes accordingly. At least that is the situation in East Africa.

In East Africa, these more equivocal cases of "mental illness" are sometimes the subject of relatively formal diagnostic procedures, in which interested parties consult a specialist in order to receive a warranted explanation for their perception that something is amiss. These interested persons usually are kinsmen of the persons whose mental status is in question, but unrelated persons who may be aggrieved by an act of the perceivedly "mentally ill" person may also be present, as may wholly unrelated and uninvolved persons who are simply interested bystanders.

In some instances, the diagnostic routine is quite rudimentary. For example, the Pokot diagnostician is likely to be an old woman who serves as a native doctor for a host of ailments. Such a doctor commands an extensive repertoire of magical treatment techniques as well as a large pharmacopeia. But she is also the specialist who is thought best able to diagnose, and hence she commands all those labels that, when applied, permit the Pokot to determine the nature of a presumed disorder, its etiology, and its preferred treatment. The doctor's labels, then, carry an authority that those of ordinary Pokot do not. Thus, where confusion or disagreement in perception or labeling exists, the native doctor may have the final word in determining whether or not a person is to be labeled mentally ill.

I worked briefly with two such native doctors among the Pokot, and while I could never fully understand the phenomenal cues to which they responded in making their diagnoses, it was a simple matter to grasp the nosology within which they worked. For severe disorders causing a person to "behave as though he had no reason," there were essentially only two labels; one referred to an aggressively dangerous person, the other to a socially harmless one. For milder emotional disorders (depression, anxiety, confusion, and the like), there was but one all-inclusive label. The procedure by which it is decided which of these labels to apply is almost entirely an empirical one, consisting of a physical and "mental" examination of the "patient" and interviews with knowledgeable persons. There are virtually no divinatory, magical, or religious elements in this recognition process.

In other African societies, however, the diagnostic routine can be complex.[9] It was certainly so among the Hehe of Tanzania. Not only do the Hehe have native doctors, they have specialists who deal only with mental illness. I knew two Hehe native psychiatrists, both of whom saw patients who came, or were brought in, from great distances. Both doctors employed complicated nosologies—fourteen major categories in the practice of one doctor and over twenty in the other. The categories, and labels, in these nosological systems ranged from major psychotic disturbances to relatively minor and specific psychosomatic disorders. The doctors worked in impressive surroundings and employed a still more impressive assortment of techniques: divination, religion, magic, and, I suspect, far-flung intelligence systems. But most important is their botanical knowledge, which gives them control over a large number of patently psychoactive drugs. These formidable drugs serve most efficiently to enforce the power of the doctors. As a result, these native doctors operate within an ambiance of great skill and authority; their diagnoses are definitive, given with the combined force of the Hehe god, the ancestors, magic, and dramatically powerful medications.

Despite all this, as we shall shortly see, even such impressively authoritative labelings are open to negotiation. *That is the critical point.* When the disorder is not both severe and chronic, even though authoritative diagnosticians may be involved, the recognition of mental illness is open to substantial negotiation.

Case 5. Sebei: Problems in recognition While traveling through an unfamiliar part of Sebei territory, I once stopped to watch a young Sebei man who was behaving strangely. With me was my Sebei interpreter and two other Sebei men whom I know only slightly—Salimu and Sayekwa. These Sebei men were also strangers in this area and did not know the young man in question.

The three Sebei men and I sat and watched this young man (who was about 18) for 20 or 30 minutes. The young man wore a "foolish" grin and occasionally giggled like a small child. He sometimes made an in-

---

[9] For examples, see Kiev (1964), Leighton (1963), Jahoda (1961), Field (1960).

effectual effort to chase some children who were playing nearby, and between these forays he would approach a group of men and utter words that were described to me as "nonsense." He appeared to be excited, and his movements were abrupt and jerky. Also, he sometimes flapped his arms like a bird, and once or twice he shook himself like a dog trying to dry off. But at times he stood quietly and conducted himself as would a perfectly "normal" Sebei.

Without direction from me, the Sebei men began to discuss him, and my interpreter gave me a running account of the conversation, approximately as follows:

Salimu: He is a strange boy.

Sayekwa: He is a foolish boy. Why does he behave that way?

Salimu: He may be mad or he may be foolish [mentally retarded].

Sayekwa: It could also be bewitchment or a fever or something like a fit.

Salimu: What is his clan? [Some clans are noted for epilepsy and mental illness.]

Sayekwa: Is he circumcised? How old is he? He should not act that way.

Interpreter: There is something wrong. People here smoke *bhang.* Perhaps he may be a *bhang* man.

Sayekwa: No. I don't think that. He is more like he is crazy.

Salimu: I think he may be a fool.

Interpreter: It is impossible to know without knowing about his family. We could ask one of these people about him.

My question: What is the difference between a fool and a madman?

Salimu: A fool was born without sense. A madman becomes senseless because of a disease or witchcraft. We would have to know his history to tell about this young man.

My question: What will happen to him if he is crazy?

Salimu: I don't know.

Sayekwa: It would depend upon many things.

My question: What do you mean?

Interpreter (answering for him): He means that so many things cannot be known. Who is his father? What clan does his mother come from? Does he have a disease or was he bewitched? Or spirits may be involved. Also it depends on what he does, whether he troubles people or is merely a silly fellow.

After some general discussion, all the Sebei men then agreed that they could not label the young man until they knew much more about his behavior, his past, and the circumstances of his family and clan. Neither could they say what action should be taken. They all perceived that something was wrong, but without additional information they could not go beyond this perception.

Case 6. Hehe: A father's disappointment and rediagnosis[10]   A 16-year-

[10] I was present during all the events related in this case, except, of course, for the midnight witch-finding episode which is always conducted in secrecy.

old Hehe boy was brought to a well-known Hehe native doctor who specialized in the diagnosis and treatment of mental disorders. The boy, who was entirely out of touch with reality, was half-carried and half-restrained by a number of his male relatives. The boy was highly agitated and would not respond to any effort at communication. The doctor had the boy tied to the centerpost of the house, then, by holding the boy's nose, he forced a liquid down his throat. In a short while, the boy was calm and the doctor began his diagnostic routine.

The doctor diagnosed by means of divination, prayer, and his accumulated empirical knowledge. The details of the diagnostic process are available elsewhere (Winans & Edgerton, 1964), and it is sufficient here to note that the process is highly dramatic, and by virtue of the simultaneous appeal to the Hehe god, to the ancestors, to magic, and to professional skill, the resulting diagnosis carries with it the force of great authority. In this case, the doctor deliberated for many minutes before he concluded that his patient was incurably psychotic (*lisaliko*), and that his psychosis was probably inherited rather than being caused by witchcraft or the will of god.

When the relatives, particularly the boy's father, recovered from the shock of this unpleasant diagnosis, a polite but vigorous protest began. The father expressed his respect for the doctor, but argued that the diagnosis simply could not be correct. After all, he insisted, the boy had been unusually successful in school and had, in fact, been sent away to an expensive school for which very few Hehe boys qualify. He had only recently graduated from this school, and his father and all his relatives were certain that he would now find lucrative employment, perhaps with the government, and bring both fame and wealth to his deserving and long-suffering family. Surely, such a boy could not be psychotic, especially not incurably so, and most obviously not from any inherited defect. The father now appeared triumphant, and, in a voice that oozed conspiracy, he suggested that he had good reason to believe that his own son was in fact bewitched by a man who had long been envious of the boy's success. The father offered to pay the doctor well if he could identify the witch and the malevolent witchcraft being used, could cure the boy, and then punish the witch.

The doctor listened gravely. Without indicating any change in his professional diagnosis, he agreed to reconsider the case by performing his very powerful witch-finding magic that night. The following day he would present his reconsidered opinion. That night the doctor went to the nearest crossroads and stood naked there, seeking the identity of the witch (the Hehe say that certain persons can see witches if they so comport themselves during the night). The next day the father and the relatives returned to the doctor's house and were told that his endeavors of the night before had indeed confirmed the suspicion of witchcraft. The boy, he announced, suffered from *mbepo,* a curable form of psychosis that is caused by witchcraft. Not only was the illness curable, but the witch was known, and could be punished. This pronouncement brought great happiness to all the relatives, who promptly pledged certain amounts of money to the doctor.

All that following day the doctor administered drugs to the boy, and by the end of the day the boy was able to sit up, eat calmly, and speak appropriately. In a few days he appeared to be completely recovered and was able to discuss his past affliction as well as show interest in the magical practices being employed to retaliate against the man who was "known" to have bewitched him. At this point, all agreed that the boy had not been psychotic, and all expressed faith in the permanency of his cure.

Three weeks later, the boy relapsed and once again appeared to be in an acute psychotic fugue state, totally out of touch with reality. Once again, this time after some eight days, a partial cure was effected, although the boy remained anxious and complained that he could not sleep. Nonetheless, the family continued to seek out the witch and to plan for the fame and wealth that the boy's expected success would bring.

When I spoke to the doctor after the relapse, he apparently confided in me, saying that the boy had, all along, been incurably psychotic. He added that the condition was inherited in that clan, and that there was really nothing he could do. He insisted that he changed his diagnosis not because of the money involved, but because it was so important to the family that he do so: "They paid me little money. It was not that. But it is very important to them that the boy not be psychotic. Do you think I have no heart?"

Here we have had a glimpse of a full-scale negotiation in which the desire of concerned relatives caused a doctor to alter his "definitive" diagnosis. The parents and relatives were determined to resist any label for the boy that would jeopardize his—and thus their—economic future. Although the Hehe doctor rarely changed his diagnoses, in this case he did so despite the fact that he actually never doubted the accuracy of his original label. It is impossible in this context to do more than hint at the complexity of the involvements in this case, but its negotiated character is obvious.[11]

[11] A detailed analysis of this case will be presented in a forthcoming publication.

Case 7. Pokot: Psychosis as a justification for execution[12]   Amalung was feared by all his Pokot neighbors. His physical prowess, his undeniable ferocity, and his willingness to implement his will with force, had made him de facto chief of his area. His power, however, did nothing to diminish his hatred for his brother, with whom he had frequently quarreled and who had inherited as many cattle from their father as Amalung had. Amalung's hatred was intense and of long standing. He often accused his brother of wrongdoing, and at least twice his accusations contained the suggestion that the brother was a dangerous psychotic who would be put to death by his neighbors. On one occasion, he accused his brother of "running mad" and burning a house down; on the other occasion he insisted that his "psychotic" brother had threatened to kill him. Despite Amalung's claims, the Pokot people did nothing. For one thing, they had no evidence that Amalung's brother had actually done any of the things he was accused of doing, and for another, apparently not everyone believed that he was psychotic. In fact, some people did not even appear to perceive him as being especially odd. All did admit, however, that he drank a great deal, even more than most Pokot men did, and that when drunk he would sometimes become aggressive or disturb the sleep of other people. It was his brother's drunkenness that Amalung finally used against him.

One night Amalung's brother was staggering home after consuming much beer. He was singing and shouting and generally raising a great din. As he reached a narrow place in the path, he was attacked by Amalung and another man. After a brief scuffle, the drunken man was murdered: while Amalung's friend sat on the fallen man's chest and choked him with a piece of wood, Amalung seized his brother's testicles and tore them from his body. Some minutes later, the neighborhood was awakened by Amalung's loud announcement that his brother had again "run mad" and that he, Amalung, had done a public service to the community by killing this dangerous "madman" who was, he alleged, once again about to set fire to a house.

The next day there was much discussion of the event, and again Amalung and his accomplice argued that it was a case of justifiable homicide because of the victim's psychosis and his intent to commit arson. The Pokot listened and argued among themselves, but none rose to accuse Amalung directly of wrongdoing. However, someone surreptitiously informed the Kenya police of the "murder." It is not known whether the

[12] This case is reconstructed from the accounts of many informants, from court records, and from conversations recorded in the field with Amalung.

police were called out of a sense of sympathy for the deceased or merely because of an urge to be rid of the feared Amalung.

The court heard evidence, but no one other than Amalung and his friend could be found who testified that the dead brother had ever been psychotic. Amalung's plea of justifiable homicide was rejected, and he was sent to prison for a brief term on the reduced sentence of manslaughter. Whether Amalung's brother was or was not mentally ill cannot, of course, be determined. And it is beside the point, for the question of whether or not Amalung's brother was "mad" cannot be separated from the welter of personal, moral, and jural considerations that attended the case. Perhaps Amalung was right and his brother was psychotic, but perhaps Amalung was merely a jealous man who used psychosis as an excuse for murder. What is certain is that many Pokot were eager to be rid of Amalung.

In this case, we lack details concerning the actual negotiations that must have taken place. We know only that a feared man attempted to impose a label in order to justify his action, and that the label—and hence the action—was rejected by his fellow Pokot who called the police and then testified against him.

Case 8.   Kamba: Murder, insanity, and reduced responsibility[13]   A few years ago, when Mutiso was about 35 years old, he killed a 6-year-old girl, not to mention two goats and a chicken. Mutiso attacked the girl and the animals in broad daylight and killed all of them with a large knife. He was in a great rage, and members of his clan finally had to tie him to a tree until he calmed down enough to explain his actions. Mutiso explained that the child was a witch who had been causing his cattle and goats to sicken and die. He claimed that he had warned the child, but when the animals continued to die, he decided to kill the "witch." Then, he killed the nearby animals "as compensation."

After hearing Mutiso's story, members of his clan met to determine their proper course. By Kamba law, the clan is responsible for paying compensation whenever one of their members harms the property or life of a member of another clan. In a murder case, they would ordinarily have considerable compensation to pay. In this instance, they were unusually reluctant to pay compensation because Mutiso was considered by his fellow clansmen to be a "worthless" person—poor, irresponsible

[13] This case is reconstructed from the accounts of many informants, from government and hospital records, and from interviews with many of the principals involved.

and a troublemaker. Mutiso's claim that the girl he killed was a witch was plausible, for even very young girls can be witches, but in this case there was no solid evidence to support his claim. Hence, Mutiso's action could not be excused, and compensation would apparently be required. However, since Mutiso previously had been in disputes that required the payment of clan compensation, his clansmen were most reluctant to pay for his misdeeds again. While the clan was debating the proper course to follow, a European police official heard of the "murder" of the child and took Mutiso into custody, saying indiscreetly that Mutiso must be "insane" to have done such a thing.

Mutiso's clansmen leaped at this interpretation with eager acceptance, for if Mutiso were found to be insane, they would be required to pay little compensation, or perhaps none at all. The clansmen agreed among themselves to testify to Mutiso's madness, and they appear to have won Mutiso's agreement to such a plea. As one old man recalled it, "We told him that if the Europeans found him guilty of murder, he would hang. But if he were only insane, he would go away to the hospital in Nairobi. He agreed that he was insane."

At the trial, Mutiso's clan members offered convincing evidence of his great psychosis, citing many explicit instances of his past psychotic misconduct. And, rather mysteriously, the age of the child who was killed was reduced from 6 to 2, making the likelihood of her being a witch even less in the eyes of the European magistrate. The deceased girl's relatives and clan argued that Mutiso was sane, but the magistrate, without benefit of psychiatric evaluation, declared him insane, referring to a speech Mutiso made before the court as evidence of his insanity. Mutiso said,

It is the custom of my people to kill people. I have killed 100. God orders this. This is done to eat meat. I eat those I kill. I want to go home and see my relations—if there are many of them, I will eat them, but if there are only a few, I will wait until there are many. My father taught me to eat people. I killed my wife and ate her breasts. Human meat is sweeter than cow meat. I would exchange 100 cows for one pound of human meat.

I visited Mutiso in the mental hospital, three years after his commitment. He occasionally spoke bizarrely, saying such things as, "You only think I am an African; actually I am English," or "I am king of the Kenya cowboys," or "This is a place for killing cows." But he was also capable of quite competent conduct, as witness the fact that he was nominally in charge of three wards of African patients. Indeed, the psychiatrist in charge stated that he was by no means certain that Mutiso was psychotic and added his own speculation that his legal insanity was contrived to escape "the noose." He quickly added, however, that he could not prove his belief, so Mutiso was still in the hospital.[14]

I asked a member of Mutiso's clan to comment upon the outcome of the case and he said, "Yes, Mutiso. A bad man, a very hot-tempered man. He was a mannerless man, always causing the clan trouble. He was not really crazy, of course, only hot-tempered. I think that things worked out well, though. We did not have to pay compensation, and Mutiso is happy because he is still alive. Only the other clan is unhappy, but after the court decided, what can they do?"

Finally, I asked Mutiso directly if he were mad. His answer, though rhetorical, is worth repeating: "Am I crazy? Of course, I am. Everyone is. You are crazy too. If everyone were not crazy, would I be here?"

In this Kamba example, a disturbed, but probably not psychotic, man became the fortunate recipient of his clan members' desire not to be further responsible for his misdeeds. European police officers and courts were the unwitting foils for the conspiracy of Mutiso's clan. The result was a one-sided negotiation, but a negotiation nonetheless.

The foregoing illustrations taken from four East African tribes have been directed toward two major points. The first is that where a person is so severely mentally ill that he cannot provide (or cause to be provided for him) an acceptable explanation for his conduct, and where he remains consistently, chronically unable to do so, then he is perceived and labeled as a psychotic. The illustrations presented could have been bolstered by a great many others, all to the same point that persons in these four societies consistently agreed in the recognition of chronic psychotics.

The second point was that when a presumably mentally ill person is not both severely and chronically psychotic, the recognition of such a person is open to negotiation. The illustrations of negotiation that were presented were not fully adequate to their purpose. No four short examples could be. Still, they served to illustrate some important points. Case 5 (Sebei) showed that the labeling of even very inappropriate behavior can be difficult. Case 6 (Hehe) gave some insight into the ways in which a label can be negotiated—so effectively negotiated in this instance that a definitive "medical" diagnosis was changed. The last two cases (Pokot and Kamba) give an intimation of the extent to which matters of personal

---

[14] The hospital authorities screened several convicted murderers each week in order to make judgments upon questions of legal insanity. Many of these murderers attempted to feign psychosis, and some, it was admitted, succeeded in doing so.

and corporate responsibility and the law can be involved in the recognition of mental illness. Although these cases both involved the European controlled police and courts, their message was nonetheless clear.

Before attempting to state the conclusions that I think ought to be drawn from this material, it would be useful to pause and ask what relevance this formulation about the recognition of mental illness has for our own society. Is there any reason to suppose that the process of recognition among native Africans is similar to the one present in the complex, highly specialized social system of modern America?

Aspects of the Recognition of Mental Illness in the United States

The first point to be made is that however much we may agree or disagree that there are strong parallels between recognition in African tribal societies and recognition by the lay public in this country, we must agree that there are few relevant data that bear upon the question. There are bits and pieces of evidence from many sources, professional and otherwise, but these fugitive materials add up to very little, and in any case they cannot be brought together within the narrow compass of this paper. Although there is some supporting evidence that the recognition of some psychotic conditions can easily be consensual, and the recognition of other mental disorders may be negotiated, the facts remain unclear.[15]

The most striking impression to be derived from materials depicting the public response is that the complex of recognition is somehow dealt with in the everyday world as though it were not a problem at all. Surely, the citizenry gives no evidence of being up-in-arms over any difficulties concerning the recognition of mental illness. Admittedly, there are certain dark forebodings and dire pronouncements issuing from some quarters, such as from the anti-mental health campaigners,[16] but such voices, though possessed of volume, hardly reflect a widespread public concern. Perhaps the public expresses no great concern with the issue because the responsibility of recognition has been handed over to specialists (obviously, psychiatrists) who possess the professional training and legal sanctions to deal with it.

---

[15] For example, *Action for Mental Health* (1961, pp. 75–76) reports findings from Shirley Star's unpublished study (based upon 3500 interviews) that asked respondents to discuss vignettes descriptive of "deviant behavior." The six vignettes included descriptions of severe and mild disorders, ranging from paranoid schizophrenia to a behavior disorder. There was as high as 75 percent recognition of the paranoid schizophrenic as being mentally ill, but recognition of mental illness in the other five vignettes ranged between 34 and 7 percent.

[16] See Auerbach (1963).

Is it true, then, that psychiatry is in an uproar over the problem of recognizing (diagnosing) mental illness? There are those within psychiatry who believe that it should be. Szasz, in his *Law, Liberty and Psychiatry* (1963), undoubtedly leads a small chorus of voices in viewing the situation with alarm.

There are, of course, some conspicuous examples of difficulties in the psychiatric diagnostic process. For instance, Jewell (1960) reports the case of a Navaho Indian who was wrongly diagnosed as a schizophrenic and was forcibly hospitalized for eighteen months before it was determined that his withdrawn and mute behavior was due to cultural reasons, not psychosis. Conversely, we have all heard of cases in which it is reported that a patently psychotic individual has repeatedly evaded diagnosis as such, until making some critical slip, as, for example, the casual admission that he is in reality Jesus Christ.

Notwithstanding such occasionally spectacular errors in diagnosis, there is no apparent sense of despair within psychiatry about the difficulties attending the recognition of mental illness. There is, rather, a general impression that the task can be difficult, especially in forensic psychiatry, but the task nevertheless proceeds as well as can be expected. After all, many might argue, the primary demand is the critical task of treatment. In general, then, both the lay public and the psychiatric specialists seem to conduct themselves as though the problem of deciding who is or is not mentally ill were being solved to their satisfaction.

But, how well do psychiatrists actually agree with each other on their recognitions—diagnoses—of mental illness? Before venturing an answer, I feel that a general observation about recognition is called for. We are all aware from our own common-sense experience, that people everywhere make astonishingly complex recognitions "at-a-glance." They do so quickly, effortlessly, and seemingly appropriately. Women "size up" other women with no more than a glance—and men surely do the same. Our everyday lives, and novels about our lives, are filled with examples of this sort of routine, high-speed recognition. Yet, we are also aware that mistakes are often made, and we surely do not always agree with each other on such "at-a-glance" recognitions. Agreement, when it is reached, is typically the product of some discussion or negotiation.

The literature on experimental studies of perception, or what is sometimes called recognition, either of persons or of visual patterns, is not completely relevant to the kind of recognition we are discussing, but it does inform us that perception and labeling are most complicated matters.[17] For example, even the recognition of color is immensely complex;

[17] For example, see Galanter (1962), Cline & Richards (1961), Mednick & Mednick (1963), Whilte (1962), Roby & Budrose (1965).

it has been estimated that a normal person can discriminate several millions of colors, but in everyday practice we label only a very limited number of colors.[18] And, we must all be aware of the difficulties that we have in deciding what color something *really* is.

If the process of recognition in general is so complex, then it would require truly oceanic credulity to believe that the recognition of so variable a phenomenon as mental illness is any less complicated.

In fact, the literature on the problem of the reliability of psychiatric diagnoses indicates that for most kinds of diagnoses, psychiatrists seldom agree with each other. For example, Ash (1949) found that agreement among three psychiatrists on major diagnostic categories ("mental deficiency," "psychopathy," "psychosis," "neurosis," and "normal") was no better than 45.7 percent with the agreement between the two possible pairs of psychiatrists only reaching 57.9 and 67.4 percent. Ash (1949) concludes as follows: "In short, in the cases under consideration, agreement between two psychiatrists in diagnoses even as high as that approaching or exceeding a fifty-fifty split of opinion was found only when diagnoses were grouped into very broad categories [p. 275]."

Similarly, Mehlman (1952) found little agreement among several psychiatrists concerning the diagnoses of a large number of psychotic patients, and Cattel (1957) found a correlation of no better than 0.25 among experienced psychiatrists in rating the symptom "anxiety" in eighty psychiatric patients. Others, such as Chodoff (1960) and Pasamanick, Dinitz, & Lefton (1959) reported similarly low agreement. Perhaps the situation is best summarized by Stoller & Geertsma (1963) who concluded on the basis of their research with 27 practising psychiatrists, " . . . that art far outweighs science when experts in the field of psychiatry try to say what they have discovered in another person, and that practitioners of the art disagree with each other much more than is commonly recognized [p. 65]."

However, there is another side to the evidence. Rosenzweig, Vandenberg, Moore, & Dukay (1961) compared the diagnoses of three psychiatrists concerning fifty chronic hospital patients. The study called for all three psychiatrists to see each one of the fifty patients at the same time to assure that all psychiatrists saw the same behavior (of course, ratings were made independently). Rosenzweig and his colleagues found that the psychiatrists agreed on their diagnoses 96 percent of the time. Zigler & Phillips (1961), in their review of the literature, support the view that there can be agreement among psychiatrists on certain broad diagnostic categories.

It may be that, while psychiatrists often, even usually, disagree on certain kinds of diagnoses, in some cases (especially those involving

[18] Compare Conklin (1964).

chronic psychotics) they can approach consensus in the application of their labels. While the data available in the literature are insufficient to support any final conclusions, it is safe to conclude that practitioners within the psychiatric edifice are not as serenely in agreement as we might have been tempted to think.

There are many reasons why this reported disagreement should exist. To mention only a few of the more common reasons, there are differing orientations, different terms, differential exposure to the patients being diagnosed, and an imperative emphasis on treatment no matter what the diagnosis. But it is also true that the diagnosis of mental illness is unlike diagnosis of most other illnesses. Not that some nonpsychiatric diagnoses, such as those concerning heart disease, are not equally difficult to make, subject to error, and intrinsically negotiable, but, as many psychiatrists have pointed out, psychiatric diagnosis involves social factors to a unique degree. Thus, Loftus (1960) in his book on diagnosis in clinical psychiatry, says that the criteria of psychiatric diagnosis, ". . . are of a social, cultural, economic and sometimes legal nature [p. 13]." Is it any wonder that negotiation is often involved?

Supporting evidence for the negotiation thesis is available in many sources, as in the work of Goffman and others,[19] but it is far outside the scope of this discussion to sort out the voluminous literature that is relevant to the negotiation process in psychiatry. This discussion is intended to be an exploration, one that takes the illustrations for its thesis from African tribal societies, not from Western psychiatry.

CONCLUSION

On the basis of the cross-cultural evidence—particularly that from Africa—part of which was presented here, I conclude that the recognition of mental illness is a social process that has fundamental moral and jural involvements. These involvements are inevitably present, because mental illness is a status—a status that carries with it a change (usually a reduction) in rights and responsibilities. Needless to say, the change affects not only the mentally ill person but also all those who must interact with him. Negotiations, therefore, must be concerned with the question of rightful entitlement to the status of being mentally ill, an entitlement that is variously claimed or denied, offered, or rejected. Although negotiations can involve all manner of persons and can hinge upon an almost limitless variety of considerations, they must always take account of these central considerations—rights and responsibilities.

With the exception of certain severe and chronic cases, the recognition

[19] See Goffman (1961). For an introduction to other material, see Greenblatt, Levinson, & Williams (1957).

of mental illness is negotiable. The labels that are applied, the actions that follow, and the perceptions that precede—all are negotiable. Because of the force of social negotiation, there can easily be perception of mental illness without consequent labeling, or labeling without consequent action, and there can even be psychosis without perception. Thus, all aspects of the recognition process can be influenced by negotiation.

That mental illness is a social and cultural phenomenon, as well as a psychological and biological one, has long been accepted. Therefore, to argue that the recognition of mental illness is a social matter is hardly original. Indeed, this view has been anticipated by many writers in a number of different disciplines. It is perhaps less widely accepted that recognition—or diagnosis—is as negotiable as I have suggested here.

If my thesis is correct, it would follow that the recognition process in contemporary psychiatry is not simply, or even primarily, a problem in medical diagnosis. It is a social transaction that often takes the form of a negotiation. And this is true not only where legal matters are concerned, such as with pleas of insanity in the courtroom, or in psychiatric deferments for military service, but also in common clinical practice where diagnoses often grow out of a prolonged interchange between the patient, his friends or relatives, and the clinician or clinicians.

Seen in this fashion, mental illness does not become merely a "myth," nor is it simply another "social problem." There are real disturbances in thought, affect, and conduct that require medical management. Moreover, this view says nothing to discredit psychiatric treatment. Neither does it suggest that psychiatric diagnosis is not essentially a sincere, empirical effort to classify symptoms or syndromes into what may someday be a scientific nosology. But more so than other forms of medical diagnosis, psychiatric diagnosis must take social factors into account.

To see psychiatric diagnosis as a process akin to a negotiation, then, helps to call attention to the moral and jural factors upon which diagnosis can depend, and it promotes increased awareness of the social basis of the diagnostic process. What is called for—what has long been called for—is a more acute analysis of these negotiations within the socio-legal systems to which they relate, and which they serve to maintain.

REFERENCES

Aberle, D. "Arctic hysteria" and Latah in Mongolia. *Transactions of the New York Academy of Sciences,* 1952, **22**, 291–297.

Action for mental health. Final Report of the Joint Commission on Mental Illness and Health, 1961. New York: Basic Books, 1961.

Ash, P. The reliability of psychiatric diagnoses. *Journal of Abnormal and Social Psychology*, 1949, 44, 271–276.

Auerbach, A. The anti-mental health movement. *American Journal of Psychiatry*, 1963, **120**, 105–111.

Bateson, G. (Ed.) *Perceval's narrative, a patient's account of his psychosis, 1830–1832.* Stanford, California: Stanford University Press, 1961.

Bowers, M. The onset of psychosis—a diary account. *Psychiatry*, 1965, **28**, 346–358.

Brelsford, W. V. Insanity among the Bemba of Northern Rhodesia. *Africa*, 1950, **20**, 46–54.

Cattel, R. B. The conceptual and test distinction of neuroticism and anxiety. *Journal of Clinical Psychology*, 1957, **13**, 221–233.

Chodoff, P. The problem of psychiatric diagnosis: can biochemistry and neurophysiology help? *Psychiatry*, 1960, **23**, 185–191.

Cline, V. B., & Richards, J. M. The generality of accuracy of interpersonal perception. *Journal of Abnormal and Social Psychology*, 1961, **62**, 446–449.

Conklin, H. C. Hanunoo color categories. In D. Hymes (Ed.), *Language in culture and society*. New York: Harper and Row, 1964.

Devereux, G. Mohave ethnopsychiatry and suicide. *Bureau of American Ethnology, Bulletin No. 175*, 1961.

Devereux, G. Primitive psychiatric diagnosis: a general theory of the diagnostic process. In I. Galdston (Ed.), *Man's image in medicine and anthropology*. New York: Universities Press, 1963.

Edgerton, R. B. Conceptions of psychosis in four East African societies. *American Anthropologist*, 1966, **68**, 408–425.

Field, M. J. *Search for security: an ethno-psychiatric study of rural Ghana*. London: Faber and Faber, 1960.

Galanter, E. Contemporary psychophysics. In T. Newcomb (Ed.), *New directions in psychology*. New York: Holt, Rinehart and Winston, 1962.

Goffman, E. *Asylums. Essays on the social situations of mental patients and other inmates*. New York: Anchor Books, 1961.

Greenblatt, M., Levinson, D., & Williams, R. *The patient and the mental hospital*. Glencoe, Ill.: The Free Press, 1957.

Jahoda, G. Traditional healers and other institutions concerned with mental illness in Ghana. *International Journal of Social Psychiatry*, 1961, **7**, 245–268.

Jewell, D. P. A case of a "psychotic" Navaho Indian male. In D. Apple (Ed.), *Social studies of health and sickness; a source book for the health professions*. New York: McGraw-Hill, 1960.

Kiev, A. *Magic, faith, and healing*. Glencoe, Ill.: The Free Press, 1964.

Langness, L. L. Hysterical psychosis in the New Guinea highlands: A Bena Bena example. *Psychiatry*, 1965, **28**, 258–277.

Lee, S. G. Some Zulu concepts of psychogenic disorder. *Journal for Social Research, Pretoria*. 1950, **1**, 9–18.

Leighton, A., et al. *Psychiatric disorder among the Yoruba*. Ithaca, N.Y.: Cornell University Press, 1963.

Linton, R. *Culture and mental disorders.* Springfield, Ill.: Charles C Thomas, 1956.

Loftus, T. A. *Meaning and methods of diagnosis in clinical psychiatry.* Philadelphia: Lea and Febiger, 1960.

Mednick, M. T., & Mednick, S. A. (Eds.). *Research in personality.* New York: Holt, Rinehart and Winston, 1963.

Mehlman, B. The reliability of psychiatric diagnoses. *Journal of Abnormal and Social Psychology,* 1952, **47,** 577–578.

Newman, P. "Wild man" behavior in a New Guinea highlands community. *American Anthropologist,* 1964, **66,** 1–19.

Opler, M. K. *Culture and mental health: Cross-cultural studies.* New York: Macmillan Co., 1959.

Pasamanick, B., Dinitz, S., & Lefton, M. Psychiatric orientation and its relation to diagnosis and treatment in a mental hospital. *American Journal of Psychiatry,* 1959, **116,** 127–132.

Roby, T., & Budrose, C. Pattern recognition in groups: Laboratory and simulation studies. *Journal of Personality and Social Psychology,* 1965, **2,** 648–653.

Rogler, L., & Hollingshead, A. *Trapped: Families and schizophrenia.* New York: Wiley, 1965.

Rosenzweig, N., S. K. Vandenberg, K. Moore, & A. Duray. A study of the reliability of the mental status examination. *American Journal of Psychiatry,* 1961, **117,** 1102–1108.

Spiro, M. E. A psychotic personality in the South Seas. *Psychiatry,* 1950, **13,** 189–204.

Stoller, R. J., & Geertsma, R. H. The consistency of psychiatrists' clinical judgments. *Journal of Nervous and Mental Disease,* 1963, **137,** 58–66.

Szasz, T. S. *Law, liberty and psychiatry.* New York: Macmillan, 1963.

Teicher, M. I. The Windigo psychosis. *Proceedings of the 1960 Annual Spring Meeting.* American Ethnological Society, 1960.

Wallace, A. F. C. *Culture and personality.* New York: Random House, 1961.

Whilte, B. W. Recognition of familiar characters under unfamiliar transformation. *Perceptual and Motor Skills,* 1962, **15,** 107–116.

Winans, E. V., & Edgerton, R. B. Hehe magical justice. *American Anthropologist,* 1964, **66,** 745–764.

Yap, P. M. The Latah reaction. *Journal of Mental Science,* 1952, **48,** 515–564.

Zigler, E., & Phillips, L. Psychiatric diagnosis and symptomatology. *Journal of Abnormal and Social Psychology,* 1961, **63,** 69–75.

chapter two

Does Culture Make
a Difference?

2.1 Introduction

None of the perennial puzzles about mental illness is more fundamental or perplexing than the nature of the relationship between culture and mental disorder. That this should be so is hardly surprising, for man does not and could not exist in a world that is noncultural, and the ways in which man's culture bears upon man's disorders are anything but simple.

Arguments over the relationship between culture and mental illness typically do not revolve around whether culture does or does not have an effect, rather the questions concern the mechanisms by which this effect occurs and the degree to which it is significant. Some opinions are universalist, holding that the effects of culture upon the etiology, incidence or, symptomatology of mental illness are minimal. A recent statement of this view is offered by E. B. Forster (1962) a psychiatrist with considerable experience in Ghana:

Psychiatric syndromes or reactions, by and large, are similar in all races throughout the world. The mental reactions seen in our African patients can be diagnosed according to Western textbook standards. The basic illness and reaction types are the same. Environmental, constitutional and tribal cultural background merely modify the symptom constellation. Basically, the disorders of thinking, feeling, willing and knowing are the same.

73

Many, perhaps even most, who have joined the study of mental illness, would probably grant culture a larger role than this. Indeed, many workers in the social sciences and psychiatry alike hold the view that culture determines both the amount and the kind of mental disorder to be found in any society. And, probably all would agree that the meaning, and hence the prognosis, of mental illness in any society is a product of that society's culture.

However, beyond these vague and general pronouncements there lies great and growing uncertainty, for we are coming to realize how little we really know about these matters. Despite a rapid accumulation of research bearing upon mental illness in various of the world's cultures, we have scarcely begun the task of careful collection of those data that may someday permit us to specify the links between "culture and mental illness." The chapters that follow provide a sense of the problem, of what we know and what we do not know, and of the complicated character of this seemingly simple relationship.

We begin this section with a general consideration of the many ways in which culture is said to be related to mental illness (Wallace). We then turn to detailed accounts of differential psychopathology in various cultural settings (Opler and Kiev). We also ask whether some cultures are more or less stressful than others (Naroll) and, still more specifically, what effect early experiences have upon adult mental health or illness (Barry). Taking another contrastive perspective, we compare mental illness in Nova Scotia and Nigeria (Leighton) and throughout Polynesia (Beaglehole). Finally, we return to the United States and examine mental illness among Mexican-Americans (Madsen), Negroes (Crawford), and Japanese-Americans (Kitano).

REFERENCE

Forster, E. B. The theory and practice of psychiatry in Ghana. *American Journal of Psychotherapy,* 1962, **16,** 35.

2.2   *Orientation*

The issues that are implied by the relationship of culture to mental illness are nowhere better raised than in the following essay by Anthony F. C. Wallace. Wallace contrasts what he calls the "psycho-social school" with the "biochemical." The psychosocial school embraces the social and psychological sciences as well as much of psychiatry. Wallace reviews the various assertions made for the critical importance of social and cultural processes in the etiology and treatment of mental illness.

As an anthropologist, and thus a member of a discipline traditionally located well within this psychosocial school, Wallace represents the arguments for the ways in which "culture makes a difference" fairly and well. Yet, he also enters a cautionary note by chiding devoted proponents of psychosocial explanations for their failure to consider existing evidence for genetic and biochemical involvements in mental illness. This balanced treatment of the issues serves well to set the stage for the chapters that follow.

2.2   Culture Change and Mental Illness[1]

A. F. C. Wallace

Social and cultural change may theoretically be expected to affect the incidence, and prevalence, of mental disorder in a number of ways. Nutritional deficiencies, life expectancy, and the spread of neurologically relevant infectious diseases will obviously affect the mental health status of a population, by increasing or reducing the frequency with which members of the population suffer from physical conditions that affect behavior, such as pellagra, senile arteriosclerosis, and syphilis and trypanosomiasis. But psychological stresses may also affect the mental health status of a population by confronting individuals with role and value conflicts, information overload, and identity challenges. Unhappily, the relative weight to be attached to such various factors in situations of social change cannot be decided on the basis of positive knowledge.

Two major schools of thought at present contend (with minimal mutual lip service) with respect to etiological and therapeutic theories: the biochemical and the psycho-social. The biochemical school primarily orients itself to the psychoses and concerns itself with identifying those currently unknown anomalies of body chemistry (in blood, endocrine secretions, neural tissue, etc.) which are responsible for psychosis, and with discovering the appropriate physical therapies for correcting such

---

[1] From *Culture and Personality,* by Anthony F. C. Wallace. © Copyright 1961 by Random House, Inc. Reprinted by permission.

anomalies (cf. Kety, 1959; Kallman, 1938). Thus, the biochemical school, in effect, expects to bring the psychoses over into the category of organically-determined mental disorders. The psycho-social school embraces the various psycho-analytic disciplines, social and clinical psychology, and (for the most part) sociology and anthropology. While this school is heterogeneous, it shares a common faith that it is in some distortion of the subject's social learning experience and current social situation that his psychopathology originates. Theories vary, however, with respect to the locus of the responsible distortion: psychoanalytic and social anthropological theories tend to emphasize early experience, particularly the parents' relationship to the child; sociologic theories tend to emphasize ecological and social class factors, and so on. With respect to cultural anthropology's participation in the scientific investigation of mental illness, the most glaring weakness has been the bland assumption that "mental disorder" (a few outstanding organic complaints apart) is caused by disorders in social, cultural, and psychological processes. This bland assumption in part has been based on failure to consider seriously the fact that the various known organic impairments can and do regularly produce symptomatologies practically indistinguishable from the whole gamut of "functional" symptomatologies, ranging from psychosis to the transient situational reactions. It has also in part been based on neglect of the existing evidence for genetic and biochemical complicity in the development of the supposedly "psychogenic" or "functional" psychoses. Since cultural anthropologists generally are consulted by, and read the works of, those psychiatrists and psychologists who are committed to the psycho-social tradition, this bias is not corrected from outside the field, but remains to stunt the development of cultural anthropological research in this important area.

In view of its importance for the theoretical orientation of students of anthropology, a brief outline is here given of a theory which attempts to relate biochemical and psycho-social processes in mental disease. Of all the psychoses, the schrizophrenic syndrome is probably the most common. It is the writer's opinion that this psychosis is precipitated and maintained by a biochemical disorder or disorders for which hereditary predisposition is common. Biochemical deficiency reduces the "semantic capacity" of the individual below the level necessary for adequate cultural participation. From the microcosmic viewpoint, this critical level is the boundary between normalcy and deviancy; from the organization viewpoint, it is the degree of diversity which the individual must be able to maintain in a state of relative orderliness, acceptable to self and others. Such a semantic decrement is experienced by the victim as a condition of relative meaninglessness or, as the psychiatrist puts it, as "feelings of unreality" and "lack of affect." These experiences of desemantication may, or may not, be accompanied by other disturbing phenomena, such as hallucination and hypochondriacal sensations. From the initial desemantication flows, inevitably, a set of consequences: a deterioration of the victim's existing personality structure; the development of increasingly desperate and generally inadequate "psychotic" defenses, intended to forestall social extrusion; and, eventually, social extrusion in some form or other. This theory recognizes that cultural differences will be reflected in the symptomatic content and the prevalence of the syndrome in various populations, but relies upon the concept of the cultural capacity of the individual to relate biochemical and psycho-social processes in the individual case (cf. Wallace, 1960).

CURRENT CONCEPTIONS OF THE RELATIONS
OF CULTURE AND MENTAL ILLNESS

Current conceptions of the relationship of culture to mental illness may be conveniently classified under four headings: cultural epidemiology; culture as providing the pathogenic process; culture as providing the therapeutic process; and culture itself, as affected by mental disorder.

Cultural Epidemiology

The epidemiology of mental disease considers the distribution of mental disorders of various kinds over a number of variables, only one of which is culture; others are sex, age, migration history, social class, education, morbidity in other disease categories, nutritional level, ecological zone, and so on. Most of these other categories are, however, not independent of culture and, consequently, are definitely relevant to culturally-oriented inquiries.

From the days of the earliest systematic ethnological fieldwork, up to the present time, anthropologists have been interested in the fact that the symptoms of mental disorder vary, depending on the cultural context of the victim. Sometimes the patterning of these symptoms is so unlike Western clinical portraits as to suggest that a new mental disease has been discovered. Familiar examples may be cited: amok and latah in Southeast Asia; piblokto among Eskimo, and arctic hysteria among northern Siberian peoples; the windigo psychosis among northwestern Algonkian forest hunters. Even within Western society, as Opler has demonstrated, the nature of the symptoms typically exhibited by members of such ethnic groups as Irish and Italians, in New York City, is sharply different: Irish male schizophrenics tend to be quiet and withdrawn, and their Italian counterparts tend to be noisy and aggressive (Opler and Singer, 1956). These differences do not, however, justify the imputation of a different disease category. Windigo psychosis, with its common pattern of somatic delusions, ideas of reference, supernatural persecution complex, and "cannibalistic panic," is a precise image of paranoid schizophrenia, as observed in Western man, except that the overt ideas of persecution or influence of Western man are apt to be oriented toward different supernatural beings or even toward other humans (such as "the men in the Kremlin" or "the FBI"), and to emphasize sex rather than food (the cannibalistic panic being replaced by the homosexual panic). Most such "ethnic psychoses," which reflect in their behavior the specific cultural content of the victim's society, are simply local varieties of a common disease process to which human beings, as such, are vulnerable. In this light, then, all mental disorders must be considered to reflect, in symptomatic content, the victim's past and present cultural environment.

Culture as Pathogenic Influence

If we conclude that the major categories of mental disorder are universal types of human affliction, even though cultural differences are responsible for conspicuous local differences in the content of symptomatology, we must still ask whether cultural differences are associated with differences in the frequency of illness in the major, and universal, diagnostic classifications. Despite semantic difficulties, and notwithstanding the scattered nature of the material, two general conclusions concerning cultural epidemiology can be made: (1) culturally differentiated populations do vary measurably in the incidence (the number of persons who contract a disease during a specified period of time, usually taken as a year) of one or another of the various disease entities, a fact which suggests that, whatever etiological factors are, in part they are culturally determined; and (2), culturally differentiated populations do vary measurably in the prevalence (the number of persons who suffer from a disease during a specified period of time) of one or another of the various disease categories. These generalizations suggest strongly that, whatever the therapeutic and chronicity factors are, their incidence and prevalence in part are culturally determined.

Epidemiological inquiries essentially are based on demographic and social survey statistics. Clinical observation, however, is the source of the data and intuitions which point to the role of culture as a pathogenic influence. Such a putative influence is considered to be direct when the very structure of human relations, and the beliefs and values commonly held in a society, are conceived to be necessarily productive of psychological conflict and anxiety in individuals who participate in the organization. The influence may be considered as indirect when the mere participation in the socio-cultural organization is not, in itself, considered sufficient to elicit psychopathology.

Culture as Indirect Pathogenic Influence

Let us consider the indirect pathogenic influence first. A particularly clear example of such an influence is given by studies of the mental disorders accompanying trypanosomiasis ("sleeping sickness"), a general infection transmitted to man by the bite of the infected tsetse fly. This disorder is said to be "the commonest cause of mental derangement throughout large areas of West Africa" (Tooth, 1950), and is difficult, if not impossible, to distinguish from schizophrenia without identification of the trypanosome micro-organism in the body fluids. The symptomatic picture in "tryps" is as variable as that in "true" schizophrenia, and the same types of behavioral disorder may be found in either. But, in line with the distinction described earlier, one (tryps) is an "organic" psychosis and the other (schizophrenia) is not.

The type of tryps to which most psychiatric attention has been paid is that carried by the flies *Glossina palpalis* and *Glossina tachinoides*. These species feed principally on human blood; they breed in shady places by the edges of streams and water holes. Human beings are bitten and infected when they visit these streams and water holes to wash and to collect water. The public health measures which are effective, in a given local area, are three: (1) clearing away undergrowth at the edge of water; (2) sterilizing the blood of infected persons; (3) prevention of migration of infected persons into the "cleansed" area from adjacent endemic areas. The first requires continuous public attention and compliance in brush-clearing. The second requires that infected persons, or their relatives, bring cases of tryps in the early stages for chemical treatment (before the pathological sleeping and schizophrenia-like symptoms begin, and when the illness is manifested chiefly by a miscellany of somatic complaints— aches and pains, fever, headache, amenorrhea, etc.). It is difficult, however, to recognize tryps in the early stages, because its early symptoms are difficult to distinguish from both malaria and yaws, which almost everyone in the region is apt to experience at one time or another; and the later stages are similar to syphilitic paresis. The third measure requires control of immigration which is impossible for various economic and political reasons: ". . . the Gold Coast is surrounded by endemic areas and there is a virtually uncontrollable migration of persons across its borders, which are only arbitrarily defined, so that, until tryps has been eradicated from tropical Africa as a whole, epidemics and sporadic cases are bound to occur [Tooth, 1960, p. 2]." Thus, we find that the incidence of tryps is affected by a host of culturally-bound factors: the technology of water use, the availability of labor supply for brush clearing, awareness of the value of chemical treatment, economic pressures affecting immigration, the location and significance of the political boundaries, various cultural factors that affect the incidence of yaws and malaria (because their incidence determines the "visibility" of early tryps), and so on.

Tryps is not an unusual example. Other "organic" psychoses—for instance, general paresis accompanying the tertiary stage of syphilis, and the mental disorders accompanying nutritional deficiencies—with equal obviousness are related to cultural factors via the mediation of the structure of sexual, economic, religious, domestic, and political relations, and of popular beliefs and attitudes relating to the disorder in question. Still other disorders, at present regarded as psychogenic, also may be caused by factors, such as nutritional and infectious disease, and thus be related indirectly, rather than directly to culture.

Culture as Direct Pathogenic Influence

We have defined the "direct pathogenic influence" of culture, in respect to mental disorder, as the result of conflict-and-anxiety-producing sets of cultural forms. The reader will note that we are concerned, here, not with culture as determinant of the content of disorder, but of its occurrence and that, for the sake of simplicity of exposition, we shall not labor a point already made: that the weaknesses of the microcosmic viewpoint afflict most of the several fairly specific types of hypotheses. Most of these hypotheses which have been offered to explain the function of culture as a direct pathogenic influence are based on one variety or another of psychoanalytic theory.

Culture per se as cause of neurosis   Freud expressed a view, common to many a humanist, that there is an unavoidable tragedy inherent in the human condition—namely, that the practical necessity of maintaining and transmitting across generations any sort of culture demands the partial, but grievous, frustration of human instincts, both sexual and aggressive. Such instinctual deprivation inevitably elicits from all human beings some sort of neurotic compromise, of greater or lesser degree, ranging from such minor phenomena as slips of the tongue and selective forgetting of unpleasant experiences, to the grand symptoms of clinical neurosis. This view is embedded, of course, in larger philosophical speculations about the universality of the Oedipus complex, castration anxiety, and self-destructive tendencies. Many anthropologists, somewhat naïvely, object that culture is a complex device for instinctual gratification rather than deprivation. It is certainly true that human instincts are usually gratified, when they are gratified, in a cultural medium; but it is also true that human instincts are frustrated, when they are frustrated, in a cultural medium.

Culture as content of neurosis Some anthropologists (e.g., Roheim, 1943) and anthropologically inclined psychoanalysts (e.g., Kardiner, 1939) have felt that major areas of the culture pattern of any given society may be conceived as widely shared and institutionalized neurotic, or even psychotic, symptomatology, arising out of particular instinctual deprivations imposed on the members, particularly in their childhood. ("Neurosis," in this usage, implies that various mechanisms of defense are employed in the building and maintenance of the personality structure; but since all human beings are such mechanisms, all have a "neurosis" in this generic sense.) This view does not necessarily include the doctrine that culture, per se, invariably produces neurosis, and some of these authors even offer recipes for non-neurotic cultures based on enlightened methods of child rearing. Usually, it is the so-called "projective systems"— religious belief and ritual, aspects of political relations, mythology, art, and so forth, which are believed to be related to particular systems of child rearing—to which the tag "neurotic" is applied. In incautious hands, such an approach is dangerous, for even professedly straightforward cultural or modal personality description may imply that an entire people is "sick," as when Benedict (1943) casually describes the Kwakiutl society as "megalomaniac paranoid." Such characterization of whole societies or cultures as mentally ill is rarely, if ever, defensible on scientific grounds; a society of psychotics is a contradiction in terms, and the use of a diagnostic label in national character evaluation expresses merely the author's hostility toward the subjects of his description. Sometimes, of course, psychiatric terms must be used to describe mental processes which occur in both sick and healthy persons as, for instance, the term for defense mechanisms, such as "repression," "sublimation," etc. When such descriptive language is used in a modal personality statement, without the use of diagnostic labels, no harm is done, unless the naïve reader wrongly infers psychopathology whenever a piece of psychiatric jargon is employed. But the use of diagnostic labels, such as "paranoid," "psychotic," and "schizophrenic," or words implying such labels, is never justified when referring to an entire society, except in cases where that society has suffered a major and identifiable trauma to which an illness, definable by the group itself as a pathological state, is a general response. Another risk in this mode of analysis is the overly free imputation of unconscious purpose to account for functional relationships in culture. Clinical psychoanalytic interpretation depends heavily upon the guess that describing the consequences of an act will define its motives. In culture-and-personality analysis, the entire culture of a society is regarded as the consequence of the acts of its members. The statement that some pattern of unconscious motives creates and maintains the culture is apt to invoke an animistic teleology which, however useful in the art of psychotherapy, is not justifiable in rigorous analysis. Furthermore, it requires the use of the dubious "cultural-deductive method" (Wallace, 1952a).

Culturally enjoined "disorders"   In many societies, religious ritual and other ceremonial protocol require individuals of certain statuses to undergo types of experiences which, in contemporary Western psychiatric tradition, often are regarded as symptomatic of mental disorder. The class of pseudo-illnesses, culturally enjoined, include such diverse phenomena as ritual dissociation (trance and possession), drug or alcohol intoxication (as, for example, in peyote), self-mortification leading to hallucination (as in the vision quest), ceremonial torture and cannibalism, and ecstatic conversion experiences. The physiological and psychological mechanisms immediately involved in the "abnormal" state in such pseudo-disorders may well be the same as those involved in symptom production in Western mental patients. Nevertheless, the consequences of such experiences are vastly different, since a "ceremonial" neurosis or psychosis, unlike the "true" disease, is voluntarily initiated, is usually reversible, and leads neither the subject nor his associates to classify him as "abnormal" and unworthy of complete social participation. Such disorders are comparable, in our own society, to the generation of dissociated states in healthy individuals by hypnosis, or the production of hallucinations by administration of lysergic acid or sensory deprivation, or the elicitation of disorganized speech in guests at a cocktail party. The subjects of such manipulations are not, as persons, classified as mentally ill, despite the fact that, under special circumstances, they have temporarily entered states which characterize chronically some mentally ill persons.

Cultural definitions of the meaning of "symptoms"   It may be taken as axiomatic that it is the concern of all human beings to maintain an image of themselves as persons competent to attain their essential goals, including maintenance of group membership. Such a self-image in part is dependent on the individual's evaluation of his own behavior, and in part on the evaluation of this behavior which is communicated to him by others. Shame—awareness of incompetence in any sphere, whether growing from self-observation or information from others—may arouse so much anxiety as to inhibit further the person's competence. In our own society, serious mental disease is conceived and recognized by law as a generalized incompetence and (not unexpectedly) the imputation of mental disease to an individual is a commonly used metaphor of insult. It is also popularly believed to be possible to "gaslight" a perfectly healthy person into psychosis by interpreting his own behavior to him as symptomatic of serious mental illness. While "gaslighting" itself may be a mythical crime, there is no question that any social attitude which interprets a given behavior or experience as symptomatic of a generalized incompetence is a powerful creator of shame, and thus of anxiety, in those who experience or behave in the "symptomatic" way. One may expect, then, that whenever a culture defines a given item of behavior as a symptom of general incompetence, the individual so behaving will suffer from shame, which elicits anxiety. This anxiety will further tend to decrease his competence, thus precipitating a reciprocal interaction between "incompetent" behaviors and anxiety. In one society, foci of anxiety over competence may center about sexual potency or attractiveness; in another, on courage in war; in still another on intelligence, and so on. Furthermore, those behaviors, such as hallucination, which Western societies generally interpret as symptoms of that generalized incompetence legally known as "insanity," may be less heavily stressed, or not be stressed at all, in others (cf. Wallace, 1959). To the extent that a society stresses failure in a given area of behavior as symptomatic of a more generalized inadequacy, and to the extent that that behavior requires minimal anxiety for successful performance, failure in such behavior probably will be repeated and will increasingly extend over other behaviors. Such reciprocal processes of shame, anxiety, and incompetent behavior are recognized today in our own mental hospitals, where patients are found to respond dramatically to almost any treatment which is carried on in an atmosphere of confidence in the ability of the patient to regain competence. Mental health associations also have worked assiduously to change popular concepts of mental disease, from the stereotype of a shameful and incurable incompetency to a respectable and curable "disease like any other." Similar contrast in social evaluation of symptomatology, and in the amount of anxiety and deterioration consequent upon them, are worthy of study in other societies.

Culture conflict and culture change   Anthropologists frequently have made note of the fact that primitive groups, who have been forced into situations of culture conflict and of partial, unorganized acculturation, seem prone to a higher frequency of the milder neurotic and personality trait disorders. Chronic anxiety and tension, psychosomatic complaints, alcoholism, narcotic addiction, delinquency and crime, witch fear, regressive or stunted personality development: such disorders apparently proliferate under the conditions produced by culture conflict acculturation.

Sociologists have reported that, among migrant groups (Malzberg and Lee, 1956), not only the incidence of such milder disorders, but also the incidence of psychosis, is measurably higher. We have discussed some of these phenomena already, in the chapter on the psychology of culture change. Although, as usual, statistical confirmation or disconfirmation of such a hypothesis is difficult to achieve, the position that culture change is associated with mental disorder has a certain obvious plausibility. But it must not be imagined that mere change in itself is so powerful a determinant that it will elicit sharply increasing incidences of psychosis. Goldhamer and Marshall (1953), for instance, studied the trends in incidence of institutionalized psychosis in America, over a hundred year period, and found that the rate of psychosis has remained constant, despite the accelerating rate of cultural change. There is, however, one socio-cultural characteristic seemingly shared by all groups which display a markedly high general incidence of mental disorders and which is often associated with culture conflict and culture change. That characteristic is relatively low social status in the larger society of which the group is a part. Semi-primitive peoples, living on the shabby fringes of Western civilization, migrants in new lands, occupants of slum areas, and lower racial, ethnic, and socio-economic classes, generally, are characterized by high incidences of both neurosis and psychosis. This suggests that a combination of physical disadvantages, such as inadequate diet, and the reciprocal process, discussed in the preceding section on social incompetence, shame and anxiety, may be major factors influencing the incidence of both the psychotic and the neurotic diseases.

Stresses produced by role and value conflicts implicit in particular sociocultural systems   Many social scientists have sought to combine epidemiological data and processual theory by the use of formulations which interpret each culture as presenting to the individual a unique spectrum of highly probable stress situations; these are determined by role or value conflicts implicit in the culture. From this standpoint, a particular sociocultural system is conceived as a congeries of roles and values, with each individual during the course of his life assuming several of these roles, some of them successively and some simultaneously, and likewise addressing himself to a number of different values, depending on the occasion. Such culture conflict can be of two kinds: role incompatibility, and value incompatibility. Whenever an individual is put in a position where two incompatible roles must be played simultaneously, he experiences stress, since he cannot succeed in both. And whenever an individual, playing one role, is faced with a situation where successful performance with respect to one value entails a high likelihood of personal loss (e.g., death) with respect to another, he experiences stress. Role incompatibility conflicts can be further divided into two sub-types: conflicts centering about role replacement, and conflicts centering about simultaneous roles. Role replacement means the dropping of one role for another; such events in the life cycle as birth, weaning, puberty, marriage, birth of child, retirement, and so on, frequently celebrated by rites de passage, are common examples of role replacement. Since role replacement entails loss of previously enjoyed rewards, the individual is apt to suffer the double stress of deprivation of past rewards and of fear of punishment if such rewards are sought again via the discontinued role. Role simultaneity conflicts are less easily noticeable, presumably because they are consciously pruned away in most societies as productive of both individual and social disturbance; at least they are avoided by scheduling role performance so as to prevent conflict, and by defining roles hierarchically, according to the relative importance of their goals. Such conflicts do, however, frequently emerge in unanticipated situations where one or another event has interfered with the normal scheduling of role behavior. This is illustrated in the role conflicts experienced by civil defense personnel during natural and man-made disasters. Another well-known category of role simultaneity conflict is provided by the phenomenon of "conflict of interest" in political organization. Value incompatibility conflicts are, again, not usually part of the ideal design of a culture, and societies attempt to forestall them by elaborate training. The classic—and an almost universal—example of value incompatibility conflicts is associated with the role of the warrior or soldier who must constantly make the choice between, in effect, being a live coward or a dead hero. Role and value conflict situations seem peculiarly apt to elicit neurotic responses; for example, in "combat fatigue" or "shell shock"; in fugues, amnesias, and a variety of phobic and neurotic compromise symptoms, in which one response to the situation is repressed, often only to be allowed to return in disguised or distorted form. It may be questioned, however, whether such situations, culturally determined insofar as the content of the conflict is determined, are to be regarded as responsible for more than the superficial content of psychoses. Psychosis, in this context, is perhaps better regarded as the result of cognitive inability to respond neurotically to a situation in which a neurotic response is the only way the "normal" individual has of avoiding a display of gross incompetence, with its consequent and crippling shame-and-anxiety cycle.

The "bad mother" theory   A special form of the internalized conflict theory has received emphasis recently in the work of psychiatrists, psychologists, and social scientists who seek to find in the parent-child, and especially the mother-child, relationship the etiology of schizophrenia. According to this view, the nuclear process in schizophrenia is withdrawal, both physical and psychological, from a world which has bombarded the victim with inconsistent communications—communications which demanded that he perform mutually incompatible roles or devote himself to antithetical values. The "schizophrenogenic" mother, for example, is supposedly prone to convey the two contradictory messages, by means of kinesic as well as linguistic communication, that her child simultaneously is loved and is rejected. The child may also be explicitly ordered to play the role of "love mommy," but be subtly rejected as unworthy or offensive when he does try to play this role. This viewpoint has received a variety of theoretical formulations, from Melanie Klein's and others' postulation of antithetical "good mother-bad mother" images (cf. Bellak, 1958), to Bateson's recent attempt to construe such ambivalent mother-child relationships as a confusion of different logical types (the "double bind" hypothesis) (Bateson et al., 1956). These and other attempts to construct formal models of schizophrenogenic family structures and communication systems are, however, in this writer's opinion, based on a somewhat sandy logical foundation. Most people, in most cultures, have to put up with a great deal of ambivalence and inconsistency in their social relationships; the "normal" response to extreme degrees of message inconsistency is neurotic rather than psychotic. Inability to cope with such poorly organized information suggests an inadequate capacity for organizing the data of experience.

In the following chapters, various positions with regard to these questions are discernible. The issues that I have outlined have not been resolved; indeed, their resolution will demand a major revolution in scientific understanding. But each of these efforts is a contribution to that enterprise.

REFERENCES

Bateson, G., Jackson, D. D., Haley, J., & Weakland, J. Toward a theory of schizophrenia. *Behavioral Science,* 1956, 1, 251–264.

Bellak, L. *Schizophrenia: A review of the syndrome.* New York: Logos Press, 1958.

Benedict, R. *Patterns of culture.* Boston: Houghton Mifflin, 1934.

Goldhamer, H., & Marshall, A. *Psychosis and civilization.* Glencoe, Ill.: Free Press, 1953.

Kallman, F. J. *The genetics of schizophrenia.* New York: J. J. Augustin, 1938.

Kardiner, A. *The individual and his society.* New York: Columbia University Press, 1939.

Kety, S. S. 1959 "Biochemical Theories of Schizophrenia," *Science,* 129: 1528–1532, 1590–1596.

Malzberg, B., & Lee, E. S. *Migration and mental disease.* New York: Social Science Research Council, 1956.

Opler, M., & Singer, J. L. Contrasting patterns of fantasy and mobility in Irish and Italian schizophrenics. *Journal of Abnormal and Social Psychology,* 1956, **53,** 42–47.

Roheim, G. *The origin and function of culture.* New York: Nervous and Mental Disease Monographs, No. 59, 1943.

Tooth, G. *Studies in mental illness in the Gold Coast.* London: H. M. Stationery Office, 1950.

Wallace, A. F. C. Cultural determinants of response to hallucinatory experience. *American Medical Association Archives of General Psychiatry,* 1959, **1,** 58–69.

Wallace, A. F. C. The bio-cultural theory of schizophrenia. *International Record of Medicine,* 1960, **173,** 700–714.

Wallace, A. F. C. *The modal personality structure of the Tuscarora Indians, as revealed by the Rorschach Test.* Washington: Bureau of American Ethnology, Bulletin 150, 1952.

2.3 Orientation

Few anthropologists have contributed more to our understanding of the influence of culture upon the expression of mental disorder than Marvin Opler. His classic account of the differences between the symptomatology of Irish and Italian "schizophrenics" exemplifies his concern with the force of culture upon the patterning of mental illness.

Opler's present chapter draws upon his own research, ranging from the Ute Indians to inhabitants of New York City, as well as the knowledge accumulated from his books concerned with culture and mental illness, to provide an unusually comprehensive account of cross-cultural research findings. The questions he asks from his broadly comparative perspective are essential ones. The answers he suggests merit our attention.

2.3   Anthropological Contributions to Psychiatry and Social Psychiatry

Marvin K. Opler

Of the various factors believed to influence the epidemiology of mental health (and, as we shall see, the forms of the illnesses themselves), culture (and, within culture, its socioeconomic classes and subcultures, its pace of urbanization and forms of culture contact, and the migration of cultures) and such life-history phenomena as age and sex roles are known to be determinants of mental illnesses. Epidemiologists construct their studies, and, indeed, organize and analyze their data in exactly such terms, not simply to make per capita age and sex corrections (though they must for accurate intergroup population comparisons), but in addition because such patterns as urban versus rural, ethnic or subcultural rates, economic groups, sex and age group rates themselves reveal differences both in rates and in types of mental disorder. Mental illnesses are never distributed at random in populations; between populations being compared, if one selects such biologically oriented variables as sex and age group rates, the same lack of randomness points to differences in the roles socially assigned to such organic classifications as age and sex.

EPIDEMIOLOGY OF ILLNESSES

How much illness of a particular *type* accords well with the terms, respectively, of epidemiology (for *how much*) and etiology (for *type*); and it is clear from our phrase linking both terms that neither of these basic considerations can be dealt with separately. There are amateur epidemiologists in psychiatry whose prime error is to miss this basic connection and, assuming that the historically derived nomenclature of the American Psychiatric Association is cross-culturally valid, to cram divergent types or forms of illness (cultural forms, really) into the preexistent mold or template of a most rudimentary diagnostic "manual." In so doing, they ignore the warnings of E. Bleuler, or even A. Meyer, Freud, Kraepelin, and phenomenologists to the effect that there are cultural differences in forms of schizophrenia and other disorders. Such notice of differences is the hallmark of the newer rapidly growing fields within psychiatry, namely social or community psychiatry, and anthropological or cross-cultural (transcultural) psychiatry.

Subsidiary to the questions of amount and form of mental disorders are, of course, the usual public health and preventive issues of prevalence and incidence rates, the former being the totality of cases amassing or piling up within a type or form of illness category, and the latter being the age and sex patterns of new cases arising in given social categories such as we have named. All these matters have been dealt with exhaustively, along with other methodological questions, in my book, *Culture and Social Psychiatry* (1956, 1967), where it is noted also that psychiatric ills are mainly disorders in the entire life history, or, as anthropologists say, life course or life cycle. While we may note such limitations of the better studies, such as the Hollingshead and Redlich New Haven Study of prevalence, which is limited to persons in treatment, or the more ambitious study of Rennie, Opler, Srole, and colleagues known as the Midtown Manhattan Mental Health Research Study, which is based on random sampling of an entire community along with treated prevalence, we can restate that the central findings of social psychiatry rest on a combination of etiology and epidemiology. The latter, attempted singly, is worthless.

In considerations of the etiology of mental illnesses, the subsciences of anthropology most useful to psychiatry are cultural anthropology, physical anthropology, and linguistics. The last has given rise to psycholinguistics, involving useful techniques for the recording, analysis, and comparison of patients' verbal and even nonverbal paratactic or emotional utterances. These have also been applied to doctor-patient and patient-doctor communications in studies of the transference and counter transference phenomena, or to other forms of patient interviewing. However, because patients may express behavior in modes other than utterance (posture, tachycardia or rapid heartbeat, dyspnea or labored breathing, sweating, neurasthenic faintness and dizzy spells, and so on), much spare human adjustice machinery does not fall even into the classification of audible paratactic utterance, and consequently must be observed through other anthropological modes. Thus, in our study contrasting the bodily motility and impulsivity of Italian male schizophrenics and a matched sample of Irish in whom fantasies of human movement operated vicariously, such psychological instruments as Porteus mazes, Time Estimation Tests, Rorschach and Thematic Apperception Tests (Murray), along with Bender-Gestalt, Sentence Completion (Lane), and seven other quantified methods, were used to establish significant differences. Anthropological psycholinguistics is therefore but a part of psychological anthropology, just as physical anthropology's studies of human growth and development, or of bodily form and function in work by Sheldon and Kretchmer, Boas, and J. Birdsell relate to human biology and such basic sciences of medicine as anatomy, neuroanatomy, and so on. Studies in human or primate physical evolution or in archaeological anatomy may tell us much about human growth and development or disease of organic etiology, but these are again part of human biology and medicine more than of social psychiatry (Opler, 1959).

The anthropological science most germane, and in fact indispensable, to social psychiatry is cultural anthropology. While not attempting here to define cultural anthropology exhaustively, we can note that most definitions emphasize a composite understanding of man and his works, usually referring to a body of custom, belief, practices, and artifacts. Some sense of this broad scope is indicated when we recall the fact that practices include child-rearing practices, infant handling, and the organization of life for adolescents, for sexual conduct, or for the aged. While early anthropologists discussed such cognitive balances in cultures by this cognitively oriented definition of *culture* itself, the pendulum has swung so that *culture* now includes emotional contents and balances as well. As a consequence, one adds today to the usual formal definitions of culture, including customs, beliefs, practices, and artifacts, or all those things engaged in and utilized by man as a member of society, the emotionally felt and creatively or negatively understood values, whether these are overtly experienced or covertly and emotionally felt. By including these unconscious or preconscious manifestations, along with conscious experiences, the anthropologist today can deal with unconscious patterning of behavior in society. I have said that the scope of anthropology has expanded to include the "total conditions of existence" meaningful to man and understandable in a science of man and culture. This definition links culture with the vicissitudes of personality in what I have called a relativistic relational system comprising both aspects.

The convergence of cultural anthropology and social psychiatry does not eliminate other interests, such as the interest in cultural evolution (how culture generically develops and changes), since the latter provides the basis for intercultural comparisons on any level including that of human behavior. Neither macroevolutionary general changes in cultures nor the microevolutionary and particular changes in specific instances and regions will be dealt with here, although I have written about cultural evolution and social psychiatry (or the psychology of peoples) elsewhere. Suffice it to say that such works as Freud's *Totem and Taboo* attempted prematurely to subordinate cultural evolution to a pan-human set of psychodynamic stages, so that, in this erroneous early effort, a *primum mobile* of cultural evolution is a psychogenetic and psychodynamic process. Freud's unsung early anthropological collaborators, from whom he derived false ideas about the nature of cultural evolution before scientific anthropology was firmly founded, were such figures as A. Lang and Atkinson, who had written luridly, if incorrectly, of primal hordes, primitive promiscuity, totemic rites, and taboos against devouring ancestral animals in the ebb and flow of the little-understood social life of such peoples as Australian tribes. An account of the errors in fact and inference would be tedious here; suffice it to say that they have been thoroughly corrected. Yet while ethnological details were straightened out for Australia, psychoanalytically inclined "anthropologists" like G. Roheim continued to exploit, with poor ethnology and poorer inferences, psychogenetic theories of culture.

More recent collaborations, while discarding the myth of *Totem and Taboo,* have nevertheless fallen into the trap of deriving "cultural forms" from psychodynamic processes. The opposite is the scientific fact, namely, that cultural forms in their evolution influence the psychology of peoples because the sociodynamic events influence psychodynamic ones. Of course, Freud understood this for the Western European instances that paralleled those of patriarchal classic Greece (Oedipal families) and for similar German family organization. The lay psychoanalyst, E. H. Erikson, in his first large work, *Childhood and Society,* collaborated with the anthropologist Scudder Mekeel of Wisconsin for analyses of Sioux Indian society and, to an extent, with A. L. Kroeber and others for work on the Yurok of California. Using a Freudian zonal theory of "anal," "oral," and other vicissitudes of personality, he derives the causes of Siouan restless movements over the plains not from their economy, their increased buffalo hunting after the introduction of the horse, or any other socioeconomic factors, but rather from their swaddling of infants in cradleboards. Similarly, the causes of their male dominance and occasional cruelties toward women he derives not from efflorescence of warfare in connection with hunting and horse raiding, or even from the facts of social organization, but from long nursing of the same infants past teething and tooth eruption stages. (Apparently, when mothers' breasts were nipped, they introjected cruelty in male offspring, though why not in female offspring?) I have steadfastly criticized Erikson and others for "zonal theories" of culture and I have studied Ute Indian society, where the identical swaddling and cradleboard usages go on even longer and where despite a much longer breast feeding past tooth eruption (and including a good deal of wet-nursing by nonrelated females), there are neither restless wanderings over the plains nor any allowed cruelties toward females. I have likewise criticized the notion that Yurok economy is due to toilet training. The Ute, for example, as a Great Basin people, followed fixed seasonal circuits and avoided marauding Plains tribes like Cheyenne and Comanche by means of hideouts in the Rocky Mountains, and they are further distinguished as being one of the most sex-egalitarian cultures in the world. After more than three years' study of Japanese, I have likewise criticized G. Gorer's toilet-training and weaning versions of Japanese culture. To these collaborations, which derive cultural forms as the epiphenomena of psychological events, could probably be added collaborations of R. Linton as anthropologist and A. Kardiner as analyst in such books as *The Individual and His Society* and *The Psychological Frontiers of Society.* More works are needed on the social frontiers of psychology (Opler, 1958, 1967).

Other interdisciplinary collaborations that were more fruitful could be mentioned. No doubt, there was cross-fertilization in the influence of Edward Sapir, an anthropologist and linguist, on the interpersonal and communication theories of Harry Stack Sullivan, Don Jackson, and others. The New Haven Study mentioned above was an interdisciplinary collaboration of A. Hollingshead, B. Roberts, F. Redlich, and J. Myers. The principal investigators of the Midtown Manhattan Mental Health Research Study in New York City were T. A. C. Rennie, psychiatrist and psychoanalytically trained anthropologist, and L. Srole, a sociologist, with dozens of others (including psychologists) in various research posts. In addition, A. Kardiner has collaborated with Cora DuBois, an anthropologist, and Emil Oberholzer, a psychologist, in Dubois's field studies of the Alorese. A collection of collaborative studies may be found in M. K. Opler (Ed.), *Culture and Mental Health* (1959).

TRANSCULTURAL STUDIES

Research in social and cross-cultural psychiatry and in psychological ethnology has its historical antecedents in the state of the sciences from which they derive. Because psychiatry is the youngest of the medical disciplines, among the clinical fields, it is inevitable that it seeks its basic science components among behavioral sciences such as anthropology, sociology, and psychology. This convergence is destined to increase because the sciences of man, with still older antecedents than the latecomer to medicine, are bound to fasten attention increasingly upon modern times and to be affected in turn by current conditions. In a modern hospital in Buffalo, New York, the last year has seen cases of mental illnesses formerly thought exotic, such as Chinese *koro,* Japanese suicidal pathology, an East Indian conversion hysteria, Italian schizo-affective disorder, Polish catatonia, and Puerto Rican homosexual panic. Because of social variables we mentioned at the outset, an entire shrinking world is apt to be affected, at different rates, by modern technology, increasing industrialization and urbanization, ethnic group migration, and modern socioeconomic processes. The Nigerian patient can be found in Glasgow, Lagos, Moscow, or Buffalo. With rapid growth of population, with spawning of new nations and rapid transportation, cultural enclaves are as characteristic of big cities as they once were of peasant society hinterlands.

Among the characteristics of urbanism encountered in the Midtown study were imbalanced sex ratios and a larger number of women in the labor force, ethnic group cultural enclaves or settlements (with increased heterogeneity for a city as a whole), social class differentiations interweaving with ethnicity factors, and a nonrandom distribution of mental health impairments which were outstandingly high for nonstabilized ethnic groups like a dwindling Hungarian, and a marginal, not yet successful, Puerto Rican community. In predictions for Midtown mental health epidemiology, these two communities were hypothesized to be in trouble because of unfavorable—that is, rapid—paces of acculturation, but more important, a kind of acculturation which destroyed basic cultural values and conditions for stabilizing.

The clinician, be he psychiatrist, general practitioner, clinical psychologist, or behavioral science researcher is caught in the web of the same conditions of existence. Cultural heterogeneity applied to human behavior manifestations makes new demands. In response, social, or environmentally oriented, psychiatry has arisen within community psychiatry. Studies that reveal the prevalence rates of various kinds of mental disorders, or even the incidence rates or the amount of healthy adaptation in a series of cultures, actually are estimates of how much malfunction can pile up, or exist, in the specific settings or milieus surveyed. As such, they are administratively useful in pointing to the scope of the problems, and in outlining factually and statistically the task of the clinician. It is at this point, however, that psychiatry in its community phase generally requires a clearer knowledge of the connections between the disorders and their cultural backgrounds if it is to proceed beyond such epidemiological cross sections to an understanding of *how* and *why* such malfunctioning has occurred. Just as the philosopher Alfred North Whitehead has called all nature a structure of evolving processes, so the social psychiatrist and anthropologist regard any epidemiological problem in the type and amount of a mental disorder that is functional or nonorganic in basis as due to a combination of social and psychodynamic processes. In my book, *Culture, Psychiatry and Human Values* (1956), I stated that epidemiological and etiological considerations in my survey of disorders, continent by continent, showed them to be processes that had changed markedly in human history. The social and cultural origins of the illnesses had changed, and only anthropological data gave control over such information. Because anthropologists study the life history, or life cycle, events for individuals, they could note that the developmental course of illness had changed. (For example, some primitive forms of simpler kinds of schizophrenias than are found in Western Europe or America are open to "spontaneous" remissions, something rare in the schizophrenias with paranoid reaction of modern societies; these forms, which I have called, following J. C. Carothers' *The African Mind,* simple psychotic confusional states, catathymic outbursts, and forms of simple schizophrenias like *latah* of Malaysia, *imu* illness of Hokkaido, Arctic hysterias—a misnomer—of northeastern Asian cultures, running amok, and so on, are all open to spontaneous remission because they are mixtures of conversion hysteria symptomatology and psychotic dissociative behavior.) In the same historical sequence, I have shown that techniques of prevention and modes of therapy have changed. Viewing the history of psychiatry and its present expansion into social psychiatry, one is forced to suggest that various new methods, theories, and directions must emerge to accommodate modern cultural heterogeneity.

Within anthropology, therefore, the fields of crucial importance for psychiatry are ethnological psychiatry (concerning the varieties of mental disorder and their etiology and change), culture and personality study (concerning the epidemiology of kinds of disorder and their etiological emergence in the life cycle), studies of folk medicine and folk psychiatry for understanding of techniques of prevention and modes of therapy, and social psychiatry, combining this information and applying it to current problems. In the latter connections, such anthropologists as William Caudill and William Stein have studied psychiatric hospitals as anthropological communities in Connecticut and Lima, Peru. Caudill's book, *The Psychiatric Hospital as a Small Community,* is based on a participant-observer technique simulating patienthood. Others, like Seymour Parker and Robert Rapoport, whose book, *Community as Doctor,* analyzes such therapeutic communities as Belmont Hospital in England, are anthropologists who have studied the organization of psychiatry in operation, ostensibly as visiting anthropologists. While sociologists have tended to study psychiatric installations historically (see, for example, the H. Warren Dunham and S. K. Weinberg study of a state hospital in Ohio), anthropologists tend to work directly in the institution in order to obtain "live" information and current reactions. The A. H. Stanton and M. S. Schwartz work, *The Mental Hospital,* by a psychiatrist and a sociologist respectively, is in the anthropological tradition, possibly because it is heavily influenced by the Harry Stack Sullivan and Edward Sapir collaboration, mentioned earlier, in interpersonal and communications interests in psychiatry. A notable compendium of works on culture and personality was gathered by Clyde Kluckhohn, Harvard anthropologist, and Henry A. Murray, physician and Harvard psychologist with analytic training, but this is now outmoded. In my *Culture and Mental Health,* psychologists like S. Sarason and G. DeVos collaborate with social scientists, like anthropologist Thomas Gladwin or sociologist Horace Miner, and with various psychiatrists, like Kardiner, Carstairs, Wittkower, Loudon, and others, contributing either anthropological or social psychiatric studies.

Such multidisciplinary studies have succeeded single-handed attempts to establish the anthropological field of culture and personality research. Thirty years ago, in her *Patterns of Culture,* Ruth Benedict described children as "the little creatures of their culture," an emphasis unfortunately disregarded in the nursing, weaning, and toilet-training theories which followed and which derived whole cultures from child-rearing practices. However, other emphases in this book were misleading. In *Patterns of Culture,* Kwakiutl Indians of the Northwest Coast of America were typified as megalomaniacal and paranoid and compared with the people of Lynd's *Middletown* as overly competitive. Franz Boas and others who had studied Kwakiutls described cooperative behavior in the *numaym* house groups of "nobles" and chiefs, commoners and slaves. Boas particularly pointed out that competitive economic rituals validating status and privileges had succeeded former patterns of warfare used to establish similar privileges like the use of favorite fishing sites, the inheritance of chiefly titles, and so on. *Patterns of Culture* further contrasted Indians of the Northwest Coast and Southwestern Pueblos on passivity and compared both with incomplete accounts of Dobuans as paranoid or obsessed with formulas for aggression. Edward Sapir promptly commented that whole cultures cannot be megalomaniacal, paranoid, or obsessed, challenging the simplicity of thematic description in Benedict's work. I too contended that such descriptions were, indeed, oversimplified, as indicated by my corrections concerning Kwakiutls, for example. But apart from the sharpness and omissions in her descriptions, Benedict raised the more important theoretical questions found in her central propositions, first, that cultural patterns are infinitely variable (anything from paranoid to obsessive may appear as so-called normative culture), and second, that a process of purely "psychological selectivity," as she termed it, determined the nature of any pattern. It is clear that the second proposition, causal in type, contains the former, more descriptive notion, since, if "psychological *selections*" produce cultures, then any psychological pattern, no matter how extreme, may evolve. In attacking the labels like "megalomaniacal," or the descriptions themselves, Sapir was objecting merely on descriptive grounds. My own criticism challenged the descriptive postulate that "anything could happen" in cultural behavior, but it added the more inclusive criticism that "psychological selectivity" must grow out of culture itself: What determines such selection, if *not* culture? Thus, in my view, child-rearing practices are part of culture; they do not "make" it. The psychology of peoples depends on culture, not the opposite.

Before anthropology could contribute in a meaningful manner to psychiatry, just such corrections in theory and presentation of data were required. It was necessary, too, that anthropology adopt more sophisticated methods of quantification, like those utilized in epidemiology, and that researchers obtain training in psychiatric observation and analysis as well. My own route, for example, was the common one of psychoanalytic training as both lecturer and student-trainee, in the Los Angeles Institute of Psychoanalysis. Others were also analytically trained, some through the auspices of a program of research-training analyses sponsored by the Russell Sage Foundation. Although epidemiological collaborations of anthropologists did not follow until the 1950s, when social psychiatry was founded and *The International Journal of Social Psychiatry* first appeared, nevertheless anthropologists working alone had earlier contributed significant field researches. Melford E. Spiro, for example, made a survey of psychiatric disorders in Ifaluk, a Micronesian island village community, which reveals extremely low rates of neurotic and psychotic disorders even after the turmoil of Japanese invasion; this work appears in M. K. Opler (Ed.), *Culture and Mental Health*. I made Ute Indian mental health and other studies in the 1930s, and in the decade following was able to make Japanese-American and Hawaiian-Japanese studies; between these two periods, from 1938 to 1943, I made etiological studies of Alaskan cases, since all hospitalized Alaskan and some Northwest Coast patients have been sent to the Morningside Clinic and Hospital since 1930. Collaborations of William Caudill and George DeVos on Japanese-Americans belong to this general period, and extensive Rorschach studies by the anthropologists, George and Louise Spindler, on acculturated Menomini Indians also. In Rorschach studies applied to Indian acculturation, the pioneer figure was A. Irving Hallowell, whose research on Ojibwa Indians was both extensive and detailed.

Thus, while studies in cross-cultural psychiatry and psychological ethnology have varied historical antecedents in the sciences from which they derive, namely anthropology, psychiatry, and psychological testing, these rather strange bedfellows have been forced to arrive at the same destination. They were born in different ages, reached by different routes, and housed in separate quarters. Today, while they sometimes live in different buildings, such as medical schools and graduate schools, the necessities of a basic sciences orientation in psychiatry, a holistic science of human behavior, has hastened the removal of artificial barriers. While practitioners in each field may, in some cases, continue to work in different buildings, observe different curricula, and produce different professionals, such as doctors of medicine and doctors of philosophy, conjoint training is increasing both in amount and in quality. The convergence of psychiatry, a medical discipline, and anthropology, a broad-based behavioral science, is increasingly due to research and training collaborations that are influencing curricula, professionals, and even language. The two most viable terms in psychiatry today, with practically identical connotations in theory and practice, are *social psychiatry* and *community psychiatry*. In anthropology, similarly, terms like *culture* and *personality study* have changed to *social* or *cultural psychiatry, ethnic psychiatry,* and the like.

While the anthropologist has always believed in cultural heterogeneity as a fact of life—affecting psychological balance or imbalance, we should add—both the notion of such influence and the variability it implies are fresh concepts for psychiatry. Yet today, the anthropologist, within his science, is forced toward new perspectives by the rapidity of cultural evolution. Not the least of these are certain uniformities, not in the perspectives on cultural differences, but in cultural processes. While 30 years ago it was possible to find in New Guinea, in remote Pacific islands, in South American jungles, or, as I found, in a remote corner of the Colorado-Utah border, people who spoke only exotic languages, who still hunted or planted with primitive implements, and who lived by customs beyond reach of mission schools or educational systems as we know them, or who had practically no involvement in cash economy, today these more remote social and psychiatric laboratories are rapidly closing. Instead, people with antecedents in "peasant societies," or ethnic groups in "the culture of poverty," and immigrant groups caught in "urbanization and acculturation processes" are more commonly in sight. Anthropologists have shifted to village and community studies geared to cultural innovation and change, technological revolution, and urban process. Studies labeled Greek, Italian, Irish, Turkish, Danish, French, or Japanese are as common today as studies from the Congo. Interest in cultural evolution, in process as well as form, or in the psychological products of a way of life have increased proportionately.

A plan of research in human behavior, as in any field of science, therefore depends in the last analysis upon the phenomena being investigated. Human behavior ranges from psychopathological states to normal ones in a continuum. While normalcy is a statistical concept in this sense, states of illness are not only maladaptive to cultural norms, but they are personally dysfunctional as well. In criticizing Ruth Benedict's *Patterns of Culture,* I have pointed out that "what is normal," or some absolutely relativistic scheme applied to this question, cannot be assumed to vary infinitely. Benedict, in fact, stated that the "normals" of one culture might seem to be "abnormals" of another in that their behavior would seem strange in alien cultural contexts. While this relativistic observation appeared plausible, she added to it the astonishing corollary that out-and-out abnormals from one cultural context could "fit in" elsewhere, something which I and my colleagues had occasion to test at the Morningside Clinic and Hospital in Oregon, with sick Kwakiutl, Tsimshian, and Tlingit Indians, finding it to be, as expected, incredibly naïve. My own position, as I have explained, is not one of *absolute* cultural relativism, but of a relativity limited by principles of cultural evolution. In this framework, neither cultures nor human adjustment and psychopathology can vary indefinitely. Mental disorder, in short, represents impairments in functioning destructive of the individual's integration in his adaptation to a context or his adjustment to *any* scene. The correct point, from one culture to the next, is not that such deviations from normative behavior can find a haven elsewhere, but that the disorder etiologically and psychodynamically can be traced to stress systems in the sociocultural background itself. Sociodynamic events produce psychodynamic ones, as I have stated. The accurate corollary is that cultural evolutionary processes induce stress systems that are comparable and, likewise, forms of psychopathology that can be found transculturally.

In contrast, psychiatry has had its historically evolved classifications of mental disorders, which date back to the last century in Europe, to Kraepelin. To men like Bleuler and Freud, this German-derived system seemed incomplete, Freud adding chiefly to the classifications of neurosis, and Bleuler modifying the terminology for schizophrenias to "a group" of variable disorders within a generic class. Apart from gross distinctions in organic and nonorganic disorders, the classification and categories of the American Psychiatric Association and the Veterans Administration are therefore fundamentally products of the nineteenth and early twentieth centuries, with little addition or modification. A similar situation in other fields of medicine would no doubt be considered scandalous. The categories are based, further, not upon etiology nor upon psychodynamics, but upon clusters of symptoms, many of which (like hallucinations, feelings of depersonalization, "asocial withdrawal," "restlessness," or "sexual identification problem") are found in illness states of varying degrees of seriousness. New etiological classifications and diagnoses connected with cultural information, within the older, more generalized and overlapping rubrics, are a prime necessity for a more mature and cross-culturally valid science of human behavior. Until such necessary distinctions are made, most studies of generic categories like schizophrenia will be, as they have been, statistically speaking, studies of mixed categories of patients and research in terms of mixed categories of illness. In statistical theory, this is category confusion of both the "thing" studied and its quantification. Social psychiatry has exactly these etiological and epidemiological interests, for it is centrally interested in the impact of culture, social environment, and family type upon the developing personality.

TYPES OF RESEARCH

In the Midtown study in Manhattan, an early stage of research sought the prevalence, treated and untreated, of mental ills throughout a whole population investigated for purposes of quantification by means of a random sample. Criteria like "impairment in life functioning," together with symptomatic or symptom-free measures, were used to determine degrees of adjustment or adaptation, or the seriousness of an illness. A psychiatrist knows such information insofar as he knows the history of a case in its total setting. Thus Rennie and Opler, as principal investigators, insisted that later stages of research continue with studies of individuals and families in their cultural and community settings, using combined methods of anthropological participant observation and psychological testing. I have used an expansion of the latter methods successfully in studies of schizophrenic samples from the area, the samples differentiating by all the quantification of measures employed according to cultural backgrounds and ethnic identities of the groups themselves (Opler, 1958).

Other researchers, using quite different methods, have been interested in cultural materials. One of Walter B. Cannon's most interesting papers, "Voodoo Death," appeared in the pages of the *American Anthropologist* for 1942. In discussing extreme anxiety reactions in different primitive cultures resulting from the breaking of social group taboos, the great physiologist adduced cases of "guilty" individuals who were impressed by the magical death sanctions in the culture for such misadventures. Cannon noted that they had, indeed, in recorded cases, literally wasted away and died. Where a taboo was broken, or the individual was convinced of bewitchment because of cultural beliefs, the extreme forms of anxiety could produce not only loss of appetite with reduced intake of foods and fluids, but in addition, loss of salts and bodily fluid through sweating. He called the effect protracted dehydration, so that indeed, literal "wasting away" resulted in authenticated instances of death.

In Nigerian folk psychiatry, our common phrase, "frightened out of his wits," has much cultural sanction, for there are very many cultural terms for cursing and bewitching. In addition, the folk medicine terminology for modes of curing contains terms for entirely psychiatric or psychological types of curative practice, for methods of therapy that are more psychological than organic, for methods that are more organically oriented than psychological, and for wholly organic methods. Since Nigerian folk psychiatry included use of such items in materia medica as *rauwolfia alkaloids* (or reserpine, also noted in Hindu folk psychiatry) and *datura* as well, the term "organic treatments" is no empty boast. Reserpine from India, as a matter of fact, in the management of hypertension and hysterical or nervous states, was the first "modern" tranquilizer to awaken interest in the so-called wonder drugs. At any rate, in Nigerian folk psychiatry, there is a good sense of dosage according to body weight (child or adult, male or female, young or old), together with such restraints as shackling the patient in initial phases of acute confusional states, catathymic outbursts, or catatonic seizures. Such effects of bewitchment, once culturally sanctioned, are no more mysterious than other cultural customs. Nigerian folk psychiatry and even its materia medica are thus well suited to the typical kinds of hysterical or schizophrenic disorder bred in the culture. Further accommodations to cultural setting are the involvement of the patient's family in his care and treatment, since both patient and family move to the healer's compound, and the family ministers to the patient's needs. If this is the analog of "family treatment"—a modern program within the ambit of social psychiatry—then the patient's later involvement in curing-group cults is a primitive form of what social psychiatry terms "therapeutic social clubs," and "aftercare" or post-hospitalization in group therapy. The Nigerian folk psychiatrist likewise uses "home treatment" (since he may, in less serious cases, make home visits rather than invite the patient to his compound), or he uses curative cult groups of patients (group therapy) directly. At any rate, elements in materia medica, modes of therapy, and organization of therapeutic services are sophisticated enough to remind us of modern methods in social and community psychiatry that have only recently emerged in Western Europe, or of Eastern European adaptations of A. Querido's "home treatment" techniques in Amsterdam, or of English and American emphases on therapeutic social clubs, group therapy, and aftercare programs. In further resemblance to psychiatry in Soviet Russia, the Nigerian folk practices include work programs whenever and wherever the patient can function productively. As one British-trained Nigerian psychiatrist, T. Adeoye Lambo, has observed, Nigerian folk practitioners are valuable allies to modern practitioners in such a setting and are now used as auxiliary or ancillary helpers where they are not actually preferred by the natives.

The anthropologist interested in styles of emotion commands a rich field for the study of human emotional life in general. There can be no doubt that such styles themselves vary with culture. A Ute Indian female will fight another as readily as any male when she is incensed at the other's flirtatious or adulterous behavior with her husband. The Tuareg nobleman (Imashek caste), although custodian of desert caravans in the Sahara and a fearless warrior, will blush furiously if the purple veil covering his face below the eyes should slip; the Imashek female, contrary to our notions of desert sheiks and modes of romance, is the one to ride over the sands in courtship or to play string instruments in love courts called *ahalns*. On the other side of Africa, a Masai warrior honors a promising and stalwart youth by spitting in his face. An Andaman Islander greets a journeying visitor or relative by sitting in his lap and weeping copiously. Navajo and Apache men and women typically lower the voice to an almost inaudible pitch as they become angry. A schoolboy in old China was expected to smile blandly and pleasantly, even when severely reprimanded by an elder or teacher. Obviously, such emotional expressions vary with culture. The Chinese schoolboy is merely showing cheerful respect. The Ute Indian women are accorded egalitarian rights with men so that they choose in partner dances, own their own products of labor, or vigorously defend their marital rights. Among Tuareg of Africa, women are not excluded from public life if they are of upper caste, while men who control caravan routes have more use for veils in sudden desert sandstorms than their wives do. To Masai warriors, saliva seems more meaningful as a sign of respect than our pallid handshake. And for Andaman Islanders, honest "tears of joy," as we call them, come more easily in their close-knit culture than in our more anonymous urban one. As for Navajo and Apache, who speak tonal languages replete with such relatively soft sounds as glottal stops, one shouts loudly across stretches of land in order to be heard, not to emphasize anger and exasperation.

Although it is clear that the functioning society affects emotional expression, the culture and personality variables likewise produce differences in the final products of emotional balance and imbalance, namely in the mental disorders themselves. Simple conversion hysterias are rarer today, undoubtedly, than they were when Freud and Breuer first undertook the case of Anna O. Reporting on the typical illnesses of hunting and gathering tribes, such as Ute and Apache, I have noted that Ute psychiatric epidemiology at one time took the form of hysterias rather than the deep-seated schizophrenias of modern urban cultures, including our own. In fact, Ute Indian shamans, using dream analysis similar to the Freudian type and enlisting family support in such treatments, actually cured many cases of hysterical blindness, lameness, and so on, according to our data. In a personal communication, Dr. J. C.

Finney of the University of Kentucky Medical School reported a high prevalence of classical conversion hysteria in islands of rural white poverty in eastern Kentucky (Southern Appalachia) where educational levels are low and one's lot, like a Ute Indian's, is cast with extended family kin. In urban midtown Manhattan, by contrast, the scientifically attestable psychosomatic disorders and schizophrenias (of various cultural types) take the place of these conversion hysterias, except among Puerto Ricans, who call their conversion symptoms "attacks" and say their schizophrenias are "organic" in origin.

Those who claim that schizophrenias (of modern type) are biogenetic in origin and therefore distributed randomly in populations are simply ignorant of the anthropological data. Variations in the form and epidemiology of mental illnesses occur transculturally. I conducted studies for five years (1938–1943) in the Morningside Clinic and Hospital in Portland, Oregon (the only federal hospital for Alaskan and Northwest Coast patients). Northwest Coast Indians, Eskimos, Whites, and northern Athabaskan tribes were represented. While the disorders were maladaptive to the human condition as well as to the cultural contexts represented, they were traceable to specific kinds of cultural stress systems. Further, while etiology of illness was similar within a group, from one case to the next, it was variable between cultural groups. In *Culture, Psychiatry and Human Values* (1956) I have discussed more fully the regional differences in mental disorders, continent by continent. If one considers a mental illness called *latah* (found in Malaysia primarily, but also in Mongolia and Micronesia), one is dealing with a confusional state psychosis, commonly with echolalia and echopraxia or negativism. These same aspects typify the so-called *imu* illness of the Ainu of Hokkaido. In both cases, and for these genetically unrelated peoples, women are more commonly affected than men. They are often women past child-bearing or near menopause, but more significantly those of poor social status. Widowed or unmarried domestics are common victims among the Ainu. A startle reaction, as in the Giles de la Tourette syndrome (which may, indeed, be a connected European form), often starts the acute symptoms. In echopraxia, simple physical imitation is sometimes varied by the opposite action (a form of negativism), and in *latah* among Javanese for example, the women may pun obscenely on words used in polite discourse. A misnamed illness, Arctic hysteria (found in northeastern Asia) is characterized chiefly by helpless imitation, or else by pathetic confusions as to the action. Sailors touching port among maritime Chukchi who had the disorder would make the victim, no matter how old and infirm, copy acts of rushing uphill or attempting feats of strength. In the same way, women who were *imu* victims were utilized as entertainers by Japanese in parody of sophisticated *geisha* dancers, singers, and conversationalists. The range of uncontrolled, confusional states may be extended to include Malaysian running amok, involving repetitive acts of violence (possibly killing innocent bystanders) and affecting males only.

Such disturbances in thinking, in affect, and especially in action modes, as well as their episodic or "seizure" characteristic, were not only reported from Mongolia down to Malaysia, but in addition, the echolalias, echopraxias, and negativisms can be found in what J. C. Carothers has called the African confusional states. They were once also found commonly in Europe, along with variations ranging from catathymic outbursts, as in Africa, to constricted catatonic behavior. I have called these primitive forms of schizophrenias, although I recognize that peasant societies, including such sophisticated forms as Javanese society, are much involved. One might also note, as in the case of catatonias, that these disorders are sometimes open to "spontaneous remissions" as the patient's social context or the conditions of his existence are changed. I have pointed out above that hysteriform behavior sometimes underlies the acute psychotic symptoms. Such illnesses are quite different from the schizophrenias with paranoid reaction encountered so frequently in modern European and American urban society. Nevertheless, as the peasant societies undergo acculturation, the rates and also the forms of illness begin to resemble those of our city culture. It was once possible to find such syndromes in places like the federal Morningside Clinic and Hospital, but this has also changed with acculturation processes.

Cultural methods of handling significant events such as birth, puberty, marriage, own and opposite sex contacts, illness and death, and, as we have seen, cross-cultural studies of drug usage, modes of therapy, and organization of therapeutic services—all these afford occasions for significant modern collaborations between psychiatry and anthropology. What we have referred to above as balances and imbalances in emotional life for the individual are the actual styles in the incessant selection of defenses and of striving and coping mechanisms. In the last analysis, these are culturally conditioned since they require a constant cognitive-emotional monitoring of inner states and outer (or remembered) happenings. In this way, the cultural loadings of particular kinds of stress become significant. If Javanese etiquette is punctilious and sophisticated, will the psychoses occur when requirements for social politeness are most exacting? Surely, the social position of women is of interest in peasant societies. And when whites in Alaskan frontiers revert regressively to wax-limb catatonias, we can see behind them the unremitting toil of a hard bargain for vigor and mobility.

Although a general relationship has been found between the independent variable of cultural background and the dependent variable of psychological disorder, descriptions of pathology in American subcultural groups have been infrequent. Further, anthropological studies of culture and personality connections in exotic societies are abundant, while those of American ethnic group subcultures in our own backyard, so to speak, are relatively rare. Perhaps there are two main reasons for this disparity. The first is that anthropologists typically go abroad and later describe remote cultures, and as a group modern anthropologists are much interested in human behavior in all of its manifestations. Further, anthropology, through such figures as Edward Sapir, Clyde Kluckhohn, Margaret Mead, and Ruth Benedict, to mention only a few, was inclined to emphasize various types of essentially psychiatric description—Sapir with his concept of "unconscious patterning," Kluckhohn with his interest both in psychoanalysis and in values orientations, Mead in child rearing, and Benedict in the styles of "psychological selectivity."

The anthropologist's frequent interest in what I have called elsewhere "the psychology of peoples" and his bold description of this specific psychology as he sees it were main factors in building up studies of cultural character and personality from remote areas of the world. The typical paraphernalia of such studies often included such tests as the Rorschach, modifications of the TAT pictures, or other projective devices.

It is a curious contrast, then, that anthropologists have typically not studied American ethnic group subcultures, which are close at hand, by the same methods. At the same time, those of us who have had years of clinical experience on the American scene would warn against tendencies to oversimplify or to stereotype a pattern of pathology for each American subcultural group. That is to say, unlike the situation in scattered and remote cultures around the world, starkly contrasting and extremely differentiated illnesses or illness types do not occur in each and every instance. At the same time, everyone knows (if he is well informed in cross-cultural epidemiology) that when an American ethnic group member is more clearly differentiated or segregated in his conditions of living, he shows related differences in pathology. Widely known and simple examples of this fact relate to the relative rarity of psychotic depression states among rural southern Negroes and the tendency for Negroes, North and South, to have very low suicide rates, although even in this group, the tendency for males to have higher rates of completed suicide than females and for females to have higher rates of attempted suicide than males gives us factors that both contrast with the American scene and resemble it concerning the differential sex rates.

REFERENCES

Cannon, W. B. Voodoo death. *American Anthropologist,* 1942, 44, 169.
Caudill, W. *The psychiatric hospital as a small society.* Cambridge, Mass.: Harvard University Press, 1958.
Dole, G., & Carneiro, R. *Essays in the science of culture.* New York: Thomas Y. Crowell Co., 1960.
Dunham, H. W., & Weinberg, S. K. *The culture of the state mental hospital.* Detroit: Wayne State University Press, 1960.
Hollingshead, A. B., & Redlich, F. C. *Social class and mental illness.* New York: John Wiley & Sons, 1958.
Kluckhohn, C., & Murray, H. A. (Eds.) *Personality in nature, society and culture.* New York: A. A. Knopf, 1949.
Opler, M. K. *Culture, psychiatry and human values.* Springfield, Ill.: C. C. Thomas Co., 1956.
Opler, M. K. (Ed.) *Culture and mental health: Cross-cultural studies.* New York: Macmillan Co., 1959.
Opler, M. K. Cultural perspectives in research on schizophrenias. *Psychiatric Quarterly,* 1959, 33, 506–524.
Opler, M. K. Cultural definitions of illness. In I. Galdston (Ed.), *Man's image in medicine and anthropology.* New York: International Universities Press, 1963. Pp. 446–473.
Opler, M. K. Epidemiological studies of mental illness: Midtown Study in New York. In *Symposium on preventive and social psychiatry.* Washington, D.C.: Walter Reed Army Institute of Research and Government Printing Office, 1958.
Opler, M. K. Anthropological and cross-cultural aspects of homosexuality. In J. Marmor (Ed.), *Sexual inversion.* New York: Basic Books, 1965.
Opler, M. K. *Culture and social psychiatry.* New York: Atherton Press, 1967.
Rapoport, R. N. *Community as doctor.* Springfield, Ill.: C. C Thomas Co., 1960.
Seward, G. (Ed.) *Clinical studies in culture conflict.* New York: Ronald Press Co., 1958.

2.4 Orientation

Ari Kiev complements Marvin Opler's anthropological orientation by addressing himself to much the same set of cross-cultural data, but from a psychiatrist's perspective. Kiev concentrates upon what he refers to as the "culture-bound" disorders, particularly the condition *bouffée delirante aigue,* an acute confusional psychosis seen among Haitian peasants.

Kiev's own field work among Haitians, West Indians, and Mexican-Americans, and his general experience in transcultural psychiatry as reflected in his books, *Magic, Faith and Healing* and *Curanderismo,* equip him unusually well for his task of evaluating the relevance of cross-cultural research for psychiatry. Of particular interest is his discussion of the means whereby the influences of culture ("culture-bound indicators") may be cut through by locating "culture-free" diagnostic indicators as provided by biochemical, neurophysiological, and behavioral measures.

2.4　Transcultural Psychiatry: Research Problems and Perspectives

Ari Kiev

THE CONCEPT OF CULTURE-BOUND SYNDROMES

Psychiatrists have for a long time turned to primitive cultures to better understand the problems of psychiatry, demonstrating an inclination no doubt to turn to simpler questions and search for simpler solutions when faced with imponderable, impenetrable, and imperative problems. A number of scholars, including Kraepelin (1909) and Bleuler (1950), have examined the influence of culture on mental illness, emphasizing, in the main, the effect of culture on the characteristics of mental illness (see also Carothers, 1953; Tooth, 1950). Others have focused on the related but different question of the effects of cultural factors on the distribution of mental illness (Berne, 1950; Opler, 1956; Seligman, 1929; Slotkin, 1955; Spiro, 1952). Even though various writers explain the effects of culture in terms of different heuristic constructs such as race, climate, constitution, and psychogenesis, in varying degrees, they all make the common assumption that cultural factors are capable of conditioning the basic form and structure of psychiatric symptoms and illness. While this hypothesis has rarely been spelled out clearly or tested in a formal way, it has come to constitute an integral part of psychiatric thinking.

This unformulated hypothesis has been reinforced by a large series of descriptive studies concerned with "culture-bound" syndromes like *amok,* the *Witiko* psychosis of the Cree, Salteaux and Ojibwa, *latah,* Arctic hysteria, and *koro* (see Cooper, 1934; Hallowell, 1934; Landes, 1938; Yap, 1951, 1952). These have been described as occurring only in specific cultural contexts, deriving their special form and content from the culture in which they occur, and as being considered distinct from the traditional nosological categories of Western psychiatry. Thus, Witiko involves a homicidal excitement associated with the not too widespread belief in possession by the *Witiko* or cannibal monster held by several North American Indian groups. *Koro,* an anxiety state associated with delusions about the retraction of the penis into the abdomen and fears of death, has been connected with certain beliefs common to the southern Chinese about improper balance between yin and yang humors. According to Yap (1965), these are "not simply pathoplastic but pathogenic in effect, much in the same way that a belief in hell-fire can help to bring about depressive states of clinical severity under certain circumstances." The bizarre acting out, denudative behavior, and mimicry seen in Arctic hysteria or *pibloktoq* has similarly been attributed to special cultural factors, as have *latah* and *imu,* both of which are characterized by echolalia and echopraxia and fright. According to Uchimura (1956), the *imu* of the Ainu is attributable to constitutional factors and the suggestibility fostered by Ainu tradition, and is to be considered as a phylogenetically intermediary state between primitive defense-reactions of lower animals and hysteria of civilized people. Writing of *latah,* Yap (1951, p. 319) has noted that certain sociocultural conditions, particularly in underdeveloped countries with little technology, may produce a "passivity of mind and an unpreparedness for sudden decision and action" which predisposes individuals to this fright reaction. In like fashion, Van Loon (1929) postulated that *amok* is an acute infectious delirium which occurs among the Malay because of their peculiar psychic nature.

An examination of the issues surrounding the study of the so-called exotic or "culture-bound" disorders serves as a useful starting point for reconsidering some important conceptual and methodological issues involved in research in transcultural psychiatry. This material is particularly important, for, along with data on the differential incidence of various conditions in different cultures, this has been to date the major body of data in the field of transcultural psychiatry.

Factors Contributing to the Concept of Culture-Bound Disorders

Differences in the content of delusions of disturbed individuals in different cultures have significantly contributed to the notion that cultural factors condition the basic form and structure of psychiatric symptoms and illness. Careful examination of the specific delusional systems, however, frequently reveals their close relationship to the belief systems in the culture, emphasizing the functional and restitutive significance of delusions, rather than their pathological significance.

In the writings of anthropologists and some psychiatrists, there has

been a great inclination to accept native notions of etiology and nosology
as having some functional significance. Thus, in that the content of an
illness such as *Witiko* relates to beliefs about taboo violation, it has
been thought likely that belief in taboo and the consequences of its
violation led to anxiety which in turn led to the illness. Such studies,
however, fail to recognize that taboo violation is a common event in the
lives of most people, so that, as in most instances, difficulties will be explained with such acceptable culturally shared explanations, which in
turn will lead to prompt diagnosis and treatment. This in itself is insufficient evidence of causation. What is crucial here is the fact that the
absence of such explanations for psychiatric symptoms leads to the neglect
of the troubled individual rather than treatment, since the culture defines, within specified limits, what patterns of disturbed mood, thought,
and behavior are to be considered as illness. Thus, among Mexican-
Americans, anxiety over a specific fright, such as may be caused by seeing
a ghost, is diagnosed as *susto* and leads to treatment, while fear and
anxiety which are not linked to a specific kind of culturally meaningful
situation are ignored or criticized and do not lead to treatment (Kiev,
1965).

Native definitions of specific entities have invariably been defined in
terms of stressful social events preceding the onset of symptoms, rather
than in terms of the specific symptoms or combination of symptoms
present. The implications of accepting native definitions are often not
adequately considered by researchers.

A case in point is Rubel's (1964) suggestions for an epidemiological
study of *susto* or magical fright among Mexican-Americans, which he
defines, as they do, in terms of the situation in which it occurs. In this
way it is not possible to determine whether, in fact, this is really a distinct clinical entity, since the presumed social etiological factors are
already built into the diagnosis. That is to say, the diagnosis is made on
the basis of the situation in which it occurs—the presence of which is
considered as essential to the definition of the syndrome. The implementation of such a study would lead to obtaining information about the
social and cultural situations in which depressive anxiety attacks occur
—a useful approach in the study of epidemiology of social causes but
not for studying the depressive-anxiety attack itself. While this proposal
is an advance from previous approaches to the problem, it nevertheless
is limited, much as previous investigations have been, in that it accepts
the culture-bound definitions of the syndromes to be studied, these definitions invariably incorporating within them the very kind of data whose
presence is to be tested.

Differences in the behavioral manifestations of psychiatric patients in different cultures have also contributed to the view of different illnesses in different cultures. Thus, such things as the berserk violence of the *amok* victim, the echolalia and echopraxia of the *latah* case, and the extraordinary fear of the victim of thanatomania have been the basis for distinguishing these entities. The dramatic nature of these behavioral manifestations has, however, distracted attention from the underlying psychopathology and from traditional methods of diagnostic procedure. Then, too, insufficient attention has been focused on the patterns of expression available to the better adapted members of these cultures, which also show marked differences from Western concepts of behavior. This point is particularly important, for it underlines the fact that cultures reward and encourage different patterns of behavior, which will undoubtedly color the external manifestations of the psychiatric disorders while not necessarily changing their basic structures.

Another factor contributing to the notion of culture-bound disorders has been the limited opportunities field workers have had to follow cases of the exotic disorders to their eventual outcome. As Kaelbling (1961, p. 18) has written:

> Most syndromes have been described only once and often back in the 19th Century, almost always by a psychiatrically untrained observer. They never could be verified sufficiently and the examiner had no occasion of comparing his experiences in one disorder directly by observation with similarly disturbed behavior in other cultural settings, including our own.

The Anthropological Study of a Culture-Bound Disorder

Focus on the dramatic has often obscured the underlying disorder as well as situational and manipulative elements contributing to the presenting of a clinical picture. The relevance of these considerations is seen in the condition of *bouffée delirante aigue,* an acute confusional psychosis seen among Haitian peasants, which in many instances progresses to a chronic schizophrenia. Native priests or *hungans* interpret such illnesses (which occur most often in individuals several generations removed from the soil) as forms of possession (spirit) due to the patient's unwillingness to accept the call of the voodoo deities to join the voodoo church. They believe that reintegration into the voodoo church will bring about the individual's recovery.

Sanseigne (1961, p. 4), who has had opportunity to treat such illnesses in a modern clinical setting, has suggested a different view:

> Clinically, the picture met most frequently is an acute psychosis, such as the "bouffée delirante aigue," sudden attack, marked confusion, psychomotor excitation, with denudative and aggressive behavior, and sometimes religious delirium, visual and auditory hallucinations; the whole thing for a short period of time,

without deterioration. We often wonder if this is not an hysterical episode, but by searching similar attacks in the histories of our chronic schizophrenic we find almost constantly such episodes have occurred many years prior to the appearance of definite schizophrenic signs.

Studies of other exotic neuroses and psychoses may similarly show that many of them will lead to more traditional disorders.

It is appropriate to consider next whether these kinds of studies answer the questions they intend to answer. In some ways they fail to answer the questions posed; in other ways they succeed. They show how culture may influence the manifestations of psychiatric illness and the treatment of various disorders and how psychoanalysis is relevant to an understanding of the content and symbols associated with illness. A particular case in point is the numerous observations of Muensterberger, Devereux, and Roheim made in support of various analytic theories. These studies do not prove that cultural factors produce illness, or even that some psychiatric entities occur only in specific cultures. They have been important, however, in demonstrating how cultural attitudes can make certain subjective experiences ego syntonic or ego dystonic, that is, how culture determines what will be felt as abnormal and unusual and how culture provides social roles which make certain ego-dystonic experiences tolerable.

The tie-in of acute psychotic behavior with learned institutionalized patterns of behavior is well demonstrated in the case of *bouffée delirante aigue*. To properly understand this condition it is necessary to understand the role-playing aspect of the possession phenomenon in Haitian culture and its characteristic manifestations in nonpsychotic individuals. As noted above, the native doctors interpret this illness in terms of spirit possession. It is of interest that this explanation and the patient's behavior correspond to the sought-after possession experience of voodoo priests and congregants. There are differences however. Ritual possession is usually characterized by a reduction of higher integrative functions such as articulate speech, social inhibitions, and muscular coordination, with a concomitant increase of reflex behavior such as trembling, convulsive movements, muscle twitching, teeth grinding, and sucking movements (see Dorsainvil, 1931; Kiev, 1961; Mars, 1955). In many instances of possession, a sensory anesthesia exists allowing the individual to expose himself to noxious stimuli that would normally be harmful. The *hungan* enters into a well-controlled, learned, complex, and refined, self-induced trance, through auto-suggestion. Possession in the *hunsi* or congregant has the quality of a dissociative state precipitated and reinforced by a highly charged emotional atmosphere accompanied by an excessive barrage of sound, light, and drug stimuli. By contrast, *bouffée delirante aigue* would seem to represent a disorganizing psychotic illness in a culturally alienated individual.

The concept of a *culturally recognized and accepted way of "going crazy"* best explains the relationship among these various behavioral patterns (Devereux, 1956; Linton, 1956). The role of the possessed is culturally sanctioned and governed, applauded in ceremonies, tolerated in public market places, and frowned upon in other contexts and when differing in degree as in forms of *folie*. It offers opportunity for the expression of repressed and suppressed ego dystonic feelings and thoughts. It allows the oppressed peasantry to act as gods in a cathartic and spiritually uplifting experience, which serves different needs. For the *hungan* it provides a flexible and recognizable set of ideas, making possible the translation of private needs into a publicly acknowledged religious chosenness. For the *hunsi* it is an opportunity for the expression of behavior and emotions. The last type of individual "possessed by a *loa*" is unable to channel his uncontrollable impulses into this acknowledged and useful role for various reasons, usually ones that have alienated him from the mainsprings of the voodoo cult.

Indeed, from an early age the peasant child is exposed to ceremonial possessions. He is made aware of the prestige of the *hungan* and the possessed. He sees how applauded are the possessed and learns of their good fortune. Observing the possessions of his elders, a Haitian peasant child grows up with the hope that some day he too will be possessed. As one well-educated Haitian told me, "Everyone in Haiti is trying to catch a *loa*." It is obvious that for the nonliterate uneducated peasant "catching a *loa*" by possession is far easier than it is for those who are more educated, intellectual, and sophisticated.

In essence, possession is a useful and culturally sanctioned form of role playing which serves public as well as private needs and is legitimized only insofar as it occurs in the context of voodoo and in the correct proportions. For those who are out of touch with voodoo or for those whose possessions last longer than the ceremonials warrant, it is not legitimized and is considered a form of *folie*. The similarity of possession phenomena and psychiatric illness plus the identical explanations for *loa* possession and supernatural *folie* suggests a strong relationship between the two and adds weight to the formulation of ritual possession as an acceptable form of "going crazy."

The Psychodynamic Study of Culture-Bound Disorders

Another approach to the study of culture-bound disorders has been to examine the relationships between two or more institutional complexes in the same culture. Such studies have been of special value in demonstrating the relationship of cultural experience and psychiatric symptom patterning. Thus, Parker (1962) has suggested that the Eskimo's cooperative social organization reinforces the expectancy of need gratification first nurtured in a permissive childhood where dependency and affectional needs were minimally frustrated, making for little conflict or repression with regard to their expression. In this setting where overt expressions of tension and anxiety attract attention and bring need gratification, there is, according to Parker, a greater prevalence of hysterical symptoms, such as convulsive hysterical attacks and conversion symptoms.

In contrast, the dependency needs of the Ojibwas are early and severely frustrated, leading them to react in a depressed or hostile way to misfortune that they interpret as the result of hostile rejection by those around them. Social institutions further curtail and negatively sanction any direct attempts to express dependency needs and repressed hostility. This creates pressure for Ojibwa men who try to seek the support of others while, at the same time, giving expression to their own masculine aggressiveness. According to Parker, the Ojibwa male fears failure to live up to the rather narrow and rigidly defined masculine role, but also fears the social rejection and envy that come with outstanding achievement and success. Failure in hunting precedes depression and anxiety in the Ojibwa male. When faced with this failure, the individual feels abandoned and worthless.

As Parker (1960, p. 620) has written:

> For the *Witiko* victim the usual masochistic devices to insure dependency satisfaction and the normative cultural channels for an oblique expression of hostility no longer suffice to relieve anxiety and depression. Under these conditions, the dam (constituted by ego defenses) is shattered and the repressed cravings for the expression of dependency and aggressive needs burst forth. The depressive conflict between the rebellious rage and the submissive fear is resolved.

The morbid depression, paranoid ideas of bewitchment, and possession by the cannibalistic and homicidal *Witiko* monster which follows is thus ultimately, according to Parker, a form of pathological adjustment of the modal Ojibwa personality to severe environmental and other pressures.

While many of these formulations make sense, they should, I believe, be viewed only as tentative and useful formulations rather than demonstrated truths. It is likely that there are many societies with the same environmental conditions and socialization experiences where this same kind of thing does not develop. Furthermore, these data do not prove that cultural factors produce illness, nor even that some psychiatric entities occur only in specific cultures. They are of importance, however, in demonstrating how cultural attitudes can make certain subjective experiences ego syntonic or ego dystonic, that is, how culture determines what will be felt as abnormal and unusual, how culture provides social roles that make certain ego dystonic experiences tolerable, and how culture influences the manifestations of psychiatric illness.

In an attempt to unify the mass of anthropological data dealing with psychological and social aspects of personality, child training, socialization experiences, and psychopathology, Devereux (1956) has formulated what is perhaps the clearest theoretical statement on the subject of the ethnic neuroses and psychoses, the essential construct of which is the notion of an ethnic unconscious.

This is that portion of the total unconscious segment of the individual psyche which is shared with most members of a given culture in that . . . Each society or culture permits certain impulses, fantasies and the like to become and to remain conscious, while requiring others to be repressed, the members of a given culture are likely to have repressed the same things and thereby to have certain unconscious conflicts in common.

It is Devereux's notion that there are emotionally disturbed persons who are not incited to wholesale rebellion against all social norms because the unconscious segment of their ethnic personality is not so disorganized. While genuinely ill, such persons tend to borrow from culture the means for implementing their subjective derangement in a conventional way. It is his idea that the classical examples of such ethnic illness are *amok, latah, imu, Witiko, koro,* and so on. Such syndromes are examples of how disturbed people in certain cultures conform to the actual behavior pattern expected in that society from disturbed people.

As Devereux has written:

We might add that the symptomatology of the ethnic psychoses conforms to cultural expectations chiefly because conventional ideas on "how to act insane" are determined by the specific nature of the conflicts prevailing in certain cultures, and also by the nature of the defense which culture provides against such culturally penalized conflicts and impulses. In other words, whereas, in view of the nature of Crow culture, the psychically traumatized Crow Indian can, because of his distinctive ethnic makeup, and the nature of his culture and culturally determined tensions, find relief by running amok. It is the cultural conformism manifested by such psychotics which often causes us to minimize the seriousness of their basic derangements.

RESEARCH APPROACHES TO THE CULTURE-BOUND DISORDERS

It thus appears that previous studies have been of value in providing a conceptual and theoretical framework for understanding the diversity of phenomena encountered in cross-cultural psychiatry. It remains now, however, to approach the basic problems and questions in such a way as to benefit from the knowledge of obstacles previously encountered. To properly evaluate some of the questions posed above it is necessary to improve research and clinical methods. Thus, better epidemiological techniques are needed to adequately study hospital usage patterns; better diagnostic skills and methods are needed to more adequately diagnose the different disorders encountered, and better follow-up and clinical methods are needed to more adequately complete the clinical picture.

Intensive Clinical Studies

One approach is to define a population of patients and to study them in great detail in the clinical situation. A good example of this is Wallace's program (Wallace & Ackerman, 1960) for studying a number of etiological hypotheses about Pibloktoq among the Polar Eskimos, including views that it is psychomotor epilepsy (kinship, genealogical, and electroencephalographic studies), psychogenic hysterical fit (depth interviewing), a chronic endemic encephalitis (cultivation of virus), a form of hypocalcemia secondary to diet, low Vitamin D3 intake in winter and mild hypoparathyroidism (Serum Ca, Serum K; studies of diet, ultraviolet radiation, food distribution patterns), food poisoning from shark meat (dietary histories, chemical studies of suspected sea creatures), and spontaneous functional hypoglycemia secondary to low carbohydrate diet and insufficient gluconeogenesis from protein (blood glucose, liver function and adrenocortical studies).

Other clinical studies can focus on the transitions from subclinical to clinical conditions by way of extending knowledge of clinical conditions in depth. This is of particular interest in those cultures that encourage and tolerate special mental states such as are seen in cult behavior, trance, and possession states. Intensive study of such phenomena extended over a long period of time may clarify the relationship of such states to clinical psychiatric conditions.

Additional benefit could accrue from the linkage of records of various social and medical agencies in order to coordinate various services individuals may use. In addition to the benefit to the individual, this may also be of value in helping to see the relationship among various kinds of behavior. It would be good, for example, to know whether the same individuals that appear in courts appear in hospitals or in the huts of native healers.

Lambo's (1962) study of "malignant anxiety" demonstrated the value for the psychiatrist of a searching clinical study of a number of individuals who were brought to attention by virtue of their unusual criminal behavior.

That native doctors can be relied on as informants and helpers in a research enterprise with a Western team has been clearly proven by Leighton and Lambo in their recent Nigerian Study (Leighton, Lambo, Hughes, Leighton, Murphy, & Macklin, 1963).

Follow-up Studies

Other techniques that could usefully be applied to the underdeveloped areas include cohort and family studies. Cohort studies would provide for the clinical follow-up of a group of individuals with a known diagnosis, or shared experience, or exposure to the same stresses to see the outcome in terms of course of an illness, or development of an illness. Of relevance here is Yap's study of "shook yang," or *koro*. According to Yap (1965), *koro* is a culture-bound acute anxiety state with "partial depersonalization leading to the conviction of penile shrinkage and to fears of dissolution." The syndrome is closely connected with the Chinese belief that masturbation and nocturnal emission prevent the healthy sex change of yin and yang humors resulting in an unbalanced loss of the yang-producing *koro*. Despite the close tie-in with Chinese beliefs and the fact that the occurrence and distribution of *koro* are determined by sociocultural factors, Yap's 15-year follow-up enabled him to diagnose these cases in terms of Western nosological categories. The nineteen typical cases he studied were categorized as follows: Passive-dependent, eleven; compulsive, four; emotionally unstable, three; and passive-aggressive, one. In addition, six cases were associated with schizophrenia, one with general paresis, and one with heroin withdrawal.

Mention should be made of the value of longitudinal studies of a single form of exotic disorder in one culture over a period of time. One such follow-up study was recently done on the *imu* reaction, a form of *latah* found among the primitive Ainu in Japan. In 1934, 111 cases of *imu* were found in a population of 17,500 Ainu. In 1958, only one case was found with *imu* symptomatology in this same area. Although the explanations for this changing frequency is undetermined, such studies offer excellent opportunity to validate the finding of earlier studies, and also to study the whole question of changing patterns of symptomatology.

The Cross-Cultural Study
of Traditional Psychiatric Disorders

Even if cross-cultural studies of exotic disorders cannot prove that cultural factors produce psychiatric illness, they are, nevertheless, of value in helping us distinguish between the minimal fundamental elements of certain psychological disorders and those aspects of these disorders that are influenced by cultural factors, that is, pathoplastic features. We have learned from such studies that even though delusional content often relates to belief systems, it cannot by itself be used for determining the severity of prognosis of an illness. The extent to which the delusions are distortions of commonly held beliefs or are wholly idiosyncratic notions may be more important considerations.

This kind of study enables us to distinguish nuclear symptoms of psychiatric illness from what may be secondary symptoms specific for a given culture. The traditional emphasis on diagnostic entities and syndromes has to some extent obscured the value of studying symptoms that are differentially distributed according to age and sex and appear in various diagnostic entities. Of further interest, they are invariably the focus of both complaints and the choice of treatment and may be at the phenomenological level most amenable to epidemiological study.

The cross-cultural difference in the symptoms of schizophrenia provide a case in point. While catatonic rigidity, negativism, and stereotypy are common in Indian schizophrenics, and aggressiveness and expressiveness are common in Southern Italian patients, African patients are reported to have a tendency to be quieter than in the Western world (Murphy, 1963). The withdrawal of Indian schizophrenics has been related to the formal, hierarchical Indian culture which fosters introversion and emotional controls, while the barrenness of the clinical picture among preliterate Africans has been tied to the paucity of their cultural and intellectual resources and their difficulties in dealing with abstractions.

Despite such cross-cultural differences, which suggest a tie-in between symptoms and culture, four out of twenty-six symptoms and signs were never reported as infrequent in schizophrenia in the McGill survey. These were social and emotional withdrawal, auditory hallucinations, delusions, and flatness of affect. The importance of these findings is that they suggest the possibility that there are nuclear features to the illness of schizophrenia which are not culturally determined and which may be distinguished from those symptoms learned in the culture.

The same kinds of considerations are applicable to depressive illness. Thus, guilt, self-reproach, and suicide have been reported as rare in the depressed in primitive societies (Murphy, 1964). Although a number of hypotheses have been advanced to explain this, it is a significant set of observations largely because it suggests the importance of studying the component parts of psychiatric syndromes.

The Cross-Cultural Study of Disability
Associated with Psychiatric Disorders

In addition to extending the clinical picture of psychiatric illness by studying the exotic disorders, it is also of value to study more familiar disorders in these settings for the relevance this might have for our understanding of the tertiary prevention of chronic breakdown and deterioration. Using the tools of epidemiological investigation (register of chronic diseases, record linkage systems, cohort studies, and family studies), one might be able to investigate factors in different cultures that contribute to or mitigate against the eventual development of chronic patterns. Such studies might be useful for studying such things as the development of chronicity in schizophrenics, suicide in depression, and the chronic social breakdown syndrome. Indeed, cultural factors may be more important in influencing psychiatric illness once they have developed than in causing them in the first place (Kiev, 1964). These considerations are demonstrated by the West Indian Pentecostal sects—which not only serve therapeutic purposes but may help decrease secondary disability in cases of psychiatric illness by providing well-defined roles and group support (see Kiev, 1964). These provide a form of social integration for West Indians in London by providing a world view and methods of attaining grace dependent on faith alone. The churches provide acceptance and a method for the emotional release. The gifts of the Spirit compensate for the lack of material gifts, while the gift of "tongues" allows the inarticulate to speak to an applauding audience. Acknowledging evil and hopelessness of the sect encourages members to transfer their hopes to the hereafter. Individuals are judged by their faith in God, as religious status is substituted for social and racial status.

The sect is authoritarian, governing members by making a particular way of life the condition for blessing. It provides several formal and informal meetings a week and exercises constraint over members by enforcing adherence to its values. Sect members can, however, act out and express themselves in an uninhibited way within traditional limits by the use of such devices as tongues, dancing, and patterned testimonials.

Although emotional instability is not necessary for participation in the services, the meetings do provide for the expression of a variety of needs and personality traits. For the depressed and guilt-ridden, the sin-cathartic basis of the ideology and services provides a useful guilt-reducing device; for the hysteric, a socially acceptable model for acting out; and for the obsessional, the encouragement of a reduction of inhibitions and increased emotionality. For such accompaniments of neurotic and real suffering as feelings of inferiority, self-consciousness, suspiciousness, and anxiety, the social aspects of the movement would seem to be of value.

Members are expected to testify periodically and when moved or touched by the Holy Ghost. The testimonies of regular members ("saints") consists of expressions of gratitude for being saved, boasts about following Jesus by means of the good life, and citations of divine intervention in everyday life. As one man said, "Someone might have had a severe temptation during the week and God's words would come back to them as Joseph was tempted to sin and he says 'how can I do this wicked thing and sin against my God!' " They will tell how God helped them through the week, of their temptation and trials. "Or if someone persecutes you —telling a terrible lie on you which you know you're not guilty of— you are able to bear it without giving way to passion or committing yourself." Backsliders report on the temptations of the Devil and their need to repent. Actual sins are not specifically cited, as the rituals are concerned more with the emotional expression of the congregation. Bible reading or hymn singing are acceptable testimonials for those who cannot express their thoughts in other ways. When individuals are disinclined to testify, the presence of the Holy Ghost in them is accepted as sufficient explanation, and they are not made to do so.

Difficulties in the Identification of Syndromes

Data on exotic diseases may also be used in the identification of syndromes, that is, the separation of clinical entities on the basis of patterns of symptoms, signs, course, prognosis, etiology, and so forth. Such study may lead to the discovery that there are two illnesses previously thought to be the same, or that two unrelated illnesses are really the same. To prove that some exotic diseases are different from known Western psychiatric disorders, it is necessary to show that they have different signs, symptoms, course, prognosis, or etiology.

Most investigators have gathered data on different signs and symptoms —often using the same data to argue for or against the hypothesis that the exotic disorders were different from known Western disorders. In general, most writers have argued that only the content was different but that the form was the same, although there are some reports that sometimes the form is different too, as in the case of confusional states, described among Africans by Carothers. It is difficult to determine which of the two views is correct, for it is hard to know whether the different signs demonstrated are really examples of form or of content. Indeed, it is difficult to make a diagnosis since, in the absence of good objective tests, it is hard to know what are the true signs present.

It would appear to be easier to examine *course* and *prognosis* as Yap and Sanseigne have done. This is particularly useful in distinguishing culture-bound forms of hysteria from chronic progressive schizophrenic illness which may present identical pictures.

These considerations suggest the need for studies to demonstrate that some exotic diseases are really not different but are the same as certain familiar or well-defined disorders. This can be done by showing that the exotic disorder is caused by a demonstrable physical agent such as the treponema pallidum or the trypanosome or by a treatable nutritional deficiency. It would also be of value to study the response of some of these disorders to modern treatments, but as yet this is not a good diagnostic tool in psychiatry since treatments are nonspecific in psychiatry as compared to treatments in medicine.

The importance of investigating such issues is underlined by findings that malaria accounted for 3.4 percent of first admissions to mental hospitals in Kenya in Carother's study, that trypanosomiasis was the most common cause of mental illness in Tooth's study of West Africa and that other parasitic, infectious, and toxic agents have been identified as productive of mental disorders in other less developed areas, suggesting that they might also be involved in some of the exotic disorders.

Difficulty in differentiating the exotic disorders from disorders that are better known to Western psychiatry may be further complicated by differences in the nature and characteristics of these better known disorders. Thus, schizophrenia in primitive people has been reported to occur frequently in acute paroxysms which may simulate the acute hallucinosis and confusional states of infective deliria with periods of normality following the paroxysm (Arieti & Meth, 1959). This observation, coupled with the suggestion that the dementia state seen in chronic schizophrenics is rare in primitive people, suggests the possibility that the form of schizophrenia experienced by the primitive is a less complex one and that various factors in Western society, perhaps in the management of the mentally ill, make for some of the complexities seen in the patients.

Difficulty in identifying the same illness or syndrome may result from the fact that different observers may have had opportunity to observe the same phenomenon at different times. This may account for such differences of opinion as have been held about a condition like *amok*. Thus, Kraepelin felt that *amok* might be a dream-state, while Van Loon thought of it as an acute, infectious delirium. Others have thought that hysterical psychopathic or schizophrenic disturbances might underlie *amok* behavior. Another explanation for such different opinions is that *amok* can occur in a variety of disorders and that each of the observers has observed basically a different entity. In this view, *amok* could then perhaps be seen as one culturally conditioned symptom which can occur in a variety of syndromes.

Much as different factors may produce the same clinical picture, the same etiological factors and psychological mechanism may produce a variety of clinical pictures. This is certainly true of the degenerative organic psychoses and the symptomatic psychoses that may be present in an extraordinary variety of ways. It is also true of hysterical disorders and, to a lesser degree, of other psychiatric illnesses. Of interest in this regard are conditions with the same underlying psychodynamic mechanisms the differing clinical manifestations and symbolic content of which reflect differences in the culture. Thus, castration fear, dependency needs, and inferiority feelings which may be expressed in the Don Juanism of Western culture or in the machismo complex of Mexican-American culture may take the form of a fear that the patient's penis will disappear into his adomen and that he will die, as in Shook Yang or *koro* in Southeast Asia.

In this connection, Devereux's (1956) formulation regarding the universality of basic psychodynamics best accounts for clinically observed differences in individuals with similar underlying psychodynamic conflicts. As he has written:

> The same defense mechanisms are present in the normal and in the abnormal personality, as well as in members of various cultures. The normal differs from the abnormal and the Eskimo differs from the Bedouin, not in terms of the presence or absence of certain defense mechanisms, but in terms of the presence or absence of the patterning of all defenses, and in terms of the relative degree of importance which culture "assigns" to the various defense mechanisms. This "assigning" of importance is not a deliberate act, but simply a more or less inevitable by-product of the prevailing cultural atmosphere.

It is this which accounts for the fact that the psychodynamic mechanisms or the patterning of behavior and defenses vary from culture to culture, which in turn will be reflected in patterns of psychiatric illnesses seen. While much work remains to be done however to validate this theory, it nevertheless has much merit in that it provides a unified view of a diverse array of data while at the same time taking account of both psychiatric and anthropological types of data.

The Problem of Clinical Diagnosis

One more basic methodological obstacle to the adequate execution of the kinds of studies we have been considering is the problem of clinical diagnosis. This problem is made up of two parts—a conceptual one, concerning the question of normality, and a technical one, concerning the development of objective indexes of mental illness.

The question of normality invariably arises in cross-cultural studies because of the marked differences in belief and behavior found in various cultures. In some instances, certain traits, considered as abnormal in the West, have been considered as normal by the members of a particular group. Thus suspiciousness has been regarded as normal for the Dobuans, while a paranoid megalomaniacal nature has been considered a modal personality trait for the Kwakiutl (Benedict, 1934). Other observers have reported on the institutionalization of certain abnormal patterns such as homosexuality in the berdache role among the Indians and the ritualization of psychotic behavior in certain shamanistic roles. It is particularly difficult in such instances to decide on just what constitutes a case, particularly as the native views are so much at variance with the Western views.

Two points which have been insufficiently recognized are relevant here. First, Devereux has suggested that even though certain patterns, considered abnormal in our own society, are institutionalized in these cultures, they are not necessarily the central thematic issues in these cultures. The individuals who fill these roles, even shamanistic roles, are often acknowledged to be on the fringes of things by the members of these societies, even though they are not limited in the performance of these roles.

Secondly, although psychiatric illnesses are defined differently from culture to culture, they are functionally similar in that the patient's symptoms are either distressing to him or to the group, so that the illness or abnormality can be operationally defined rather than judged against an absolute standard. This is not to take a cultural relativist stand, but to suggest that it is not so much the content or character of the behavior —which even if abnormal from our point of view can be taken as a modal personality trait in a particular culture—but its compatibility with the individual or his group. This view of illness or disease should be carefully distinguished from those views that take as their criterion of mental illness an idealistic, valued state of mental health, making anything that deviates from perfect mental health an example of maladjustment, irrespective of the culture in which it occurs. To overcome the difficulties inherent in the transcultural study of psychiatric illnesses, it is desirable to develop methods for distinguishing normal from abnormal, and one diagnostic entity from another. This involves, first of all, more intensive studies within single cultures. At the same time, investigations should be carried out for the purpose not only of making distinctions between syndromes but for finding common elements in apparently different syndromes. Such studies will be greatly aided by recourse to improved diagnostic methods, both clinical and experimental.

Along these lines, Zubin has suggested a useful distinction between culture-bound indicators, wherein diagnoses are based on observed deviations from sociocultural norms, culture-fair diagnostic indicators, which are the cross-cultural invariant deviations from expectation that characterize mental disorders, and such culture-free indicators as can be provided by biochemical, neurophysiological, and behavioral measures (Zubin & Kietzman, 1964). The first 1000 milliseconds of a patient's response to stimulation in various sense modalities has been suggested by him as a suitable testing ground for the culture-free or culture-fair indicators, on the presumption that the effects of learning may not be expressed quickly enough to influence the response in this phase. Although culture undoubtedly influences an individual's attitude to the taking of tests, these tests are less readily influenced by cultural factors than are conceptual tests like the IQ.

According to Zubin, the various culture-fair tests have been constructed to minimize the contamination of testing by variables such as the subject's understanding of the test, his motivation, attention, and cooperation; which variables also contaminate comparisons of schizophrenics and normals even from the same culture.

Insofar as conceptual, and therefore cultural, elements appear to enter into most physiological responses as is seen in conditioning, perceptual, placebo, and other studies, there are a number of kinds of study that may minimize these elements.

Techniques that are little dependent on socio-cultural norms include pupillography, cross-modality reaction time, and measures of temporal resolution in vision and audition. In one well-documented study, schizophrenic subjects displayed longer and more variable reaction times than did normal subjects. Venables (1960) reported on the periodicity of reaction times in which normals and schizophrenics demonstrated 100 millisecond periodicities that were out of place with each other by 10 milliseconds. King (1962) demonstrated that schizophrenic and normal subjects differ in their ability to tap in synchrony with a repetitive click presented 1 to 3 seconds apart. Normal subjects tend to anticipate or respond before the synchronizing stimulus is given. Other behavioral studies of phenomena that occur in the 1000 milliseconds range include critical flicker frequency, apparent movement, two-pulse thresholds, auditory localizations, and masking. The culture-free indicators derived from laboratory experiments appear to be more objective than culture-dependent techniques, such as systematic interviewing schedules and accompanying inventories for evaluating mental status and social adaptation. In addition the results obtained from them are not dependent on the trained judgment of the operator or technician as in culture-dependent techniques but only on his skill at operating the apparatus. In these indicators according to Zubin (1964): "The speed, accuracy and temporal or spatial integration of responses to specified types of stimuli can be measured and contrasted in patients and controls."

SUMMARY

Cross-cultural studies are of great value for modern psychiatry, since they afford considerable opportunity to see the effects of a variety of social and environmental forces in the production, perpetuation, and management of psychiatric illness and enable us to understand with greater clarity which aspects of the illnesses we ordinarily see are central to them and which are grafted on by situational and environmental factors.

Examination of studies of culture-bound disorders reveals numerous factors that have contributed to the acceptance of this concept. One such factor has been the difference found in the content of delusions of disturbed individuals in different cultures, although closer examination reveals not only a close relationship of delusions to belief systems in a culture, but also no basic difference in the form of such illnesses. It appears also that there has been too great an inclination to accept native notions of etiology and nosology. The exotic disorders have invariably been defined in terms of culturally defined stressful social events preceding the onset of symptoms, rather than in terms of specific clinical groupings of symptoms which in their basic components are largely invariant from culture to culture. Differences in the behavioral manifestations of psychiatric patients in different cultures have also contributed to the view of different illnesses in different cultures. Closer examination, however, reveals the fact that cultures reward and encourage different patterns of behavior that undoubtedly color the external manifestations of mental disorders without necessarily changing their basic structures. It becomes clear that the behavioral manifestations of psychotic illnesses are related to learned institutionalized patterns of behavior, as is shown in the study of *bouffée delirante aigue* and spirit possession in Haiti.

Spirit possession is seen as a culturally recognized and accepted way of "going crazy" which influences the behavior of the "bouffée" patient. For others it offers a useful and culturally sanctioned form of role playing for the expression of repressed and suppressed ego dystonic feelings and thoughts which are legitimized only insofar as they occur in the context of voodoo and in correct proportions. Studies of the relationship of two or more institutional complexes in the same culture have been of special value in demonstrating the relationship of cultural experience to psychiatric symptom patterning. Studies such as Parker's of the Ojibwa witiko psychosis and Eskimo hysteria demonstrate how cultural attitudes can make certain subjective experiences ego syntonic or ego dystonic, that is, how culture determines what will be felt as abnormal and unusual (Parker, 1960).

A variety of research approaches to the culture-bound disorders would appear to be appropriate at the present stage of our technological knowledge. We now can approach the basic problems and questions in such a way as to benefit from the knowledge of previously encountered obstacles. One approach involves the intensive clinical study of a population of patients supplemented by studies of kinship, a genealogy, electroencephalography, and biochemistry. Additional benefits would accrue from the linkage of records of various social and medical agencies in order to obtain a broader picture of patients by studying the various services they may use. Other epidemiological techniques that can usefully be applied to the underdeveloped areas are cohort and family studies which can provide for the clinical follow-up of a group of individuals with a known diagnosis or shared experience of exposure to the same stresses to see the outcome in terms of the course of illness and/or the development of secondary symptoms of disability. Related to these are longitudinal studies of a single form of exotic disorders in one culture over a period of time. Such studies would be of value in distinguishing between the minimal fundamental elements of certain psychological disorders and those aspects of these disorders that are influenced by cultural factors, that is, pathoplastic features. Similarly the cross-cultural study of such disorders as schizophrenia and endogenous depression may help in differentiating the nuclear features of these illnesses that are not culturally determined from these symptoms grafted on by different cultures. It is also of value to study more familiar disorders in underdeveloped societies for the relevance this might have for understanding of the tertiary prevention of chronic social breakdown and deterioration. Using the tools of epidemiological investigation (register of chronic diseases, record linkage system, cohort studies, and family studies) one might be able to investigate factors in different cultures that contribute to or militate against eventual development of chronic patterns. Indeed, cultural factors may be more important in influencing psychiatric illnesses once they have developed than in causing them. In this regard, it is of value to study naturalistic forms of psychotherapy such as are found in certain religious sects and certain forms of primitive medicine. Not only may these serve therapeutic purposes, but they may help to decrease secondary disabilities in psychiatric cases by providing well-defined roles and group support.

Data on exotic diseases may also be used in the identification of syndromes, that is, the separation of clinical entities on the basis of patterns of symptoms, signs, course prognosis, and etiology. Such studies may lead to the discovery that there are two illnesses now thought to be the same one, or that two apparently unrelated illnesses are really the same. It is likely that some exotic diseases are really not different but are the same as certain familiar and well-defined disorders. To be of value, such studies should take account of differences between culture-bound diagnostic indicators where diagnoses are based on observed deviations from sociocultural norms, culture-fair diagnostic indicators, which are the cross-cultural invariant deviations from expectations that characterize mental disorders, and such culture-free diagnostic methods as can be provided by biochemical, neurophysiological, and behavioral techniques such as pupillography, cross-modality reaction time, and measures of temporal resolutions of vision and audition.

This essay has reviewed some of the crucial aspects of the various forms of psychiatric illness in various cultures. The reasons for these studies and for some of the observations repeatedly made by different workers were examined in the light of the relevance of these studies for a scientific psychiatry. Special attention was focused on the issue of whether these studies did indeed demonstrate what they intended to demonstrate and the reasons why they did not. Some of the data were examined to see if other questions were answered.

It appears that previous studies have been sidetracked by questions of etiology when the approaches used were not designed for this. Previous studies have often relied on inadequately gathered incidence and/or prevalence data, in making remarks about the effects of culture on psychiatric disorders. Previous studies have, in using a variety of methods, led to much confusion between native diagnostic groupings and Western nosological categories and have led to the notion of culture-bound disorders. This concept and the data have been reviewed, and suggestions have been made for the study of such conditions by way of extending the clinical picture of them and similar disorders, and by way of more adequately identifying existing syndromes.

REFERENCES

Arieti, S., & Meth, J. M. Rare, unclassifiable, collective, and exotic psychotic syndromes. In Silvano Arieti (Ed.), *American handbook of psychiatry*. New York: Basic Books, 1959. Pp. 546–563.

Benedict, R. *Patterns of culture*. Boston: Houghton Mifflin, 1934.

Berne, E. Some Oriental mental hospitals. *American Journal of Psychiatry*, 1950, **106**, 376–383.

Bleuler, E. *Dementia praecox or the group of schizophrenias.* New York: International Universities Press, 1950.

Carothers, J. C. *The African mind in health and disease.* Geneva: World Health Organization, Monograph Series No. 17, 1953.

Cooper, J. M. Mental disease situations in certain cultures. *Journal of Abnormal and Social Psychology,* 1934, **29,** 10–17.

Devereux, G. "Normal and abnormal," the key problem of psychiatric anthropology. *Some Uses of Anthropology, Theoretical and Applied.* The Anthropological Society of Washington, D.C., 1956.

Dorsainvil, J. C. *Vodou et nevrose.* Port-au-Prince: Imprimerie La Press, 1931.

Hallowell, A. I. Culture and mental disorder. *Journal of Abnormal and Social Psychology,* 1934, **29,** 1–9.

Kaelbling, R. Comparative psychopathology and psychotherapy. *Acta Psychotherapeutica,* 1961, **9,** 10–28.

Kiev, A. *Curanderismo: Mexican-American folk psychiatry.* New York: Free Press, 1968.

Kiev, A. Psychotherapeutic aspects of Pentecostal sects among West Indian immigrants to England. *The British Journal of Sociology,* 1964, **15,** 129–138.

Kiev, A. *Spirit possession in Haiti. American Journal of Psychiatry,* 1961, **118,** 133–141.

Kiev, A. *Magic, faith and healing; Studies in primitive psychiatry today.* New York: Free Press, 1964.

King, H. E. Anticipatory behavior: Temporal matching by normal and psychotic subjects. *Journal of Psychology,* 1962, **53,** 425–440.

Kraepelin, E. *Psychiatrie,* Vol. I. (8th ed.) Leipzig: Barth, 1909.

Lambo, T. A. Malignant Anxiety. *The Journal of Mental Science,* 1962, **108,** 256–264.

Landes, R. The abnormal among the Ojibwa Indians. *Journal of Abnormal and Social Psychology,* 1938, **33,** 14–33.

Leighton, A. H., Lambo, T. A., Hughes, C. C., Leighton, D. C., Murphy, J. M., & Macklin, D. P. *Psychiatric disorder among the Yoruba.* New York: Cornell University Press, 1963.

Linton, R. D. *Culture and mental disorders.* Springfield: Charles C Thomas, 1956.

Mars, L. *La Crise de possession.* Port-au-Prince: Imprimerie de l'Etat, 1955.

Murphy, H. B., Wittkower, E. D., & Chance, N. A. Cross-cultural inquiry into the symptomatology of depression. *Transcultural Psychiatric Research Review and Newsletter,* 1964, **1,** 5–18.

Murphy, H. B., Wittkower, E. D., Fried, J., & Ellenberger, H. A cross-cultural survey of schizophrenic symptomatology. *International Journal of Social Psychiatry,* 1963.

Opler, M. K. *Culture, psychiatry and human values.* Springfield: Charles C Thomas, 1956.

Parker, S. Eskimo psychopathology in the context of Eskimo personality and culture. *American Anthropologist,* 1962, **64.**

Parker, S. The Witiko psychosis in the context of Ojibwa personality and culture. *American Anthropologist*, 1960, **62**, 603–623.

Rubel, A. J. The epidemiology of a folk illness: *susto* in Hispanic America. *Ethnology*, 1964, 268–283.

Sanseigne, A., & Desrosiers, M. The evaluation of psychopharmaceuticals in an underdeveloped country. In N. S. Kline (Ed.), *Psychiatry in the underdeveloped countries*. Washington, D.C.: American Psychiatric Association, 1961, 52–58.

Seligman, C. G. Sex, temperament, conflict and psychosis in a Stone Age population, *British Journal of Medical Psychology*, 1929, **9**, 187–202.

Slotkin, J. S. Peyotism, 1521–1891. *American Anthropologist*, 1955, **57**, 202–230.

Spiro, M. E. Ghosts, Ifaluk and teleological functionalism. *American Anthropologist*, 1952, 54, 497–503.

Suwa, N., et al. "Imu and recent findings of it. *Seishinigaku*, 1963, 5, 397–493. Quoted in Kumasaka, Y. *A Culturally Determined Mental Reaction Among the Ainu.*

Tooth, G. C. *Studies in mental illness in the Gold Coast*. London: H. M. Stationery Office, 1950.

Uchimura, Y. Imu, eine psychoreacktive Erscheinung der Ainu-Frauen. *Nervenarzt*, 1956, **27**, 535–540. Cited in Kaelbling (1961), ref. 20.

Van Loon, H. G. Protopathic instinctive phenomena in normal and pathologic Malay life. *British Journal of Medical Psychology*, 1929, **8**, 264–276.

Venables, P. H. Periodicity in Reaction Time. *British Journal of Psychology*, 1960, **51**, 37–48.

Wallace, A. F. C., & Ackerman, R. E. An interdisciplinary approach to mental disorder among the polar Eskimos of northwest Greenland. *Anthropologica*, 1960, 2.

Yap, P. M. Koro—a culture-bound depersonalization syndrome. Reprinted from *The British Journal of Psychiatry*, Vol. 111, No. 170, January, 1965.

Yap, P. M. Mental diseases peculiar to certain cultures: A survey of comparative psychiatry. *Journal of Mental Science*, 1951, **97**, 313–327.

Yap, P. M. The latah reaction. *Journal of Mental Science*, 1952, **8**, 515–564.

Zubin, J., & Kietzman, M. A cross-cultural approach to classification in schizophrenia and other mental disorders. Paper presented at American Psychopathological Association Annual Meeting, New York, February, 1964.

2.5 Orientation

Those who await the millennium, or hope to engineer yet another utopia, seem to be convinced that some ways of life are better, or worse, than others. One version of this belief has sustained the long-standing search for the basis of the "healthy" or "sick" society.

Anthropologist Raoul Naroll faces this question squarely when he asks whether some societies are more stressful to live in than others.

In his search for indicators of stress, Naroll considers many—rates of mental illness, stuttering, homicide, witchcraft accusation, and so on—before he concludes that given the present state of our ethnographic knowledge, the best indicator of the sickness or health of a society is its suicide rate. Naroll's development of his thesis is intriguing and controversial, as is his conclusion that some societies are indeed more stressful to live in than others.

2.5 Cultural Determinants and the Concept of the Sick Society[1]

Raoul Naroll

SUICIDE AS A MEASURE OF SOCIETAL SICKNESS

Can "culture" determine the amount or kind of mental illness in a society? Are some societies sick, or at least sicker than others? The evidence at hand is not yet conclusive, but it certainly points strongly in the direction of a "yes" answer. The main difficulty about a rigorous test of this hypothesis is the difficulty in getting accurate statistics on mental illness incidence from large populations. In our own society, where accurate statistics are difficult enough to obtain, we know that mental hospital admissions are influenced by the relative status of psychiatrist and patient, and by the attitude of the patient's family toward whatever stigma may be attached to mental hospitalization. But in other societies, where formal institutional care for mentally ill may be rare, or absent altogether, and where concepts of normal and abnormal behavior may vary considerably from

[1] This research was supported primarily by grant M-3821 from the National Institute of Public Health, United States Public Health Service. The work was facilitated by pooling much of it with that of other projects supported by grants G-13141 and G-21584, National Science Foundation, and by a series of contracts under Project Michelson, United States Naval Ordnance Test Station, China Lake, California. Space does not permit listing here the dozens of colleagues and students who contributed materially to the work; payment of that debt of gratitude must be deferred to a later time and another place.

those in our own, it may be very much harder to assemble accurate statistics on mental illness.

Nearly a decade ago, I combed the Human Relations Area Files for data on nine supposed symptoms of culture stress. Neither on mental illness, nor on stuttering, nor on psychosomatic illness, nor on use of narcotics, nor on crimes or offenses against the mores (except homicide) were there enough data to provide a basis for any sort of meaningful analysis. In other words, the existing books and papers written by anthropologists and missionaries do not say enough about any of these five types of stress symptoms even to *suggest* conclusions about relative frequency (see Naroll, 1962).

However, considerable data was found on suicide, homicide, drunken brawling, and witchcraft accusations. These four hypothetical symptoms of culture stress along with some others were made the basis of a subsequent cross-cultural test of the frustration-aggression hypothesis. This test was at the same time a test of the "sick society" hypothesis. For if it became clear that in some societies people were systematically frustrated by their culture patterns to a high degree, and manifested this frustration in much aggressive activity, we could term such societies "sick." Calling these societies "sick" would make more sense if we could likewise call a society "well" or "healthy" when it became clear that, in contrast to the "sick" societies, its people were systematically frustrated by their culture patterns only to a relatively moderate degree and consequently did not manifest much aggressive activity. But of the four symptoms mentioned above, our cross-cultural test disclosed that only the suicide rate provided a dependable index for the "sick society" hypothesis.

To be sure, we must not presume that all frustration is bad or unhealthy. On the contrary, it seems clear that all human cultures must frustrate their culture bearers to some extent. Incest taboos are universal and constitute clear frustrations, and, according to Freud and his followers, these frustrations are of great importance in personality formation. Furthermore, all human culture contains some sort of socialization patterns inhibiting many other specific behavior patterns deemed undesirable. All cultures have toilet training patterns, for example.

Furthermore, the validation of a frustration-aggression hypothesis would not in itself be enough to settle conclusively the existence of a variance in relative mental "sickness" or "health" among culture patterns. Suppose we definitely showed that cultures varied in their manifestations of aggressions, that this variation went hand in hand with a highly correlated variation in extent and severity of individual frustrations, and that whenever individual frustrations were first varied by outside circumstances, then manifestations of aggression usually followed suit—we still would have no answer to Li An-che (1937). Li, a Chinese anthropologist, wrote a celebrated critique of American studies of Pueblo Indian culture. American anthropologists like Benedict (1946) had made much of the peaceful orientation of many of these Southwestern farming tribes. The two westernmost pueblo peoples of Zuni and Hopi were taken as special cases in point. The very name *Hopi* means "peaceful," and any sort of overt manifestation of aggressive feeling is frowned upon by them. However, Li felt that these peace-loving attitudes were no evidence of a lack of aggressive feelings, but only a cover-up for them. The Pueblo peoples, not being conversant with modern psychological theory, did not perceive malicious gossip or accusations of witchcraft as manifestations of aggression. Li An-che felt intuitively that the Zuni people he visited were suffused with feelings of hostility toward their friends, relatives, and neighbors. I myself, having spent a scant couple of weeks among the Hopi of the third mesa, find Li's views easy to believe. The Hopi seem to me, by comparison with our own war-oriented and aggressive culture or the equally war-oriented and aggressive culture of Tyrolean peasants, to be quite distrustful, suspicious, and hostile toward one another. (I am not referring to their attitude toward outsiders—rather only their attitude toward each other.) Thus, there is here some support for Herbert Kelman's argument, set forth in a letter he wrote me some years ago, that symptoms of aggressive behavior might well indicate lower frustration levels. Kelman's idea is that, given a constant level of frustration, those cultures that provide for their people's blowing off steam in aggressive activities, have by and large less frustrated people than those cultures that inhibit aggressive activities—which keeps the steam pent up.

In light of this consideration, I wish to propose that for the time being one of our best indications of the sickness or health of a society is its suicide rate. Suicide is always rare. Those countries keeping good statistical records show no higher suicide rates for any country as a whole than thirty or forty suicides per 100,000 population per year. We may take Japanese statistics to be especially trustworthy for two reasons. First, they have long had a tradition of meticulous government records on individuals. This tradition was well developed during Japan's "hermit" centuries under the Tokugawas and so is no recent innovation. Second, the Japanese do not attach any stigma to suicide, indeed often take pride in it. Thus, in Japan there seems to be no special motive to conceal or disguise the fact of a suicide. (However, I must admit that I do not know about Japanese life insurance affairs which might perhaps create such a motive.) The Japanese government statistical bureau reports a suicide rate of 17.3 per 100,000 per year for 1962. If that is the reported rate in Japan, where suicide is notoriously frequent, where the people often take pride in it, and where record-keeping is excellent, we may well conclude that suicide is almost always a comparatively rare and unusual event. (In Naroll, 1962, pp. 144–146, I offer a great deal more data about the extent of variance of suicide rates among human societies.) If suicide then is a rare and unusual event, it does not have enough of the "safety valve" or "blowing off steam" effect to worry about. Consider two imaginary societies with the same sorts and amounts of frustration, the Abazaba people and the Wampiwampi people. Suppose the Abazabas have ten times the suicide rate of the Wampiwampi—say twenty per 100,000 per year for the Abazaba but only two per 100,000 for the Wampiwampi. Suppose that in both tribes all suicides reflect severe frustration: people kill themselves because they cannot stand the unhappiness of their lives. The difference in suicide rates, extreme though it is, would not lower the total frustration level of the Abazaba enough to matter, since even twenty suicides per 100,000 leaves 99,980 people just as frustrated as before, compared with 99,998 Wampiwampis. While the difference between two and twenty is impressive, the difference between 99,980 and 99,998 is not worth bothering with.

However, it seems a reasonable assumption that for every person who actually kills himself there are dozens, perhaps even hundreds or thousands of others who are in similar trouble but are not quite that desperate. For instance, we know that in the United States and Europe, a higher proportion of divorced people kill themselves than married people. For reasons which will be clear to the reader later, we suspect that this difference comes from the greater loneliness and sexual frustration of divorced people. It seems reasonable to suppose that for every American divorced woman who kills herself in a mood of depression arising out of loneliness and sexual frustration, there are a thousand other such women also suffering loneliness and sexual frustration, who are able somehow to cope and to carry on.

Thus, although suicide seems a useful thermometer for societal "sickness," it is hardly ideal. In most societies where Christian or Jewish ethics have been influential, suicide is felt to be more or less shameful. Wherever a potential suicide carries life insurance that pays his survivors more if his death is believed to be accidental, he and his survivors have a motive to conceal or disguise the nature of his death. Thus, we have two strong objections to the use of suicide as a societal thermometer. First, its frequency presumably is influenced to some extent by the attitude of the people toward it. Second, statistics on suicide are always subject to a greater or lesser degree of doubt, even in countries with the most efficient and conscientious methods of record keeping.

The fact remains that *for the time being* one of the best cross-cultural "thermometers" we have to measure social "sickness" is the suicide rate. Not that this approach is completely free of difficulties, but any other approach involves even greater difficulties. The suicide rate is *not* a good measure of societal "sickness," it is a poor measure. But it is one of the best measures we have available today.

In the best of all possible worlds, societal "sickness" would, I suspect, be measured by the incidence of psychoneurosis and certain sorts of psychosis. These in turn would be measured by studies of probability samples for large societies or by complete censuses for small societies. Each person studied would be interviewed at length, not only by a trained psychiatrist, but also by a cultural anthropologist, as part of a team. Both these workers would have in mind clear taxonomies of mental illness—taxonomies yet to be worked out by psychiatrists and psychologists. Until such taxonomies are discerned and validated, and until there is enough money and enough governmental cooperation and public acceptance to make this sort of measurement possible, we will have to make do with second rate, inferior measures of societal "sickness."

I take as a working hypothesis the notion that suicide and many kinds of mental illness reflect frustration and are alike symptoms of personal unhappiness. Such is the common-sense "folk wisdom" view. Such is the view widely held by psychiatrists and psychologists today. This view is certainly supported by the well-known fact that suicide is much more common among mental hospital patients than in the society at large.

But my main reasons for preferring suicide rate as a crude measure of societal sickness today are three. First, as already said, suicide, because of its absolute rarity, does not appreciably *lower* the frustration level of the society by "letting off steam." Second, there is reason to suspect that suicide is a sort of quintessential stress symptom. Aggressive behavior like witchcraft attribution, wife beating, child beating, homicide, and warfare seems in turn to create stresses that raise the suicide rate. Third, and most important, there are copious data on suicide in a wide variety of societies, primitive and civilized, all over the world. These data include a wide variety of case reports. They also include extensive discussions of suicide in societies where it is thought to be rare or absent altogether, as well as in societies where it is thought to be frequent—although we cannot be sure that we have accurate statistics on suicide rates among these people. In my book, *Data Quality Control,* I offered a few examples in which ethnographers in effect made some statement about suicide rate. Rarely do they even do that. For most primitive tribes, no one even pretends to estimate the suicide rate. Far from having accurate statistics, we usually do not even have informed guesses.

Now I wish to make the apparently outrageous proposal that we attempt to measure accurately what data we do have. What we do have are the reactions of ethnographers to suicide among the people they study, and these reactions can be measured in several ways. They can be measured by noting the number of suicide cases mentioned or discussed by the ethnographer. They can be measured by noting the number of suicide circumstances (alleged or suggested causes or causal factors) mentioned or discussed by the ethnographer. Or they can be measured most directly and, I believe, most effectively in another way: by simply counting the number of words devoted to the topic of suicide by an ethnographer. Divide that number by the total number of words in his report and we get what I call the suicide source wordage ratio—a measure of an author's relative attention to suicide as a topic.

Clearly this measure will be influenced—and strongly influenced—by a factor entirely irrelevant to the relative "sickness" or "health" of the society studied: the author's own personal attitude toward suicide. Does it fascinate him? Does he love to dwell upon it? Does it repel him? Does he view it with distaste? Is he indifferent to it? Some authors are chiefly interested in formal social structure, some in pot-making, some in dancing, some in folk tales. Some are interested in the life cycle, in happiness and unhappiness, in frustration and satisfaction. Clearly, half a dozen authors could visit a single tribe with a constant suicide rate and write reports with half a dozen widely differing suicide source wordage ratios.

This measure will probably be further influenced by another confounding factor which further distorts its readings—the attitude of the people studied toward suicide. Are they proud of it or ashamed? Do they flaunt it or conceal it? Among primitive tribes uninfluenced by Judeo-Christian moral traditions, there is good reason to doubt the importance of this second confounding factor. In the study whose results I am about to report, of fifty-one societies with data on suicide, only seven had any indication of a moral attitude toward suicide on the part of the people studied. In other words, most ethnographers did not mention either approval or disapproval of suicide by the people they studied. This finding confirms an earlier finding by Jakob Wisse. Wisse (1933) studied a much larger sample—several hundred tribes. He came to the tentative conclusion that most primitive people seemed to view suicide with moral and ethical indifference. They thought it neither good nor evil. Thus, there is reason to suspect that this second confounding factor may be far less important than the first. Still, I do not doubt for a moment that suicide source wordage ratio variance from tribe to tribe is affected to some extent by the attitude toward suicide of the people being studied as well as by the attitude of the ethnographer.

Let us consider for a moment the analogy of the fever thermometer. That thermometer measures precisely the body temperature. But body temperature is only a crude and approximate measure of the seriousness of bodily illness. Some fatal diseases or injuries may produce little or no fever. Some trifling illnesses may for a day or two induce a burning fever, yet pass away harmlessly even if not treated. The fever thermometer is the physician's servant, not his master. The physician uses its data on bodily temperature for what it is worth, depending upon the circumstances of the case.

So I would suggest that the suicide source wordage ratio is a useful measure of social "sickness"—useful as a servant rather than a master. It is useful in some situations and for some purposes. It is more useful surely in cross-cultural surveys, where whole arrays of societies are studied, than in individual tribal studies, where particular circumstances may make it irrelevant.

The working hypothesis tested by the present study is simply that *one* of the factors affecting suicide source wordage ratio is the actual suicide rate among the people studied. The present study uses suicide source wordage as a dependent variable. It uses seven hypothetical causes of suicide as independent variables. A skeptical reader will study the reported relationships among these seven hypothetical causes of suicide on one hand and suicide source wordage on the other. In looking at these relationships, he will have two questions to consider. *First,* is an association or correlation between such things as marriage arrangement practices or divorce rules on one hand and suicide *rate* on the other hand best explained by considering the former as the cause and the latter as the effect? Or is this association best explained in some other way? *Second,* is an association or correlation between such things as marriage arrangement practices or divorce rules on one hand and *suicide source wordage* on the other hand best explained by supposing that suicide source wordage reflects suicide rate? Or is this association best explained in some other way?

These are two distinct questions. The first question is the interesting question of theory, and gets at the validity of suicide rate as a fever thermometer of societal sickness. The second question is the interesting question of method, and gets at the validity of gauging a society's suicide rate by the extent of the ethnographer's reaction to it.

The implications of the answer could be important. If suicide source wordage is indeed a useful measure of suicide rate, at some times in some circumstances, then, much of the attention of comparative ethnological studies may be extended from the tribe alone to its ethnographer also.

Even more important, if suicide rate, and hence suicide source wordage, is a reflection of a general type of social frustration—here to be called "thwarting disorientation"—then we must conclude that from the point of view of the culture bearers, at least, some cultures are better than others. Some cultures, we must then conclude, literally make their people sick; others keep them well.

But please notice a sharp difference between this sort of value judgment about a culture and the sort common in social science writing a hundred years ago.

Classical nineteenth-century views of cultural evolution evaluated a culture studied according to the standards of the observer's culture. For example, an English ethnologist evaluated Zulu culture according to English cultural values. This kind of judgment was the cultural absolutism rejected by twentieth-century social science. The present study offers no comfort to this kind of cultural absolutism. Rather, in its use of suicide as an evaluating yardstick, it tends to make the culture bearers themselves the evaluators of their own culture. It is the Zulus themselves who in effect "vote" to stay with the Zulu way of life or to pull out by killing themselves.

SUICIDE THEORY AND THE THWARTING DISORIENTATION CONCEPT

In the opening chapter of his great sociological classic, Emile Durkheim (1951) began a controversy over a false problem. Durkheim held that psychiatric factors were not relevant to the study of suicide. Psychiatrists are still disputing this question (Jackson, 1957; Schneider, 1954). Yet, as many of Durkheim's followers have since pointed out, psychiatric and sociological explanations of suicide are not contradictory but complementary (see Durkheim, 1951, Introduction; Halbwachs, 1930; Schneidman & Farberow, 1960). Both are needed for a full understanding.

More recent research by sociologists has produced much empirical evidence supporting one of Durkheim's basic propositions—suicide is especially likely to occur among socially disoriented individuals, those who lack or who lose basic social ties. For example, suicide is more frequent among single people than among married people; it is more frequent among childless couples than among those with children; it is more frequent among divorced people than among either married people or among bachelors and spinsters; it is more frequent in times of depression than in times of prosperity and, in the United States at least, is more frequent among upper class people (who risk greater loss of status in times of depression) than among the general population; it is more frequent among downwardly mobile people than among lower class people; it is also apparently more frequent among people whose statuses are less integrated with one another than among those with more integrated statuses (see Breed, 1963; Dublin, 1933, 1963; Gibbs & Martin, 1964; Halbwachs, 1930; Henry & Short, 1954; Kruijt, 1960). A recent survey by a group of anthropologists of suicide among seven tribes of Central Africa reports similar findings: suicide among these tribesmen was classified by Bohannan (1960) into three types: jural, domestic, and status-linked. Jural suicides are committed by offenders against public mores, who thus assuage whatever guilt feelings they may have and who also thus avoid shame and punishment. Domestic suicides are committed by people in serious trouble with close relatives, especially spouses. Status-linked suicides are committed by people who have recently suffered a serious sociological dislocation, involving a major change in status. All three of Bohannan's types of African suicide may be classified as types of social disorientation. The offender against the mores has by his offense seriously jeopardized his normal social relationships with the community in which he lives. The person in serious family trouble necessarily finds his social relationships with the family member(s) concerned likewise in serious jeopardy. Thus, jural and family suicides no less than status-linked suicides involve serious social disorientation.

These findings all support the hypothesis that social disorientation influences the suicide rate—the more socially disoriented he becomes, the more likely is it that a person will kill himself. Yet, granted all this, suicide still remains a psychological problem. The fact remains that suicide is always a rare event. Even among so suicide-prone a population as the depressive cases in mental hospitals, we still find that most people however socially disoriented cling to life and that only a minority take their own lives, or try to. As Simpson (Durkheim, 1951, Introduction) has insisted, sociological explanations are not enough; psychological explanations are needed also.

According to Simpson, "the most widely accepted view today in psycho-analysis is that suicide is most often a form of displacement; that is, the desire to kill someone who has thwarted the individual is turned back upon the individual himself" (p. 24). A more elaborate version of this view is that of Karl Menninger (1938), which has been widely quoted. Menninger sees three basic elements in the emotional makeup of a suicide: the wish to kill (reflecting anger against another person), the wish to be killed (reflecting feelings of guilt), and the wish to die (reflecting the "death instinct," widely posited in psychoanalytic theory).

Many of these psychoanalytic explanations can readily be integrated with the sociological ones just discussed by means of an examination of the emotional implications of sociological contexts. Does a social situation commonly involve the thwarting of one individual by another? Does this thwarting mean such severe frustration of the thwarted person that in anger he would strongly wish to kill the thwarter? If so, then according to the generally held psychoanalytic view, that anger alone might produce feelings of guilt about the wish to kill strong enough to engender a wish to be killed. Finally, without positing any "death instinct," does this thwarting involve a social catastrophe of an apparently lasting or long-term sort, such a catastrophe as might lead a person to wish to die because life no longer seemed to offer its usual satisfactions?

I propose to consider some such sociological contexts. Let us call them contexts of *thwarting disorientation*. These contexts involve two major components: (1) they are situations in which a person's social ties are broken, weakened, or threatened; and (2) they are also situations involving the thwarting of the disoriented person by some person. By thwarting I mean behavior by the thwarter in strong conflict with the wishes of the thwarted. Thwarting takes place if a person withholds desired and expected satisfactions from someone; thwarting also takes place if a person inflicts injuries upon someone. Such thwarting disorientation situations are those in which sociological and psychoanalytic theory alike predict an increase in the probability of suicide.

Such a theory of suicide would predict stronger impact upon suicide rates of social disorientation when the disorientation was personified by a thwarting individual than when it merely reflected the general impersonal situation. However, since suicide is a rare event anyway, the personification to be hypothesized need not be an invariable component of the sociological situation but only a common one. Furthermore, where the social disorientation is in considerable part a result of the discretionary act of the thwarted individual, he might well consider *himself* the thwarter as well as the one thwarted. For example, if a wealthy American loses his fortune in a stock market crash, would he not be likely to think, "If only I had not bought on margin," "If only I had sold out sooner," or the like. Similarly, if a person violates community mores, and sees himself faced with the consequent shame and punishment, would he not be likely to think, "If only I had not killed her," or "If only I had not stolen it."

A *thwarting disorientation* situation, then, is one in which social disorientation is produced by a discretionary act of some person, either the thwarted person himself or another, and contrasts with disorientation produced by the action of impersonal natural, social, or cultural events. Thus, a widow of a cancer victim and an unwilling divorcée are socially disoriented; but only the divorcée is a victim of thwarting disorientation.

A *thwarting disorientation* theory of suicide is not inconsistent with most sociological findings on suicide, in that most types of social disorientation studied can often plausibly be supposed to involve some sort of discretionary act or omission on the part of some person. In other words, a *thwarting disorientation* theory makes sense wherever the social situation offers some person whom the suicide can plausibly blame for his troubles, whether the suicide himself or someone else. But the *thwarting disorientation* theory makes no sense where the suicide cannot see any person at all to blame for his situation.

For example, the thwarting disorientation theory does not at all help to explain the finding by Durkheim (1951) that in most European countries Roman Catholics reportedly have lower suicide rates than Protestants (see also Halbwachs, 1930). Durkheim explains this difference in reported suicide rates as a reflection of the greater degree of social integration in a Roman Catholic religious congregation than in a Protestant one. This difference in integration is not established by Durkheim through any kind of statistical study but is merely asserted by him as a hypothesis. Waldstein (1934) presented evidence tending to explain this difference as a mere artifact of statistical reporting. Waldstein shows that in Switzerland accidental deaths are disproportionately more frequent in predominantly Catholic cantons, while suicides are disproportionately less. As Schneider (1954) says, "One may ask whether suicides in Catholic districts are not simply disguised as accidents, a fact which would completely discredit all the conclusions which have been drawn about these differences" (pp. 90ff). Schneider's own clinical data on suicide attempters treated in Vaud, Lausanne, and Basel showed no significant difference according to religion between the proportion of Catholics and Protestants treated and their proportions in the populations at large of the respective cantons.

The thwarting disorientation hypothesis, however, is not at all inconsistent with the large body of research on suicide linking suicide with mental illness, particularly acute depression. Several studies have shown a high association between suicide and mental illness. In a study of all suicides reported in St. Louis during a one-year period—134 suicides—evidence of mental illness was found in all but eight; nearly half were diagnosed as manic depressives in the depressed phase at time of suicide (Robins, Murphy, Wilkinson, Gassner, & Kayes, 1959). Yessler, Gibbs and Becker (1961) studied 272 suicides in the armed forces, diagnosing 22 percent as psychotic, 43 percent as neurotic and the remaining 35 percent as "character and behavior disorders." Their finding of only 22 percent psychotic is in conflict with the work of the Robins group; according to Yessler et al., many St. Louis suicides diagnosed as psychotic depressive by the Robins group should have been diagnosed as neurotic depressives. Not wishing to involve myself in this taxonomic dispute, I am content to point out that both these careful studies provide considerable evidence that suicide is often associated with mental illness. Schneider's (1954) studies of Swiss suicide attempts led him to a similar conclusion—that most suicides were mentally ill persons.

How can this finding be reconciled with the thwarting disorientation hypothesis? Thwarting disorientation situations may conceivably lead to mental illness, particularly psychotic, manic, or neurotic depression, and likewise may also lead to suicide. Or, alternately, depressed states may arise from other causes, not related to thwarting disorientation; but depressed patients may be particularly sensitive to thwarting disorientation and hence particularly likely to commit suicide when they experience it.

METHOD OF STUDY

Tables 1 and 2 present data from a cross-cultural survey of some fifty-eight societies, mostly primitive tribes. These tables show high correlations between each thwarting disorientation trait and suicide source wordage. They show low correlations or no correlations at all among the seven thwarting disorientation traits. It is this combination of correlation patterns which I argue is most parsimoniously explained by the supposition that thwarting disorientation situations tend to cause suicide— that an increase in the former will tend to be followed by an increase in the latter, but not vice versa. Of course, the correlational pattern does not of itself demonstrate any such thing. But it can be most easily explained in that way.

The manner of collecting and coding these data cannot be described here because of the limitations of space. The cross-cultural survey method of anthropology involves many challenging technical difficulties. These difficulties have been ably reviewed by Köbben (1952). The present study used five new techniques, trying to overcome these technical difficulties of method. These techniques were (1) probability, rather than judgmental, selection of tribes to be studied (see Naroll, 1961); (2) rigorous use of a new concept of the primitive tribe, the so-called *cultunit* (see Naroll, 1964a); (3) the control factor method of data quality control, by which evidence of systematic bias in the data collection process (informants, ethnographers, comparativists) is searched for (see Naroll, 1962); (4) the linked pair method of interdependence control, checking to see whether the correlations between suicide wordage and thwarting disorientation traits could be explained merely by joint diffusion through borrowing or migration (see Naroll, 1964a); and (5) content analysis scales or indexes measuring ethnographers' statements rather than attempting to directly measure behavior of tribe concerned. This last procedure involves rigorous and detailed definitions of the basic concepts, detailed answers to questions like "Exactly what do you mean by the term *suicide?*"

TABLE 1. Thwarting Disorientation Data

Society	Sample[a]	Suicide wordage[b]	Wife beat-ing[c]	Marriage restric-tions	Men's divorce freedom	Witchcraft accusations	Drunken brawling	Defiant homi-cide	Warfare frequency
19 Hottentot	DA	59	0	A	A	P	0	0	0
41 Thonga	WES	34	0	A	A	P	P	0	0
38 Ila	DA	55	0	P	0	P	0	P	P
58 Chagga	WES	54	0	A	0	P	0	P	0
16 Mongo	DA	49	0	A	0	0	P	A	0
62 Mende	WES	44	0	P	A	P	0	0	0
09 Tallensi	WES	48	0	P	A	P	A	P	0
55 Tiv	WES	51	0	A	A	P	0	P	0
42 Azande	1957	38	0	A	A	P	P	0	0
54 Luo	WES	70	P	P	A	P	P	P	0
66 Amhara	WES		A	P	A	0	0	A	0
27 Fur	DA	29	0	A	A	0	P	0	0
05 Kababish	DA	52	0	P	0	0	A	0	P
04 Egypt	WES	41	0	P	A	P	A	P	0
59 Italy (Calabria)	WES		P	A	A	P	0	0	0
03 Irish	DA		P	A	0	P	0	0	0
08 Dutch	DA	49	0	A	A	0	0	0	0
30 Austrians	DA	45	0	A	A	0	0	0	0
02 Turks	DA		P	A	A	0	P	0	0
33 Iraqi	DA		0	A	0	0	0	0	0
14 Kafir	DA	41	0	P	0	0	A	A	P
65 Kazaks	WES	53	P	A	A	0	0	0	0
29 Chukchi	DA	64	P	P	P	P	P	0	P
24 Gilyak	DA	57	P	P	0	0	A	P	A
15 Korea	DA	64	P	P	A	0	P	A	0
36 Gond	DA	72	P	0	P	P	P	P	0
23 Andamans	DA	45	0	A	0	P	0	P	A
48 Burmese	WES	48	A	A	A	P	P	A	0
45 Semang	DA	37	0	A	A	A	0	A	0

[a] DA—Diffusion Arc sample (all probability sample).

1957—World Ethnograph Sample subsample, culture areas represented by societies in 1957 study

WES—World Ethnographic Sample (probability sampling choices)

[b] Entry is value of Z where X = number of words on suicide in ethnographic sources consulted on a given society; Y = square root of [natural logarithm of $(X + 1.001)$], producing a quasi-normal transformation; S = standard deviation of all the Ys; $\overline{X}$ = Arithmetic average (mean) of all the Ys; $Z = 50 - 10[(X - \overline{X})/S]$. Where suicide is not discussed at all, no score is given and society is ignored in computing suicide correlations.

[c] P = trait present; A = trait absent; 0 = no data on trait.

TABLE 1 (*continued*)

Society	Sample^a	Suicide wordage^b	Wife beating^c	Marriage restrictions	Men's divorce freedom	Witchcraft accusations	Drunken brawling	Defiant homicide	Warfare frequency
52 Apayao	1957	51	0	A	A	P	P	A	0
12 Land Dyak	DA	48	0	A	A	P	A	A	P
34 Toradja	DA	49	0	A	A	P	P	P	P
06 Kapauku	DA		P	A	A	P	0	P	P
28 Crokaiva	DA	56	0	P	0	P	0	P	P
51 Ifaluk	1957	34	0	A	0	A	A	0	0
17 Malaita	DA	42	0	A	0	P	0	0	0
56 Malekula	WES	48	0	P	0	P	0	0	P
39 Tikopia	DA	62	0	A	A	0	0	P	0
20 Tonga	DA	56	P	A	P	P	0	P	P
31 Mangareva	DA	55	0	P	0	P	0	0	0
53 Copper Eskimo	1957	45	0	A	A	P	0	P	0
07 Eyak	DA	52	0	P	A	P	0	0	A
40 Klallam	DA	50	0	P	0	P	0	A	P
46 Wintun	WES	62	0	A	P	P	0	P	0
18 Southern Paiute	DA	34	0	A	A	P	0	0	A
50 Cheyenne	WES	65	0	A	A	P	0	P	P
49 Ojibwa	1957	55	P	0	P	P	P	0	P
50 Iroquois	1957	74	0	P	P	P	P	0	P
11 Coyotero	WES	57	0	A	P	P	P	P	P
37 Papago	DA	45	A	0	A	P	P	0	0
15 Nahua	DA	42	P	A	A	0	P	0	0
26 Mosquito	DA	42	0	P	A	P	0	0	0
35 Callinago	WES	42	0	P	0	P	A	0	0
32 Yagua	DA	38	A	A	A	P	0	A	A
43 Araucanians	DA	60	P	P	A	P	0	0	P
21 Ona	DA	44	0	A	0	P	0	0	P
10 Mataco	DA	38	0	A	0	P	P	A	0
57 Aweikoma	WES		0	A	0	A	P	P	P

I plan to discuss these problems in the forthcoming *A Handbook of Method in Cultural Anthropology*. And more to the point being discussed, I plan to describe in full detail the method of study that produced the data of Tables 1 and 2 in a forthcoming monograph.

In coding these traits, content analysis classifications of ethnographers' statements were used to reduce subjective interpretation by comparativists to a minimum. At times this practice made me skip societies that intuitively seemed clearly classifiable but which could not be coded by the rules. For example, I could not code warfare frequency among the Aztecs, a notoriously warlike society, simply because none of the sources examined said that the Aztecs fought wars frequently; and I had similar difficulties with peoples like the Austrians, the Turks, and the Dutch, whose history of war and peace was readily available.

Suicide   The basic suicide concept used is that of *protest suicide,* discussed more fully in my book on data quality control (Naroll, 1962). Protest suicide is defined as voluntary suicide committed in such a way as to come to public notice. This definition excludes suicides to avoid capital punishment, suicides whose victim is designated by custom (for example, *suttee*) or by another person, suicides disguised as some other kind of death (for example, by the suicide himself or his relatives), and suicides not consciously intended but only unconsciously precipitated through an avoidable fatal accident.

Wife beating   Only societies in which ethnographers explicitly report the occurrence of wife-beating husbands (whether or not it was considered proper) are coded as practicing wife beating; only societies in which ethnographers explicitly deny the occurrence of wife beating are coded as not practicing wife beating; other discussions of wife beating that suggest its presence or absence without explicitly asserting or denying it are ignored.

Marriage restrictions   This trait is coded as present if young people are not free to select their own spouses, but instead are presented with marriage partners chosen by other people (usually their parents) or preferred by custom. Even where the consent of the young person is required to the marriage proposed by others or by custom, the trait is still coded as "Restriction Present." The trait is only coded as "Restriction Absent" where the young people (being of marriageable age as locally defined) are entirely free to make their own marriage choice from among the general category of eligible candidates.

Men's divorce freedom   This trait is coded present if a society permits a man to divorce his wife at will, without requiring grounds for divorce or approval of others.

Witchcraft accusation   In this study, witchcraft accusation disorientation is coded as present in any society in which people are reported to have been executed as witches or in any society that is explicitly reported to offer a diagnosis of death due to witchcraft more frequently than a diagnosis of death due to the actions of spirits; it is also coded present where nothing is said in the ethnographic reports either about executions for witchcraft or diagnoses of death due to spirits but where diagnoses of death due to witchcraft are reported. Witchcraft attribution disorientation is coded absent where execution for witchcraft is denied or not reported and where, furthermore, diagnosis of death due to spirits is reportedly made more often than that of death due to witches, or where the first diagnosis is reported as present but nothing is said about the second diagnosis.

Drunken brawling The trait is coded present only in societies where it is explicitly reported; it is coded absent only in societies where alcoholic beverages are drunk but brawling is explicitly denied or characterized as rare or uncommon. Societies in which alcohol is not drunk or in which nothing is said about brawling are ignored.

Defiant homicide This concept, also discussed more fully in my book on data quality control (Naroll, 1962), is defined as deliberate homicide committed in such a way as to come to public notice despite disapproval not only by a majority of the kin of the slayer but also by a majority of the members of the society involved. This definition excludes homicides resulting from negligence, accident, blood revenge (where locally approved), and such publicly sanctioned activities as warfare, human sacrifice, and judicial executions.

The coding of Table 1 is a dichotomized count of the number of cases of defiant homicide mentioned by ethnographers. The trait was coded present if two or more such cases were mentioned; the trait was coded absent if fewer than two such cases were mentioned in the discussions of defiant homicide; if nothing at all was said about defiant homicide, the society was ignored.

Frequent warfare Frequent warfare is coded "Present" where ethnographers use words that explicitly report that war is frequent rather than rare, common rather than unusual (for example, "perpetual," "frequent," "not infrequent," "chronic," "periodic," "numerous," "three hundred years of fighting," "continually," "regularly," "annually," "at war for generations"). Frequent warfare is coded "Absent" where ethnographers explicitly report wars so (for example, "not often," "only three wars," "brief and far from bloody," "occasional," "rare").

INFLUENCE ANALYSIS

Each of the seven thwarting disorientation traits shown in Table 2 is positively correlated with suicide source wordage. Let us consider whether the other correlations shown in the table—those among the thwarting disorientation traits themselves—tell us anything at all about the plausibility of our hypotheses (1) that thwarting disorientation situations tend to cause suicide and (2) that suicide source wordage is correlated with thwarting disorientation situation reports because suicide source wordage reflects—among other things—the actual suicide rate (and because thwarting disorientation situation reports likewise reflect actual thwarting disorientation situations).

Let us agree to call the seven correlation coefficients between each of the seven thwarting disorientation traits (the hypothetical causal influences)

TABLE 2. THWARTING DISORIENTATION CORRELATION MATRIX

Entries in upper right portion of table, in roman type, are coefficients of correlation. Those between suicide wordage and other traits are point biserials; other correlation coefficients are *phi* coefficients. Entries in lower left portion of table, in italic type, are two-tailed probabilities. Those between suicide wordage and other traits are *t* test values; others are *chi*-square test values (with Yates's correction).

	Suicide wordage	Wife beating	Marriage restrictions	Men's divorce freedom	Witchcraft accusations	Drunken brawling	Defiant homicide cases	Warfare frequency
Suicide wordage		.69	.34	.60	.34	.30	.45	.41
Wife beating (B224)	.01		.05	.05	0.0	−.08	.36	.25
Marriage restrictions (B201)	.01	.75		0.0	.06	−.39	.04	0.0
Men's divorce freedom (A210)	.02	.75	1.0		.06	.02	.17	.18
Witchcraft accusations (A222)	.02	1.0	.70	.75		−.01	−.03	−.05
Drunken brawling (B223)	.10	.75	.06	.90	.90		.05	.13
Defiant homicide cases (A221)	.01	.25	.75	.45	.90	.90		−.14
Warfare frequency (C615)	.05	.50	1.0	.50	.75	.70	.60	

and Suicide Source Wordage (the hypothetical effect) *encorrelations*. Let us agree to call the remaining twenty-one correlation coefficients of Table 2 (those among the Thwarting Disorientation traits themselves) *intercorrelations*.

My case rests upon two pillars. First, the seven thwarting disorientation traits all reflect situations in which a person's social ties are broken or threatened by the act of some human being. Second, the encorrelations are much greater than the intercorrelations. These two facts, taken together, lead to only one simple explanation. All twenty-eight correlation coefficients (the seven high encorrelations and the twenty-one low intercorrelations) make sense if thwarting disorientation causes suicide. They make sense if suicide source wordage reflects, at least in part, the actual suicide rate.

Of course, these two facts taken together do not demonstrate the validity of our two main hypotheses. These two facts can be explained in other ways. But they cannot be explained in other equally simple ways; the other acceptable ways get complicated and intricate. Therefore, the researcher tends to prefer the simpler explanation. This preference is one of the three fundamental axioms of scientific thinking (the other two are the canon of skepticism and the canon of empirical observation). This preference goes under the name of the canon of parsimony—Occam's razor.

As I have said, my case, even at its best, falls short of a true demonstration. It does not shut the door on rival explanations. But it takes us somewhat farther than simple association. On the one hand, it does not leave us with any feeling that we *know* thwarting disorientation practices cause suicide. On the other hand, it does leave us with a preference for that explanation over any other. It creates a leaning in our minds toward that theory. It establishes a mild presumption in its favor. That presumption could easily be overcome by other evidence, of course. It could even be overcome by mere argument; or it could be overcome merely by suggesting some other equally simple explanation. But until some such evidence or some such argument is put forward, the presumption is there. Let us then look more closely at my facts and my argument.

Seven Thwarting Disorientation Traits

I now review each of the seven thwarting disorientation traits in turn. In each there is an element of threat or rupture to a social tie. In each there is some human being to be blamed. (It goes without saying that many other traits than these seven might likewise have both these elements and thus likewise be thwarting disorientation traits.) It is also well to note that four of the seven traits involve personal violence (as does suicide itself). Two of the remaining three involve direct sexual frustration.

Wife beating clearly affords a social situation in which wife and young children may often be frustrated and angered and given a plausible person to blame for these feelings. Presumably in such a situation the wife and children often would feel a severe strain in the social ties binding them to the wife-beating husband and father and thus feel disoriented from the nuclear family.

Marriage restriction situations presumably often involve young people in undesired marriage or bar them from preferred marriages. Case data from societies like Korea and the Jivaro suggest that wives trapped in unhappy marriages often resort to suicide. According to unpublished field work verbally reported by Robert Edgerton, young girls among the Suk of East Central Africa often hang themselves when their parents arrange marriages with unwanted bridegrooms. In either the betrothal or the unhappy marriage situation, the social tie between the dissatisfied one and his nuclear family is severely strained, and his parents are plausible candidates for blame.

Since *divorce freedom* is defined as freedom for men to divorce their wives, in this context presumably divorces often take place against the wishes of the wife and minor children involved. These then would suffer severe social disorientation against their will and would have in the husband and father a plausible person to blame.

Societies where *witchcraft accusations* are present offer two kinds of thwarting disorientation situations not present in societies where witchcraft accusations are unknown. First, from the point of view of a person accused of committing witchcraft: Such a person is commonly subject to capital punishment, and certainly would usually be feared and shunned by those of his associates who credit the accusation. The spouse and children of a person executed for witchcraft would suffer social disorientation from the death. Second, from the point of view of the family of a person who in fact died of disease: In societies where witchcraft attribution is a common explanation of illness, people would often explain the natural death of a loved family member as the effect of witchcraft by some suspected witch. *They* would then perceive their situation as a thwarting disorientation context, even though a person believing, for example, in the germ theory of infectious disease would not.

The *drunken brawling* situation is that of violent brawling among people immediately after taking alcoholic drinks. Brawling among any members of the local community or acquaintance circle involves weakening and threatening the social ties among the participants; and persons feeling thus injured often can readily identify particular brawlers to blame.

In the *defiant homicide* situation, the close relatives of both the slayer and his victim suffer social disorientation and have in the slayer an obvious person to blame.

In *warfare,* finally, war casualties involve their relatives in social disorientation; the casualties are victims of particular enemy warriors, even though the warrior to blame would rarely be known to the relatives of the victim.

Encorrelations and Intercorrelations

The mean of the seven encorrelations of Table 2 is .447. That of the twenty-one intercorrelations is only .036. But some of this difference may be attributable to the fact that the seven encorrelations are the more sensitive point biserials while the twenty-one intercorrelations are the less sensitive φ coefficients. If we recompute the seven encorrelations by dichotomizing suicide source wordage and classifying each society as either "High Wordage" or "Low Wordage," the mean of the seven φ coefficients comes to .2552. The nonparametric U test between the seven φ encorrelations and the twenty-one φ intercorrelations shows that this difference is significant at the .001 level.

Another way of looking at the same situation is to take first-order partial correlations. As Table 3 shows, most first-order partial correlations between suicide source wordage, each one of the thwarting disorientation traits, and all the other thwarting disorientation traits in turn, far from vanishing, remain high or even increase. Such a result is no more than what we would expect mathematically from a matrix with high encorrelations and low or even zero or negative intercorrelations.

Finally, Table 4 shows the results of a factor analysis of the matrix of Table 2. (The factor loadings shown came from an orthogonal rotation to a varimax criterion. Analysis was done with a computer, using the MESA 2 program, written at the University of Chicago by Ben Wright.) While the usual purpose of a factor analysis is to explain a correlation matrix by reducing a large number of variables to a much smaller number of factors, its purpose here is the contrary—to show that the correlation matrix *cannot* plausibly be explained by less than seven factors, and thus to show that the seven thwarting disorientation traits are independently related to suicide source wordage. The results of this analysis are supportive, but not conclusive. They show the expected pattern of factor loadings. Seven factors appear, each identifiable as one of the thwarting disorientation traits. Suicide source wordage has a moderate loading on all seven. The question remains whether with such small

TABLE 3. PARTIAL CORRELATIONS WITH SUICIDE WORDAGE

Each column shows the first-order partial correlations between suicide wordage and the captioned trait controlled for the trait shown in the stub. Thus column one, line two, shows a coefficient of .71, being $r_{ab.c}$ where trait a is suicide wordage, trait b is wife beating, and trait c is marriage restrictions while column two, line one shows a coefficient of .43, being $r_{ac.b}$. These partial coefficients assume linearity of relationship of the underlying variables.

	Correlates						
Controls	Wife beating (B224)	Marriage restrictions (B201)	Men's divorce freedom (A210)	Witchcraft accusations (A222)	Drunken brawling (B223)	Defiant homicide cases (A221)	Warfare frequency (C615)
Wife beating (B224)		.43	.86	.47	.49	.28	.33
Marriage restrictions (B201)	.71		.63	.34	.18	.50	.44
Men's divorce freedom (A210)	.89	.42		.38	.39	.69	.64
Witchcraft accusations (A222)	.73	.34	.61		.32	.49	.46
Drunken brawling (B223)	.75	.26	.63	.36		.49	.39
Defiant homicide cases (A221)	.63	.41	.76	.40	.36		.53
Warfare frequency (C615)	.66	.37	.75	.40	.28	.56	
Suicide source wordage (423)	.64	.35	.66	.36	.26	.43	.41

samples any factor analysis is meaningful. The average number of societies involved in the seven encorrelations is only thirty. The problem of validating factors is still a vexing one. For small samples, Fruchter (1954) suggests Humphrey's rule. A product moment correlation of sample size thirty has a standard error of 0.186 (for $r = 0$). Humphrey's rule would require the product of the two highest loadings on each factor to exceed twice that amount, or 0.372. Only the first two of the seven factors do so. With the loadings shown in Table 4, a sample size of at least ninety would be required to achieve significance by Humphrey's rule. On the other hand, Guilford and Lacey (1947) and Dudek (1948) would accept as a factor any one the product of whose two highest loadings exceed the standard error of zero r at all. All seven factors of Table 4 do so (see also Vernon, 1949). What it amounts to is that the five questionable fac-

TABLE 4. ROTATED FACTOR LOADINGS

The highest factor loading in each column is shown in boldface type, thus **0.977**. These loadings, all greater than 0.971, are taken to identify the factor with the variable so loaded. Thus factor 1 is identified as Divorce freedom, factor 2 as Wife beating, factor 3 as Drunken brawling, factor 4 as Marriage restrictions, factor 5 as Witchcraft attribution, factor 6 as Defiant homicide, and factor 7 as Warfare frequency. The second highest factor loading in each column is shown in italic type, thus *−0.659*. These invariably turn out to be Suicide wordage, and range between 0.216 and 0.659. This loading pattern is interpreted as evidence that all seven thwarting disorientation traits are associated with suicide wordage but *not* with one another. (Some relationship between homicide and wife beating is suggested, but not nearly enough to reduce the two variables to a single factor.)

Variables	Communality	1	2	3	4	5	6	7	8
Suicide wordage	1.086	*−0.659*	*0.583*	*0.240*	*0.289*	*0.263*	*0.232*	*0.216*	0.0
Wife beating	1.012	−0.038	**0.977**	−0.051	0.010	−0.010	0.190	0.136	0.0
Marriage restriction	1.025	−0.003	0.042	−0.171	**0.996**	0.039	0.032	0.014	0.0
Men's divorce freedom	0.979	**−0.981**	−0.009	−0.105	0.049	0.010	0.038	0.043	0.0
Witchcraft attribution	1.013	−0.055	0.022	0.011	0.038	**1.004**	−0.019	−0.026	0.0
Drunken brawling	1.099	0.058	−0.016	**1.026**	−0.177	0.013	0.048	0.090	0.0
Defiant homicide	1.008	−0.084	0.210	0.048	0.034	−0.020	**0.972**	−0.091	0.0
Warfare frequency	1.004	−0.084	0.152	0.087	0.016	−0.027	−0.087	**0.978**	0.0

tors exceed chance expectation in the product of their two highest loadings, but not by enough of a margin to be impressive.

RIVAL HYPOTHESES

Take all three of these statistical measures together. They accord more easily with the hypothesis that thwarting disorientation situations tend to cause suicide than with any other equally simple rival hypothesis I am acquainted with.

Ethnographer's Orientation as Underlying Cause

No doubt some authors are more interested in suicide and hence write more about it; other authors are less interested and write less. Perhaps authors interested in suicide are also interested in warfare, in homicide, in brawling, and in wife beating, since these are all likewise manifestations of violent aggression. But if the correlation between suicide wordage and warfare reports is merely a reflection of an interest in violent affairs by ethnographers, and if the correlation between homicide reports and suicide reports again merely reflects a like interest, why is the correlation between warfare and homicide so low? Would we not in that case expect a similar correlation? I am calling attention here to the encorrelation-intercorrelation difference. Furthermore, how in that case are we to explain the very high ($r = .60$) correlation between divorce freedom and suicide wordage? Divorce freedom *reports* seem unlikely to be sensitive to the same sort of bias that would lead ethnographers to pay attention to or withhold attention from suicide. A similar argument holds for marriage restrictions.

Societal Orientation as Underlying Cause

Here we ignore whatever distortions in our data are produced by ethnographers' biases and consider our reports as reflections of the actual behavior they purport to measure. But our argument repeats itself. Just as we would not expect a generalized interest by ethnographers in aggression to produce high encorrelations but low intercorrelations, neither would we expect a generalized orientation toward aggressive activities on the part of the societies studied to produce high encorrelations but low intercorrelations. Both these rival hypotheses are single-factor hypotheses; they would predict that the societal orientation factor would account for all the correlations. But our factor analysis (Table 4) shows with confidence at least two factors, the divorce factor and the wife-beating factor. If we lump together even four traits as reflecting violent aggression, and conclude that societies oriented toward violent aggression are likely to be given also to warfare, homicide, wife beating, and suicide, we still have not explained the encorrelations of marriage restrictions, divorce freedom, witchcraft attribution, or drunken brawling. At the very least, then, our factor analysis permits the collapsing of our seven-factor model into a five-factor model.

We could, however, explain the factor analysis and the encorrelation-intercorrelation differences in terms of violence orientation if we adduce some additional complications. We could suppose that in certain as yet unidentified circumstances, violently oriented societies restrict marriage arrangements, that in certain other unrelated circumstances they permit divorce freedom, that in certain still other unrelated circumstances they develop witchcraft attribution, in still other ones drunken brawling, and in still other ones wife beating–homicide–warfare. There are surely an infinite number of conceivable circumstances that *might* produce such a situation. For this reason, my line of argument is uncompelling and leaves the door open to proper doubt. On the other hand, such a five factor explanation, involving five hypothetical unknown and unidentified vague "circumstances" is certainly less parsimonious and less elegant than the thwarting disorientation hypothesis.

Are These Correlations Mere Combing Artifacts?

A scientist can collect data on a large number of traits and run these data through a computer, generating hundreds of coefficients of correlation. Even if in fact the traits are entirely unrelated, he could expect through mere chance to pick up five correlations per hundred "significant" at the 5 percent level, one per hundred "significant" at the 1 percent level, and so on. The correlations of Table 2 were in fact selected from a much larger matrix. We can call this practice *combing* a large correlation matrix for a small number of nominally significant correlation coefficients. Of course, the nominal significance levels of such combinings mean very little by themselves.

However, three of these seven thwarting disorientation correlations were implied in earlier research by other students of suicide. A correlation between divorce *frequency* and suicide is noticed by the Durkheim (1951), Dublin (1963), and Dublin & Burzel (1933) studies. A linkage between marriage restrictions and suicide was found by me in a previous study of another sample. Bohannan (1960) found linkages between homicide and suicide in Africa, as did Wolfgang (1958) in the United States, and Vigil (1956) in Great Britain.

However, the question is still troublesome; the combing hypothesis is still plausible; after all, the remaining four encorrelations were not predicted in advance. There is, however, a way we can test its plausibility statistically. This test requires the working hypothesis that thwarting disorientation influences are cumulative. In other words, the test is a test to see if suicide wordage is especially great where several thwarting disorientation traits occur together.

If the combing hypothesis is valid (or if it is not, but nevertheless the thwarting disorientation influences are not cumulative), then in either case the suicide source wordage score (standard score computed by transform states in Table 1) of a given tribe should be predictable from the "Present" or "Absent" codings of its seven thwarting disorientation traits, as follows: If a given trait is coded "Present," then note the mean wordage score among all tribes where that trait is coded "Present"; if a given trait is coded "Absent," then note the mean wordage score among all traits where that trait is coded "Absent." Predicted wordage score is then given by the mean of these seven means. (If a trait is coded "No Data," omit it from the computation.) If the combing hypothesis is valid, no pattern should occur in the differences between the wordage scores thus predicted and the observed scores; these differences should vary randomly, regardless of the pattern of "Presence" and "Absence" among all seven

TABLE 5. Influence Cumulation Computation

Mean Suicide Wordage Scores

Trait	Trait Present	Trait Absent
Wife beating	59.3000	43.6667
Marriage restrictions	53.7368	46.8276
Men's divorce freedom	62.8571	48.1786
Witchcraft attribution	50.9737	35.5000
Drunken brawling	51.7059	45.3750
Defiant homicide	55.5882	46.4000
Warfare frequency	54.6250	45.2000

A Society	B Number of TD traits present	C Number of TD traits absent	D Observed suicide wordage	E Expected suicide wordage	F[a] Difference in predicted direction

Thwarting Disorientation (TD) High: Ratio of Present/Absent at least 4 to 1

					D–E
Chukchi	6	0	63.5637	55.5330	8.0307
Gond	5	0	71.6483	56.0850	15.5633
Ojibwa	5	0	54.5137	55.8923	−1.3786
Iroquois	5	0	73.9599	54.7797	19.1802
Ila	4	0	54.6171	53.7309	.8862
Orokaiva	4	0	55.7121	53.7309	1.9812
Malekula	3	0	47.6156	53.1118	−5.4962
Mangareva	2	0	55.4606	52.3553	3.1053
Luo	5	1	69.9038	53.2472	16.6566
Tonga	5	1	55.5459	55.0286	.5173
Coyotero	5	1	56.8679	53.7629	3.1050
Araucanians	4	1	59.5354	53.3628	6.1726

Thwarting Disorientation Low: Ratio of Absent/Present at least 4 to 1

					E–D
Yagua	1	5	38.0180	47.0411	9.0231
Austrians	0	2	45.1425	47.5031	2.3606
Dutch	0	2	49.3098	47.5031	−1.8067
Ifaluk	0	3	34.1987	42.5675	8.3688
Semang	0	4	37.1362	43.9766	6.8404
Total Column F					93.1098

[a] Null hypothesis predicts zero total for Column F. Standard deviation of Column F: 6.8175. Mean of Column F = 5.477. Standard error of the mean = 1.65348; $t = 3.3124$; $df = 16$; $p < .005$.

traits. If, however, the combing hypothesis is invalid, and the correlations between the thwarting disorientation traits actually reflect a true cumulative correlation in the universe, then the underlying causal factor (whatever it is, whether thwarting disorientation or some other unidentified set of lurking variables) should be unusually strong when most of the seven thwarting disorientation traits are present, but should be unusually weak when most are absent. Consequently, the observed suicide wordage should differ consistently in the appropriate direction from the wordage predicted by the combing hypothesis. As Table 5 shows, these differences clearly occur. Hence, there appears to be some underlying causal element common to all seven thwarting disorientation traits that exerts a cumulative influence.

SUMMARY

Some cultures (ways of life) seem more stressful to their culture bearers than others. Suicide is suggested as a possible useful measure of this culture stress. For cross-cultural studies of primitive tribes today, the relative attention paid to suicide by ethnographers is considered the best measure of suicide rate available, despite the obvious distortions that such a measure inflicts. The measure is used in a test of the thwarting disorientation hypothesis—the hypothesis that suicide rates tend to be higher in cultures where rules or practices involve rupture or strain on social ties in conditions where the victim believes that a particular person (himself or another) is to blame.

REFERENCES

Benedict, R. *Patterns of culture*. New York: Mentor Books, 1946.

Bohannan, P. J. *African homicide and suicide*. Princeton: Princeton University Press, 1960. Pp. 253–263.

Breed, W. Occupational mobility and suicide. *American Sociological Review*, 1963, **28**, 179–188.

Dublin, L. I. *Suicide: A sociological and statistical study*. New York: Ronald Press, 1963.

Dublin, L. I., & Bunzel, B. *To be or not to be*. New York: Smith and Haas, 1933. Pp. 125–134.

Dudek, F. J. The dependence of factorial composition of aptitude tests upon population differences among pilot trainees. I. The isolation of factors. *Educational and Psychological Measurement*, 1948, **8**, 613–633.

Durkheim, E. *Suicide*. Transl. by J. A. Spaulding & G. Simpson. Glencoe, Ill.: The Free Press, 1951. Pp. 57–81, 152–156, 259–276.

Fruchter, B. *Introduction to factor analysis*. Princeton: Van Nostrand, 1954. P. 79.

Gibbs, J. P., & Martin, W. T. *Status integration and suicide: A sociological study*. Eugene, Ore.: University of Oregon Press, 1964.

Guilford, J. P., & Lacey, J. I. *Printed classification tests*. Army Air Forces Aviation Psychology Program, Research Report No. 5. Washington: Government Printing Office, 1947.

Halbwachs, M. *Les causes du suicide*. Paris: Alcan, 1930. Pp. 197–286, 403–450.

Henry, A. F., & Short, J. F., Jr. *Suicide and homicide*. Glencoe, Ill.: The Free Press, 1954. Pp. 23–44.

Jackson, D. D. Theories of suicide. In E. S. Schneidman & N. L. Farberow (Eds.), *Clues to suicide*. New York: McGraw-Hill, 1957. Pp. 11–21.

Köbben, A. J. New ways of presenting an old idea: The statistical method in social anthropology. *Journal of the Royal Anthropological Institute*, 1952, **82,** 129–146.

Kruijt, C. S. *Zelfmoord*. Utrecht: Van Gorcum, 1960. Pp. 416–437.

Li, An-che. Zuni: Some observations and queries. *American Anthropologist*, 1937, **39,** 62–76.

Menninger, K. *Man against himself*. New York: Harcourt Brace, 1938. Pp. 24–71.

Naroll, R. Two stratified random samples for a cross-cultural survey. Unpublished manuscript, 1961.

Naroll, R. *Data quality control*. New York: Free Press, 1962. Pp. 48, 56*f*, 61–65, 142.

Narroll, R. A fifth solution to Galton's problem. *American Anthropologist*, 1964, **66,** 863–87. (a)

Naroll, R. On ethnic unit classification. *Current Anthropology*, 1964, **5,** 283–312. (b)

Naroll, R., & Cohen, R. (Eds.) *A handbook of method in cultural anthropology*. New York: Natural History, in press.

Parsons, T. *The structure of social action*. New York, 1937. P. 326.

Robins, E., Murphy, G., Wilkinson, R. H., Jr., Gassner, S., & Kayes, J. Some clinical considerations in the prevention of suicide based on a study of 134 successful suicides. *American Journal of Public Health*, 1959, **49,** 888–899.

Schneider, P.-B. *La tentative du suicide*. Paris: Delachaux and Niestlé, 1954. Pp. 48–50, 90–92, 267–269.

Schneidman, E. S., & Farberow, N. L. A sociopsychological investigation of suicide. In H. P. David and J. C. Brengelmann (Eds.), *Perspective in personality research*. New York: Springer, 1960.

Simpson, G. Introduction. In E. Durkheim, *Suicide*. Transl. by J. A. Spaulding & G. Simpson. Glencoe, Ill.: The Free Press, 1951. P. 17.

Vernon, P. E. How many factors? Unpublished manuscript, 1949.

"Vigil." Patterns of murder. London, 1949. *Observer*, 1956 (pamphlet).

Waldstein, E. *Der Selbstmord in der Schweiz*. Basel: Philographischer Verlag, 1934.

Wisse, J. *Selbstmord und Todesfurcht bei den Naturvölkern*. Zutphen: W. J. Thieme, 1933. Pp. 508–519.

Wolfgang, M. E. *Patterns of criminal homicide*. Philadelphia: University of Pennsylvania Press, 1958. Chapter XV.

Yessler, P. G., Gibbs, J. I., & Becker, H. A. On the communication of suicidal ideas. *Archives of General Psychiatry*, 1961, 5, 12–29.

2.6   Orientation

No questions are more basic or more difficult to answer than those concerning the relationship of early experience to mental illness. Basing his analysis upon the voluminous data of ethnographic literature, the psychologist Herbert Barry, III provides a thorough review of this and related questions. Although Barry admits that no single study he examines is conclusive, he believes that many studies point toward the same conclusion—that early experience is critically relevant. Specifically, Barry notes the relationship between indulgence in early infancy, the development of trust, and mental health. Barry also examines the biologically oriented Freudian theory of psycho-sexual development and finds the evidence negative; however, Barry finds support for Erikson's interpersonal theory of development.

Many anthropologists have been critical of the kind of correlational research that Barry reviews—and there *is* reason to be cautious—yet he rests his case not upon any single study, but upon an over-all consistency in pattern that he finds in many studies. His conclusions are likely to please some, and annoy others, but they should not be ignored.

2.6   Cultural Variations in the Development of Mental Illness[1]

Herbert Barry, III

Experience with psychiatric patients has provided much information on the events in early childhood that may lead to the development of mental

[1] The author wishes to acknowledge helpful suggestions from Roger V. Burton and Irvin L. Child. Preparation of the Chapter was also aided by the author's experience in directing the 1965 Summer Institute in Cross-Cultural Research, conducted at the University of Pittsburgh Anthropology Department and supported by the National Science Foundation's Advanced Science Seminar Program Grant GE-7785.

illness. Blum (1953) has written an excellent summary of theories by Sigmund Freud, Erikson, and other clinicians, relating childhood events to variations in type and severity of adult pathology. However, the clinical findings are limited to the cultural customs that prevail in a particular society. Some childhood conditions may appear to be universally related to adult illness only because of the influence of the particular cultural setting. For example, death of the mother during early childhood is a traumatic event which may give rise to mental illness or other pathology (Barry, Barry, & Lindemann, 1965), but this might be due to the monogamous nuclear family structure which often fails to provide an adequate mother substitute. Other events might have an ambiguous interpretation in a particular society because they represent several factors; for example, fatherless families tend to give rise to delinquency in our society, but it is not clear whether this is because of the lack of the father's influence or because such families are usually disrupted and associated with low socioeconomic status in our society. Some important childhood determinants of mental illness might be overlooked because they are held at a constant level in our society. The use of a worldwide sample of societies makes it possible to overcome these limitations, so that the effect of childhood experiences on development of mental health or illness can be studied under a much wider range of cultural conditions than is possible in studies limited to a single society.

The use of a worldwide sample of societies, representing a substantial part of the range of known human cultural variation, permits greater universality of conclusions. This provides a safeguard against drawing spurious conclusions based on an unusual combination of circumstances in a particular society. Most of the studies reviewed in the present chapter report on cross-cultural comparisons of a sizable sample of societies, with cultural variations in child training practices being correlated with variations in other cultural customs. Ethnographic information available in the literature is coded in a quantitative form to obtain usable measures of child training practices and other features of culture. Tests of statistical significance show the degree of likelihood that the findings are not due to chance alone. This chapter generally cites only the relationships between variables that are consistent enough, or are based on a large enough number of societies, to have a probability of less than one in twenty of being due to chance alone.

CULTURAL UNIVERSALS AND VARIATIONS

Any comparison among societies shows many features that all have in common, and many features in which they differ. Thus, universals and variations are both prominent characteristics in cross-cultural comparisons. Either of these characteristics may be emphasized, but neither of them should be ignored. From the point of view of studying determinants of mental illness, an important and severely limiting cultural universal is the fact that all of the societies have shown a sufficiently good adaptation to the environment, and to the needs of the members, to become established and to survive. Severe mental illness must necessarily be restricted to a minority of the people, if the culture is to survive. A cross-cultural sample of societies may include a few that have had a recent shattering or disrupting event, resulting in pervasive pathology of the individuals, but most of the societies are relatively stable and have been functioning for a long period of time.

If all societies offered the best possible opportunities for mental health, the variations among them would merely identify those characteristics that have no influence on the development of mental health or illness. However, universal adequate functioning of societies does not necessarily mean universal optimal functioning. Other chapters in this book give examples of the great variations among societies with respect to the incidence of various types of mental illness. There may be corresponding variations among societies in the degree to which their child training and other customs establish an environment favorable for the mental health of the individuals.

A fundamental purpose of culture is to provide satisfactions for the needs and motives of the individuals. These needs include not only biological drives, such as hunger, shelter, and sex, but also social motives, such as love, aggression, and ambition, which are largely learned and shaped by the cultural influences. Each individual's motives are strong and diverse, and they come into conflict with each other as well as with the environmental conditions and with the motives of other people. Cultural customs that satisfy one motive may leave others unresolved.

Certain conflicts are universal, but there are great variations in the severity of the different components of each conflict aroused, and in the methods for dealing with them. The present chapter emphasizes these cultural variations, relating the child training determinants of the conflicts to the adulthood expressions of them. The universal tendency for adequate cultural adjustment sets a limit on the destructive expression of the conflicts in adult life, and hence on the degree of pathological development in childhood, but the great diversity among societies gives a wide scope for variations in the development and expression of conflicts and pathological tendencies.

Mental illness is an expression of the individual's failure to make an adequate adjustment to his biological and social needs. This failure generally occurs because the conflicting motives are dealt with in a pathological way, beginning with traumatic events, and responses to these events, in early childhood. The present chapter reviews cross-cultural evidence about determinants of mental illness in terms of four major conflicts: (1) trust versus fear of other people, (2) love versus hatred, (3) independence versus dependence, and (4) expression versus control of bodily functions. This classification of conflicts is based on Freud's and Erikson's theories of personality development, with some modifications necessitated by the nature of the available cross-cultural information.

Conflict between Trust and Fear

The first few months of life are described by psychoanalytic theorists as the oral stage of development. In keeping with the undifferentiated nature of the infant's responses, a pervasive attitude of trust or distrust toward oneself and other people may persist throughout life, depending on whether the initial oral needs have been satisfied or frustrated. There is evidence for the development of severe pathology as a result of deprivation of contact with a nurturant figure, even without any denial of the nutritional needs. Spitz (1949) reported a syndrome of "hospitalism," including severe apathy and retardation of development, in babies who were reared in a foundling home with each nurse responsible for a number of infants. Harlow (1962) reported that rhesus macaque monkeys raised on a cloth dummy "mother surrogate" showed severe deficits in adult social behavior; they were almost completely incapable of normal sexual or maternal behavior. However, even the tactual stimulation provided by the cloth had some beneficial effect, because these monkeys were less severely affected than other monkeys that were raised on a wire frame (Harlow, 1958).

Such extreme deprivations during infancy are not likely to be prevalent in any existing societies. Cultural survival requires not only the physical survival of the individuals but also an adequate degree of trust and friendliness in their social behavior. Accordingly, one of the cultural universals is a high degree of oral satisfactions during infancy, with an attitude of trust and self-confidence being strongly developed. However, delays and deprivations of the initial oral satisfactions are inevitable, and their effects are heightened by the infant's helplessness and strongly aroused emotions (Dollard & Miller, 1950, p. 130). Therefore, fear and distrust are universally aroused during the initial infancy period; the degree and immediacy of oral satisfactions may be expected to influence the intensity of the conflict between trust and fear.

Whiting and Child (1953), in a large-scale cross-cultural study, included a quantitative rating of initial satisfaction of dependence. This is a measure of the degree to which the infant is fondly and continuously cared for. Societies with low initial satisfaction of dependence tended strongly to explain illness as being caused by soul loss or spirit possession. Thus, a conflictful, fearful concern about dependence on supernatural agents appears to be characteristic of the theories of illness in societies with relatively low satisfaction of the initial dependence needs during infancy The same conclusion may be drawn from the finding by Spiro and D'Andrade (1958) that societies with low initial satisfaction of dependence tended to believe that the supernatural beings could not be influenced to be nurturant by means of compulsive ritual.

Barry, Bacon, and Child (1957) used a similar but independently rated measure of over-all infancy indulgence. Whiting (1959) reported that societies with low infancy indulgence tended to express a high degree of fear of the ghosts of the dead at funerals. Lambert, Triandis, and Wolf (1959) reported that societies with low infancy indulgence also tended to believe that the supernatural figures (gods or spirits) were predominantly malevolent, whereas those with high infancy indulgence usually believed that the supernatural figures were benevolent. Supernatural malevolence was even more closely related to the occurrence of frequent or intense painful procedures inflicted upon the infants; this measure was one of the components of the more general measure of over-all indulgence. Lambert et al. (1959) noted that in most societies with frequent or intense painful procedures during infancy, the deities were believed to be capricious, not controllable by humans. This specific characteristic of the deities may be an expression of the infant's inability to understand or predict the painful experiences to which he is subjected.

Adult behavior with regard to drinking alcoholic beverages is also related to infancy indulgence. Bacon, Barry, and Child (1965) reported that societies with high over-all consumption of alcoholic beverages tended to be low in over-all infancy indulgence. The possible meaning of the negative correlation between these two variables may be indicated by relationships of infancy indulgence with other measures of alcohol consumption. Societies with low infancy indulgence were preponderantly characterized by high ritualization of drinking and low intensity of sociability expressed by the drinkers. Alcoholic beverages in these societies were drunk in a wide variety of situations, as shown by high negative correlations between infancy indulgence and frequency of drinking in household, party, religious, and segmented contexts. Societies with low infancy indulgence may thus be described as drinking large quantities of alcoholic beverages in varied situations, but with a spirit of formality and restraint. This may indicate conflict between desire for the effects of alcohol and fear of the uninhibited emotional expressions which tend to be aroused.

Cultural variations in treatment of infants are limited by a universal cultural tendency toward highly indulgent treatment of the infants. More than half of the societies were given high ratings in over-all infancy indulgence (Barry, Bacon, & Child, 1957) and in initial dependence and oral satisfaction (Whiting & Child, 1953). In a separate study, Cohen (1961, p. 319) reported that in fifty-nine out of sixty-four societies (92 percent) the infants are fed whenever they cry for food. The United States was rated by Whiting and Child (1953) as being unusually low with respect to initial satisfaction, because of the widespread custom of feeding infants on a prescribed schedule and leaving the baby alone in the crib most of the time. Ethnographic accounts of most cultures generally emphasize that the infant is welcomed and cherished, not only by the parents but also by the entire community. The few societies with very low ratings of infancy indulgence show conspicuous pathological features in adult personalities beyond those reported in this section as being associated with relatively low infancy indulgence. Notable examples are found in the highly suspicious and fearful adult social relationships among the Alorese (Kardiner, 1963), Marquesans (Linton, 1939), and Trukese (Gladwin and Sarason, 1959). Kardiner (1963, p. 253) stated that the Alorese survive as a culture only because of their isolated, island location, with the absence of challenge from any external enemies. This interpretation is also appropriate for the Marquesans and Trukese. Cohen (1961) reported that nonsharing of food or money characterized the adult culture in all five societies where infants were not always fed when they cried for food but in only one of the fifty-nine societies where food was never withheld.

Conflict between Love and Hatred

Following the initial stage of infancy, the young child's emotions become more differentiated and directed toward other humans. According to Freud, the Oedipal conflict ensues, with the mother being the primary love-object and the father being the target of the boy's feelings of rivalry and hatred. However, these emotions are not completely segregated. The child also experiences feelings of hatred for the mother and love for the father; conflicting love and hatred are likewise directed toward siblings and other people. The child identifies to some degree with both parents and thus turns the conflicting emotions of love and hatred upon himself. Thus, aggression may be expressed not only against other people, as by murder or fighting, but may also be turned against oneself, in suicide or depression. The aggressive feelings also may be attributed to others by the mechanism of projection, as in paranoid fantasies, or they may be displaced onto other objects. Such indirect expressions of hostility are often prominent features in the symptoms of mental illness.

Severe punishment for aggression in childhood might be especially likely to lead to indirect expressions of aggression, because such punishments would arouse further the child's aggressive feelings while inhibiting their direct expression. Whiting and Child (1953) reported that fear of human beings, a measure of the cultural belief that illness is caused by sorcerers, was highly correlated with aggression socialization anxiety (severity of punishment for aggressive behavior). A measure of fear of ghosts of the dead at funerals (Whiting, 1959) likewise showed a high positive relationship with aggression socialization anxiety. Wright (1954) reported that in societies with high aggression socialization anxiety, the folk tale themes expressed a higher over-all intensity of aggression, the agent and object of this aggression tended to be a stranger rather than being a friend of the hero, and the hero was less likely to be triumphant.

Aggression socialization anxiety thus gives evidence of being related to a wide variety of cultural beliefs and practices, expressing aggression or aggression-related anxiety. Some of the findings have been interpreted as indicating that anxiety about direct expression of aggression caused the aggressive response to be displaced to objects more remote from the source of the hatred (Whiting, 1961). On the other hand, Bacon et al. (1963) have introduced measures of criminal behavior that represent more direct expressions of aggression by individuals against the society's standards of conduct. These measures of crime are not correlated significantly with aggression socialization anxiety, but they are correlated with other measures of socialization anxiety that would be expected to intensify the conflict between love and hatred. Frequency of personal crime was positively correlated with Whiting and Child's (1953) measure of dependence socialization anxiety, and frequency of theft was negatively correlated with Barry, Bacon, and Child's (1957) measure of childhood indulgence. Thus, certain aspects of child training that would be expected to arouse aggression give evidence of increasing the incidence of directly hostile, antisocial acts by individuals.

Whiting and Child (1953) included a measure of oral socialization anxiety, aroused by the process of weaning. This may be an important determinant of hostility aroused during the transition from infancy to childhood. There was a very high positive correlation between oral socialization anxiety and the belief that illness is caused by eating or drinking food or poison or by verbal spells and incantations. These "oral explanations" of illness usually imply a belief in malicious action, such as by witches. Therefore, arousal of strong feelings of hatred by severe weaning, as well as by severe punishment of aggression during childhood, is apparently related to a cultural tendency for people to attribute hostility to others by the mechanism of projection.

In contrast with the almost universally high degree of infancy indulgence, large cultural variations have been found in the severity of child-training practices that may be expected to arouse strong conflict between love and hatred. Severe conflict of this type is thus apparently compatible with the survival and adequate functioning of the society. However, the great potential destructiveness of this conflict makes it likely that important cultural institutions may be found to express and alleviate severe conflict between love and hatred. The next section of this chapter reviews studies on cultural variations in household composition and in expression of sex role that may be related to the conflict between love and hatred. This is followed by a section on features of social structure that contribute further to the identification of a pattern of meaningfully interrelated variables.

Household and sex role In several studies, the experiences of the infants and young children have not been measured directly but have instead been assumed to be determined by the prevailing type of household. Particular attention has been directed to the mother-child household, in which the mother shares a dwelling alone with her nursing infant. This custom is generally associated with a post-partum sex taboo longer than 1½ years. Throughout this prolonged time, the infant is suckled by the mother and generally sleeps in the same bed with her. In most of these societies the mother is one of several wives, each of whom lives in a separate establishment, and the husband stays away from his infant and its mother until weaning ends the post-partum sex taboo.

According to a theory propounded by Whiting, Kluckhohn, and Anthony (1958) and elaborated by Stephens (1962), this type of living arrangement results in a heightened erotic attachment between mother and child. It should also be noted that the father's return and the birth of a younger sibling typically occur when the child is several years old, at an age when strong Oedipal and sibling rivalries may be most readily aroused. LeVine (1961) stated that sibling rivalry is intense in African societies; many of them have mother-child households. At the opposite extreme is the monogamous nuclear household, where typically the post-partum sex taboo lasts only a few weeks or months and the infant lives in the same dwelling with both parents, generally sleeping alone in the same room with both parents but in a separate bed. The infant's emotional attachment to the mother is likely to be less intense because of the less close and less exclusive contact with her; the presence of the father and younger siblings from a very early age would be expected to counteract the arousal of hostile feelings toward them. However, a severe conflict between love and hate may develop in this type of household also, as indicated by Freud's clinical observations of Oedipal rivalry in individuals raised in monogamous nuclear households.

Whiting, Kluckhohn, and Anthony (1958) reported that almost every society with mother-child sleeping arrangements and long post-partum sex taboos had initiation ceremonies for adolescent boys, characterized by at least one of the following features: painful hazing, genital operations, seclusion from women, and tests of manliness; societies without initiation ceremonies for boys almost all had other sleeping arrangements and a short post-partum sex taboo. Brown (1963) reported that painful initiation ceremonies for girls tended to be found in societies with mother-child households, whereas the initiation rites for girls were generally nonpainful in societies with other types of households. These findings might be interpreted as expressions of heightened interpersonal rivalry in societies with mother-child households. Stephens (1961) and Young and Bacdayan (1965) found that extensive menstrual taboos were prevalent in societies with a long duration of post-partum sex taboo. Stephens (1962) found that long post-partum sex taboo was also related to kin avoidances, change of residence for adolescent boys, and exclusion of breasts as sexual stimuli; he interpreted these cultural practices as being defenses against sexual anxiety aroused by the prolonged mother-child contact.

There is also evidence that the mother-child household is associated with the custom of couvade, which typically includes a taboo against the father's indulging in certain foods or activities in conjunction with the birth of his child (Burton & Whiting, 1961). Flugel (1929) has pointed out that the magical, phobic characteristics of the couvade, with the belief that the child will be harmed if the taboos are violated, suggest that it functions as a defense against the parents' unconscious hostility toward the child for restricting their freedom. A high incidence of crime, characteristic of societies with mother-child households (Bacon, Child, & Barry, 1963), indicates a more direct expression of hatred aroused in societies with this household type.

Freud's conception of the Oedipus conflict emphasizes the child's differential feelings toward masculine and feminine figures. The cultural conditions that intensify the conflict between love and hatred may be expected to arouse conflict in the child concerning his or her sex-typed role. The status-envy theory of sex identification, proposed by Burton and Whiting (1961), states that the child, when feeling deprived of food, love, or other desired resources, tends to imitate, and thus to identify with, the person who is perceived as being in the privileged position of controlling the resources. In societies with mother-child households, the infant will thus form an initial feminine identification, because the mother is likely to be the only adult figure in the household. The child will subsequently form a secondary masculine identification when the father returns and expresses his superior authority, especially because of the polygyny and patrilocality which characterize most societies with mother-child households. This sequence of events should result in a severe conflict between feminine and masculine sex identification.

Many of the cultural features related to mother-child household have been interpreted as expressions of this conflict. Male initiation rites are regarded as a mechanism for symbolic rebirth, renouncing the primary feminine identification (Burton & Whiting, 1961). Brown (1963) likewise interpreted the presence of painful female initiation rites as a means of resolving the girl's conflicts about her sex identification. Bacon, Child, and Barry (1963) interpreted high frequency of crime as an exaggerated assertion of masculinity, motivated by the need of males to deny their primary, unacceptable feminine identification. Other effects of sexual identification are predicted for other household types. Burton and Whiting (1961) interpreted the couvade as an expression of nonconflictful feminine identification in males; they reported that this custom is found mostly in societies with exclusive mother-child sleeping arrangements and matrilocal residence. The monogamous nuclear family may be expected to produce a nonconflictful masculine identification, because the father is continuously present and dominant in this type of household.

The mother-child household, which is assumed to arouse strong conflict between masculine and feminine identification, is the same situation that has been described as arousing strong conflict between love and hatred. These different conflicts are compatible with each other, and, indeed, the sex identification hypothesis may be regarded as a more detailed formulation of the same conflict. The status-envy theory of identification implies conflicting feelings of love and hatred toward the person perceived as controlling the desired resources. The primary feminine identification and the secondary masculine identification are both ambivalent, and the secondary identification requires a conflicting rejection of the earlier sex identification. The cultural features associated with mother-child household, and explained as expressions of conflict between masculine and feminine identification, seem to be adequately explained also as expressions of the more general conflict between love and hate. The explanation in terms of sex identification has the disadvantage that very little is known about the process of identification, especially sex identification. It seems doubtful that a very clear-cut distinction between masculine and feminine identification is formed in the infant or young child because of the primitive stage of its sexual development and the variety of important attributes, other than sex, that characterize the adults in the child's environment.

Features of social organization The pattern of cultural variables that link together male initiation ceremonies, mother-child households, menstrual taboos, and other cultural customs, has been shown to include additional features of social organization. Young (1965) reported that societies with male initiation rites tend to have a high degree of male solidarity in the adult culture. Cohen (1964) reported that in societies with male initiation ceremonies, the children are generally trained by members of the child's descent group rather than by nonmembers of the descent group. These variables are also positively related to the custom of collective kin-group responsibility in adult life ("joint liability"), to unilineal rather than bilateral descent, and to the custom of either "extrusion" of boys from their childhood home or brother-sister avoidance. Sorcery is also related to this pattern of cultural features. Beatrice Whiting (1950) reported that societies that attribute illness to sorcery generally lack an effective governmental authority. Swanson (1960) similarly found that witchcraft tends to be prevalent in societies characterized by unlegitimized or uncontrolled relationships, either within the society or with other societies.

Cohen (1964) and Young (1965) argued that the presence of male initiation rites is satisfactorily explained by the features of adult social organization with which they are shown to be related; these authors rejected the child-training practices and their effects on human motives as a causal factor. However, the widespread pattern of cultural features included in these relationships may be expected to have effects on child training and thus may influence the motivations of the next generation of adults, leading to certain directions in the evolution of social structure. For example, one such possibility is that the intensified conflict between love and hatred, aroused in mother-child households, may contribute to the formation of male and female solidarities, and collective kin responsibilities, as a defense against disruptive aggressions within the group and as an expression of hostility toward outsiders. Likewise, the conflict between love and hatred might tend to prevent the formation of stable, effective governmental authority, thus contributing to the unlegitimized and uncontrolled relationships which Swanson (1960) proposed as the explanation for sorcery.

Whiting (1964) has shown that his interpretation of child training as a determinant of features of social organization may be supported and supplemented rather than contradicted by relationships of social organization to characteristics of the physical environment. He reported that a long duration of post-partum sex taboo, and the presence of polygyny, patrilocal residence, and male initiation ceremonies, are preponderantly found in societies located in the tropics, with a low amount of protein in their subsistence diet. It seems likely that under these climatic and nutritional conditions, a prolonged nursing period is essential for the survival of the infant. This physiological requirement may be met by the custom of prolonged post-partum sex taboo, which in turn gives rise to the related customs of male initiation rites, polygyny, and patrilocal residence. In South America, however, male initiation rites are absent, and there is a low frequency of the other variables associated with initiation rites, although a tropical climate and protein deficiency are prevalent. This exceptional circumstance was explained by the fact that these societies apparently provide the necessary prolonged nursing period for infants by means of abortions instead of by a long post-partum sex taboo. These findings give evidence for a direct causative effect of long duration of post-partum sex taboo on the presence of male initiation rites and other related cultural customs.

Other child training practices have also been shown to be related to features of social organization. Whiting (1961) showed that over-all infancy indulgence (Barry, Bacon, & Child, 1957) tends to be highest in societies where extended families comprising three or more generations customarily live in the same household, almost as high in societies with polygynous households where the husband lives in the same dwelling with all his wives, much lower in societies with monogamous, nuclear families, and even lower in societies with polygynous, mother-child households, where each wife lives in a separate dwelling with her children. These differences were interpreted as indicating that infancy indulgence was related to the number of caretakers available in the household. Fear of ghosts at funerals was shown to be related to low infancy indulgence, independent of type of household, whereas the relationship of type of household to fear of ghosts was weaker and apparently attributable entirely to the common relationship of both variables to infancy indulgence.

Another pattern of interrelated, diverse variables is found in the positive correlations of complex design in pictorial art with Whiting and Child's (1953) measures of severe socialization (Barry, 1957) and with adult cultural measures of high social stratification and male superiority in social solidarity and status (Fischer, 1961).

When a particular child training practice is related to an adult custom, it is often reasonable to assume that the child training variable causes the adult custom rather than vice versa, but it is always possible that a third cultural feature, with a causative relationship to both variables, accounts for their correlation with each other. A clear-cut distinction between psychogenic and sociogenic determinants of cultural customs is sometimes attempted, but it seems likely that a wide variety of cultural features tend to be organized into a meaningful pattern of interrelationships by the process of cultural evolution. Therefore a comprehensive explanation of correlations among cultural practices would probably need to include both psychogenic and sociogenic variables in the chains of cause-and-effect relationships.

Conflict between Independence and Dependence

A universal conflict arises from the necessity for a profound change in behavior during the course of childhood. The infant is completely dependent on others for food and physical care. The process of development includes a gradual increase in the child's capability and motivation to provide for his own needs, but a conflict inevitably arises between the capability and motivation for self-reliance and the motivations and behaviors that have been strongly learned during the earlier infancy stage of dependence. A forbidden craving for succorance and security is clearly evident in many neurotic symptoms of adults. The development of a mental illness that requires hospitalization represents in part an acting out of the need for dependence.

There is great cultural variation in the severity of the demands for independence. In some societies the transition from infancy dependence to childhood self-reliance is sudden and drastic, as indicated by the distinction sometimes made between "lap child" and "yard child." In other societies the child's development of self-reliance is accompanied by a continuation of close contact with the mother or other nurturant agents. An over-all measure of severity of independence training (Barry, Child, & Bacon, 1959) consisted of the strength of socialization pressure toward assertion, measured by ratings of pressures toward achievement and self-reliance, relative to the pressure toward compliance, measured by ratings of pressures toward responsibility and obedience. Bacon, Barry, and Child (1965) reported that frequency of drunkenness is positively correlated with pressure toward assertion, in support of their hypothesis that an important motivation for drunkenness is the need to express the forbidden dependence needs in a manner acceptable to oneself and to others. Societies with high frequency of drunkenness also tend strongly to be characterized by a low degree of encouragement of needs for dependence and cooperation in adult life. High frequency of divorce, which was found to be associated with high frequency of drunkenness and strong socialization pressures toward achievement, in an unpublished study by Penny Addiss and Carol Friedman, gives further evidence of conflictful social behavior in societies with severe demands for independent behavior.

In some societies little or no difference is reported between socialization of boys and girls, but in those societies where a sex difference is found, the boys are trained more strongly in responsibility, obedience, and nurturance (Barry, Bacon, & Child, 1957). The universal differentiation in adult sex roles, based on universal biological differences, apparently results in a tendency for the society to train boys to develop assertive behavior while girls are trained to be compliant (Barry, Child, & Bacon, 1959). A cross-cultural tendency for a lower frequency of drunkenness among women than men (Child, Barry, & Bacon, 1965) gives support to the hypothesis that drunkenness may be a consequence of severe independence training and denial of dependency needs, which are imposed more often and more strongly in the socialization of boys than girls.

The child training practices that give rise to a conflict between independence and dependence also show evidence for relationships with cultural beliefs that seem to express conflicting dependence and fear toward the supernatural. Lambert, Triandis, and Wolf (1959) reported that the gods tend to be malevolent rather than benevolent in societies with strong child training pressure toward self-reliance and general independence, especially in societies with severe punishment for the child's failures to act self-reliantly and independently. D'Andrade (1961) reported that the use of dreams to seek and control supernatural powers is positively correlated with high socialization pressure toward assertion.

Whiting and Child (1953) included a rating of the severity of independence training in early childhood. This measure of dependence socialization anxiety was found by Spiro and D'Andrade (1958) to be highly correlated with the belief that it is necessary to obey the gods and to perform propitiatory ritual toward them in order to obtain their good will and avoid punishments. Whiting and Child (1953) found a high positive correlation between severe dependence socialization anxiety and presence of dependence avoidance therapies for illness, measured by the custom of either isolating the patient or removing him from his home. Illness generally requires dependent behavior, and the treatment of sick people apparently expresses conflicting, fearful avoidance of dependence in societies where the dependence motivation is severely punished in early childhood. Conflict about dependence is also indicated in a positive correlation between dependence socialization anxiety and the belief that illness is caused by soul loss or spirit possession (dependence explanations).

The cultural customs found to be correlated with conflict between independence and dependence are subject to other interpretations. Field (1962) gave a sociogenic rather than psychogenic interpretation of drunkenness in reporting evidence that insobriety tends to occur only in societies with egalitarian and informal interpersonal relationships among adults. However, psychogenic factors are involved; these cultural conditions might be expected to represent socially insecure and unstable relationships, thus enhancing the conflict between independence and dependence. These unsatisfactory relationships might originate in childhood experiences; Barry, Buchwald, Child, and Bacon (1965) showed that frequency of drunkenness is more closely related to child training pressure toward assertion than to the measures of social organization.

Barry, Child, and Bacon (1959) showed that the socialization pressure toward assertion or compliance was related to type of subsistence economy, with high accumulation of food (agriculture or herding rather than gathering, fishing, or hunting) being associated with compliance rather than assertion. The authors suggested that the subsistence economy leads to the selection of child training practices that provide training in the motives and behavior necessary for the adult role. However, an alternative possibility is that strong socialization pressure toward assertion rather than compliance produces strong conflict between independence and dependence motivation, giving rise to traits that are incompatible with the patient, cooperative, and compliant behavior required for successful agriculture and care of livestock. It seems probable that the child training practices and the subsistence economy mutually affect each other during a continual process of cultural adjustment and evolution.

In spite of the wide variation among societies in pressures toward assertion, there seems to be an upper limit on the severity of independence training. Cohen (1964) has presented data on a widespread custom of physical dislodgement of the young child from his household (extrusion). In most of these societies, socialization is the responsibility of members of the child's linear descent group in addition to the parents. Any effects of the greater separation of the child from his family are counteracted by the strong kinship bonds in these societies. The custom of sending boys away to a boarding school to be educated by strangers, prevalent in the English upper class, is very rarely found in a cross-cultural sample. Perhaps this demand for early independence tends to be excessive for the healthy development of the individual or for the stability of the society.

Conflicts about Body Functions

There is a universal cultural necessity for regulating the elimination of the body's waste products and the expression of sexual behavior. Bladder and bowel control must be imposed for hygienic reasons wherever a sizable number of people live in close proximity. Sexual controls are required for the maintenance of stable, harmonious social relationships.

Incest taboos universally prohibit sexual relations within the nuclear family except for husband and wife; Murdock has written (1949, p. 260), "Possibly in man's long history there have been peoples who have failed to subject the sexual impulse to regulation. If so, none has survived, for the social control of sex is today a cultural universal."

Elimination and erotic behavior are universally regulated, beginning at an early age. According to Freud, excessively severe training of bladder and bowel control may give rise to a syndrome of neurotically exaggerated traits of obstinacy, orderliness, and parsimony, termed the "anal personality." Severe punishments for childhood erotic behavior may disrupt the normal psycho-sexual development and produce widespread symptoms of neurotic conflict, such as hysteria and anxiety.

The child training practices rated in Whiting and Child's (1953) cross-cultural study included measures of anal socialization anxiety and sex socialization anxiety. There was little evidence for any strong or generalized effects of severe childhood training in bowel and bladder control or severe punishments for childhood erotic behavior. Relationships of anal and sexual socialization anxiety to corresponding anal and sexual features in explanations of illness, avoidance therapies, and performance therapies were slight and mostly short of statistical significance.

A factor analysis of Whiting and Child's data by Prothro (1960) gives suggestive evidence that any possible pathological effects of severe toilet training and punishment of childhood erotic behavior are mitigated by the association of these variables with beneficial child training practices. One of Prothro's factors, with a high loading on severe anal socialization anxiety and early age of onset of training in bladder and bowel control, is related to mild dependence socialization anxiety. Thus, any pathological effect of severe training in bladder and bowel control may be outweighed by the satisfaction of dependence needs, associated with this form of attention on the part of the mother or other socializing agent. A negative correlation between anal socialization anxiety and frequency of drunkenness, reported by Bacon, Barry, and Child (1965), was interpreted as indicating that the precise, clean, neat, and orderly anal personality would avoid getting drunk. However, a reasonable alternative explanation might be that the mild dependence socialization anxiety, associated with severe anal socialization anxiety, reduces the conflict between independence and dependence which motivates drunkenness.

Another factor reported by Prothro (1960), with a high loading on severe sexual socialization anxiety, was related to low oral socialization anxiety, late age of weaning, and high oral initial satisfaction. Therefore, the pathological effect of severe sex socialization anxiety may be outweighed by the beneficial effect of low oral socialization anxiety associated with it. Whiting and Child (1953) reported a positive correlation between severe sex socialization anxiety and a measure of belief that illness is caused by sorcery (fear of human beings). This finding, which is consistent with Freud's theory that paranoid fantasies may represent a projection of sexual conflicts, seems to be largely explainable by the relationships of both variables to prolonged post-partum sex taboo (Whiting, 1959), with sorcery being more closely related to prolonged post-partum sex taboo than to severe sex socialization. However, a weak relationship of severe sex training to belief in sorcery apparently remained when the effect of length of post-partum sex taboo was held constant. Another, somewhat limited effect of sex socialization anxiety on adult behavior is indicated by Shirley and Romney's (1962) report that the use of love magic is associated with severe sex socialization anxiety.

There is no doubt that the child's development can be pathologically affected by excessively severe training in bladder and bowel control or in modesty. Such excessively severe socialization practices have apparently seldom if ever become established as the prevalent custom of a society, presumably owing to the influence of natural selection of customs in the process of cultural evolution. The acceptable levels of severity seem to include a wide range of variation among societies, although Whiting and Child (1953) found that in comparison with the United States, almost all societies are more lenient in bladder and bowel training and the majority of societies are more lenient in modesty training.

EVALUATION OF CROSS-CULTURAL RESEARCH METHODS

The studies reviewed in this chapter are based on data that have considerable limitations and imperfections. The ethnographic accounts were written by anthropologists, or in some cases by missionaries or explorers, who varied greatly in their skill, experience, and points of view. Many of the ethnographers were not primarily interested in child training, and the routine care of infants and children in the home is less easily accessible to observation than are the more public cultural activities. The quantitative coding of the ethnographic accounts requires subjective judgments which introduce a further source of error and variation in the data. Most of the cross-cultural studies should be described as being exploratory, preliminary research, with the use of a limited sample of societies and only a few quantitatively coded variables. Statistical analysis is hampered by the fact that many societies and variables are closely related to each other instead of being completely independent cases. Different studies have often used different samples and different measures, so that their findings are isolated and fragmentary rather than contributing to an accumulative advance of knowledge.

These limitations and shortcomings are counteracted by some important advantages of the cross-cultural research material. The wide range of cultural variation, and the use of a worldwide sample of several dozen societies in most studies, mitigate the effects of inaccuracies in ethnographic accounts and of misclassifications in the quantitative coding. The use of statistical significance tests provides some degree of protection against making conclusions based on findings that are due to chance association between variables. A general trustworthiness and accuracy of the ethnographic accounts is assured by the fact that most ethnographers have a sincere desire to report the cultural customs accurately and comprehensively. Their role as observers of an alien culture gives the advantages of a more detached position and a more objective point of view.

The materials available for cross-cultural research are improving rapidly. There is greater standardization of techniques of field work by ethnographers, and an increased interest in child training practices. The books *Six Cultures* (Whiting, 1963) and *Mothers of Six Cultures* (Minturn & Lambert, 1964) are notable examples of a trend toward applying a comprehensive and uniform set of concepts and interview questions to the study of different societies. The Human Relations Area Files, available at a number of universities, provide a conveniently organized and comprehensive source of ethnographic literature on more than 200 societies. A large number of variables, coded for more than 1100 societies, are published in the Ethnographic Atlas in the journal *Ethnology,* with new codes and societies being added periodically. A book by Textor (1967) presents correlational findings and the codings of each of 400 societies on many of these variables and also a wide variety of other codes, including Whiting and Child's (1953) ratings of child training practices and beliefs about illness for seventy-five societies and Barry, Bacon, and Child's (1957) socialization ratings for 110 societies. Bacon, Barry, Child, and Snyder (1965) make available a number of ratings of alcohol use for 139 societies. Whiting (1968) has recently reviewed materials and methods used in cross-cultural research.

The most severe limitation of cross-cultural research is probably the fact that it is a correlational, observational technique, which does not permit experimental manipulation of the variables. Cultures are complex entities, with a wide variety of interrelated features. When a socialization measure is found to be correlated with an adult cultural custom, various causative relationships are possible. The child training practices might have an effect on personality and thus on adult behavior, the adult cultural features may influence the child training practices, or some sociological, environmental, or other feature may influence both of these aspects of culture. The controversy between psychogenic and sociogenic explanations indicates the difficulty of interpreting correlational findings. It seems likely that each of these causal mechanisms generally influences cultural evolution, leading to a coherent, mutually consistent pattern of interrelationships among cultural customs.

One of the principal necessities for future cross-cultural research seems to be the use of multivariate analyses for structuring and simplifying the separate interrelated variables. One such technique is partial correlation, testing for the relationship between two variables while holding constant the effects of a third variable. Whiting (1959, 1961) has shown some tests of the relationship between two variables, separately for the cultures at each level of a third variable. However, the effective use of this technique requires a larger number of societies than have been available in most samples. If two variables are positively correlated with each other, it is possible to use only the minority of the societies (those having a high score on one variable and a low score on the other) for holding constant the effect of one of these two variables in a test of the relationship of the other variable to a third variable.

Multivariate analysis is not limited to testing the interrelationships among three variables. The technique of factor analysis has been used in cross-cultural research to reduce a large number of variables to a few independent factors (Prothro, 1960; Child, Bacon, & Barry, 1965; Sawyer & LeVine, 1966). Other techniques available for descriptive analysis of multivariate data include discriminant analysis and canonical correlation. Analysis of variance may be used for testing statistical significance of multivariate data.

A different method for identifying cause-and-effect relationships is to select societies that have changed in a particular feature, observing which other variables have changed and which have remained the same. This technique is efficient, requiring a relatively small sample of societies for reliable findings, because each society is observed in two stages which differ with respect to the feature suspected of causing variations in other features. This has the same purpose as the experimental method of isolating and manipulating one variable to observe its effects, but it is necessary to rely on nature or other agents to provide the manipulation of cultural variables. Cohen (1961, pp. 339–346) and Young (1965, pp. 128–137) made some use of this technique, but in most cross-cultural studies the customs have been measured in a static manner, fixed at a time that is usually specified as being aboriginal or else shortly after contact with the enthnographer's civilization.

Another potentially useful technique is to compare cultural customs associated with different social stratifications, castes, subcultures, or regions within the same society. This resembles the experimental method of isolating a particular variable by holding constant other sources of variation. Cohen (1961, pp. 335–339) has suggested the use of this technique in cross-cultural research, but in most studies each society has been treated as if it were a homogeneous entity.

Cross-cultural research has suffered from a restricted number and variety of quantitatively coded variables. Variations in human development have nearly always been measured by Whiting and Child's (1953) or Barry, Bacon, and Child's (1957) socialization ratings, or else by categories of household type, which are assumed to influence child training. More measures of child training practices should be identified and rated. In many of the studies, the socialization variables have been related to very indirect and inferential measures of adult pathology, such as initiation ceremonies and beliefs about the supernatural and about illness. In some studies adult pathology has been measured by culturally approved or prevalent behavior that is presumed to be pathological, such as frequent drunkenness and belief in sorcery, or else by a high incidence of crime, suicide, or other deviations from culturally approved behavior. Several such variables have been included in more comprehensive measures of cultural ego strength (Allen, 1962, 1967), and in the measures of cultural pathology that Naroll, in the preceding chapter of the present book, proposes as causes of suicide or other deviations from culturally approved behavior. Other measures of cultural variations in mental health need to be developed and related to child training practices.

CONCLUSIONS FROM CROSS-CULTURAL FINDINGS

Even with all their shortcomings, the cross-cultural data seem to give meaningful information about relationships of child training to cultural health and pathology. None of the studies by itself is highly convincing, but in the aggregate they point to a consistent pattern. Societies where child training practices lead to intensified conflict in certain specified motivational areas tend to show cultural features symptomatic of the conflict. The findings reviewed in the present chapter are organized according to these basic conflicts.

The cross-cultural findings are interpreted as giving evidence that early infancy indulgence, resulting in the development of a basic social attitude of trust, is an extremely important determinant of mental health in adulthood. This is indicated by the universal cultural tendency for indulgent, loving care of the infant, and also by pathological features of the few societies where the care of infants is not highly indulgent. Diffusion of nurturance among other caretakers in addition to the mother seems to be beneficial rather than detrimental. The large cultural variations found in severity and other aspects of socialization after the infancy period indicate that a functioning society, with most of its members being adequately adjusted, seems to be compatible with a very wide variety of child training practices. The conditions hypothesized to maximize conflict between masculine and feminine identification seem to be almost identical to the conditions that are assumed to maximize the conflict between love and hatred. Cultural variations in the intensity of the conflicts between love and hatred and between independence and dependence, aroused by child training, seem to have greater effects on personality development than the cultural variations in the intensity of the conflicts engendered by training in bladder and bowel control and by punishments for sexual behavior.

The cross-cultural data fail to support some of the relationships that Freud suggested between biological universals in development and mental illness. There is little evidence for a universal sequence of anal and phallic stages of development in early childhood, followed by the latency period and then adolescent stress in later childhood. Freud's hypothesis that pathological fixation at a particular stage of development may result from either excessive deprivation or gratification at that stage (Allen, 1964) was not supported by Whiting and Child (1953, p. 217), nor in a recent article by Allen (1967); both studies found evidence for pathological effects of deprivations but no indication that gratifications could be excessive. In general, the cross-cultural data are more consistent with Erikson's theory of development, which emphasizes interpersonal relationships, than with Freud's more biological conception. Freud's theories of the Oedipus conflict and sexual identification, which have been applied to cross-cultural data (Stephens, 1962; Burton & Whiting, 1961), seem to be socially rather than biologically oriented.

The cross-cultural data on relationships between human development and mental illness are limited by the fact that the subjects of investigation are preponderantly surviving and functioning rather than sick societies. Many of the cultural customs that give evidence of expressing intense conflict are not themselves severely pathological. For example, in a sample of preliterate societies (Child, Bacon, & Barry, 1965), even those with the highest frequency of drunkenness generally showed little or no incidence of chronic alcoholics. The cultural customs with apparently pathological effects may have compensating features that are beneficial. For example, societies with monogamous nuclear families have a low incidence of crime (Bacon, Child, & Barry, 1963), but Whiting (1959) has shown that these cultural features are accompanied by strong feelings of guilt, measured by Whiting and Child's (1953) rating of patient responsibility for illness. Thus, societies with mother-child households, which have a high frequency of crime, do not necessarily give rise to a greater degree of hostility, but instead may cause the aggression to be expressed extra-punitively against other people rather than intrapunitively in the form of guilt. A compensatory high degree of affectionate behavior in adult-hood, following emotional deprivation in infancy, is a possible interpreta-tion for a recent finding by Rosenblatt (1967) that romantic love as a basis for marriage tended to be found in societies with low initial oral indulgence and high severity of oral socialization.

Some cultural universals have been identified as outcomes of uni-versal biological and social needs, in conjunction with the universally adequate adjustment of surviving societies. However, cultural variations are given greater emphasis in cross-cultural research and in the present chapter. All of the cross-cultural research on relationships of child training practices to other features of culture, reviewed in this chapter, is very recent (the first study was Whiting and Child, 1953). Rapid advances in materials and techniques make it likely that the cross-cultural research findings in the coming years will prove increasingly valuable.

REFERENCES

Allen, M. G. The development of universal criteria for the measurement of the health of a society. *Journal of Social Psychology*, 1962, **57**, 363–382.

Allen, M. G. Psychoanalytic theory on infant gratification and adult personality. *Journal of Genetic Psychology*, 1964, **104**, 265–274.

Allen, M. G. Childhood experience and adult personality—a cross-cultural study using the concept of ego strength. *Journal of Social Psychology*, 1967, **71**, 53–68.

Bacon, M. K., Barry, H., III, & Child, I. L. A cross-cultural study of drinking: II. Relations to other features of culture. *Quarterly Journal of Studies on Alcohol*, Suppl. No. 3, pp. 29–48, 1965.

Bacon, M. K., Barry, H., III, Child, I. L., & Snyder, C. R. A cross-cultural study of drinking: V. Detailed definitions and data. *Quarterly Journal of Studies on Alcohol*, Suppl. No. 3, pp. 78–111, 1965.

Bacon, M. K., Child, I. L., & Barry, H., III. A cross-cultural study of correlates of crime. *Journal of Abnormal and Social Psychology*, 1963, **66**, 291–300.

Barry, H., Jr., Barry, H., III, & Lindemann, E. Dependency in adult patients following early maternal bereavement. *Journal of Nervous and Mental Dis-eases*, 1965, **140**, 196–206.

Barry, H., III. Relationships between child training and the pictorial arts. *Journal of Abnormal and Social Psychology*, 1957, **54**, 380–383.

Barry, H., III, Bacon, M. K., & Child, I. L. A cross-cultural survey of some sex differences in socialization. *Journal of Abnormal and Social Psychology*, 1957, **55**, 327–332.

Barry, H., III, Buchwald, C., Child, I. L., & Bacon, M. K. A cross-cultural study of drinking: IV. Comparisons with Horton ratings. *Quarterly Journal of Studies on Alcohol,* Suppl. No. 3, pp. 62–77, 1965.

Barry, H., III, Child, I. L., & Bacon, M. K. Relation of child training to subsistence economy. *American Anthropologist,* 1959, **61,** 51–63.

Blum, G. S. *Psychoanalytic theories of personality.* New York: McGraw-Hill, 1953.

Brown, J. K. A cross-cultural study of female initiation rites. *American Anthropologist,* 1963, **65,** 837–853.

Burton, R. V., & Whiting, J. W. M. The absent father and cross-sex identity. *Merrill-Palmer Quarterly of Behavior and Development,* 1961, **7,** 85–95.

Child, I. L., Bacon, M. K., & Barry, H., III. A cross-cultural study of drinking: I. Descriptive measurements of drinking customs. *Quarterly Journal of Studies on Alcohol,* Suppl. No. 3, pp. 1-28, 1965.

Child, I. L., Barry, H., III, & Bacon, M. K. A cross-cultural study of drinking: III. Sex differences. *Quarterly Journal of Studies on Alcohol,* Suppl. No. 3, pp. 49–61, 1965.

Cohen, Y. A. *Social structure and personality: A casebook.* New York: Holt, Rinehart and Winston, 1961.

Cohen, Y. A. *The transition from childhood to adolescence.* Chicago: Aldine, 1964.

D'Andrade, R. G. Anthropological studies of dreams. In F. L. K. Hsu (Ed.), *Psychological anthropology: Approaches to culture and personality.* Homewood, Ill.: The Dorsey Press, 1961. Pp. 296–332.

Dollard, J., & Miller, N. E. *Personality and psychotherapy.* New York: McGraw-Hill, 1950.

Field, P. B. A new cross-cultural study of drunkenness. In D. J. Pittman & C. R. Snyder (Eds.), *Society, culture, and drinking patterns.* New York: Wiley, 1962. Pp. 48–74.

Fischer, J. L. Art styles as cultural cognitive maps. *American Anthropologist,* 1961, **63,** 79–93.

Flügel, J. C. *The psycho-analytic study of the family.* (3rd ed.) London: Hogarth Press, 1929.

Gladwin, T., & Sarason, S. B. Culture and individual personality integration in Truk. In M. K. Opler (Ed.), *Culture and mental health.* New York: Macmillan, 1959. Pp. 173–210.

Harlow, H. F. The nature of love. *American Psychologist,* 1958, **13,** 673–685.

Harlow, H. F. The heterosexual affectional system in monkeys. *American Psychologist,* 1962, **17,** 1–9.

Kardiner, A. *The psychological frontiers of society.* (Paperback ed.) New York: Columbia University Press, 1963.

Lambert, W. W., Triandis, L. M., & Wolf, M. Some correlates of beliefs in the malevolence and benevolence of supernatural beings: A cross-cultural study. *Journal of Abnormal and Social Psychology,* 1959, **58,** 162–169.

LeVine, R. A. Africa. In F. L. K. Hsu (Ed.), *Psychological anthropology: Approaches to culture and personality.* Homewood, Ill.: The Dorsey Press, 1961. Pp. 48–92.

Linton, R. Marquesan culture. In A. Kardiner, *The individual and his society*. New York: Columbia University Press, 1939. Pp. 137–196.

Minturn, L., & Lambert, W. W. *Mothers of six cultures*. New York: Wiley, 1964.

Murdock, G. P. *Social structure*. New York: Macmillan, 1949.

Prothro, E. T. .Patterns of permissiveness among preliterate people. *Journal of Abnormal and Social Psychology*, 1960, **61**, 151–154.

Rosenblatt, P. C. A cross-cultural study of child-rearing and romantic love. *Journal of Personality and Social Psychology*, 1967, 4, 336–338.

Sawyer, J., and LeVine, R. A. Cultural dimensions: A factor analysis of the world ethnographic sample. *American Anthropologist*, 1966, **68**, 708–731.

Shirley, R. W., & Romney, A. K. Love magic and socialization anxiety: A cross-cultural study. *American Anthropologist*, 1962, **64**, 1028–1031.

Spiro, M. E., & D'Andrade, R. G. A cross-cultural study of some supernatural beliefs. *American Anthropologist*, 1958, **60**, 456–466.

Spitz, R. A. Motherless infants. *Child Development*, 1949, **20**, 145–155.

Stephens, W. N. A cross-cultural study of menstrual taboos. *Genetic Psychology Monographs,* 1961, **64**, 385–416.

Stephens, W. N. *The Oedipus complex*. Glencoe, Ill.: The Free Press, 1962.

Swanson, G. E. *The birth of the gods*. Ann Arbor: University of Michigan Press, 1960.

Textor, R. B. *A cross-cultural summary*. New York: Taplinger, 1967.

Whiting, B. B. *Paiute sorcery*. New York: Viking Fund Publications in Anthropology, No. 15, 1950.

Whiting, B. B. (Ed.) *Six cultures: Studies of child rearing*. New York: Wiley, 1963.

Whiting, J. W. M. Sorcery, sin, and the superego: A cross-cultural study of some mechanisms of social control. In M. R. Jones (Ed.), *Nebraska Symposium on motivation*. Lincoln, Nebraska: Nebraska University Press, 1959. Pp. 174–195.

Whiting, J. W. M. Socialization process and personality. In F. L. K. Hsu (Ed.), *Psychological anthropology: Approaches to culture and personality*. Homewood, Ill.: Dorsey Press, 1961. Pp. 355–380.

Whiting, J. W. M. Methods and problems in cross-cultural research. In G. Lindzey & E. Aronson (Eds.), *Handbook of social psychology*. (2nd ed.) Cambridge, Mass.: Addison-Wesley, 1968. Vol. 2, pp. 693–728.

Whiting, J. W. M. Methods and problems in cross-cultural research. In E. Aronson and G. Lindzey (Eds.), *Handbook of social psychology*. (2nd ed.) Cambridge, Mass.: Addison-Wesley, 1967.

Whiting, J. W. M., & Child, I. L. *Child training and personality: A cross-cultural study*. New Haven: Yale University Press, 1953.

Whiting, J. W. M., Kluckhohn, R., & Anthony, A. The function of male initiation ceremonies at puberty. In E. E. Maccoby, T. M. Newcomb, & E. L. Hartley (Eds.), *Readings in social psychology*. (3rd ed.) New York: Holt, Rinehart and Winston, 1958. Pp. 359–370.

Wright, G. O. Projection and displacement: A cross-cultural study of folk-tale aggression. *Journal of Abnormal and Social Psychology*, 1954, **49**, 523–528.

Young, F. W. *Initiation ceremonies.* Indianapolis, Indiana: Bobbs-Merrill, 1965.

Young, F. W., & Bacdayan, A. A. Menstrual taboos and social rigidity. *Ethnology,* 1965, 4, 225–240.

2.7 Orientation

This article by the psychiatrist Alexander Leighton offers us a rare opportunity to examine social psychiatric data from two radically different areas of the world with the knowledge that in both areas, the data were collected by similar techniques, were analyzed in a consistent manner by the same investigators, and are consequently comparable to an unusual degree.

The research by Leighton and his colleagues—in Nova Scotia and later in Nigeria—is perhaps the most extensive comparative research yet undertaken in social psychiatry. It may also be the most significant. Leighton and his associates have developed a methodology of data collection and of diagnosis that they believe to be as applicable in Nigeria as in rural Nova Scotia. Even more important is their general finding that both the amount and the kind of mental illness in rural Nova Scotia and in Nigeria are much more similar than they are different. The implications of Leighton's work are far-reaching, for his data speak directly to the question of the extent to which culture does affect mental illness.

2.7 A Comparative Study of Psychiatric Disorder in Nigeria and Rural North America

Alexander H. Leighton

PRELIMINARY NOTE ON THE PROBLEM OF CULTURAL DIFFERENCE[1]

"Psychiatry" is a medical specialty that is a cultural sub-pattern within Western cultures. The phenomena with which it deals, namely "psychi-

[1] The first part of this chapter—The Problem of Cultural Difference—was written in collaboration with Jane M. Murphy, who conducted most of the field investigation.

Grateful acknowledgment is also made to Professor T. A. Lambo of the Department of Psychiatry, University of Ibadan, and Dr. T. A. Asuni, Medical Super-

atric disorders," are patterns of behavior and feeling that are out of keeping with cultural expectations and that bother the person who acts
and feels them, or bother others around him, or both.[2] Since different
cultures, by definition, have different systems of standards and expectation, it follows that what may be disturbing in one is not necessarily so
in another.

An extreme proponent of cultural relativity could push this line of
argument to the point of denying the possibility of ever identifying and
counting the same kinds of psychiatric disorder in markedly different
cultures. This is because any pattern of behavior is well or ill only to the
extent that it is so defined by a given culture. The greater the contrast
between cultures, the more radically different these definitions are apt to
be. To speak, therefore, of "the same psychiatric disorder in two different
cultures," is to utter a contradiction.

Such cultural relativity embodies two rather doubtful assumptions.
One is that cultural patterns are infinitely variable, and the other is
that personality is infinitely plastic. It seems more probable that there
are common limiting factors at work the world over in both cultures and
personalities. Nevertheless, cultural differences must, to some extent,
enter into the definitions and perceptions of psychiatric disorders. A
problem of interest, then, is this: If we start with our Western subcultural definitions and the criteria by which we recognize disorders, to
what extent is it possible to identify comparable phenomena in other
cultures?

An attempt to explore this problem among members of the Yoruba
tribe in Nigeria was made by the Cornell-Aro Mental Health Research
Project in 1961. Inasmuch as a detailed report has already been published
(Leighton et al., 1963, Ch. VI), what follows will be an overview of the
main results.

After finding that the Yoruba do have a general conception of "mental
illness," we posed for ourselves this question: What kind of subdivisions

---

intendent of the Aro Hospital for Nervous Diseases, who provided help in
explaining Yoruba concepts of mental illness. Additional comment and advice
was provided by Dr. Dorothea C. Leighton of the University of North Carolina,
Dr. Raymond H. Prince of McGill University, and Dr. Charles Savage of Spring
Grove State Hospital, Maryland.

Some of the material in this chapter appeared in an earlier version in A.
Leighton et al., 1963, © Cornell University Press. It is used by permission of
Cornell University Press.

[2] Summary statement suggested by Professor John S. Harding in personal communication.

of psychiatric disorder do the Yoruba make? Some illustrations from discussion with our informants may be summarized as follows:[3]

1. There is a kind of dwindling or sapping of a person's inner self that is caused by someone making an image of him and putting it on a fire.

2. Witchcraft is a cause of many types of symptoms, but particularly characteristic are bad dreams, sleeplessness, worries, sterility, stomach pains, headache, and skin sores.

3. If the god of smallpox, Sanponna, is about to trouble a man, and the man does not have the usual skin eruptions, often the god will run into his brain and make him insane.

Many other descriptions of this sort were given, with few showing any correspondence to the diagnostic categories of psychiatry. Evidently there is a world of difference in the way various kinds of disorders are defined in the two cultures under consideration.

If, however, one moves back from diagnosis and considers the topic at a more abstract level, a number of similarities becomes apparent. In both cultures people are said to have this or that illness according to symptoms and degree of impairment, according to theories about causations in mental illness, and according to response to treatment. Our recognition of this makes it possible for us to examine the particulars of each type of Yoruba criterion for correspondence with, or difference from, particulars employed by psychiatrists.

Symptoms

By "symptoms" we mean complaints and behaviors that are *thought by Yoruba people* to indicate or constitute mental and emotional illness. The following are some of the symptom types volunteered by our Yoruba informants when asked to describe the Yoruba view of mental disorder.

1. *Wèrè* is a general term for all forms of insanity.[4] Examples are talking to oneself, hearing voices and seeing people not seen or heard by those around one, refusing food because of belief that it is poisoned,

[3] The central vein of information reported here was obtained by interviewing three native healers, Mr. Oladipo Obafemi, Mr. J. O. Shoyinka, and Mr. Michael Amoleghe. Additional information was provided by Dr. Lambo and Dr. Asuni, and by Mrs. D. M. Davies, Mr. A. Erha Imohiosen, Mr. B. B. Johnson, Mr. Ogunbayo Akinode, Mr. Daniel D. Shodipo, and Mr. Jola Showemimo.

[4] Tone and vowel sounds are necessary for correct identification of Yoruba words. A note on the Yoruba language and the orthography employed here can be found on page xi of *Psychiatric Disorder Among the Yoruba* (A. Leighton *et al.*, 1963).

inappropriate defecation, and sudden attacks on people, with loss of memory afterward.

2. *Wèrè alaso* refers to a person who is normal most of the time, but then exhibits odd behavior for an hour or two, as for instance gathering up things from traders or hawkers without paying for them, and giving them away.

3. *Wárápá* is a condition that gets hold of the stomach and then the body, feet, and brains. The person falls to the ground, and foam comes out of his mouth. He may bite his tongue, stretch out his body, begin to shake his arms and legs. It lasts 15 to 20 minutes, and there is no recollection of the event afterward.

4. *Apòdà* means "fool" or "village idiot." Such a person merely lives; talking comes hard to him, especially giving a sensible answer to questions. He is "cloggish in his tongue," and does not know how to take care of himself.

So far, then, we have not come upon any symptom patterns noted by the Yoruba that are not also recognized in psychiatry. Our Yoruba informants spoke easily of delusions, such as fearing poisoned food, and of hallucinations, especially hearing voices. This eliminated the general question of whether or not delusions and hallucinations can be identified among the Yoruba. Plainly, in some instances they can.

If we ask whether the descriptions given cover all the main categories of symptom patterns employed in psychiatry, it is at once apparent that they do not. The examples we have presented so far, as well as the remaining data, pertain mainly to symptoms associated with mental deficiency, schizophrenia, epilepsy, paresis, and other organic brain disorders. For the most part, mention of symptoms characteristic of psychophysiologic, psychoneurotic, personality, and sociopathic disorders is absent, and so too with regard to symptoms found in the commonest brain syndrome—senile change. When we described these to our informants and asked about them, we found they were known, but not generally considered an illness in the same sense as the conditions mentioned in the volunteered information. Some examples:

1. *Senility:* it is well known that older people become "childish," do not answer questions properly, cannot remember things, and in general lose their mental capacities. This is the natural course of events, is incurable, and is not treated by native healers.[5]

2. *Airi-orunsùn* refers to "unrest of the mind" and sleeplessness.

---

[5] Although the condition is easily recognized and described, there is no specific Yoruba label for senility.

3. A person may have an emotional reaction involving loss of appetite and loss of interest in life as a result of the death of a family member.

4. *Itijú* means a sense of shame expected of all normal people. It is also used, however, to refer to extreme bashfulness, a fear of being among people.

5. *Iwárá* refers to a person who is tense and overeager, always wanting things done in a hurry. He may do five religious rituals instead of one, in order to speed up the results he desires.

6. *Sociopathic:* all the main characteristics of this category are familiar to the Yoruba—dyssocial and antisocial behavior and addiction.

It appears, then, that the symptoms of senility, some of the psychoneurotic symptoms, certain manifestations of depression, and a good many kinds of personality disorder are remarked in the Yoruba cultural system. They were not, however, elicited by general questions regarding mental and emotional illness and are evidently not consistently perceived as belonging in such a category, *although they are considered to be uncomfortable, undesirable, impairing and, in some instances, unusual.*[6]

While our understanding of the range of symptom patterns of which the Yoruba are aware is now augmented, we are still left with certain omissions as compared to psychiatric categories.

1. *Phobic* symptoms were virtually unknown to our informants, although we were told that fear of closed space is sometimes observed.

2. *Obsessive-compulsive* symptoms were also not known, except insofar as this might be implied under *Iwárá* above.

3. Depressive symptoms as such—psychotic or psychoneurotic—were not volunteered by our informants and when described were not accepted immediately as something familiar. On the other hand, many of the component symptoms of depression came up in one context or another: sapped vitality, a sense of "dwindling," crying continuously, extreme worry, loss of appetite, and loss of interest in life.

[6] In planning our discussion of psychiatric symptoms with our informants, we drew on the work of Forrest E. Clements, *Primitive Concepts of Disease,* University of California Publications in American Archaeology and Ethnology, Volume XXXII, No. 2, 1932; and John M. Whiting and Irvin L. Child, *Child Training and Personality: A Cross-Cultural Study,* New Haven: Yale University Press, 1953. Particularly valuable guidance and help was also obtained from William Bascom's list of Yoruba terms for mental symptoms in "Social Status, Wealth and Individual Differences Among the Yoruba," in *American Anthropologist,* Volume 53, pp. 490–505, 1951.

It seems possible, therefore, that we have now come upon cultural differences of some importance for psychiatric assessment. Depression appears to be an unfamiliar concept to the Yoruba, and there is linguistic difficulty in finding Yoruba words with which to describe the subjective feelings meant by the term. It is likely that these circumstances could have a distorting influence, from the psychiatric point of view, on the responses obtained from patients and their families in the course of examination and history taking.

Impairment

The Yoruba see a person as handicapped by his mental and emotional illness to the degree that his symptoms interfere with his relationships to parents, husband, wife, or child; with his ability to earn a living; and with his participation in the common activities of the community. The idea of "impairment" also includes the individual's suffering, even though he may be able to carry on his economic and interpersonal functions despite this.

Ideas of Cause

It is here that the views of healers and other Yorubas part most widely from the ideas of psychiatrists. As we listened to our informants discuss cases and case types, a large number of causes emerged. While some of these would be accepted by psychiatrists, many would not, especially those which the Yoruba emphasize. In what follows we have organized the various causes into a limited number of categories, and present them in order of the importance the Yoruba attach to them.

Malignant influences   These may be superhuman attacks from gods, spirits, and ghosts and may be occasioned by breaking taboos or failing in ceremonial duties. Influences may also come from human agents through witchcraft, curses, and the practice of magic (or *"juju"* as it is called throughout West Africa).

Drugs and medicines   Certain substances, if taken into the body, have tremendous power. Some can produce illness, others can cure.

Heredity   Some people suffer illness because they are born with it. Also, to the Yoruba an illness is a being; it has life and a volition of its own. As such, it can exist for a time in one person, or it may continue for several generations in the family, lying hidden part of the time.

Contagion   Although there is no theory of germs, it is believed that many illnesses can be acquired from a sick person, and some disturbances of the mind and emotions are thought to be transmitted in this way. The prime instance of this belief that came to our attention is the idea that foam from the mouth of a person with epilepsy can produce seizures and accompanying mental disturbances in one who touches it.

Violation of one's destiny   The thought here is that each person has his own destined life pattern fixed by a contract made before he was born. If wittingly or unwittingly he departs from this, the results may be mental or emotional illness.[7]

Cosmic forces   Illness may be influenced by the moon, by the sun, or by dry season.

Physical traumata   A blow on the head is the paradigm for this, but Yoruba people also think that other kinds of accidents, loss of blood, or serious sickness can, on occasion, affect thinking and emotions.

Psychological traumata   It is believed that severely distressing experiences can sometimes produce acute or chronic disturbances that may properly be called illness. It is also believed that such experience can produce those feelings and behaviors which psychiatry regards as indicative of psychoneurotic and other disorders, but which the Yoruba do not classify as illness. On the whole, however, belief in psychological experience as a cause is weak.

It is now apparent why there is so little correspondence between Yoruba and psychiatric diagnostic categories. In each the main outlook on the nature of cause, despite certain similarities in mode of thought, is radically different. The Yoruba group together symptoms and causal ideas in ways that have no counterpart in psychiatry, and this makes comparisons based on etiological typology impossible.

On the other hand, if attention is limited to the comparison of symptom patterns, rather than diagnostic categories, a great part of the cross-cultural obstacle disappears. What is left points to the need to ask about some symptoms under headings other than illness, and to realize that for a study of the Yoruba there are special problems regarding the symptom patterns represented by the psychiatric words "phobic," "obsessive-compulsive," and especially "depressed."

This conclusion is, of course, limited to the Yoruba. It suggests, however, a way of conceptualizing psychiatric phenomena and an approach

---

[7] For an account of Yoruba ideas of soul, fate, and destiny see: William Bascom, "Yoruba Concepts of the Soul," in *Selected Papers of the Fifth International Congress of Anthropological and Ethnological Sciences,* Philadelphia, September 1–9, 1956, edited under the Chairmanship of A. F. C. Wallace, Philadelphia: University of Pennsylvania Press, pp. 401–410.

to cross-cultural comparison that may have much wider use. A framework is provided for making and comparing observations that promises sufficient objectivity to permit replication and validity checks by independent observers. The separation of phenomena (symptoms) from notions of cause strengthens the possibility of discovering—rather than assuming—etiological relationships. Thus, cultural perceptions and influences are not ignored, but remain alive as questions to be explored step by step.

THE STIRLING COUNTY STUDY

The conclusions outlined in the previous section are congruent with the methods employed in a number of investigations in psychiatric epidemiology among people of Western culture. Thus, the Stirling County Study (Hughes, 1960; A. H. Leighton, 1959; D. Leighton, 1963), which may be taken as an example, has used symptom patterns as a basis for estimating the prevalence of psychiatric disorder in community populations.

This study was made in a rural and small-town county in one of the Atlantic provinces of Canada. The population of 20,000 is about half English and half Acadian French and is distributed in small communities of a few hundred or less, with one town of 3000 people. A major means of data collection was a questionnaire survey of a probability sample of the adults of the county. A systematic sample of households was made, and the interviewers took alternately the male and the female household head. These data were supplemented by interviews with local key informants regarding all the individuals surveyed. In addition, hospital records pertaining to county residents were collected both locally and from the nearest large metropolitan hospitals.

The psychiatric data obtained regarding each individual in the sample consisted of a review of the systems of the body for physical symptoms, and a series of questions about psychiatric symptoms. For evaluating these data, we used independent ratings by two or more psychiatrists who then prepared a joint evaluation of the person stating whether he did or did not show significant psychiatric symptoms, how much his functioning was impaired by such symptoms, and the degree of confidence felt that he was or was not a psychiatric "case."

With a few modifications, it was possible to use the terminology of the *Diagnostic and Statistical Manual* (American Psychological Association, 1952) for codification purposes, but we did not try to make diagnoses. Instead, we employed the terms descriptively and recorded for each person as many different symptom patterns as he showed. With this method, it was possible to achieve a workable degree of agreement between psychiatrists on each of the required judgments.

A first task of the social scientists was to select communities showing low and high levels of sociocultural integration. This was done initially by interviewing knowledgeable local informants. These communities were then studied intensively by participant observers, who usually lived in them. The social scientists also analyzed questionnaire survey data according to various sociocultural criteria, which included occupational position, education, migration, extent of French or English cultural commitment, and religious involvement.

THE YORUBA STUDY

The research area consisted of about 100 square miles around the Aro Hospital for Nervous Diseases, which is located near the city of Abeokuta (population approximately 80,000), in the western part of Nigeria. The people in this area are almost exclusively of the Yoruba tribe (whose membership numbers about 5,000,000), and Abeokuta is the headquarters for the Egba subtribe.

Within the area, a preliminary selection of twenty-five villages, and from these a final selection of fifteen, was made to provide a range in size, in modernization, and in state of sociocultural integration. Eight segments of Abeokuta were also chosen for study.

Psychiatric interviewing was done with a male and a female adult in each selected household in the villages and towns. The households were chosen according to sampling principles. Anthropological data were gathered concomitantly, again using samples, and had as a main focus the detecting of cultural change and determining of various levels of integration. A team of four full-time and two part-time psychiatrists and three social scientists made up the behavioral research group, together with numbers of interpreters and assistants, and a medical team that provided treatment for all comers in the villages while the interviewing was going on. It should be noted that two of the psychiatrists, Lambo and Asuni, are themselves members of the Yoruba tribe.

Working intensively for three months, psychiatric data were collected on 262 villagers and 64 residents of Abeokuta. Interviews lasted 1½ to 2 hours each. Also, during the three-month period, 152 social science questionnaire interviews were obtained from the same sample of people in the villages and in Abeokuta, as well as more free ranging interviews with headmen and elders.

Evaluations following the Stirling technique were then carried out on the 326 psychiatric interviews.

TABLE 1. ALL SURVEY RESPONDENTS BY AGE, SEX, AND PLACE OF STUDY
(IN PERCENTAGES)

	39 or under	40–59	60 and over	Total	No.
Yoruba villages (Africa)					
Men	32	40	28	100	(138)
Women	46	28	26	100	(124)
Total	38	35	27	100	(262)
Abeokuta (Africa)					
Men	28	47	25	100	(32)
Women	37	44	19	100	(32)
Total	33	45	22	100	(64)
Stirling County (North America)					
Men	30	40	30	100	(463)
Women	40	36	24	100	(547)
Total	35	38	27	100	(1010)

COMPARISON OF FINDINGS

The distribution of respondents by age and sex for the two Nigerian and one North American sample is shown in Table 1. The limitation to three age groups is due chiefly to the difficulty of ascertaining the exact age of Yoruba respondents.

The similarity of the sex and age distribution in the Yoruba villages to that in Stirling County is striking. We had anticipated that early deaths would leave a lower percentage of Yoruba in the middle and especially the older age groups. Abeokuta women differ somewhat from the village pattern, but not significantly.

Table 2 shows the percent of A, B, C, and D or "caseness" ratings and the percent of significant impairment.

The Yoruba villages show the smallest percentage of A's (almost certainly psychiatric disorder) and the second smallest percentage of B's (or probables). If these two are added together, and compared across the three groups, the result is a steady rise from the villages through Abeokuta to Stirling County. The differences between villages and Stirling in both A and A + B is significant at the 1 percent level. The D percentage (or "well" people) is higher for both groups of Yoruba than for Stirling, a difference that is significant at the 5 percent level of confidence.

The percent showing impairment also rises from left to right, with twice as large a proportion in Stirling as in the Nigerian villages (a difference with statistical significance at the 1 percent level). In both

TABLE 2. MAIN PSYCHIATRIC RATING AND IMPAIRMENT IN SURVEY RESPONDENTS (IN PERCENTAGES)[a]

	Villages	Abeokuta	Stirling County
Number of respondents	262	64	1,010
A	21	31	31
B	19	14	26
A + B	40	45	57
C	35	30	26
D	25	25	17
Total	100	100	100
Significantly impaired	15	19	33

[a] A = almost certainly an instance of psychiatric disorder; B = probably an instance of psychiatric disorder; C = doubtful; D = almost certainly a psychiatrically well individual.

samples, the great bulk of this impairment is mild. The excess in percent of A + B ratings over the percent with mild or greater impairment emphasizes the fact that a person can exhibit psychiatric symptoms without being impaired by them throughout the greater part of his life.

At this point, we wish to introduce a statistical score called the "ridit," which has certain advantages over the percentage. The term "ridit" stands for "index relative to an identified distribution." Bross (1958), its originator, applied the index first to the measurement of severity of injury sustained in automobile accidents (Bross & Feldman, 1956). In the field of psychiatric epidemiology, it has been used in both the Midtown and Stirling County studies.

Some of the characteristics of the ridit are as follows: It has a range from 0 to 1 with a mean of .50 in the identified distribution which serves as a standard of reference. The meaning of a "high" ridit—that is, one larger than .50—is determined by the nature of the variable being measured. As applied to mental health ratings, the higher the ridit number, the poorer is the mental health condition. The ridit of a single individual is interpreted as the probability that he is worse off than an individual selected at random from the reference distribution group. The average ridit of a subgroup is interpreted as the probability that an individual selected at random from this group is worse off than another individual selected at random from the reference distribution group. One advantage of the ridit as compared to percent is that in ratings such as ABCD and impairment, it combines in a single index number both the influence of frequency and the influence of degree. That is to say, it

TABLE 3. ABCD Ridits by Age and Sex, Yoruba Villages, Abeokuta, and Stirling County (Stirling-based Ridit)[a]

	Villages	Abeokuta	Stirling County
Men			
Under 40	.45	.46	.40
40–59	.41	.43	.45
Over 60	.44	.39	.47
Total	.43	.43	.44
Women			
Under 40	.38	.52	.45
40–59	.43	.38	.62
Over 60	.37	.71	.61
Total	.39	.49	.55
Men and Women	.41	.46	.50

[a] These ridits are calculated, for all three samples, without weighting for differences in sampling rates.

registers not only the prevalence of A, B, C, or D in relation to the whole sample but also their combined effect. If, for instance, a subgroup of the sample had a high frequency of A's but also a high frequency of D's, the modifying effect of the D's registers in the subgroup's ridit. Another subgroup with the same proportion of A's but with fewer D's and hence more C's and B's would have a higher ridit.

The ABCD ridits for the villages, Abeokuta, and Stirling are shown on Table 3. As noted above, the ridit of any individual expresses his probable degree of mental illness or health in relation to a particular reference population. In this table only, the reference population is that of the Stirling County Study, in order to make comparisons from the two cultures clearer.

A review of the tables that show the A and B ratings, impairment, and the ABCD ridits (Tables 2 and 3) makes evident a general trend among the totals. This is the rise in psychiatric disorder, as reflected in these measures, from the villages through Abeokuta to Stirling County. Although the differences in psychiatric ratings between the villages and Abeokuta are not striking, they are nonetheless worth noting. The psychiatric findings are in keeping with what is suspected to be the difference of influence in social environments portrayed by the villages and Abeokuta. Abeokuta is a more complex competitive milieu than the villages; Western influences are noticeable, and the changes that they imply have occurred with greater intensity and in more rapid sequence. A further point

TABLE 4. Current Symptom Patterns Among Survey Respondents, Yoruba Villages, Abeokuta, and Stirling County

	Villages	Abeokuta	Stirling County[a]
Number of respondents	262	64	1,010
Symptom Patterns[b]			
Psychophysiologic	81%	95%	59%
Gastrointestinal	42	50	33
Musculoskeletal	34	52	22
Cardiovascular	20	33	15
Headaches	42	55	12
Respiratory	8	16	3
Genitourinary	24	47	4
Skin	18	28	1
Endocrine	3		2
Overweight	c		6
Subjective body sensations	38	41	not used
Psychoneurotic	71	77	52
Anxiety	27	36	10
Depressive	30	27	7
Hypochondriacal			4
Other	53	61	41
Personality disorder	7		6
Passive-aggressive	3		1
Emotionally unstable	2		2
Compulsive			c
Inadequate	c		1
Other	3		3
Sociopathic behavior	2		6
Alcohol	2		3
Dyssocial			2
Antisocial	1		1
Drug addiction			c
Mental deficiency	2		5
Psychosis	2		1
Affective			c
Schizophrenic	1		1
Other	c		c
Brain syndrome	5	8	3
Chronic	5	6	2
Convulsive	1	3	c
Other		2	1

[a] In this table the percentages for Stirling County are figured on the basis of a weighted sample.

[b] Some symptom patterns described in the handbook are not listed here because we found no examples.

c More than zero but less than 0.5 percent.

of note is that the ABCD ridit for men is virtually the same in all three groups. This means that the marked group differences are due to the women. In the Yoruba villages, the women are, if anything, healthier than the men. The reverse appears true in Abeokuta and Stirling.

The symptoms for the villages, Abeokuta, and Stirling County are shown in Table 4.

Although the actual percentage of respondents showing symptoms in a major symptom category (psychophysiologic, psychoneurotic, and so on) varies considerably between groups, it is nonetheless interesting that the over-all patterning is similar—there are many psychophysiologic and psychoneurotic symptom patterns and very few of the other categories.

Probably more revealing than the direct comparison or percentages between Yoruba and Stirling samples is the comparison of rank order. The major symptom categories of psychophysiologic, psychoneurotic, and personality disorder have the same rank order in the villages and in Stirling. Under psychophysiologic, moreover, the villages and Stirling County have the same rank order for gastrointestinal, musculoskeletal, and cardiovascular. Under psychoneurotic, the "other" category is much the most common in all three groups, with anxiety or depression coming next. Hypochondriasis was not definable by our methods in the Yoruba sample because of the large overlay of organic disorder. The total absence of persons showing symptoms in four categories in Abeokuta (personality disorder, sociopathic, mental deficiency, and psychosis) is probably a function of the small size of the sample (64). It should be noted, however, that in the psychophysiologic and psychoneurotic categories a trend upward is discernible from the villages to Abeokuta. This follows the same pattern as the A + B ratings, impairment, and total ABCD ridits mentioned earlier as being congruent with the environmental picture.

With regard to points where there are major differences in rank order, it can be seen that under psychophysiologic the Yoruba stand out for apparently having more headaches, respiratory difficulty, genitourinary disturbance, and skin trouble. We attribute most of this to the generally higher prevalence of organic disorder which affects the percentage figures of this whole major symptom category.

In view of the literature on depression in Africa, it is interesting to observe that our percentage figures suggest that the Yoruba have a greater prevalence of depressive symptoms than was found in the North American sample. Not only were these symptoms present in our respondents, but they were common and easily detected in response to the same questions employed in Stirling County.

Two categories that are found more frequently in Stirling County are sociopathic behavior and mental deficiency. It seems reasonable to suppose that there was actually more sociopathic behavior in the comparatively more complex, less intimate group in North America than in the face-to-face African village.

In the case of mental deficiency, it seems likely that the apparent lower percentages in Nigeria constitute an artifact. Without the measure of school achievement, this symptom pattern is not easy to detect in its milder forms, and most of the interviewers and evaluators were probably not sufficiently familiar with the culture to pick up indications of mild subnormal mental functioning.

Even though people with sociopathic symptoms are few, it is clear that they consist chiefly of abusers of alcohol, as was the case in Stirling. It seems quite likely that if we had known more details about the social structure and standards, we might have detected at least some dyssocial individuals.

The increased amount of brain syndrome among the Yoruba as compared to Stirling County may be an indirect effect of the commoner occurrence of disease. Since Table 4 shows only current symptom patterns, and since the sample did not include any persons suffering from an acute brain syndrome, it is worth reporting that the addition of past symptoms would raise the brain syndrome percentage 1.1 percent for the villages and 4.7 percent for Abeokuta, while it would not change the Stirling County figures at all. On the whole, however, it was surprising that we did not encounter more evidence of brain syndrome.

In the Stirling County study, a high association was found between a community's level of sociocultural integration and the prevalence of

TABLE 5. ABCD Ridit and Level of Integration in the Yoruba Villages and Stirling County, for Men and Women

	Yoruba Villages		
	Integrated	Intermediate	Disintegrated
Men	.50	.53	.51
Women	.30	.53	.55
Both sexes	.40	.53	.53
	Stirling County		
Men	.45	.44[a]	.68
Women	.52	.55[a]	.65
Both sexes	.48	.50[a]	.66

[a] Average for the whole county.

psychiatric disorder. In the Yoruba study, we hoped to get some idea whether the same kind of association would be found among the Yoruba —that is, in a cultural context that is markedly different from Stirling County. The most convenient figure to use for this comparison is the ABCD ridit. Table 5 shows how the ridit varies with sociocultural integration both in the Yoruba villages and in Stirling County, for men, for women, and with both sexes averaged.

The ridits in this table are simple averages; for example, the sum of ridit scores for all men and all women in integrated villages divided by the total number of respondents in those villages. A similar convention is used in presenting Stirling County ridit data in this context.[8]

In the comparison of Stirling and the Yoruba, it is evident that, over all, the figures show a similar trend: the best mental health is found in the best integrated communities. However, two rather striking differences are evident. In Stirling, the best integrated communities and the county average are rather close together in ridit values, while the disintegrated communities stand apart. With the Yoruba villages, the converse is true— the well integrated communities stand apart, while the intermediate and disintegrated have identical ridit values. This may simply mean that the "county average" and "intermediate" are not comparable. On the other hand, it may imply a sociocultural difference of major importance in the two populations, and as such deserves further investigation.

The other point of contrast is that the Stirling men show a good deal more variation in mental health between integrated and disintegrated communities than do the Stirling women. Among the Yoruba, the women show a high degree of variation, and the men show almost none.

In the case of Stirling County, we are satisfied that the differences are statistically and theoretically significant, but this question needs to be examined more closely in the case of the Yoruba. As a partial control on age, mean ridits were calculated for each of the age divisions that were broken down according to integrated, intermediate, and disintegrated villages. The results are shown in Table 6.

These figures continue to suggest no integration effect on mental health for men but a strong one for women, especially for those under 60. An analysis of variance, employing controls on sex and three age classes, showed that integration has an effect that is significant at the .01 level of confidence.

[8] The complete report on Stirling ridits may be found in D. Leighton et al., (1963). In both Stirling and Nigeria, statistical tests of significance are reported on ridit data corrected for extraneous-to-community influences such as sex and age differences. In addition, statistical controls were used to equalize the distributions of sex and age across community types. See also Snedecor (1956).

TABLE 6. ABCD Ridit and Level of Integration for the
Yoruba Men and Women, by Age Groups

Villages	39 or less	40–59	60 or over
Integrated			
Men	.51 (15)[a]	.53 (13)	.42 (5)
Women	.28 (18)	.33 (7)	.30 (7)
Intermediate			
Men	.58 (20)	.48 (24)	.55 (19)
Women	.56 (25)	.52 (14)	.50 (18)
Disintegrated			
Men	.47 (9)	.56 (14)	.49 (10)
Women	.55 (11)	.62 (10)	.45 (6)

[a] Figures in parentheses are numbers of individuals.

Our interpretation of these findings is that they reflect a difference in the quality of the village environment as it affects men and women. The women of the integrated villages live in a sociocultural environment that fits well with the way their personalities have been conditioned by their upbringing. In other words, there are no major discontinuities between child preparation and adult achievement. While their world is in many ways limited, it is relatively predictable, providing numerous psychological satisfactions and relatively little in the way of uncertainty, confusion, disorientation, role conflict, or other similar sources of anxiety. The women of the disintegrated villages, however, live in an environment that presents them with nearly all the above difficulties.

Yet, the variation in health ridit of the women of the different age groups in the disintegrated villages gives grounds for pause. If the environment, as it affects women in these villages, were uniformly noxious, this variability should not be so apparent. Perhaps its presence is due to the vagaries of sampling, perhaps to selective resistance, or perhaps to other, currently unknown factors. Our general interpretation remains: Traditional sources of security are failing and are not yet replaced by functionally effective new patterns.

With men the situation is different. Because of the very nature of the male role they are more exposed to the turmoil, uncertainties, and frustrations of the general change going on in Yoruba society as part of West Africa. Even in the most integrated villages, the men are thoroughly touched by the changes of the larger society and by difficulties of adjustment and of knowing what to expect and how to conduct themselves. This effect is sufficiently strong and pervasive to render the sociocultural environment of men not drastically different as one moves along the range from integrated to intermediate to disintegrated villages.

A comparison of the integrated and disintegrated columns of Table 6 brings out the male-female differences rather clearly. At all ages in the integrated column, the groups of women have much lower ridits than the groups of men. This is particularly marked in those under 60. However, in the disintegrated column, the women under 60 have a higher ridit (worse mental health) than the men, while those over 60 are almost the same as the men.

We are reminded here of somewhat parallel differences noted among communities in Stirling County. The one community in which the findings suggested that mental health was better among women than men, was one in which a strong traditional (French Acadian) culture gave the women a protected position, while the men were left more exposed to adjustment difficulties emanating from the larger society. In another community, the sociocultural environment appeared more favorable to men than to women, and the situation was reflected not only in the lower ridit of the men but in a wider difference between the sexes than seen in the county average. In the disintegrated communities of Stirling, where the effects of social malfunction are presumably strong on both men and women, the ridits of both sexes were high, but approximately equal.

MAIN POINTS AND INTERPRETATION

The fact of cultural differences between groups poses serious difficulties for cross-cultural studies of psychiatric disorders. This is particularly so when typologies based on etiology are employed. If, however, psychiatric disorders are conceptualized in terms of symptom typologies, a number of avenues are opened for cross-cultural comparison.

A trial of this approach among people of the Yoruba tribe in Nigeria indicated that Yoruba healers are familiar with most of the symptom patterns known to Western psychiatry and regard them either as illness or at least as undesirable behavior. Three exceptions to this generalization were, however, encountered. Our informants were not acquainted with either phobic or obsessive compulsive symptom patterns. Depression as a unified pattern was also unfamiliar, but here the component elements such as excessive crying, loss of appetite, worry, and so on, were recognized as manifestations of trouble. We detected no indication that the Yoruba are familiar with symptom patterns that are unfamiliar to psychiatry. But their concepts and typology of causes are in a framework so different from that of psychiatry as to make comparison largely impossible.

On the basis of discussion with Yoruba informants, it appears that if the clinical investigator focuses on symptom patterns rather than diagnostic categories a great many of the obstacles inherent in cultural relativity disappear. While such a conclusion is of necessity limited to the Yoruba in this instance, it seems likely that the approach does have a much wider use. The separation of phenomena (symptoms) from ideas of cause not only facilitates cross-cultural comparisons, but also avoids built-in correlations and enhances the chances of discovering various cultural and environmental factors of importance that otherwise might remain imputed rather than demonstrated.

Employing a method based on symptoms, our research group made a comparison of psychiatric disorder prevalence between rural Yorubas and the inhabitants of a small town and rural area in North America. Probability samples of both populations were employed as subjects for investigation, and the full range of psychiatric disorders were considered. This last means that the statistics refer mainly to milder types of psychoneurotic disturbances rather than to sweeping impairments such as psychoses.

Interpreting the results, it appears that the two populations are fairly similar in the kinds and general proportions of the disorders manifested. Despite various factors that could have entered to distort comparisons, it seems likely that the rural Yorubas studied have a lower prevalence rate of impairing psychiatric disorders than their North American counterparts. Further, an investigation of a small sample of urban Yorubas suggests that here the prevalence rate is higher, approaching more the North American level.

Of particular interest are male-female differences. In the Western group, women generally have a higher prevalence rate than men. Among the Yoruba the women appear to have the same or a lower rate than the men. It is plausible to suppose that this is a matter of role and role change. In most of the villages that were the subjects of this study, the Yoruba women were living according to highly stable (so far) traditions, in a world pretty well apart from men and with a minimum of discontinuity between the conditioning experienced in childhood and the fulfillments of adult life. The men on the other hand, whether Yoruba or Western, were living much more in a changing and uncertain environment, with many consequent psychological difficulties, and especially the experience of discontinuities in the course of their lives. The women of the Western group, finally, are even more exposed to environmental turmoil than either group of men because they are undergoing a double set of changes. They are exposed to all the main factors affecting Western men, and in addition they have the particular problems and uncertainties characteristic of the well-known alterations in feminine role that have been an outstanding feature of these times in the West.

Some credence to these interpretations is given by the fact that in the one village studied in the Western group which had a highly stable social environment for women, their mental health picture approached that of the Yoruba group. Conversely, in the socioculturally disintegrated Yoruba villages, the mental health of the women is, if anything, worse than that of the men.

The study of sociocultural disintegration among both Yoruba and Western groups shows a high over-all correlation between sociocultural disintegration and the prevalence of psychiatric disorders. A breakdown according to sex reveals that among the Western group this difference is mainly due to the men, while among the Yoruba it is entirely due to the women. In line with what has already been said above about sex differences, this can be explained by saying that the noxious effects of sociocultural disintegration are more evident in a group that has good mental health than in one that has bad. Possibly in the latter case the susceptible individuals are for the most part already affected, so that additional environmental malignant influences do not alter the group prevalence very much.

The apparent relationship of sociocultural disintegration to psychiatric disorder has a number of implications. One of these is that in situations of cultural change it is the disintegration, and not cultural change in and of itself, that is damaging to mental health. If this is so, one would expect to find that communities that undergo cultural change, but do so while maintaining a functional social system, would not show a high prevalence rate of psychiatric disorder. This consideration led our research into the comparative study of traditional versus "modern" Yoruba communities with and without sociocultural disintegration. The results are tentative, but, such as they are, they do point to poor group mental health being associated with disintegration whether it occurs in a traditional or a modern setting. Comparatively low prevalence is found in communities that are modern and well integrated. Apparently, the worst position of all is to be traditional and disintegrated.

In concluding this chapter, I would like to suggest that a reciprocal or circular relationship between sociocultural disintegration and psychiatric disorder seems exceedingly likely. Thus, it would seem that preventive psychiatry has a stake in preventing and correcting sociocultural disintegration as a form of mental hygiene. On the other hand, development programs, with their inherent tendency to alter and so disrupt social systems, have a stake in having as low a prevalence of psychiatric disorder as possible in the population being developed. Apathies, depressions, and anxieties can reduce motivation and increase the occurrence of program failures. The best kind of active intervention, therefore, is one in which the development program is supported by projects concerned with maintaining both the functioning of the social system and the mental health of the constituent members. The phrase "congruent programming" might be used to designate such an approach.

REFERENCES

American Psychiatric Association, *Diagnostic and Statistical Manual: Mental Disorder.* APA Mental Hospital Service, 1952.

Bross, I. D. J. & Feldman, R. *Ridit Analysis of Automotive Crash Injuries,* New York, Cornell University Medical College, 1956.

————, "How to Use Ridit Analysis" in *Biometrics,* Vol. 14, No. 1, pp. 18–38, 1958.

Hughes, C. C., *et al., People of Cove and Woodlot; Communities from the Viewpoint of Social Psychiatry.* New York: Basic Books, 1960.

Leighton, A. H., *My Name Is Legion: Foundations for a Theory of a Man in Relation to Culture.* New York: Basic Books, 1959.

Leighton, A. H., *et. al., Psychiatric Disorder Among the Yoruba; A* Report from the Cornell-Aro Mental Health Research Project in the Western Region, Nigeria, Cornell University Press, 1963.

Leighton, D., *et al., The Character of Danger: Psychiatric Symptoms in Selected Communities.* New York: Basic Books, 1963.

Snedecor, G. W. *Statistical Methods Applied to Experiments in Agriculture and Biology.* Ames, Iowa: Iowa State College Press, 1956.

2.8   Orientation

Polynesia has often been referred to as a natural laboratory for the study of mental illness, a place where the gene pool, the language, and the culture are all constant and only the stress of culture change varies from island to island. Alas, the realities of modern Polynesia are immensely complex, as this chapter, completed shortly before his death by the late Professor Ernest Beaglehole, demonstrates. In attempting to determine what the life stresses in Polynesia are, and how they are reflected in differential rates of mental illness, Beaglehole introduces us to the complications of social psychiatric research —to uncorrected hospital data, to diagnostic categories that may vary in meaning from place to place, to omnipresent change that resists simple measurement, and to the pressing need for carefully designed research.

Polynesia is ethnically complex, and it is changing. Understanding

the psychological impact of change in ethnically different populations is a fundamental concern of all who are concerned with mental
illness. As Ernest Beaglehole shows us, this understanding is not
easily purchased.

2.8   Pathology among Peoples of the Pacific

Ernest Beaglehole

Two classes of variables must be studied in any attempt to establish
hypotheses explaining the determination of mental disorder: genetic-
physiological influences and environmental-stress influences. Much ingenuity in experiment and research design has been devoted to the impossible task of disentangling these two interoperating influences. Students
of mental health early decided that that part of the Pacific known as
Polynesia (roughly, all those island groups between Hawaii in the north,
Easter Island to the east, New Zealand to the south, and skirting the east-
tern boundaries of Fiji in the west) constituted an almost perfect natural
laboratory for the study of the determinants of mental disorder.

THE GENETIC BASIS OF POLYNESIAN CULTURE

In Polynesia, so the preamble ran, the social scientist finds a people of
one basic and similar ethnic stock, language, and culture—genotypes, if
you will—split, by migrations and subsequent cultural and ecological
determinants, into a number of different sociocultural or phenotypical
units. The genotype has been held constant. The phenotypes differ in
definable, anthropological ways. A study, therefore, of mental disorders
among these different Oceanic communities should enable us to say with
some precision what is the role of environmental stresses in the causation
of mental disorder in Oceania. All the likenesses are largely genotypical;
all the differences phenotypical.

The design is neat, the laboratory is ready. Then secondary questions
intrude. How uncontaminated today is our genotype, genetically and
culturally? The biological answer now seems to be that Oceania and
Polynesia, far from being an ethnically pure and stable population, really
consists of a native population which from 1521 (when Magellan first
discovered the South Seas for the Western world) up to the present has
been subject to continuous intermixture with European immigrants,
whether as beachcombers, missionaries, whalers, traders, planters, or
government officials. The number of immigrants involved at any partic-

ular time is hard to estimate, but Maude, for example, suggests that in 1818 there were as many as 200 escaped convicts from New South Wales enjoying the life idyllic in the Sandwich Islands (Maude, 1964, p. 259). At about the same period, Maude also suggests that of Polynesian beach-combers in general, 75 percent of them were British and American seamen, 20 percent were convicts (mostly Irish), the remainder a handful of Ne-groes, Lascars, and Red Indians.

Even if the number of immigrants is hard to estimate, we can be sure that the amount of intermixture was considerable. Maude indicates that many inhabitants of the Gilbert Islands today are of part-European de-scent. When Maude knew him, one European beachcomber in the Gilberts had reduced his wives from seven to three, but at last fifty of his known children could be listed by the conscientious district officer. Whichever way one looks in Oceania, whether to Tahiti, Hawaii, the Marquesas, Fiji, Melanesia, or New Zealand, it is doubtful that one can see many pure-blooded natives (Maude, 1964, p. 274; Harre, 1962, p. 20). This point would not need emphasis but for the fact that the 1961 census for New Zealand implies that 62 percent of the Maori population today is of pure Maori blood. It is most probable that such statistics on the propor-tion of full-blooded Maori in the New Zealand population are inaccurate. New Zealanders not only consider it indelicate to question a person— Maori or European—about his ethnic origin, but some social and minor financial advantages still accrue today to any New Zealander, and to his children or his grandchildren, who can claim half or more "Maori blood." Thus, Maori census returns tend to be weighted, almost unconsciously and in good faith, in favor of full-bloodedness.

In addition to this extensive cross-cultural mating between Europeans and Polynesians, there has always been within Oceania a large amount of intraregional cross-cultural migration and contact. In pre-European days, this migration was due to drift and possible intentional voyages. After European contact, much of this intraregional contact resulted from the fact that whaling and trading vessels, missionary and slaving vessels, from time to time landed natives from one part of Oceania on the faraway islands of another part: thus Hawaiians could be found on Tahiti, Tonga, and Rotuma; Maori on Rotuma, Rarotonga, and Ponape; and more recently (as indentured laborers), Tonkinese in New Caledonia, Chinese and Melanesians in Samoa. Filipinos, Portuguese, Chinese, and Japanese have also added to the biological mixture in Hawaii.

Some of this intraregional migration may have had minimal effect upon genotypes. Other aspects of it have undoubtedly left behind sufficient traces that materially alter phenotypical forms of structure and function-ing.

Far from possessing a genotypically stable population, then, Oceania and Polynesia may probably be said to encompass one of the most diverse populations in the world. Only in isolated islands or hidden hinterlands may there still exist today pockets of pure-blooded Polynesians who are usable as controls for genetic investigations.

It may, of course, be supposed that the important variable for study is not the relation of ethnic genetic types to mental disorder, but rather the effects of culture in the production of behavioral disorder. Thus, the argument would run, we must try to show how a presumed universal Polynesian genetic stock has responded to the stresses and strains of a similar but not identical culture, as Polynesian peoples have historically migrated from island to atoll, from tiny atoll to large land mass. One hundred and fifty years ago this program of study for Polynesia might have been viable. Today, after long years of acculturation, New Zealand Maori culture no longer imposes its Polynesian-like stresses upon the dark-skinned Maori-speaking New Zealander in quite the same fashion that Hawaiian American culture imposes its patterns upon Americans of Hawaiian ancestry in Hawaii. Acculturation has proceeded at such different rates in response to different sociocultural stresses that comparisons, in order to be meaningful, can be made only in the most general terms, and in terms that, perhaps, suggest hypotheses, rather than empirical definitions.

One aspect of this problem may be illustrated from New Zealand experience in trying to define who is a Maori. Since there is in New Zealand today some legislation that discriminates in favor of the Maori as compared with his European fellow-citizen, administrative and census definition is of considerable import. Some definitions, for census or electoral purposes, for example, allow a person to state whether he elects to be a Maori and what percentage of Maori blood he claims to possess. It is generally conceded by anthropologists that there are many persons on the Maori electoral roll who possess less than half or more Maori ancestry that is the criterion for admission to this roll (Harre, 1965, p. 20). Again, a recent adminstrative survey (Hunn, 1961, pp. 19, 85–86) states that there are at least ten different statutory definitions of what constitutes being a Maori.

In these troubled waters, psychologists have also been fishing. A study by Williams (1960, pp. 22–50) following up earlier suggestions by Ritchie (1963, pp. 36–38), applied a modest scale of "Maoriness" to Maori teacher-trainees. An item analysis and a factor analysis of the results showed that there were two kinds of "Maoriness"—that is, of Maori cultural self-identity—the two being negatively correlated with each other. They can be termed "Maoriness by enculturation" and "Maoriness by choice." Some Maori today consciously attempt to accumulate Maori culture, knowledge, lore, and practice. They are Maori by conscious choice and learning. Other Maori are Maori because of childhood training and up-bringing—enculturation, if you will. Finally, there are persons who look like, and call themselves, Maori although they are in fact rapidly ac-culturating to New Zealand European culture. With at least these three kinds of psychologically defined Maori and the ten different statutory definitions of a Maori (the latter basically reducible to definitions empha-sizing either half-blood or more descent from a Maori), it can hardly be expected that there will be in New Zealand a clear-cut relationship be-tween ethnic affiliation (or culture) and mental disorder. Doubtless, a comparable contemporary analysis of the Hawaiian scene would result in the same conclusion and confusion about the Hawaiian population in Hawaii.

This introduction, then, purports to argue that data on the differential incidence of mental disorder in Polynesia are suspect. They cannot be taken at their face value. They must be regarded, at least, as indicating possible, and perhaps even probable, relationships between culture and mental disorder that may now serve as hypothesis-generators to be tested by other means in other parts of the world.

I can best indicate these relationships by considering in turn two closely related problems: what in general is the nature of Polynesian cultural stresses? and secondly, employing Western psychiatric diagnostic categories, how do subcultural areas in Polynesia differ in the incidence of mental disorders? In this field one cannot systematically review and compare data from one island after another. One can only follow rather limited data, wherever available, and draw whatever conclusions seem appropriate from these data trails.

POLYNESIAN CULTURAL STRESS

That Polynesian culture, like any other, inevitably causes stress con-ditions that lead to behavioral conflicts and often to outright psychotic conditions, is well documented both by contemporary qualitative reports and also by the historical record. Stress conditions, metaphorically de-scribed by Kroeber (1948, p. 404) as "cultural fatigue," were apparently responsible for the dramatic overthrow of the Hawaiian *tapu* system of social controls in November 1819, when women ate forbidden foods in public and the semi-divine King-chief also broke another prohibition by sitting and eating food with them (Webb, 1965, p. 22). We have no record of Hawaiian mental disorders at or about this time. However, it is not improbable that the social order of the day was seen as so oppressive and frustrating that only a sudden break with the past could adequately relieve the abnormal banking-up of excessive tension.

Contemporary accounts of stress are less dramatic but perhaps more reliable. Margaret Mead informs us that in her study of the Samoan society of Manu'a, she could diagnose in a population of just over 2000 persons at least five cases of behavioral abnormality: one idiot, one imbecile, one feeble-minded boy of 14 years with catatonic dementia, one person with delusions of grandeur, and one sexual invert. On the neighboring island of Tutuila, Mead records at least four additional cases of manic depressive insanity, together with five or six other cases with diagnoses varying from epilepsy to neurasthenia (Mead, 1939, pp. 278–281). Naturally, there were other girls on Manu'a showing abnormal behavioral responses to the physiological and other stresses of growing up (Mead, 1939, pp. 158–184). I have not counted the number of these Samoan "girls in conflict." They were relatively few, but their existence stresses the fact that even in the benign Samoan society described by Mead, some stresses occurred and were likely to result in behavioral disorders. Winston (1934, pp. 236–237) has reexamined Mead's data and produces a figures of 100 cases per 100,000 of population as the Samoan incidence, which, she claims, was about equal to the United States rural data for 1922.

A second qualitative account comes from Tonga, another Polynesian society, with a culture that seems to be tougher and more dour in its values than Samoa. The life of the Tongan (Beaglehole, 1939a, p. 51) is today organized around the tenets and religious practices of contemporary Wesleyan Protestantism: church-going four times each Sunday and three additional times each week, plus a whole week of church-going, with two services each day, to celebrate each New Year. Behind these beliefs rests the power of the Tongan state, which has officially established this religion and implements its morality with secular authority. Stresses in this society can be traced through a study of dreams and an interpretation with common-sense symbolism that emphasizes the behavioral stress of the persons, often young persons of both sexes between 18 and 36 years of age, caught in conflicts caused by clashes in behavioral norms of Puritanism or of intradoctrinal differences, with more easygoing Polynesian moral frames of reference. In the four or five cases of psychosis known in this Tongan island group, mostly manic-depressives, symptoms were for the most part organized about beliefs in the grimmer aspects of a punishing afterlife, and the literal concepts of sinfulness and the symbols of Wesleyan Christianity.

Tongan society changed rapidly in the nineteenth century. Today it appears to have achieved a new social and cultural integration. Significantly, therefore, it is not possible to consider that all Pacific behavioral abnormality is due to the stresses of acculturation (though much can rightfully be ascribed to such strains). When acculturation stabilizes itself in a new and unique cultural form (as has probably now occurred in both Samoa and Tonga), stresses built by chance into this culture and interacting with a contemporary physical phenotype may create the conditions for a development of mental disorder.

In another Polynesian island, the coral atoll of Pukapuka in the Northern Cook Islands, there are historical records that suggest earlier forms of tension release, this time in a violence which does not seem alien to Polynesian character structure (Beaglehole, 1937, p. 1938).

NEW ZEALAND

Contemporary New Zealand and Hawaii offer us opportunities, within the limitations on the data implied by the earlier statements in this chapter, for comparing the incidence of gross forms of mental disorder between Polynesians and peoples of other "racial" stock apparently living together in the same socioeconomic environment. One must emphasize the adverbial qualification *apparently,* since it is probably difficult to establish the fact that the person of Hawaiian Polynesian stock and culture has the same access to power and the other good things of life as the white (*haole*) banker of downtown Honolulu, or that the isolated and rural-dwelling Maori can look forward to the same kind of education as his city Maori or European counterpart. Nonetheless, the general climate of tolerance and understanding for all racial groups is comparable in both countries and acts in such fashion as to offer people of all ethnic stocks reasonably adequate and competent medical or psychiatric help. An examination made some years ago (Beaglehole, 1939c) of the New Zealand mental hospital population showed that over an 11-year period, for psychosis in general, the incidence for Maori males was definitely lower than for males of European stock, while the incidence for Maori females was below that of European females. The total incidence for both sexes is consistently lower among Maori (31 cases per 100,000 of population) than among Europeans (57.7 per 100,000). More exact figures were obtained for the year 1926 by excluding in both populations persons under the age of 16 years, among whom one might expect to find few hospitalized psychotics. These "weighted" figures give an incidence of 83.7 per 100,000 among Europeans and 41.9 per 100,000 among the Maori population. However one looks at these figures and whatever weight one attaches to such variables as socioeconomic status (Maori definitely lower), rural versus city dwelling (Maori predominantly rural dwelling), that operated at the time of analysis and which have sometimes been thought to affect the incidence of psychosis, one can only arrive at the conclusion that the incidence of severe psychosis is definitely lower among the Maori than in the European cultural group.

The first-admission figures for New Zealand mental hospitals may provide unsatisfactory comparisons because of small Maori numbers. Even so, the figures indicate that manic depressive psychoses have a relatively high incidence among Maori females (much higher than for Europeans: an average for three random sample periods, Europeans, 25.8 percent of first admissions, Maori males 26.1 percent, and Maori females 61.0 percent of first admissions). For schizophrenia the European first-admission percentage was 17.6, while that of the Maori was 13.0. Over an 11-year period, and with slightly different calculations, Maori intra-cultural comparisons show that the incidence of manic depression is about twice as high among Maori females as among Maori males, whereas the incidence of schizophrenia is from two or three times as high among Maori males as it is among Maori females.

The figures just quoted are now almost 30 years old. They may therefore be compared with statistical data more recently collected and published by Foster (1962; but see also New Zealand, Department of Health, 1963). Taking as his definition of a Maori a person of half or more Maori blood, and using as cases Maori people admitted to, discharged from, or dying in New Zealand mental hospitals (but for first admissions using only data collected three months after admissions, when a firm, final diagnosis of a case was made), Foster (1962, p. 3) shows that the over-all picture of Maori admission rates from 1953 to 1960 is one of ever-increasing admissions. During 1953–1957 the mean annual rate was 68.1 first admissions per 100,000 Maori population, increasing to 73.8 per 100,000 for the following three years, and reaching a figure of 123.5 per 100,000 mean Maori population in 1963. These and subsequent Maori figures are significantly higher than those recorded for 1939, and therefore cannot but serve to re-emphasize the fact that growing acculturation pressures bring their cost in mental health casualties.

For the major psychoses, schizophrenia has become by 1958–1960, the leading diagnosis in Maori first admissions: thus, whereas the rate for 1953–1957 was 23.4 per 100,000 and perhaps abnormally low, this rate has increased to 40.9 per 100,000 by 1958–1960. About one case in every three new Maori admissions is now diagnosed as schizophrenia. The rates for manic depressive reactions for 1958–1960, 17.5 per 100,000, show a decrease compared with 1953–1957 (46.9 per 100,000). The possibly correlated changes in schizophrenia and manic depression may be due to differences or changes of fashion in diagnosis over the period studied.

Foster has also studied change in admissions for the group he calls "other psychoses" (small numbers but large decreases in 1958–1960), alcoholism (few cases but small increases for 1958–1960), psychoneurosis (few cases serious enough to be hospitalized, but the 1958–1960 rates substantially higher than for the earlier period), and mental deficiency (a general increase of about 10 percent in rates for the 1958–1960 period).

So much for Maori incidence and for those changes (since this incidence was first studied in 1926) that appear most plausibly to be explained by reference to the pressures of acculturation on the one hand, and to the growing sophistication of the Maori in learning about hospitals (for instance) and their uses, on the other hand.

It now remains to compare Maori and European incidence for this later period, 1958–1960. A significant difference in incidence will still be explainable only by cultural or constitutional-cultural differences between the two populations. In 1958–1960 (or more exactly, the mean population figures for 1959), the diagnosis of schizophrenia accounted for 35.2 percent, or a third of all Maori first admissions, but only for 16.5 percent of European admissions (less than half the Maori figure). For Maoris, there were nearly as many females as males (males 50.8 percent, females 49.2 percent), but for Europeans the relationship was males 43.0 percent, females 57.0 percent. Within the schizophrenic disorder types there were interesting ethnic variations: paraphrenia accounted for 3 percent of Maori cases and 9 percent of European, while catatonia accounted for 9 percent of Maori cases and 4 percent of Europeans (Foster, 1962, pp. 6–7).

For manic depressive reactions, the European rates were generally higher than the Maori rates: European rate is 55.6 per 100,000 for 60–69 year group, contrasted with a comparable Maori rate of 39.1. More European females were manic-depressive than European males, but there were more Maori males than females, thus apparently reversing a trend of earlier statistics (however, the Maori rates for the subgroup of mania were much higher for Maori than for European patients). "States of excitement" could almost be claimed as a Maori mental disorder, with the proviso, however, that in Fiji the spectacular major psychoses account for the majority of hospital admissions. It is not improbable that a relatively unsophisticated people, like Maori or Fijians, are more likely to hospitalize persons who more nearly conform to a popular stereotype of a "madman" or "lunatic," than those numerous cases of neurotics or mental deficients (see Wilson, 1965, p. 366).

For all other psychoses (except alcoholism), the Maori first-admission numbers are small and the ratio correspondingly low: 2.1 percent for Maori and 20.4 percent for Europeans. The Maori rate for hospitalized alcoholism is also very low compared with the European rate, even though the New Zealand public is not infrequently informed that an excessive consumption of alcohol is today a grave Maori social problem. It is doubtless a grave social problem, but for Europeans in New Zealand as well as Maori.

The only conclusion that can be reached by this cross-cultural analysis within New Zealand is that there are marked differences in *hospitalized* psychotic incidence between Maori and European. The emphasis here may need to be placed on the term hospitalized, since there are probably marked cultural differences between Maori and European over the use made of hospitals, whether for physical or mental disorders, or even for Maori births. There are signs that Maori mothers are now making more use of maternity hospitals: in 1937, 16.8 percent of Maori births were in maternity hospitals; in 1960, 91.5 percent of Maori babies were born in hospitals (Foster, 1962, p. 12). Increases in Maori hospital figures for mental disorder may reflect both an increased use of hospitals in general and an increased acculturative stress. One more complication must be introduced before confusion is complete; in New Zealand today, Europeans themselves are making a freer, less emotional, more voluntary use of mental hospitals, as the stigma attached to mental disorder slowly dissipates. Perhaps Maori patients are not unaffected by this process of education.

To arrive at a tentative immediate conclusion, one can make a number of positive statements that hold true, after allowances are made for differences in the age structure of Maori and European populations. These statements imply valid ethnic differences between Maori and European populations. They can be inferred from a slow percentage increase in Maori first admissions to mental hospitals. The differences may be due to differences in the genetic structure of the two populations (although both structures must by now be quite mixed and in the midst of rapid change), differences in cultural adjustment (however one looks at the Maori today, he is still a Maori culturally and not just a colored European), differences (now narrowing, but still significant perhaps for psychoneuroses and mental deficiency) in the use of community health facilities. All in all, the differences appear to be due more to a cultural than to a constitutional variable, and to a cultural variable that must be viewed mainly as an acculturative stress.

Before going on to the case of Hawaii, one might mention in passing that some additional evidence to support the low New Zealand hospital figures for psychoneurosis is contained in official histories of Maori battle casualties during the second world war. New Zealand histories of the various war theaters in which New Zealanders were engaged show that the incidence of war neurosis among Maori soldiers was minimal and absolutely lower than the incidence for New Zealand European soldiers. Also, subsequent Maori claims for war pensions were likewise definitely lower than the pension claims of European soldiers (Stout, 1954, p. 636, 1956, p. 485). Maori soldiers appear to have been matter-of-fact and resilient fighters during war service (not unlikely a cultural variable), and to have readjusted, rather simply and easily, to subsequent civilian peacetime life.

Their women, however, may be undergoing a more difficult adjustment. A recent study of Maori housewives who have migrated with their husbands and families from rural districts to one major New Zealand town (J. Ritchie, 1964, pp. 95–146) indicates that the level of neurotic-like anxiety is definitely high among these Maori women. The women were tested with TAT, the Maudsley Personality Inventory, and a Sentence Completion test derived in part from Kaplan and Plaut's (1956) Hutterite personality study. Adding some of the results of this careful study to previous work by J. E. Ritchie (1956) on Rorschach testing of a rural Maori sample, we would seem to have reasonably valid data and documentation for the existence of a neurotic tendency among Maori subjects at a surprisingly high rate (about twice Eysenck's English norms). In fact, Ritchie dismisses the earlier popular concept of the Maori as a happy-go-lucky person with no neurotic anxieties or worries as a "piece of wishful pseudo-scientific folklore." She argues that her data show, in fact, that a serious mental health problem exists among urban, acculturating Maori women, among whom tension is exacting a high toll. Whether this Maori neurotic tension is similar to western European neurotic anxiety is probably a question that has to be answered along two different lines. One is that the "pure" anxiety responsible for both Maori and European neuroticism is probably identical, but that there is in Maori society today "less structure and fewer models for the generation of differentiated neurotic states" (J. Ritchie, 1964, p. 103). Rephrased, this statement probably means that, genotypically, Maori and European anxiety is the same, whereas its phenotypical expression varies in amount, structure, and content. European neuroticism, for instance, may be complicated by expressions of guilt. Maori neuroticism, according to the Ritchie study, is a compound of fluctuating mood states, feelings of anxiety, and low morale, but with an absence of guilt feelings. In terms of an increase in the on-going Maori urban migration, the dominant Maori psychoneurosis of the near future may be a syndrome compounded of loneliness, anxiety, and deep and profound misery. It may escape the notice of the European psychiatrists.

It will exist nonetheless and represent one of the less obvious but real overhead expenses of New Zealand Polynesian acculturation (J. Ritchie, 1964, pp. 144–146; J. E. Ritchie, 1963, p. 150; McDonald, 1958, p. 58).

HAWAII

But for the cautions over the raw Polynesian data mentioned in the first section of this chapter, one might be prepared to regard Hawaii as Polynesia's prime social laboratory. But the data must be considered a little suspect. Even so, implications from them seem to be consistent with other Polynesian data. Hence it is worth considering the Hawaiian data in some detail. These data have been analyzed for the nine major ethnic or "racial" groups in Hawaii for the period 1920–1936. One can roughly establish a "ratio of psychosis" for each ethnic group by relating the number of ethnic inmates in the hospital to the proportion that each ethnic group constituted in the total population of the then territory of Hawaii for the various years studied (a figure of 100 shows that a given group has its "correct" proportionate share of psychosis). This ratio gives an extraordinary range and variety of figures: the Filipinos, Japanese and part-Hawaiians, have less than their share of psychosis; all the other ethnic groups have consistently more than their share of psychosis—the "full-blood" Hawaiian about twice his share, the Puerto Rican about three times, and the Korean over five times his share. This "ratio incidence," as it may be termed, when established for first admissions, confirms the picture just outlined. The Hawaiian ratio is still very high (range 161 to 268), as compared with Japanese (range 50 to 65). Filipinos and Puerto Ricans are still at a high rate—higher than Hawaiians (range 46 to 99), but lower than Chinese (73 to 114)—but note that by 1952, a report on Okinawan migrants to Hawaii shows that they have a rate for psychosis higher than any other major group in Hawaii (Wedge, 1952).

The range of variation is probably explainable by reference to the operation of such variables as age composition, sex composition, marital status, socioeconomic status, and other variables among the nine ethnic groups. It is unnecessary to annotate the role of each of these variables in any detail. One only may be considered for illustrative purposes: The sex composition of the population of Hawaii in 1930, a midpoint in the range of years covered, shows that of the four ethnic groups just mentioned (Hawaiian, Puerto Rican, Korean, and Filipino), the sex proportion of the population 15 years and over was 10:10, 10:13, 10:20, and 10:96, respectively. At least some of the ethnic differences in Hawaii are probably attributable to a sex imbalance of population. Whenever it is possible to make corrections for this imbalance, the conclusion seems to be that the incidence of psychosis is about the same for Hawaiian and Polynesian men and women, but that more part-Hawaiian women are psychotic than part-Hawaiian men.

It is possible to study the differential incidence of schizophrenia and of manic depression from the data. Schizophrenia has a relatively high incidence among all ethnic groups in the state. Part-Hawaiians and Puerto Ricans claim the most patients, Hawaiians the fewest. For manic-depression the Filipinos, Koreans, and Japanese stand at the top, with the part-Hawaiians showing the least incidence, the Hawaiian a significant incidence. Where cases are classified as preponderatingly manic or depressive, the manic condition is high among the Hawaiians and Portugese; depression is relatively low among Hawaiians, relatively low among Portugese, and very high among the Koreans, Chinese, and Filipino groups.

There exist some data that make possible a rough comparison between the incidence of major psychoses among Chinese and Japanese in Hawaii and mainland China or Japan. In rough figures, these comparisons suggest that whereas about 50 percent of psychotics in Japan are schizophrenics, 43–55 percent of Japanese psychotics in Hawaii are schizophrenic. There also seems to be more of a tendency toward manic depression among Japanese in Hawaii than in Japan. The Chinese in Hawaii appear to suffer about the same amount of schizophrenic psychoses as the Chinese in Soochow, but somewhat less from manic-depressive psychoses.

One of the methodological difficulties that has troubled cross-cultural investigators of mental disorder in the Pacific has been an uncertainty as to whether similar diagnostic categories have the same meaning for dissimilar ethnic groups. Many of these categories are in reality little other than blanket generalizations that may disguise more than they reveal about cultural differences. A test case to disentangle similarities and differences has recently been studied in Hawaii, which is peculiarly fitted for such a study by virtue of the fact that all hospitalized ethnic groups are judged "mentally ill" by substantially the same social and psychiatric criteria in the same state hospital by the same psychiatrists. Nonetheless, as Enright and Jaeckle (1961–1962, p. 72) argue, a similar diagnostic category (in this instance "schizophrenia, paranoid type") applied to all male Filipino and Japanese first admissions to Hawaii State Hospital in the 6-year period beginning in July 1954 (123 subjects in all, from the two groups that together made up 47 percent of the total population of the state in 1960) may unwittingly conceal the fact that there are clear and important differences, verified by χ^2 statistical analysis of presenting symptoms, between the two groups, ostensibly similar in diagnostic classification. For instance, Japanese show more disturbance of thinking in the form of confusion, obsession, and preoccupation; Filipinos are more likely to have delusions that persons are wishing to kill them, whereas the Japanese are content with less drastic forms of persecution; again, Japanese are more likely to have ideas of reference, with delusions that they are being influenced, hypnotized, or controlled; finally, Filipinos are more prone than Japanese to indulge in wild, violent, and uncontrollable behaviour. In more general and summary terms, Japanese patients are more restrained and inhibited, with marked autoplastic behavior, than their Filipino counterparts, who are noticeably less constrained and conforming, and more alloplastic in their behavior.

This demonstration that similar diagnostic labels conceal valid and significant cultural differences of behavior represents a valuable corrective to the more usual global and molar ethnic studies of Pacific mental disorder; symptom-study may very well be more rewarding at the cross-cultural level than diagnostic-category reporting. In Hawaii, for instance, we may infer that "schizophrenia, paranoid type," has different behavioral emphasis in the two cultural groups, even though the two groups live in a shared society and participate in a common but not identical culture. Further studies are urgently required to test the validity of this "difference in similarity" hypothesis. They are all the more urgently required in the face of the remorseless march of Euro-American acculturation across the Pacific, which threatens to stamp out valid cultural differences and thus close one laboratory for the detailed study of the cultural phrasing of abnormality.

Any attempt to outline the picture of the incidence of mental disorder in Hawaii is almost inevitably bound to produce either an impressionistic or an abstract portrait. There are many conflicting and interrelated genotypical or constitutional variables. There is the fact that each ethnic group is not only acculturating to a dominant American culture but is also in acculturative competition with at least eight other ethnic groups. The resulting stresses and strains are likely to be continuous and severe. What the figures I have summarized for Hawaii are worth is almost anyone's guess. At a minimum, however, they do most strongly imply that the process of acculturation in Hawaii is an extremely difficult one. Enculturation and socialization by themselves are partly sufficient to produce psychoses among white persons of mainland American descent now living in Hawaii. If enculturation in an amalgam of Hawaiian-American or Hawaiian-Chinese-American culture is now added to this stress, then the miracle seems to lie in the fact that there are so many nonpsychotic persons in Hawaii, not that there are a detectable proportion of psychotics.

FIJI

There is one further Pacific island group, Fiji, for which we have not only cross-cultural mental health data, but also material with sufficient time depth to suggest stability or change in disorder patterns. Unfortunately, the ethnic grouping in Fiji cannot offer any clear-cut comparisons with Polynesian data from Hawaii or New Zealand.

The Fiji Islands are today a meeting place for three or more very different peoples and cultures. In 1962 the population of these islands was estimated to include 213,000 persons of Indian descent (their ancestors were indentured laborers from mainland India), 178,000 Fijians (generally a "racial" and cultural mixture of Polynesians and darker, more Negroid Melanesians), 10,553 Europeans, 9226 part-Europeans (mainly a mixture of Europeans and Fijians), 5177 Chinese, 5300 Rotumans, and 6800 other Pacific islanders. The Fijians are mainly rural-dwelling agriculturalists, the Indians either rural sugarcane growers or small-town businessmen. The Europeans are usually in business, in executive positions in administration or technology (Wilson, 1965, p. 364). In 1936 comparative data were collected for the five ethnic groups of European, Fijian, East Indian, Chinese, and "half-caste" populations (Beaglehole, 1939c, p. 151). By 1965 a single mental hospital of 150 beds, for all the islands in the Fijian group, had been established in Suva, and a flourishing out-patient service was in operation. The 1936 data made possible only approximate statements, to the effect that European and half-caste incidence of psychosis is relatively high and Chinese very high. By 1964 a more refined cross-ethnic analysis was possible, so that Wilson states that despite enormous fluctuation in yearly rates, linear interpolation indicates a hospitalization rate for the confused "others" rate that is consistently higher than that of the Indians and about twice as high as the Fijian rate. Probably part of the reason for the high "others" rate is an older age-grouping of this population and its being composed of that small-family urban population which is everywhere most likely to seek hospitalization.

It is also probable that some of the differences between the Fijian and Indian groups may be due to different degrees of acculturation. Indians are more Europeanized and upwardly class mobile, and therefore more apt to use European hospitals, whereas Fijians, still tribally organized, for the most part, prefer to handle sickness at the rural personal tribal level than by hospitalization in what is still to many Fijians a strange urban institutional culture. That this explanation, though plausible, may not be the whole one is shown by the fact that almost 30 years ago there was still a wide disparity between Indian and Fijian incidence (1936, incidence per 100,000 population: Fijian 16, Indian 67.3, Chinese 201.8). In the light of both 1936 and 1965 figures, it is a little difficult to agree with the conclusion of Berne (1959) that the actual rate of gross psychopathology is probably the same for Fijians and Indians (Wilson, 1965, p. 366). When one reviews the strikingly different cultures of Fiji and India and recalls the attempts of both to adjust to each other and to the dominant European power-culture of the islands, one may well feel it reasonable to expect different cultural incidence and to give high priority in explanation to cultural differences in susceptibility to mental disorder.

This cultural explanation (however it is ultimately phrased in detail —conflicts of value, business worries, economic insecurities, changes in status and role) is given wider plausibility when a comparison is made between specific psychoses in, say, Fiji and New Zealand. Thus, in Fiji, in 1963, schizophrenia and mania together account for 77 percent of admissions to mental hospitals, whereas in New Zealand as a whole in 1962, they account for no more than 20 percent of first admissions (Wilson, 1965, p. 366; see also Foster, 1962).

No reports from Pacific island groups, with the exception of New Zealand figures and speculations already referred to, give any information about the incidence of psychoneuroses. In one very real sense psychoneurosis is a luxury response to stress that only relatively affluent members of the contemporary world can afford to display. For those peoples and cultures closer to the breadline of mere economic existence, psychoneurosis may cause misery and distress, but the people concerned all learn to live with both the misery and the symptoms displayed. Most significantly, in New Zealand, statisticians and psychologists are now beginning to ask questions about the incidence of psychoneurotic disorders among the Maori—a sure sign of increasing Maori integration away from a Polynesian heritage and toward a European cultural future, an integration that displays itself *inter alia* in an increased use by Maori psychoneurotics of New Zealand mental hospital facilities. The position of the Maori in this respect may well remind us of those Oceanic Chamorro women in Saipan of whom Joseph and Murray (1951, p. 289) comment that, although a psychiatric survey detected little unequivocal neurotic illness, many of the younger women making great effort to conform to American cultural patterns were suffering from profound emotional disturbances and were nearing the limits of their capacity for normal functioning.

CONCLUSION

The picture that emerges from this brief survey of mental disorder in Polynesia is, to say the least, smudgy and distorted. There are few undisputed facts that remain undisputed over, say, a decade or two of study. There are apparently no cases in which one can plausibly nominate a C.N.S.–physiological variable responsible for disorder as Wallace can for Eskimo "Arctic hysteria" (Wallace, 1961, pp. 262–270) or the investigators of the New Guinea Fore district can for *kuru* (Harrison, 1964, p. 287). For the most part, Polynesian generalizations can be only temporary stopping places in an on-going process of social, personal, and behavioral change that results from the tendency of an indigenous people, no longer genotypically stable, and no longer culturally similar, to acculturate itself at dissimilar rates to a dominant changing European culture and value system (which is itself sometimes an amalgam of strictly indigenous and strictly imported European values).

The scientific value of the study of mental disorder in Polynesia must lie not in the search for absolutely certain data (the soul that looks for these can receive only a dusty answer), but in the study of social and personal process, the study, in this context, of how Polynesian or Oceanic peoples are meeting the stresses and strains of acculturation. We are probably no longer able from these data to disentangle by comparative study the relative effects of constitutional, genetic, and cultural pressures. But as we study the movement of indexes of incidence of mental disorder among Polynesians, Oceanians, and Europeans in the major island groups of Hawaii, New Zealand, Fiji, and perhaps Tahiti, and secondly, in the (for this purpose) minor groups of Samoa, Tonga, and the Cook Islands, we will at least have some inferential data that we can use to evaluate the sociocultural change that is going on, and the personal cost of this change.

REFERENCES

Beaglehole, E. Emotional release in a Polynesian community. *Journal of Abnormal and Social Psychology.* 1937, **32**, 319–328.

Beaglehole, E. A note on cultural compensation. *Journal of Abnormal and Social Psychology.* 1938, **33**, 121–123.

Beaglehole, E. Psychic stress in a Tongan village. *Sixth Pacific Science Congress, Proceedings,* 1939, 4, 43–52. (a)

Beaglehole, E. *Some modern Hawaiians.* Honolulu: University of Hawaii Research Publications, No. 19, 1939. (b)

Beaglehole, E. Culture and psychosis in New Zealand. *Journal of Polynesian Society,* 1939, **48**, 144–155. (c)

Berne, E. Difficulties of comparative psychiatry: The Fiji Islands. *American Journal of Psychiatry,* 1959, **116**, 104–109.

Enright, J. B. & Jaeckle, W. R. Ethnic differences in psychopathology. *Social Process,* 1961–1962, **25,** 71–77.

Foster, F. H. *Maori patients in mental hospitals.* Wellington, New Zealand: Department of Health, Medical Statistics Branch Special Report No. 8, 1962.

Harrison, G. A., Tanner, J. M., & Barnicot, N. A. *Human biology.* Oxford: Clarendon Press, 1964.

Hunn, J. K. *Report on department of Maori affairs.* Wellington, New Zealand: Government Printer, 1961.

Joseph, A. & Murray, V. F. *Chamorros and Carolinians of Saipan.* Cambridge, Mass.: Harvard University Press, 1951.

Kaplan, B. & Plaut, T. F. A. *Personality in a communal society.* University of Kansas, 1956.

Kimmich, R. A. Ethnic aspects of schizophrenia in Hawaii. *Psychiat.* 1960, **23,** 97–102.

Kroeber, A. L. *Anthropology.* New York, 1948.

McDonald, F. Mental health of the Maori. *Te Ao Hou,* 1958, **6** (4), 57–59.

Maude, H. E. Beachcombers and castaways. *Journal of Polynesian Society,* 1964, **73,** 254–293.

Mead, M. *Coming of age in Samoa* in *From the South Seas.* New York: Morrow, 1939.

New Zealand Department of Health *Annual report of the medical statistician, 1963.* Wellington Department of Health, 1963.

Ritchie, J. E. *Basic personality in Rakau.* Wellington, New Zealand: Victoria University Publications in Psychology, No. 8, 1956.

Ritchie, J. E. *The making of a Maori.* Wellington, New Zealand: Victoria University Publications in Psychology, No. 15, 1963.

Ritchie, Jane. *Maori families.* Wellington, New Zealand: Victoria University Publications in Psychology, No. 28, 1964.

Schmidt, R. C. Psychosis and race in Hawaii. *Hawaii Medical Journal,* 1956, **16,** 144–146.

Stout, T. D. M. *Official history of New Zealand in the Second World War, 1939–45. War Surgery and Medicine.* Wellington, New Zealand: War History Branch, Department of Internal Affairs, 1954.

Stout, T. D. M. *New Zealand medical services in Middle East and Italy.* Wellington, 1956.

Wallace, A. F. C. Mental illness, biology and culture in F. L. K. Hsu (ed.), *Psychological Anthropology,* Homewood, Ill. Dorsey Press, 1961, pp. 255–295.

Webb, M. C. The abolition of the taboo system in Hawaii. *Journal of Polynesian Society,* 1965, **74** (1), 21–39.

Wedge, B. M. Occurrence of psychosis among Okinawans in Hawaii. *American Journal of Psychiatry,* 1952, **109,** 255–258.

Wedge B. & Abe, S. Racial incidence of mental disease in Hawaii. *Hawaii Medical Journal,* 1949, **8,** 337–338.

Williams, J. S. *Maori Achievement Motivation.* Wellington, New Zealand: Victoria University Publications in Psychology, No. 13, 1960.

Wilson, G. S. D. Europeanisation and admission to mental hospital in the Fiji Islands. *New Zealand Medical Journal,* 1965, **64,** 364–367.

Winston, E. Alleged lack of mental disease among primitive groups. *American Anthropologist,* 1934, **36,** 234–238.

2.9   *Orientation*

The influence of culture upon the patterning of mental illness is as apparent in the ethnic heterogeneity of our own society as it is in Africa or Oceania. For example, Mexican-Americans, in Texas, California, and throughout the Southwest, are noted for their remarkably low rates of hospitalization for mental illness. However, the explanation of this anomaly is as elusive as it is intriguing.

In this chapter, William Madsen, an anthropologist with extensive research experience in Mexico and among the Mexican-Americans of South Texas, offers a vivid glimpse into the life circumstances of Mexican-Americans and Anglo-Americans of Hidalgo County, Texas. He discusses their differing concepts of propriety, of masculinity and femininity, of the nature and origin of disease, and, of the etiology and prognosis of mental illness.

Although Madsen makes no claims to epidemiological precision, he believes that there may in fact be less mental disorder among Mexican-Americans than among Anglo-Americans. In explanation, he suggests that stress falls more heavily upon the Anglo because it falls upon him as an individual, whereas stress among Mexican-Americans is shared and relieved by the family.

2.9   Mexican-Americans and Anglo-Americans: A Comparative Study of Mental Health in Texas[1]

William Madsen

This paper presents a comparative analysis of the relationship between culture and mental health among the Mexican-Americans and Anglo-

[1] This paper is based on research carried out by the staff of the Hidalgo Project on Differential Culture Change and Mental Health during the four-year period from 1957 to 1961. The staff included Antonieta Espejo, Octavio

Americans of South Texas.[2] Its purpose is to examine the sociocultural determinants of mental health and mental illness in two ethnic groups belonging to the same society but maintaining different ways of life.

Following contemporary psychiatric theory, it will be assumed that anxiety-producing stress is the predisposing factor in most mental illness (Horney, 1937, p. 41; Honigmann, 1954, pp. 371, 404). It will attempt to show that differences in the mental health of Mexican-Americans and Anglo-Americans are related to differences in the stresses and anxieties produced within the two ethnic groups.

Jaco (1959, p. 474) presented the provocative proposition that Mexican-Americans suffer less mental illness than Anglo-Americans. His findings were based on a sociological study of the comparative incidence of mental illness in these populations. A comparison of the sociological and anthropological approaches to the same problem is essential because of the different premises and methodologies used by the two disciplines. In a very general way, we may say that sociology, on the one hand, depends upon the quantification of a few meaningful variables in the problem area. Anthropology, on the other hand, tends to demand a consideration of the total sociocultural setting of the problem, thus making adequate quantification difficult. When the two disciplines reach similar results in the same area of investigation, the probability of accurate reporting and interpretation is greatly increased.

As an index of psychological ill health in the Texas populations, Jaco (1957) used the relative occurrence of treated psychosis in each group.

The study was designed to include all inhabitants of the state of Texas who sought psychiatric treatment for a psychosis for the first time in their lives during the two-year period of 1951 and 1952. Data were obtained from all psychiatrists in private practice in Texas during this time, and from all private, Veterans Administration, city-county, and state mental hospitals in the state. The

Romano, Arthur Rubel, Albino Fantini, and William Madsen (director). The project was supported by the Hogg Foundation for Mental Health, University of Texas. The following members of the Department of Sociology at Purdue University provided me with many helpful ideas and leads, and I wish to express my appreciation to them: Edward Dager, Katherine Johnsen, and Eugene Kanin. I also wish to thank my wife Claudia for her invaluable aid.

[2] The terms "Anglo-American" and "Anglo" are sometimes used in reference to all Texans who are not Latins. More common in Hidalgo County is the triple classification of Anglos, Negroes, and "Mexicans." The Negro population is comparatively small. Jaco uses the term "Spanish-American" for the Latins to include the non-Mexican derived Spanish-speaking peoples. However, such non-Mexican-derived Spanish speakers in Hidalgo County make up but an infinitesimal part of the population.

states bordering Texas were also canvassed and many cases were picked up who had received treatment out of state [p. 322].

On an adjusted rate per 100,000 population, Jaco found the Mexican-American to have almost 50 percent less psychosis than the Anglo-American (Jaco, 1959, p. 474). On the basis of this difference, Jaco concludes that the Mexican-American is mentally healthier than the Anglo-American.

Jaco's findings raise an important question: Can the total picture of mental health in any ethnic group be obtained by counting patients treated for mental illness?[3] Some authorities think not. The Midtown Manhattan Study (Srole, Langer, Michael, Opler, Rennie, & Thomas, 1962) states that ". . . the patient prevalence measure is itself an inadequate foundation of evidence about over-all (untreated and treated) prevalence of mental illness [p. 382]." Opler (1959) concludes from the findings of the Manhattan Study that ". . . both the ethnic groups and the lower classes who received the least treatment had the most serious disorders both in quantity and quality [p. 13]." For example, the percentage of mentally "well" first-generation Puerto Ricans was rated as 0.0 percent and the sum of first, second, and third generation Puerto Ricans as only 3.7 percent (Srole et al., 1962, pp. 290–291).

One reason for the reported differences in the mental health of minority ethnic groups in Manhattan and Texas is the difference in the total historical and sociocultural settings of the two areas. Perhaps equally important, however, are the criteria used to define mental health and illness. Jaco uses the frequency of the psychiatric diagnosis of psychoses as a key to the total picture of mental illness within a population. The Midtown Manhattan Study also used the occurrence of a number of psychologically defined malfunctions in the untreated population (Srole et al., pp. 388–394). Valuable as the attempt may be to set up psychological absolutes for all subgroups to measure the effective functioning of the larger society, I doubt whether this technique has any great value for cross-cultural comparison. For example, I do not believe that cross-cultural measurement of mental illness can be validly based on responses to concepts such as "one drink is one too many," "never show feelings to others," "never change mind," "always be on guard with people," and "often, old ways are best ways" (Srole et al., p. 389).

[3] After this paper had been completed, Dohrenwend published a significant evaluation of the techniques for measuring psychological disorder in different groups with specific references to the Midtown Manhattan Study. (Bruce P. Dohrenwend, Social status and psychological disorder: An issue of substance and an issue of method. *American Sociological Review*, 1966, **31**, pp. 14–34).

The Midtown Manhattan Study implies that the behavior of the "Old Americans (Generation IV)" is the standard for mental health, although the percentage of the mentally "well" in this group is only 28.0 percent. However, this percentage is considerably higher than the 18.5 percent "well" found for the total Midtown sample (Srole *et al.*, p. 290). Another indication that the Old Americans are used as a standard to define mental health is the implied effect of acculturation on the New York ethnic groups. As stated above, mental health among Puerto Ricans increases from the first generation to the third. As opposed to the Midtown Manhattan findings, Jaco (1957) writes of the Texas Mexican-Americans, ". . . as this sub-culture becomes assimilated into the dominant culture of the Anglos, one can predict that the incidence of mental illness will increase correspondingly and become more like that of the Anglos in form as well as frequence [p. 328]."

Both studies face the problem of avoiding a cultural bias in the measurement of mental illness. Various studies have attempted to define a culture-free method of defining mental illness (for example, Honigmann, 1954, pp. 370–376; Wegrocki, 1948). Today, it is generally accepted that no form of behavior can be judged as abnormal outside of its cultural context. More importantly, however, as stated by Wegrocki (1948), "It is not the mechanism that is abnormal; it is its function which determines its abnormality [p. 561]."

Within the context of any one society, therefore, behavior can be judged as mentally healthy or ill according to its function. In the case of the minority groups studied by Jaco and the Manhattan Study, however, another dimension is added. These groups operate within the larger national society of which they are a part. The determination of the comparative mental health of an ethnic group can be made in terms of its own values or those of the dominant society. What is functional behavior in one group may be dysfunctional in terms of the other. Major differences in the interpretation of data in the mental health of United States ethnic groups may depend on the point of reference. In an attempt to avoid the pitfall of using a single reference, I will examine the probability of dysfunctional behavior resulting from anxiety-producing stresses (1) within the context of traditional Mexican-American society, (2) within the context of Anglo-American society, and (3) in contexts where the values of the two groups meet.

HILDAGO COUNTY: ANGLOS AND CHICANOS

Most of the ethnographic data used in the following discussion were collected in Hidalgo County, Texas between 1957 and 1961. This county is located in the lower Rio Grande Valley and is bordered on the south by the Rio Grande River and the Mexican state of Tamaulipas. The county's proximity to Mexico facilitates reinforcement of Mexican-derived patterns of behavior. Hidalgo County is one of the strongholds of Mexican-American folk culture. Many Mexican-Americans who, through anglicization, deviate from traditional Latin patterns for other parts of Texas or other states. Their ranks are refilled by legal and illegal immigrants from Mexico.

It is interesting to note that south Texas is listed by Jaco (1957b, pp.3–4) as one of the regions with the lowest incidence of Mexican-American psychoses and the highest of Anglo-American psychoses. These facts would seem to reinforce Jaco's theory that the more conservative Mexican-American will be mentally healthier than the Anglo-American and that the acculturating Mexican-American will fall between these two extremes.

However, a psychological comparison of the Mexican-American and Anglo-American populations of Hidalgo County requires some historical perspective. The area was originally settled from Mexico, and the Anglo-American population remained small until the beginning of land improvement by real estate firms in 1910. The newly cleared and irrigated land was sold primarily to Midwesterners, some of whom migrated to the area, while others hired Texas Anglo-Americans to run their properties. Labor was provided by the local Mexican-Americans and by Mexican immigrants (many of the latter were fleeing from the revolution in Mexico). Thus, the present class structure of the area was established: a lower class composed almost exclusively of individuals of Mexican ancestry and a middle and upper class that is primarily Anglo-American. The towns laid out by land companies in the twentieth century were planned to maintain the ethnic separateness of the population. Each town is clearly divided into a Mexican-American and an Anglo-American section. Until the terminal part of World War II, each section was self-contained with its own schools, churches, and stores. Today, shopping areas are open to Mexican-Americans, and schools are integrated.

Assimilation of the Mexican-Americans has been impeded by stereotypical and unflattering images which each ethnic group has of the other, and by the fact that each group clearly distinguishes between "we" and "they." The Anglo refers to himself as "white," "Anglo," or "American" and refers to the Mexican-American as "Mexican" (pronounced "Meskin"). Occasionally, an Anglo uses the very derogatory word "greaser" for Mexican-American. The Mexican-Americans refer to themselves as "Mexicanos" ("Mexican") when no Anglo is present, or as

"Chicanos" (from "Mexicano"), or "Tejanos" ("Texan"). Mexican-Americans use the respectful "Anglo" and "Americano" for the Anglo-American or the derogatory terms *"bolillo"* and *"gringo."*

The Anglo sees the Chicano as basically "lazy," "unreliable," "immoral," "superstitious," "ignorant," and in need of the guidance of a firm Anglo hand. The Chicano views the Anglo as being grossly materialistic, lacking in sophisticated intelligence, crafty in money matters, lax in sexual morality, and irreligious. Each group regards the other as a foreign element on its own native soil. The Chicano knows he was here before the Anglo whom he sometimes calls an *extranjero* ("foreigner"). The Anglo knows he owns the land and associates the Chicano with the foreigners of Mexico.

WORLD VIEWS

The Anglo and the Chicano see existence and the meaning of life differently. The Chicano views the natural and the supernatural as blending intimately into an integrated and significant unity. His real world is populated by ghosts, spirits, saints, and witches, as well as by the mundane and objective things of everyday life. God and the Virgin are not strangers to the Chicano but are Beings who can and do influence his life for better or for worse. Although the Hidalgo Anglo usually belongs to a church, his everyday activities are in a natural world that the supernatural cannot touch. The typical Anglo refers to God on Sundays, in profanity, and in great need, desperation, or fear. The Anglo God lives in a world apart from man and in a world the Anglo has trouble conceiving and sometimes even believing.

The Anglo sees the material world as something he should dominate, control, and rearrange. The Mexican-American sees his ideal role in life as living in harmony with others and fitting into an existing order rather than rearranging things to suit his will.

The Anglo sees himself as an individual with a free will which he should use to increase his well-being, usually defined in terms of material possessions, power, or popularity. The Mexican-American sees himself controlled primarily by fate, and therefore he is more willing to accept things as they come. The Chicano does not give up all individual effort because of a fatalistic philosophy. Rather, he sees the possible rewards of his efforts as more limited than does the Anglo.

The concept of limited success is probably due in part to the frustrations that come with belonging to a subordinate group. Before World War II, the lower-class Chicano saw nearly all Anglo goals as completely beyond his own means. Today, the Chicano still sees most Anglo goals as being denied him. Mexican-American fatalism, historically derived from

Mexico, prevents the individual from undertaking endeavors doomed to failure by Anglo society. Although it softens the necessity of accepting inferior position, the concept of fatalism is not enough to convince the Chicano that this is a just or friendly world. As is true for the Negro (Kardiner & Ovesey, 1951, p. 308), the Mexican-American sees the world as primarily hostile. Romano (1960) describes the Chicano view as follows: ". . . the most basic premise which governs behavior holds that the world is fickle and undependable. Individuals outside the kin group are almost invariably suspect, and quite normally a stranger is judged guilty until proven innocent [p. 971]."

In contrast, most Anglos see the world as a friendly place waiting to reward their efforts. Basic optimism combined with the value placed on effort leads the Anglo to look for his rewards in the future. The Mexican-American looks for his pleasures today. Knutson (1965) sees the Anglo as "future-oriented" and would describe the Chicano as "present-oriented." He states that those who are ". . . future-oriented tend to be also achievement-oriented, eager to 'get going' on things, anxious to 'get things done'; whereas those oriented toward the present may find greater satisfaction in spontaneous activities less oriented toward future goals [p. 283]."

While the Anglo is optimistic and future-oriented, he does not see the future as being free of threat. But a concrete threat is something he thinks he can handle and overcome. Vague anxieties about the future are generated in the successful Anglo by the accelerated sociocultural change in contemporary America. Unable to pinpoint the enemy as change itself, the Anglo tries to safeguard his future by fighting what he conceives as the concrete "un-American" forces of Communism, "leftists," the United Nations, labor, and social welfare. Many of the more reactionary Anglos are convinced that the mental health and civil rights movements are weapons of Russian Communism.

While the Anglo thinks of himself as a striving individual in something he calls "the American Way of Life," the Mexican-American usually classifies himself first as a member of "La Raza" and secondly as a United States citizen. La Raza is literally translated as "the race" and refers to all those of Latin descent who are bound together by a common spirituality and fate. La Raza, it is believed, was originally given great destiny by God, but the Mexican-Americans destroyed this promising fate by producing traitors, thieves, and prostitutes within their own ranks. Thus, all of La Raza are held back by the faults of a few. It is considered sinful for a Chicano to seek self-advancement by abandoning La Raza.

In general, then, the Anglo sees the world as an optimal place in which to prove himself by his own efforts. The Chicano sees himself existing in a hostile world as a member of a group condemned by the actions of its own members. Ultimately, the Anglo must blame himself for failure, while the Mexican-American has every reason to attribute his failures to external forces beyond his control. In Mexico and Texas, Mexican-Americans like to tell the following anecdote: "I am never late for a bus, but buses often depart before I arrive at the station."

THE INDIVIDUAL, THE FAMILY, AND SOCIETY

When an Anglo fails, he thinks first of how this failure will affect him and his status in society. When a Chicano fails, his first evaluation of the failure is in terms of what it will do to his family and how it will affect his relationship to other family members. The Anglo [child] is prepared and trained for the day when he will remove himself from parental authority and face the world as an individual. The Mexican-American is raised to think of himself foremost and forever as a member of the family and only secondly as an individual. The Anglo reference point is "I." The Chicano reference point is "we."

The Anglo family is unclear, and relatives frequently are not known. When relatives are known, they may be regarded as nuisances unless they are in a higher socioeconomic bracket. The Mexican-American recognizes all relatives on both sides of the family and acknowledges reciprocal rights and duties toward all of them. The family is fictively extended by the custom of *compadrazco* ("co-parenthood"), by which the godparents of a child become the *compadres* of the parents. *Compadres* must be reliable people who can be counted on and trusted. However, primary concern is with parents, siblings, grandparents, and offspring. Although ideally parents and children live in a separate household, it is considered good and wise to live near other family members. As Fantini (1962) writes of this area, "Families live near each other and it is common to see numerous one or two-room frame houses huddled together on one small property lot [p. 33]."

The Chicano is raised in the belief that a family should be a self-sufficient unit in an unstable world. The family should provide for all its members and be the source of assistance in time of trouble. The individual's dependency on the family is instilled in the child from his earliest years. When a Chicano seeks aid from another source, it reflects discredit on the family, which is seen as being unable to provide for its members. For this reason, Mexican-Americans rarely resort to credit associations, mutual aid groups, or unions. The reluctance to seek non-familial aid is reinforced by the concept that no one outside the family is really to be trusted.

Because of the Chicano's concept of familial sufficiency, he is not a joiner. Moreover, to affiliate with another group would be regarded as a possible strain on his loyalty to the family. By contrast, the Anglo appears to be almost a compulsive joiner. Writing of the 6000 Anglos in one Hidalgo town, Rubel (1960) notes that they

are organized into more than 70 social, civic, and fraternal organizations. What remains of their time is further devoted to the social and religious activities of 16 major churches, which include within their framework many study groups, women's circles, and other types of formal organizations. The lives of Anglo-American children are mirror images of their parents, and the youngsters are trained in the group way of life by a succession of organized activities which range from school clubs to associations such as Girl Scouts, Boy Scouts, Sea Scouts, 4-H Clubs, Future Farmers of America, and Little League baseball clubs, to name a few [p. 796].

The Mexican-American has a sharper sense of identity than the Anglo and has fewer role conflicts. In any situation, the Chicano is a representative of his family, and he avoids involvement by maintaining social distance. The Anglo has a number of roles, many of them conflicting, and his self-image shifts as he moves from one social situation to another. The Chicano need remain loyal to only one institution, the family, while the Anglo's loyalties are fragmented among multiple organizations and his own self-interests.

MALE AND FEMALE

Behavior in male and female roles is more explicitly defined for Mexican-Americans than for Anglos. As a Mexican-American college student described it to me, "A Chicano male is more masculine and the female is more feminine than the Anglo counterparts." The clean-cut division between what a male may do and what a female may do in Mexican-American society is lacking in Anglo society.

The prime value for the Mexican-American male is *machismo* ("manliness"). *Machismo* requires the development of a powerful self-image similar to the *egoismo* of Spain. The Latin male sees himself as capable of accomplishing almost anything he tries and dismisses as undesirable those areas of behavior in which he does not try to prove himself. He must be indebted to no one outside the family in financial matters or other obligations. He must maintain dignity at all times. To avoid situations that might compromise him, he maintains social distance outside the home and mentally pictures himself as superior to male peers with whom he is interacting.

The need to maintain superiority while not giving overt offense in relationships between males is resolved through the institution of verbal dueling. As Romano (1960) describes it, an individual must also learn to cope with the daily onslaughts of verbal dueling. This dueling consists of a complex use of everyday words as metaphors which contain insinuations, innuendos, and outright accusations of effeminacy and lack of courage. For example, seemingly innocent remarks which contain the word "leche," or milk, may constitute a veiled reference to sperm. Words such as "key," "whip," or "walnut" may refer to male genitalia. A statement with the word "eye" may refer to the anus, as might the word "pocket." In short, the intended metaphorical significance is derived from common everyday words and one must be wary enough to distinguish between the common usage and verbal thrusts. In addition, there are refinements to verbal dueling. The fully competent opponent is expected neither to reveal his intentions and meanings, nor his reactions during an exchange. Furthermore, it is generally believed that the highest refinement in verbal duelings is achieved when the implied meaning is phrased in such a manner as to convince the victim that he has been greatly complimented and flattered [p. 972].

Due to the vagueness of the associated word meanings in verbal dueling, each participant can leave a duel with the feeling that he has downgraded the opponent and proven his own superiority.

The Chicano must be able to defend himself in ways other than verbal dueling. Any overt insult must be avenged and it is considered the very negation of *machismo* to run away from a fight. In avenging oneself, intelligence is regarded as perhaps more important than physical might. It is considered intelligent to delay the attack until the enemy is drunk or otherwise incapacitated. It is also considered wise to seek revenge when backed up by a brother or other ally. The enmity is not ended with the fight, despite its outcome. An enemy is always an enemy for life.

A major arena for proving one's superiority and manliness is sex. The Mexican-American pursues the subject of sex with abandon. A man's reputation in male society rests to a large extent upon his actual or claimed seductions. The sexual act itself is regarded as right and proper, and no guilt is experienced by the male after premarital or extramarital intercourse.

Samuel Ramos (1962) theorizes that the Mexican *machismo* complex is probably the reflection of a repressed inferiority complex. The subordinate social condition of the Mexican-American in Texas would tend to intensify feelings of inferiority masked by *machismo*.

Anglo society raises its males to feel self-confidence and acquire the ability to prove their worth by socioeconomic advancement. Failure is cushioned to some extent by the concept of the "second chance." The respect that the Chicano seeks by proving his *machismo*, the Anglo pursues by display of his economic worth. Conspicuous consumption is most evident in the Texas Anglo community.

While the Chicano male seeks to maintain his identity through social distance outside the family, the Anglo male seeks to establish his through popularity. While the Chicano wants to be respected, the Anglo wants to be liked. Next to dollars, friendship is the most pursued commodity in the Anglo community.

Like the Chicano, the Anglo is interested in sex and likes to think of himself as desirable to the female. Unlike the Chicano, the Anglo usually is indoctrinated with the fundamentalist concept that "sex is sin." This ambivalent attitude leads the Anglo to dally with sex but block its completion in the sexual act. The Anglo likes to look at girls, "girlie magazines," and strip acts. He also enjoys necking in the proper setting. But premarital or extramarital coitus arouses a deep sense of guilt within him. It is significant that in the Mexican red-light district called "Boy's Town," Latin customers are usually sober while Anglos are usually drunk.

The Anglo female also has mixed reactions to sex. Before marriage, her self-esteem is largely measured by her popularity with the opposite sex, which involves a certain amount of sexual access to the boys she dates. However, she shares the Anglo male's fear of completion and is expected to resist full seduction. She knows that once she acquires the reputation of availability her chances of a good marriage decline. And it is a husband of higher socioeconomic position that is the ultimate goal of the Anglo woman.

The Mexican-American girl who comes from a proper family is guarded against the possibility of sexual experience before marriage. It is believed that a woman lacks the intelligence of a man and, if left alone with him, will be tricked into bed and shamed. Respected families never allow their teen-age daughters to be alone with a male or even indulge in the physical contact of holding hands. A good marriage for a Mexican-American girl depends on her sexual ignorance and purity. Not to marry would be a tragedy for her that should not even be contemplated. She would never marry without the consent of her parents, and frequently the marriage is arranged for her. It is considered a good thing for a Chicana to marry a man richer than she is, but it is far more important that the husband be of a good family and have a good name.

Ideally, an Anglo marriage limits the sexual experience to the two spouses. It is considered part of the marriage obligation for each mate to assure complete sexual satisfaction for the other. The husband who pursues extramarital sex experiences guilt and anxiety. A man is usually so sure of his wife that, should she have an affair, he may be "the last to hear about it." After marriage, the social activities of the wife are supposed to increase in number. Most Anglo husbands view marriage as a curtailment of their freedom.

Marriage moves the Mexican-American bride from the home of her parents into the household of her husband. Here her social isolation continues, for her husband replaces her parents as the watchdog of her morality. In contrast, he is expected to continue his pursuit of females outside the home. The ultimate in proving *machismo* is the ability to maintain a mistress in a separate household or *casa chica*. The husband is not supposed to allow his wife to fully enjoy the pleasure of his experienced sexual technique. The wife who develops an appreciation for sexual pleasure, it is believed, may seek variation in her sexual partners, and the worst scandal that can befall a family is one involving the purity of the wife.

Isolated from possible sexual contacts outside the home, the Chicana wife is also denied the right to visit in the homes of unrelated women. Rubel (1960) states, in relation to his work in one of the Hidalgo towns, that

during the two years in which [I] was in Mecca only two cases were discovered in which a woman regularly visited the home of another to whom she was not related. In both instances the visiting was non-reciprocal, i.e., only one of the pair was the visitor; the other was always the visited. Neither of the visitors had any kin in town other than affinals; one of the visitors had been deserted by her husband many years ago. Each of the visitors conceived of herself as a social isolate for whom life was meaningless, hopeless, and without order; one of these anomic women was contemplating suicide at the time of our acquaintanceship [pp. 810–811].

The proper Mexican-American wife, however, finds much companionship in the homes of her parents, sisters-in-law, cousins, aunts, and nieces, as well as in her own home.

The Mexican-American husband is the undisputed ruler of his home. It is unthinkable for his wife or children to question him or show him disrespect. The Mexican-American wife is expected to accept his extramarital affairs and submit to mistreatment when her husband is annoyed. Ideally, the wife serves as a reservoir of serenity and love for the entire family. It is considered unbecoming for a woman to display anger or to withhold affection from her husband. She is idealized as an earthly double of the Virgin, a repository of purity and love.

Within the Anglo household, the question of authority is confused. Most Anglo couples spend years improvising a method of decision-making and may never succeed. Both husband and wife are determined to protect their individuality and defend their "rights," and the results are rarely peaceful. Contemporary Anglo culture lacks a clear-cut definition of marital roles, which are beginning to blur and merge in many contexts.

While the Anglos suffer from the nebulousness of sex-defined roles, the Mexican-Americans know exactly what is expected of them to maintain their male or female images. The Chicano faces the task of maintaining his masculinity in a seemingly hostile world, but his anxieties can be relieved by male interaction, drinking, and sex. Moreover, the Mexican-American male can use the ego-inflating techniques of mentally denigrating others and being the monarch within his own household. The Mexican-American woman, however, has the difficult goal of living up to the model of the Virgin while realizing that she would fall to sordid depths if she were not protected, since women are weak and less intelligent than men. The Chicana wife frequently suffers sexual frustration while her husband seeks his sexual fulfillment. While the Chicano is free of sexual guilt despite his indulgence, his wife is supposed to feel guilt at the very thought of sex. Their Anglo counterparts may each have abundant sexual experiences, but both suffer guilt from deviant fantasies or forbidden sexual behavior.

PARENTS AND CHILDREN

As the male rules the female, so, within the Mexican-American home, the elders rule the young. At no time is a Chicano child allowed to disobey or doubt his parents. The ultimate authority is always the father, but the mother is to be promptly obeyed as well. Among the children, the older have authority over the younger, especially among the boys.

As infants and young children, the Chicanos are exposed to great love and overt affection. Open demonstrations of affection are reduced as the child ages and especially as new babies appear. The diminishing of open expressions of love are accompanied by the assignment of household tasks to the child. This is not an intentional relationship, but it undoubtedly leaves an impression on the growing child that love is associated with dependency.

With the onset of puberty, daughters are restricted to the household and outside activities that are carefully supervised by adults. Boys are expected to begin their explorations of the outside world, especially in the informal gangs known as *palomillas* ("moths"). Here they learn the facts of life and the ways to defend themselves.

At adolescence, the child's relationship to the father becomes formalized and distant. The son must now be especially careful to show respect to his father and accept without question all paternal restrictions placed on his behavior. At the same time, the boy's affective ties to his mother are strengthened. He is now placed in a double bind in respect to his developing *machismo*. His sexual activities may be unconsciously felt as possibly contaminating in respect to the purity of his mother and her close relationship to him. At any rate, sex and sexual problems must never even be hinted at in the presence of the mother. The adolescent boy may feel that his masculinity is being compromised by his father. The independent and self-reliant ways that the boy has learned to display within the *palomilla* must be replaced by a submissive, childlike obedience before the father. He tends to develop a hostility toward the father which is suppressed at home and manifested toward authority figures outside the home. The Chicano only reluctantly accepts the authority of the teacher or employer and tries to terminate the relationship at the first hint that his autonomy is being violated.

The Anglo child is reared to expect an ultimate break from the parents that is unknown to the Mexican-Americans. Controls over the Anglo child are greatly relaxed when he enters high school. If he goes on to college, the only effective form of parental control is financial. The self-reliance which the Anglo child is expected to cultivate is described by Hsu (1961) as "the American core value . . . , the most persistent psychological expression of which is the fear of dependence [p. 217]." The dependency of children is not given up lightly by the parents, and strained relations between the two generations frequently mark the child's entrance into the world of adulthood. The desire for a child's dependency is probably an unconscious quest for the emotional security of a tight-knit and enduring family.

The emotional satisfactions that a child obtains from the relationship with his parents are different for the Anglo and the Chicano. These differences are reflected in the terms by which the parents are addressed directly or referred to when speaking to others. Throughout life, the Chicano refers to his mother with affection, usually calling her *mamá* or the affectionate diminutive *mamicita* ("little mama"). Among the Texas Anglos, the term of affection is used for the other parent. Throughout his life, an Anglo refers to his father as "daddy." This difference in address reflects a difference in authority and affection. The Mexican-American father commands, while the mother provides affection. In the Anglo family, the father tries to play the role of "buddy" with his children.

The emotional basis of social conformity also differs in the Mexican-American and Anglo-American systems of child raising. The difference is comparable to Benedict's contrast between guilt and shame cultures. Mexican-Americans tend to be controlled by "shame," while Anglos tend to be controlled by "guilt," although these distinctions are not always mutually exclusive. Benedict (1946) differentiates between the two by saying,

True shame cultures rely on external sanctions for good behavior, not, as true guilt cultures do, on an internalized conviction of sin. Shame is a reaction to other people's criticism. A man is shamed either by being openly ridiculed and rejected or by fantasying to himself that he has been made ridiculous [p. 223].

Hsu (1949) discusses social control with practically the same reference, roughly equating the function of suppression to shame and that of repression to guilt.

The concept of *vergüenza*, found in Spain, Mexico, and among the Mexican-Americans, means susceptibility to shame. It is best described by Pitt-Rivers (1954) in its Spanish setting, where its use is precisely the same as among the Mexican-Americans:

The code of ethics to which "vergüenza" is related is that which incurs the moral stricture of the community. To use Marrett's distinction, it relates to "external moral sanctions" not to "internal moral sanctions" or conscience. Thus, to do a thing blatantly makes a person a "sin vergüenza" (shameless one); but to have done it discreetly would only have been wrong. This, then, is the difference. Shamelessness faces the world, faces people in particular situations. Wrong faces one's conscience. Let us now try a definition.

"Vergüenza" is the regard for the moral values of society, for the rules whereby social intercourse takes place, for the opinion which others have of one. But this, not purely out of calculation. True "vergüenza" is a mode of feeling which makes one sensitive to one's reputation and thereby causes one to accept the sanctions of public opinion.

Thus a "sin vergüenza" is a person who either does not accept or who abuses those rules. And this may be either through a lack of understanding or through a lack of sensitivity. One can perceive these two aspects of it.

First as the result of understanding, upbringing, education. "Lack of education" is a polite way of saying "lack of vergüenza." It is sometimes necessary to beat a child to give him "vergüenza," and it is the only justifiable excuse for doing so. Failure to inculcate "vergüenza" into one's children brings doubts to bear upon one's own "vergüenza."

But, in its second aspect as sensitivity, it is truly hereditary. A person of bad heredity cannot have it since he has not been endowed with it. He can only behave out of calculation as though he had it, simulating what to others comes naturally. A normal child has it in the form of shyness, before education has developed it. When a two-year-old hides its face from a visitor it is because of its "vergüenza" [pp. 113–114].

The Anglo tradition began as a guilt culture but shame is becoming increasingly important. As Benedict (1946) states, "The early Puritans who settled the United States tried to base their whole morality on guilt and all psychiatrists know what trouble contemporary Americans have with their consciences. But shame is an increasingly heavy burden in the United States and guilt is less extremely felt than in early generations [pp. 223–224]." Honigmann (1954) interprets Riesman as also indicating an American shift from guilt to shame: "If we interpret Riesman correctly, as America moves to an outer-directed personality we are reducing the role of guilt in favor of increasing sensitivity to shame [p. 293]." Texas, like the Midwest as a whole, has been slow in following the shame trends of the East and West Coasts. The guilt component is stronger in Texas than on the two coastal areas.

Obviously, both guilt and shame can be felt in either Mexican-American or Anglo-American culture. The Chicano, as a lifetime member of a tradition-oriented family and of La Raza, thinks of a deviant act primarily in terms of how it will shame him in the eyes of others. Guilt feelings may also accompany or follow his first reaction. The Anglo, raised in the ethics of rugged individualism, feels guilty about a deviant act even if it is not known to others. If his deviant behavior is exposed, however, the Anglo also feels shame. The Texas Anglo thinks primarily in terms of self-righteousness, while the Chicano thinks in terms of traditional rightness as viewed by others.

These differences are manifested in relations between the two ethnic groups. When the Anglo is dealing with Mexican-Americans, he maintains his Angloness. He knows that his way is right and superior to the Chicano way. When the Chicano is operating in an Anglo group, he tries to show no sign of Mexican behavior for fear of shaming himself in the eyes of Anglos who disapprove of Mexican ways.

Within traditional Mexican-American society, guilt is felt most strongly in regard to acts involving disloyalty to the family. Anglo guilt is felt primarily in connection with socioeconomic failure, lack of popularity, and sexual aberrance.

SICKNESS AND DEATH

Sickness means dependency during the period of treatment. Attitudes toward such dependency differ for the Anglo and the Mexican-American. For the Anglo, dependency violates his value of self-sufficiency. Although the Anglo patient receives the sympathy of his family and friends, his recovery depends mainly on the attending physician. The situation is different for the Mexican-American. As Fantini (1962) states,

Illness involves the immediate family, the extended family and sometimes the entire community. As long as the Latin patient is surrounded by his family and relatives, the illness is shared. Definite roles are assumed by corresponding family members until circumstances are brought back to normal. Of all these members, the mother is by far the most important [pp. 35–36].

The team working for the Chicano patient's recovery also includes the saints who are asked to intercede with God. If the services of a folk curer, or *curandero,* are utilized, he establishes a close affective relationship with the family. Family affiliation, therefore, makes the dependent Chicano patient more comfortable than his Anglo counterpart. A Chicana woman feels little anxiety about the dependency of illness. However a man's *machismo* is almost completely destroyed if he is crippled. A cripple may receive pity and great affection from his family, but he feels humiliation outside the home.

Concepts of the etiology of disease also differ in Anglo and Mexican-American culture. The Mexican-American sees illness as a lack of balance in the parts of the body or in the relationship between the individual and his socioreligious environment. For the Anglo, recovery involves restoration of his ability to be self-sufficient in his struggle to achieve success. For the Mexican-American, recovery involves restoration of a harmonious relationship with society and the supernatural powers controlling the universe. Psychosomatic ailments serve as an escape from social crises among the Mexican-Americans. When role conflicts develop or role achievement is blocked, the Chicano frequently avoids the crises by the development of *susto* ("fright"), *mal malo* ("bewitchment"), or another one of the Mexican-American folk diseases (Rubel, 1960, 1964; Madsen, 1964, pp. 97–99). The patient receives social support which helps maintain his self-image and thereby avoids the crisis. He is ultimately returned to society as a balanced and functioning person.

In Anglo society, the social function and usefulness of the individual are seen as declining during the period of old age. The aged are often regarded as being so dependent that they are classified in the same category as the ill. Anglo families fear being burdened with old parents who may be placed in old folks' homes or mental institutions until they die. The aged react with feelings of uselessness, loneliness, and despair.

The Mexican-American gains status with age if he has lived up to the dictates of La Raza. He still maintains a position of authority and respect in the family and the community. Mexican-Americans believe that the worth of an individual increases with experience, and the aged are the most experienced of all.

The elderly Mexican-American accepts death as a valued experience, a thing of beauty, and an entrance into another world that is real. For him, death is an inevitable event that takes place in the presence of his entire family. For the Anglo, death is the ultimate horror, usually experienced in the sterility of a hospital room. It is a lonely voyage fraught with fear of total extinction.

So far, I have been comparing two cultures in regard to the determinants of sickness and health. This comparison has focused on cultural differences between the lower-class Mexican-Americans and middle-class Anglo-Americans. The increasing anglicization of Mexican-Americans since World War II has complicated this simple picture of two separate cultures operating within a single society. Some Anglo values are penetrating Mexican-American culture and producing value conflicts that are related to mental illness.

ANGLICIZATION AND THE AGRINGADO

Generally speaking, the older generation of Mexican-Americans clings to traditional culture while the younger generation is caught between two conflicting cultures. Mexican-American children are indoctrinated in Anglo culture through the system of compulsory education. Anglo schools teach them new ideas and values which contradict those learned in the home. Fantini (1962, p. 36) cites the example of a teen-age Chicana girl who had learned something about modern medicine in school. The girl said,

I told my mother that I believed many people die because they insist on consulting curanderos, and they seek one after another until it becomes too late to go to a doctor to be treated properly. I suggested this to her because she had already taken my sister to five folk curers and no improvement was noted. My mother told me to keep quiet because I didn't know what I was talking about. She became very angry with me and called me impudent and disrespectful. I became very angry too but of course I could not answer her back and so I had to go out of the house. I could say no more about it [p. 36].

After a few such experiences, most Mexican-American children learn to compartmentalize their lives so that ideas from one cultural world do not intrude into the other. There is a growing tendency for Mexican-American youths to accept as true what they learn in school, but they keep controversial ideas away from their parents and conform to the values of La Raza at home.

Increased education and opportunity have opened white collar positions for many Mexican-Americans in the Anglo part of the community. During working hours, these Chicanos must act like Anglos. Upon returning home from work, the Chicanos switch from English to Spanish and operate by Mexican-American values and customs.

In general, the higher the educational level achieved by lower-class Mexican-Americans, the greater are the value conflicts and the anxiety involved in maintaining an integrated identity. The majority continue to think of themselves as Chicanos and as loyal members of La Raza.

Traditional Mexican-American values internalized in early childhood constitute major determinants of behavior, sentiment, and attitudes. Anglo-defined roles are consciously acted out as an expedient solution to the social situation. Anglo discrimination excludes most Chicanos from Anglo social activities and helps reinforce the Chicano's identity as a member of La Raza.

The Anglo value that has produced the most friction in Mexican-American society is the goal of economic advancement. As a member of La Raza, the Chicano learns that the Latins should advance only as a group. As a member of American society, he has acquired a desire for the material benefits of economic advancement. Although the Chicano desires economic advancement, he sees the attainment of this goal as something that will meet a negative reaction within his community. A parallel situation exists among American Negroes. "Every Negro who is higher than lower class has a sense of guilt . . . because he considers success a betrayal of his group and a piece of aggression against them [Kardiner & Ovesey, 1951, p. 316]."

In an attempt to resolve the conflict between conformity and material gain, many Chicanos practice inconspicuous consumption. The desired refrigerator is purchased when economic resources are available, but it is put in a back room to avoid arousing the envy of the neighbors. The Chicano fears arousing envy (*envidia*) in his neighbors because they may try to bring him down to their own level. The most common leveling technique is witchcraft. The lower-class Chicano striving for upward social mobility lives with the fear that he and his family will be bewitched.

Internalization of Anglo values induces some Chicanos to rebel against the restraints felt from Mexican-American society. They attempt cultural transfer by turning their backs on the traditions of their parents and seeking identification with Anglo culture. Conservative Chicanos look upon such individuals as traitors to La Raza who are *sin vergüenza*. The person who deserts La Raza is labeled with the derogatory term *inglesado* ("anglicized") or *agringado* ("gringoized"). The *agringado* is not accepted by Anglo society unless he attains the economic affluence to rise above his lower-class background. Thus, anglicization produces a multiplicity of conflicting values and anxieties (Madsen, 1964a). Escape may be sought through alcohol (Madsen, 1964), drugs, or migration to another part of the country. Sometimes, the stress of attempted cultural transfer precipitates rebellion that is manifested in criminal acts. The *agringado* who remains in Texas and avoids alcohol, drugs, and crime still suffers from guilt for deserting La Raza and shame when he sees fellow Mexican-Americans. His sense of inferiority is heightened and his protecting shield of *machismo* is cracked.

MENTAL ILLNESS

The concept of mental illness is narrower in Mexican-American culture than in Anglo culture. Among Mexican-Americans, the primary categories of disease are "natural" and "unnatural" rather than mental and physical. *Males naturales* ("natural illnesses") occur by the will of God, whereas *males artificiales* ("unnatural, contrived illnesses") are the result of witchcraft (Rubel, 1960, p. 797). Mental illness falls mainly within the category of unnatural sickness associated with bewitchment. Chicanos make a distinction between mental illness and emotional illness. Diseases resulting from emotional imbalance are categorized as natural illnesses.

Locura ("insanity") is the main form of mental illness recognized by Mexican-Americans. The principal cause of insanity is thought to be witchcraft. However, mental illness is only one of many types of illness attributed to witchcraft. Others include paralysis, constant headaches, and severe pains in the stomach. In fact, almost any prolonged illness or other misfortune of inexplicable origin may be identified as bewitchment.

The concept of *locura* may be illustrated by a case history. Within a few weeks, Juanita had experienced two traumatic crises. She had been caught shoplifting by an Anglo store manager who berated her for being a "thieving Mexican" and threatened her with arrest. He did not carry out his threat and the girl's family apparently knew nothing about this incident. The second crisis occurred when Juanita refused the hand of her suitor. Shortly thereafter, her behavior became odd. She said a demon was following her in an attempt to destroy her soul. She was afraid to be by herself and afraid to look out of windows. If left alone she became hysterical. No matter what room she was in, she insisted on having all the doors locked. Frequently, she slumped down in a corner and gave way to unconsolable crying.

Juanita's family diagnosed her illness as bewitchment sent by her rejected suitor to obtain revenge for her affront. Unquestionable evidence of bewitchment was supplied by Juanita's conviction that she was being followed by a demon.

Most cases of suspected witchcraft are not so easily diagnosed. Symptoms such as crying, fear, nervousness, pains, and headaches can be produced by natural illnesses as well as by bewitchment. When proof of witchcraft is lacking, the family usually consults a *curandero* ("folk healer") who tries to reconstruct the events preceding the illness in order to determine whether the patient has offended a neighbor, a suitor, or even one of his in-laws.

Juanita's illness was precipitated by two stressful situations in which she failed to fulfill the role demands of society. The first situation involved value conflict. Juanita valued material possessions which she could not afford to buy. By attempting to steal them, she violated both Anglo and Mexican-American values. Her behavior as a member of La Raza contradicted the expectations of her people. In the second situation, her sex role behavior was irregular because she humiliated her suitor. By the standards of Mexican-American culture, she should not have encouraged Pedro's courtship unless she intended to accept his offer of marriage.

Unfortunately, Juanita's case history does not indicate what kind of medical treatment she received. Such cases are usually treated by *curanderos,* since Mexican-Americans believe that bewitchment cannot be cured by modern medicine.

Although witchcraft is viewed as the main cause of mental illness among Mexican-Americans, it is not considered the only possible cause. In some cases, severe mental illness is considered to be *castigo de Dios* ("punishment from God") for immoral behavior. In another publication (Madsen, 1964, p. 104), I cited the case of a Mexican-American girl who was committed to a state mental hospital as a paranoid patient. After two years of unsuccessful treatment she was released to the custody of her parents who took her to a *curandera.* The *curandera* diagnosed the illness as *castigo de Dios* after learning from the patient that she had committed a sexual perversion with an Anglo boy during her teens. The treatment has been described elsewhere (Madsen, 1964, pp. 104–105).

Mental retardation is accepted by Mexican-Americans as an unavoidable product of fate. The mentally retarded are thought to be "born that way," and there is nothing to be done about their condition. They are cared for by their families. As Fantini (1962) states,

Defects of many kinds and even mental retardation are ignored by the Mexican-American. . . . The mentally retarded may be described as "flojo" (lazy, weak) or "distraído" (inattentive, absent-minded). Seldom does one consider that the "flojo" and the "distraído" both might be helped. Seldom is therapy or rehabilitation considered. The afflicted must learn to fare as he can with emotional illnesses [p. 55].

As mentioned above, the Anglo concept of mental illness differs from the Mexican-American concept in that the latter does not include emotional illnesses. The Mexican-Americans believe that powerful emotions such as anger and fear can cause natural physical illnesses. Extreme anger is said to cause an overproduction of bile resulting in the condition known as *bilis.* The sick person suffers from exhaustion, general aches and pains, nervousness, irritability, and sometimes nausea. *Susto* ("fright") causes irregular heart beat, loss of appetite, insomnia, and complete lethargy. Both *susto* and *bilis* are precipitated by stressful inter-

personal relationships. Treatment by a *curandero* or members of the
family is designed to restore the balance of the body. When equilibrium
of the body parts and fluids has been restored, the nervous and emotional
symptoms disappear.

Mental illness, as defined by Mexican-American culture, belongs to the
group of folk diseases that are most resistant to modern medical treatment. Even if mental illness among Mexican-Americans is defined by
broader Anglo standards, it seldom receives psychiatric treatment except
among those individuals who have adopted Anglo values in the process
of cultural transfer.

Recognition of mental abnormality depends on different criteria established by the two cultures. Mexican-Americans tend to have a higher
tolerance of idiosyncratic behavior than Anglos. An Anglo who claimed
to have had long conversations with angels would certainly be deemed
mentally ill, but the Mexican-American *curandero* who converses with
angels and a host of other supernatural beings is regarded as being mentally superior to others.

DISCUSSION

A comparative study of the extent of mental illness among Anglos and
Mexican-Americans presents many difficulties. Jaco's technique of counting patients treated for psychosis has a number of shortcomings. The first
concerns cultural differences in the concept of mental illness described
above. It has been shown here that mental illness is not considered
amenable to psychiatric therapy, according to the value premises of
Mexican-American folk culture.

Jaco (1957a) takes this factor into account when he states that "the
frequency of practicing 'witch-doctors' in Latin American communities of
the Southwest indicates lesser acceptance of 'Anglo medicine' [pp. 327–
328]." Elsewhere (Jaco, 1959), he states, "However, the fact that such patients eventually come to the Anglo psychiatrist for aid, particularly
those with more severe mental disturbances, indicates the lack of influence of such practitioners in minimizing the known psychotic rate of this
group [p. 483]." I believe Jaco has underestimated both the resistance
to psychiatry among conservative Mexican-Americans and the therapeutic
success of the treatment given by *curanderos*.

The Mexican-American cultural aversion to hospitals supports the
contention that members of La Raza seldom seek treatment for mental
illness in these institutions. The hospital is seen as a place to die. It is
also a place of isolation from La Raza. Fantini (1962) writes, "More ter-
rifying than any illness to the Mexican-American mind is the idea of
entering a hospital for treatment. When the patient is hospitalized, he is

separated from ordinary life and withdrawn from his family and friends [p. 39]."

If Jaco's figures do not provide an adequate measurement, the question remains: How can mental illness be measured accurately among Mexican-Americans? I am not sure that it can. Because witchcraft is thought to be the main cause of mental illness, the subject is shrouded in secrecy. The conservative Mexican-American never discusses current cases of bewitchment with strangers, particularly if they are Anglos. He may even deny his belief in witchcraft because he is quite aware that Anglos ridicule Mexican-Americans for holding onto such "backward superstitions."

Despite my doubts about Jaco's use of statistical methods in this case, I agree with his basic conclusion that there is less mental illness among the Mexican-Americans than among the Anglo-Americans in Texas. It has been argued here that Mexican-Americans have a sharper sense of identity than Anglos and fewer role conflicts. The conservative Mexican-American is a proud representative of his family and La Raza. He and the members of his family share the same values and know exactly what to expect of each other. The rules of behavior are spelled out in Mexican-American culture.

The family also serves as an anxiety-sharing and anxiety-reducing mechanism in stressful situations. The Chicano seldom faces a crisis alone. Even when a man fails to prove his *machismo,* his family stands behind him and finds external causes for his inability to fulfill the male sex role.

Their world view enables Mexican-Americans to blame failure on witchcraft or fate without suffering the feelings of guilt and self-doubt which plague the Anglos when they experience failure.

Although anxiety-producing stresses are abundant in both ethnic groups, these stresses tend to produce different kinds of anxiety. Anglo stresses fall squarely on the shoulders of the individual, who has only himself to blame. Stress situations among Mexican-Americans are less likely to produce mental illness because they are shared by the family group. Moreover, it may be an important fact that Mexican-Americans do not worry about the possibility of mental illness as much as Anglos do.

The highest area of anxiety occurs among Mexican-Americans who are striving for cultural transfer but have not yet been accepted by the Anglos. Fear of bewitchment also seems to be greater among these individuals than among conservative members of La Raza. Respected Mexican-Americans who avoid offensive or envy-eliciting behavior have little fear of witchcraft. However, the *agringados* who have accepted the Anglo goal of economic advancement fear that they will be envied for having better clothes, food, and houses than other Mexican-Americans. The *agringado* seeks psychiatric treatment only when he has fully accepted Anglo values and discarded his belief in witchcraft. Adoption of the Anglo value system depends in part on social acceptance of Mexican-Americans by Anglos.

The discussion presented here on mental illness attributed to witchcraft shows that fear of bewitchment serves as a powerful social sanction against anglicization and other forms of proscribed behavior. It is predictable that belief in witchcraft as a primary cause of mental illness will be sustained and psychiatric treatment rejected by conservative members of La Raza.

In conclusion, it is hypothesized that anxiety-producing stress seldom precipitates mental illness when the anxiety is shared and relieved by a tightly knit, primary group. It could even be argued that a certain amount of anxiety is required for successful performance of occupational roles in the highly competitive society of Texas Anglos. However, anxiety associated with guilt and fear of social isolation tends to be a predisposing factor in the etiology of mental illness.

REFERENCES

Benedict, R. *The chrysanthemum and the sword*. Cambridge: The Riverside Press, 1946.

Clark, M. *Health in the Mexican-American culture*. Berkeley: University of California Press, 1959.

Fantini, A. E. *Illness and curing among Mexican-Americans of Mission, Texas*. Unpublished M.A. thesis University of Texas, 1962.

Honigmann, J. J. *Culture and personality*. New York: Harper and Brothers, 1954.

Horney, K. *The neurotic personality of our time*. New York: W. W. Norton and Company, 1937.

Hsu, Francis L. K. Suppression versus repression. *Psychiatry*, 1949, **12**, 223–239.

Hsu, F. L. K. American core value and national character. In F. L. K. Hsu (Ed.), *Psychological anthropology: Approaches to culture and personality*. Homewood, Ill.: The Dorsey Press, 1961. Pp. 209–230.

Jaco, E. G. Social factors in mental disorders in Texas. *Social Problems*, 1957, **4**, 322–328. (a)

Jaco, E. G. Incidence of psychoses in Texas, 1951–1952. *Texas State Journal of Medicine*, 1957, **53**, 86–91. (b)

Jaco, E. G. Attitudes toward, and incidence of, mental disorder: A research note. *Southwestern Social Science Quarterly*, 1957, June, 27–38. (c)

Jaco, E. G. Mental health of the Spanish-American in Texas. In M. K. Opler (Ed.), *Culture and mental health*. New York: The Macmillan Company, 1959. Pp. 467–485.

Jaco, E. G. *The social epidemiology of mental disorders—A psychiatric survey of Texas*. New York: The Russell Sage Foundation, 1960.

Kardiner, A. & Ovesey L., *The mark of oppression: A psychosocial study of the American Negro*. New York: W. W. Norton and Company, 1951.

Knutson, A. L. *The individual, society, and health behavior*. New York: Russell Sage Foundation, 1965.

Madsen, W. *Society and health in the lower Rio Grande Valley*. Austin, Texas: The University of Texas Press, 1961 (Published by the Hogg Foundation for Mental Health).

Madsen, W. Value conflicts in cultural transfer. In P. Worchel & D. Byrne (Eds.), *Personality change*. New York: John Wiley and Sons, 1964. (a)

Madsen, W. The alcoholic agringado. *American Anthropologist*, 1964, **66**, 355–361. (b)

Madsen, W. *The Mexican-Americans of South Texas*. In series, *Case studies in cultural anthropology*, ed. by George and Louise Spindler. New York: Holt, Rinehart and Winston, 1964. (c)

Opler, M. K. The cultural backgrounds of mental health. In M. K. Opler (Ed.), *Culture and mental health*. New York: The Macmillan Company, 1959.

Pitt-Rivers, J. A. *The people of the Sierra*. New York: Criterion Books, 1954.

Ramos, S. *Profile of man and culture in Mexico* (transl. by P. G. Earle). Austin, Texas: The University of Texas Press, 1962.

Romano, O. Donship in a Mexican-American community in Texas. *American Anthropologist*, 1960, **62**, 966–967.

Romano, O. Charismatic medicine, folk-healing and folk sainthood. *American Anthropologist*, 1965, **67**, 1151–1173.

Rubel, A. J. Concepts of disease in Mexican-American culture. *American Anthropologist*, 1960, **62**, 795–814.

Rubel, A. J. The epidemiology of a folk illness: Susto in Hispanic America. *Ethnology*, 1964, **3**, 268–283.

Srole, L., Langer, T. S., Michael, S. T., Opler, M. K., Rennie, T. A. C. *Mental health in the metropolis: the midtown Manhattan study*. New York: McGraw-Hill, 1962.

Wegrocki, H. J. A critique of cultural and statistical concepts of abnormality. In C. Kluckhohn and H. A. Murray (Eds.), *Personality in nature, society, and culture*. New York: Alfred A. Knopf. Pp. 551–561.

2.10   Orientation

Of all ethnic or social groups within the United States, the Negro has received the greatest amount of attention and concern in recent years. Since the Supreme Court decision of 1954 that banned continuation of the "separate but equal" principle of segregation, world-wide headline material has been provided by the Negro's attempts to achieve equality.

Fred R. Crawford presents a sophisticated analysis of research on the mental health and illness of the American Negro. His review is focused on whether or not there are differences in rates of psychosis between Negroes and whites in the North and the South, and whether or not there are differences in the ability of either group to remain in the community after hospitalization.

Recognizing that there may be differences in rates based on advantages gained since the Supreme Court ruling, Crawford separates his analysis into two major time periods, differentials in rates prior to 1959 and differentials in rates after that period. His operating assumption is that if Negroes are achieving greater equality in larger areas of their daily lives, then any rate differentials should have gradually begun to disappear since 1959.

The analysis is sophisticated and takes account of differences that can be attributed to social class membership in both groups. He presents a clear picture of the difficulties encountered in arriving at conclusions because of the lack of comparability in research methods and approaches among various investigators. His presentation focuses on three important questions:

1. Are there variations in prevalence and incidence rates between Negroes and whites?

2. Are there variations in quality of mental hospital care for both groups?

3. Are there variations in values and expectations within and between both groups that affect both preceding questions?

2.10   Variations between Negroes and Whites in Concepts of Mental Illness, Its Treatment and Prevalence

Fred R. Crawford

Mental health experts have grappled for many years with such questions as whether Negroes have higher rates of mental illnesses than whites, whether the kinds of mental illnesses diagnosed among Negroes differ from those diagnosed among whites, and whether Negroes receive a different quality of treatment for mental illnesses than do whites.

In 1959, difficulties in comparing and interpreting available studies of mental illnesses among Negroes and whites were described along with an effort to summarize the findings from such studies. With caution, four general "conclusions" were identified about which there was little apparent disagreement in the literature (Crawford, Rollins, & Sutherland, 1960). The first held that among residents of the northern part of the United States, Negroes had higher incidence rates of mental illnesses than did whites; that among residents of the southern part of this nation, Negroes had lower incidence rates than whites; and that these differences in incidence rates were *not* associated with differences in physiological (racial) characteristics. Second, the reported admissions to state mental hospitals of Negroes occurred at a higher rate than for whites. Third, Negroes received a lower quality of care while under treatment than whites, and proportionately fewer Negroes were released from state mental hospitals than whites. Fourth, when separated from state mental hospitals, Negroes had the higher rate of successfully remaining in their communities even though the "attitudes and knowledge" of the Negro population concerning the mentally ill were "less accepting and less understanding" than those attributed to the white population.

Each of these generalized conclusions was reexamined in the 1959 study. Although additional evidence presented in the 1959 study did tend to support the conclusion that Negroes, as a minority group, "had a somewhat lower level of understanding of the current theories of mental illness than did whites," Negroes in Texas were found to be more accepting of former mental patients than were whites. A number of studies have established that education is probably the key to differences in knowledge about mental illnesses and sources of treatment (Freeman & Kassebaum, 1960; Nunnally, 1959). Such a conclusion is certainly logical. As equality of education becomes more universal in this nation, then at least in theory this difference should tend to disappear; and, in fact, it is disappearing, as will be shown later.

The ability of a former mental patient, whether Negro or white, to survive in his community was equated not only with attitudes and opinions of his family, friends, and associates, but with economic opportunities available to him. Certainly today the various sources of possible economic support through expanded vocational rehabilitation programs, more adequate welfare coverage, and the many resources established under the mantle of the Office of Economic Opportunity, are changing the odds facing the former mental patient to find gainful employment, whether his skin be black or white or some shade in between.

As the civil rights social movement progresses, the inequalities in quality of treatment should also disappear. Federal laws now make illegal such inequalities, and even provide channels and procedures through which any reported inequalities are investigated. There is still much to be accomplished in this area of treatment, however, as will be described later. But the constantly changing pattern of human interrelationships bound up in the civil rights movement has other overtones as well. A small but vocal element under the banner of "Black Power" calls for the end of any joint Negro-white effort to bring about equality. Under all of the many different kinds of pressures, the Negro minority is changing. If the suggestion presented as part of an official report from the United States Department of Labor (*The Negro Family,* 1965) is correct, the Negro society and particularly its institutions of the family are deteriorating, and this "is the single most important social fact of the United States today" (p. 4). On this basis it could be predicted that the future will see a rise in the rates of mental illnesses among Negroes, coupled with their increasing utilization of treatment resources because of new knowledge about such resources and the lack of barriers to the services that these resources are making available.

This same official document claims that "There is no very satisfactory way, at present, to measure social health or social pathology within an ethnic, or religious, or geographical community. Data are few and uncertain, and conclusions drawn from them . . . are subject to the grossest error." In spite of case registers, expanded patient data reporting systems, computerized analytical procedures, and even new theoretical approaches, this same charge can be made against current measures of mental illness. Studies of the distribution of mental illnesses among the American population remain largely uncoordinated and produce data that are, at best, difficult to interpret and compare. Long lapses of time still occur between the collection of patient data and the publication of findings. The idea of testing the significance of such data statistically is reflected in few studies, as is the reporting of error potentials or magnitudes in any series of patient data. Of all inadequacies in current efforts, the lack of coordination looms largest. Not only do methodologies differ widely, but, most importantly, definitions and methods of identifying and classifying the mentally ill also differ. These lacks preclude comparisons. Conclusions drawn from them well may be subject "to the grossest error."

Unfortunately, these lacks exist because of the failure of professionals to exercise their scientific dedication, and not because of the absence of opportunities to carry out comparable studies. At least four major opportunities to bring about coordinated and comparable studies characterize the 1960s. The year 1963 saw all fifty states initiate comprehensive mental health planning efforts with the help of funds and guidelines established by Public Law 88-164. This magnificent chance to develop and bring together valid data about the mentally ill in all states was not utilized. Comprehensive mental retardation planning efforts are currently being completed in all fifty states, and again there has been no coordination

among them. Shortly, a third major comprehensive planning effort will
be initiated in the fifty states, dealing with vocational rehabilitation services which now include the mentally ill as part of the responsibility carried by these services. Again, coordination and comparability among the
states in these studies will not occur unless some attempt is made immediately to bring this about. A few pilot studies are also under way
to study people living in depressed housing areas. If this program is put
into operation, hundreds of such neighborhoods all over the country will
be surveyed, and information about the presence of mentally ill persons
in each population group studied will be gathered. The one example of
this type of study available, although it reports some data about mental
health problems and treatment, fails to describe even simple facts about
differences between Negroes and whites in rates of mental illnesses (Greenleigh Associates, 1965).

Perhaps, from one viewpoint, this lack of any effort to contrast Negroes
and whites is realistic. Who can prove that the diagnosing of mental illnesses is performed in a uniform, standardized way across this nation?
Has not enough been written about Negroes, including the 960-page *The
American Negro Reference Book* (Davis, 1966), to establish that there
is no single Negro culture? Have demographers not documented the
transfer of racial identification through "passing" (Guptill, 1950)? Is it
not time to challenge the census definition of Negro, and in that one act
destroy the basis for official discrimination?

From a different viewpoint, diagnosed mental illnesses still represent
the only hope for studying the magnitude and distribution of this pandemic pathology among the American people. Past failures to take into
consideration variations among Negroes can point the direction to more
valid studies, based upon these recognized variations. Finally, the United
States census represents the only consistent and comprehensive source of
information about the American people. What is needed is more specific
information about each individual, and ethnicity (or race) remains as an
important characteristic. The stigma of the identifying label should be
removed, not the label itself. The following interpretations have been
written from this second viewpoint.

NEW APPROACHES IN THE STUDY OF INCIDENCE AND PREVALENCE

Of the four "tentative conclusions" identified in the 1959 study, the
differences in frequency of appearance of mental illnesses among Negroes
and whites has received the most attention in subsequent studies.
Through the development of new research procedures, a more valid
answer could be made available soon. Two important publications appearing in 1960 set the stage for the new research procedures in studies

of records of mental patients. E. G. Jaco conducted social epidemiological studies of the mentally ill as early as 1954, culminating his work in *The Social Epidemiology of Mental Disorders* (1960). R. J. Plunkett and J. E. Gordon, outstanding names in medical epidemiology, applied their knowledge to the field of mental disorders in a report prepared for the Joint Commission on Mental Illness and Health (Plunkett & Gordon, 1960). Their definition of epidemiology states that it is "a body of knowledge about the occurrence and behavior of disease in populations and, also, a method of study to determine causes and courses of diseases affecting the individual and community."

Although it is generally accepted that mental illnesses are pandemic rather than epidemic, the study techniques of the epidemiologist have proven to be of great importance, and correctly belong under the more general field of human ecology, the study of man-environment relationships. The meaning of "environment" in this new theoretical approach has been expanded toward the holistic position that any and all possibly influencing conditions—social, physical, cultural, political, economic, and so on—must be considered (Crawford, 1960, 1963; Jaco, 1957). Of even greater utility in clarifying differences in rates of mental illnesses among population groups are studies that have begun to examine, if only in limited detail, the social processes that select out certain persons for admission to treatment for mental illnesses (Crawford, 1964; Crawford *et al.,* 1961).

These processes, at least as reflected in partial descriptions, have differed between certain groups of Negroes and certain groups of whites, resulting in variations in admission rates so diligently reported over the years and not infrequently interpreted as demonstrating Negroes have "higher rates" than whites. Legal commitments, alcoholic admissions, and criminal arrests are three types of processes which Negroes reportedly have been involved in more frequently than whites.

There are other benefits that hopefully may arise from the application of epidemiological techniques to the study of mental illnesses. One is the derivation of accurate incidence and prevalence rates of admission for defined populations. In general terms, incidence refers to the rate (or number) of new cases of mental illnesses that occur during an extended time period. Prevalence is a measure of active cases present in a defined population at a particular moment. Both measures are necessary before accurate descriptions of the distribution of known cases of mental illnesses are possible.

Another benefit that may grow from epidemiological studies is the further refinement of labels and terms applied to the mentally ill, a process that belongs in the field of nosology. Such studies should permit increasing clarification of the nature and dynamics of illness-producing forces within the environment-organism relationship, a probe into etiological factors still greatly needed which will point the way to new treatment techniques. Epidemiologically developed data also are superior when projections of future numbers or rates of mental illnesses have to be developed. Thus, planning for future needs in treatment, the location of psychiatric facilities, staffing, case loads, and even rehabilitation services would become more practical if such projections were available. Finally, epidemiological reporting systems operating on a permanent and continuous basis provide evidence through which the effectiveness of treatment, control, rehabilitation, and preventive measures applied to a patient group and defined population might be measured. This is one of the keys to comprehensive mental health services required under many new state plans for combatting the mental illnesses.

There are two major types of epidemiological studies. The first, studies of patient records, clarifies and describes the visible part of the iceberg of "the mentally ill." As individuals appear for treatment, information is obtained and started on its way to becoming a reported admission to treatment. Most studies of the distribution of mentally ill persons within population groups have been based upon some kind of patient records, usually developed by the treatment facilities for other purposes. Many of the dubious findings that plague the field of mental health have grown out of such data replete with all the weaknesses thus far identified, such as the lack of common definitions and classifications and the lack of patient data from all treatment sources, whether public or private, in clinic or hospital. Because state mental hospital records are the one source that has been readily available over the years, most studies have been made of such records with the conclusion that "northern Negroes were admitted to state mental hospitals more frequently than whites." In some southern states, such as Virginia, this has also been reported (Wilson & Lantz, 1963), but certainly not in all southern states (Crawford, 1965).

The second handicap in using admission records exists because of the inability of researchers to unduplicate these records. If one person were admitted several times to psychiatric treatment facilities during the period of study, there was no practical way the *person* could be counted rather than his *admissions*. Duplication of admissions distorted the true picture, resulting in incorrect conclusions by some writers.

Recognizing the crucial importance of accurate patient data reporting and interpretation, Morton Kramer of the National Institute of Mental Health and his staff became involved in the development of case registers. The first exists for Monroe County, New York. The second is now operative for the whole state of Maryland. A third has been established recently for the state of Hawaii. Data originating from these sources are gathered under standardized definitions on a continuous basis. For the first time, unduplication of patient records is possible, longitudinal studies of large numbers of patients' service experiences are occurring, and various kinds of "specific rates" can be computed.

The second type of epidemiological study seeks information about the "unseen part of the iceberg," the mentally ill persons in a population who are not seen for treatment. Hutterites, rural Canadians, and even 110,000 residents of midtown Manhattan have been studied in this way.

For years, the estimate "one in ten" has been used to refer to the number of mentally ill persons in the nation's population. There is certainly no evidence of magnitude to support this estimate, although it is less suspicious than the Midtown study's finding that only 19 percent of their random sample of 1660 cases was without some degree of mental disturbance (Srole, Opler, & Langman, 1962).

Differences in diagnostic concepts and interpretations in the populations studied, in the location of these populations, in research techniques, and even in the moments in our developing history when the many studies have been made, preclude many valid comparisons and specific conclusions that apply beyond each study itself. The search must go on, however, hopefully through both types of endeavors.

VARIATIONS IN PREVALENCE AND INCIDENCE RATES

What evidence is now appearing that may begin to establish the different rates of mental illnesses, if such exist, between Negroes and whites? In 1963, Martin Grossack edited a volume which brought together a number of important studies dealing with Negroes and mental health (Grossack, 1963). A 1949 study by Helen McLean reprinted in this volume drew upon first admissions to state mental hospitals in Illinois for data. McLean said that there was no discrimination or segregation of Negroes in these hospitals, and the chances of Negroes being admitted were equal to the chances of whites. By dealing with only one diagnostic group, she was able to conclude that "there is no greater incidence of psychosis in Negroes than in whites" (p. 134).

In another article reprinted in this same volume, Benjamin Pasamanick (1963) brought to light some of the first definitive data about comparative rates:

The findings based on a community survey and state, private, and V.A. hospital rates indicate that the white population has the higher rates for the psychoses, psychoneuroses, and the psycophysiologic-autonomic-visceral disorders. Nonwhite rates are higher for the acute brain syndrome and for mental deficiency.

As a conclusion to the 1959 summary study mentioned previously, it could be stated that "Although great cultural and demographic differences exist between Texas Negroes and whites, the 'known-case' rates of mental illness for the two population segments are similar [Crawford *et al.*, 1960, p. 935]."

Early reports from the Monroe County case register indicated a prevalence rate, unadjusted, of 7.38 per 1000 population for nonwhites and 8.50 for whites (Gardner & Associates, 1962). These rates, when adjusted for age and applied to the total Monroe County population, changed to 10.80 for nonwhites and 8.37 for whites. This case register includes all patients not only seen by public and private hospitals and clinics, but patients treated by psychiatrists in private practice as well. The incidence rates for Monroe County during 1960 were also slightly higher for nonwhites than whites (10.17 to 8.46). This difference was further extended when adjusted for age (11.55 for nonwhites, 8.39 for whites). These figures, however, must be considered in their context. Monroe County is not typical of most counties in this country. It has unusually comprehensive and accessible psychiatric services and a very small proportion of nonwhite citizens. Specifically, there were only 185 nonwhites under care on January 1, 1960, and 255 entrances into care during 1960. The comparable numbers for whites are 4773 under care and 4748 coming into care during 1960.

A profound criticism can be levelled at this and other comparisons of data developed through case registers, because even simple statistical tests for significance of differences between rates have not been made. There certainly is no parametric test that will establish an acceptable level of significance for differences in rates of 10.17 per 1000, and 8.46 per 1000, or even for the age-adjusted rates of 11.55 and 8.39 per 1000. The numerical difference is only 3.16 per 1000, and few statisticians would hold this to be significant. Thus what does the "higher rate" really mean?

By 1964, Kurt Gorwitz was cautious enough to seek a more definitive explanation, using the word "substantially" rather than "significantly" in reporting findings from the Maryland case register data:

A comparison of white and nonwhite rates indicates that (in Maryland) the latter are substantially higher, both for males and females. It is not known at the present time whether this data reflects a true greater incidence of mental illness or whether this is merely a result of a combination of such factors as:

1. Socio-economic and cultural differences. A study in Ohio comparing whites and Negroes of the same socio-economic levels showed similarities in treatment rates.

2. Variations in the availability of other treatment services. Most patients seen by private psychiatrists are white.

3. The relatively greater concentration of Negroes in the crowded central urban core areas. Two-thirds of Maryland's Negroes and twenty percent of those white live in Baltimore. . . .

Nearly all Negro females who went to inpatient facilities were seen in State hospitals only and Negro males who were not seen in State hospitals were seen mainly in the V.A. hospital [Gorwitz, 1964, p. 6].

Other recent evidence available in comparing prevalence rates of Negroes and whites was developed by Morton Kramer, Gorwitz, and Anita Bahn, who were involved in the case register studies. In 1964, age adjusted rates combined for both Monroe County and Maryland reveal a gross pattern of 10.3 per 1000 for Negroes and 8.7 for whites, now a difference of only 1.6 per 1000. As Kramer describes these findings, verification of some previous conclusions with additional cautions are presented:

Male rates were consistently higher than female until late in life for both the white and nonwhite population. Nonwhite rates were higher than white rates for almost all age and sex groups. To some extent, this difference by race is accounted for by the fact that a much higher proportion of the nonwhite population of Maryland lives in the large urban area of Baltimore City as compared with the white population (62 and 24% respectively). Further, Baltimore City age-specific rates were generally higher than comparable rates for other areas of the state probably reflecting the greater availability and use of psychiatric services in urban core areas. The Baltimore City age-adjusted prevalence rate was about the same for whites and nonwhites (10.5 and 10.4 respectively), but there were differences in age-specific rates. In making these comparisons it should be borne in mind that the data in the Maryland register do not include reports from private psychiatrists [Bahn, Gorwitz, & Kramer, 1964, p. 2].

It is generally accepted that few nonwhites are treated by psychiatrists in private practice.

During 1964, as part of the comprehensive mental health planning effort in Texas, patient data were obtained from 90 percent of the psychiatric treatment facilities in the state, excluding psychiatrists in private practice. Although 13 percent of the Texas population was classified by the 1960 census as Negro, only 10 percent of all reported admissions were for Negroes (Crawford, 1965). As has been reported by other states, the majority of Negro mental patients in Texas were treated in state mental hospitals (59 percent) as contrasted to white mental patients (39 percent).

The only conclusion that is logically defensible at this time for the nation as a whole is simply that *adjusted incidence and prevalence rates of "mental illnesses" between Negroes and whites are more similar than different.* Differences that are reported are explainable on the basis of the region of the nation in which the population studied is located, on the basis of different sex ratios, age distributions, what is defined as "mental illness," and other nonphysiological characteristics.

VARIATIONS IN QUALITY OF CARE

Although the evidence was overwhelmingly in support of the 1959 conclusion that "Following commitment the Negro patients receive less treatment and care than do their white counterparts," restrictions to integration in all state mental hospitals have since been removed, as previously mentioned. Health insurance is more readily available to Negroes now than in previous years, and in many policies written today mental illnesses are covered. The Veterans Administration hospitals, which provide the same quality of care for all patients under their jurisdiction, are also recognized now as an important source of treatment for a Negro veteran who is mentally ill, as Gorwitz (1964) points out. Even outpatient clinics are reporting increasing numbers of Negroes who learn of these services and attempt to use them.

Equality in care is still some time away, however. Jan Howard (1965, p. 203), describes the general pattern succinctly:

The differential social and economic status of Negroes and whites in the United States almost certainly results in whites receiving the better medical care. Available data suggest that whites have had the greater medical insurance coverage than nonwhites; that white patients have made relatively greater use of hospitals than Negro patients; and that whites have had access to more physicians in general, and to more board-certified specialists in particular than Negroes have had.

Helen McLean, in her 1949 article referred to earlier, stated that at that time there were only five Negro members of the American Psychiatric Association. The NIMH report (Bahn et al., 1964) on the case registers includes this statement: "Studies on private practice in other areas have shown that white persons use these resources at a much greater rate than nonwhite persons" (p. 2).

Gorwitz, also using case register data, established that the average number of days of care for mental illnesses is lower for Negroes than whites. Also, the Negro patients are proportionally more heavily concentrated among those who receive only limited care. Finally, on the basis of information concerning longitudinal studies of services experienced by mental patients, Gorwitz (1964), concludes that "In general, white residents had a higher percentage of multiple services than Negroes" (p. 9).

From these various pieces of information, the conclusion that can be defended at this time is simply that Negroes still have less chance of receiving the full range of services utilized by whites, that Negroes are not kept under treatment as long as are white patients, that Negroes do not utilize multiple sources of help as frequently as whites, and consequently *inequality of care still exists.*

VARIATIONS IN VALUES AND EXPECTATIONS

Studies of Negroes and rates of mental illnesses too frequently have been approached under the implied assumption that Negroes in America constitute a homogeneous group. The reverse assumption can also be misleading. In an effort to dispel the idea that major differences exist between Negroes and whites, Benjamin Pasamanick (Grossack, 1963) states "the Negro . . . shares the same cultural heritage as other Americans" (p. 151). A brief reminder that the Emancipation Proclamation is only slightly more than 100 years old, and that expanded civil rights laws had to be enacted in the 1950s, should reinforce the truth that this heritage has been different for the two population groups (Jeff, 1965; Smith, 1962). Also different has been the heritage of the Mexican-American, the Chinese-American, and many other subpopulations with distinct cultural ties to other nations.

In spite of the disadvantaged position the majority of Negroes have occupied during the history of this nation, significant differences do exist among them on any characteristic that is studied, be it income, education, occupation, goals in life, and so on. In fact, the ranges of these characteristics are as wide among Negroes as among whites. At some point, researchers will focus their attention on measuring rates of mental illnesses over these wide ranges rather than simply overlooking this important difference with such statements (Pasamanick, 1963) as "Since the Negro population, relative to the white, is overwhelmingly lower class, it follows that nonwhites will be proportionately over-institutionalized" (p. 155). The concept of "class" applied to rates of mental illness has been challenged elsewhere (Crawford, 1966).

If this assumption concerning class and admissions to state mental hospitals were true, the rates of admission for the 16 percent of the Texas population with Spanish surnames would rank highest, above Negroes and Anglos. As a matter of fact, the reverse is true. Whether Hollingshead's two-factor index of social position is used or whether any of the other commonly accepted distinguishing characteristics of class differences are employed, the Spanish surname population in Texas ranks *lower* than does the Texas Negro population. There is no doubt about the fact that the lowest rates of admissions to any and all psychiatric treatment facilities in Texas occur among the Spanish surname population

(Crawford, 1965, 1966). Explanations of this lack of use of mental health facilities by Spanish surname people have been made over the years and consistently are explained through the values held by this minority group (Crawford, 1961; Jaco, 1959; Madsen, 1962). Madsen again discusses these values elsewhere in this volume.

To Pasamanick's credit, he does point out the fact that Negroes in the North are primarily urban dwellers, while in the South, Negroes have been primarily rural dwellers. Even this one difference offers a clue to differences in reported rates of admission to certain kinds of psychiatric facilities, as Kramer and others have demonstrated.

Exploratory studies carried out in Texas suggest that rural dwellers may be admitted to state mental hospitals for reasons somewhat different than urban dwellers (Crawford, 1966; Crawford et al., 1961). If these few data are representative, rural dwellers (and this would include southern rural Negroes) are admitted at higher rates than are urban dwellers. The reverse of this pattern, as suggested by interpretations of the Maryland case register data, might be explained by the migration of southern rural Negroes to the slum areas of major eastern cities. The disintegration of the family, as pointed out in the United States Department of Labor's official statement, growing out of urban pressures as well as the pressures of social change in all aspects of American life could certainly be expected to increase admissions to state mental hospitals serving these urban populations. A definitive explanation, however, must await further research.

The interpreters of the American Negro culture are numerous. Because of the rapid changes occurring as integration continues, about all that can safely be said at this moment is that wide variations exist. At one end of this pattern are values strongly similar to those in the dominant culture, stratum by stratum. At the other end are values that reject any semblance of the dominant culture, striving for a completely different identification such as that sought by the Black Muslims.

Thus, the need is for more careful research into the attitudes and values held by different social levels and unique groups of both Negroes and whites, for more specific studies of the different social processes experienced by persons in these various social levels as they seek and find treatment for mental illnesses, studies of the methods and definitions through which diagnoses of the many kinds of mental illnesses are determined, and finally, studies of differences that occur as the various kinds of treatment are provided.

Again, a conclusion can be offered and defended that if the available data concerning incidence and prevalence of mental illnesses could be standardized for Negroes and whites and subjected to statistical verification, differences in rates would tend to disappear; and those remaining could be explained more adequately.

REFERENCES

Bahn, A. K., Gorwitz, K., & Kramer, M. A cross-sectional picture of psychiatric care in an entire state. Psychiatric Studies and Projects Series, published by the Mental Hospital Service of the American Psychiatric Association, Volume 2, Number 3, February, 1964.

Boone, M. C. A study of the need for mental health services in Atlanta, Georgia. Unpublished M.A. thesis, Atlanta University, 1962.

Crawford, F. R. The forgotten egg. Austin, Texas: Texas State Department of Health, 1961.

Crawford, F. R. Brief description of data gathering and processing plans and procedures. Austin, Texas: Office of Mental Health Planning, Texas State Department of Health, 1963.

Crawford, F. R. Are these the unwanted? Austin, Texas: Texas Governor's Committee on Aging, 1964.

Crawford, F. R. Lower class values and attitudes relevant to mental health. In K. S. Miller & C. M. Grigg (Eds.), Mental Health and the Lower Social Classes. Tallahassee, Florida: Florida State University Studies, No. 49, 1966. Pp. 23–41.

Crawford, F. R. Data for planning—A series of technical reports to aid Texas communities and agencies in their planning for comprehensive mental health and mental retardation services. Austin, Texas: Texas Department of Mental Health and Mental Retardation, 1966.

Crawford, F. R. Mental Illness in Texas, A Morbidity Report for 1964. Austin, Texas: Office of Mental Health Planning, Texas State Department of Health, 1965.

Crawford, F. R., Rollins, G. W., & Sutherland, R. L. Variations between Negroes and whites in concepts of mental illness and its treatment. Annals of the New York Academy of Sciences, 1960, 84, 918–937.

Crawford, F. R. Proposal for the development of a mental illness epidemiological information center in the Division of Mental Health, Texas State Department of Health. Austin, Texas: Texas State Department of Health, 1960.

Crawford, F. R., Rollins, G. W., & Sutherland, R. L. Four Texas communities look at the mentally ill. Unpublished manuscript prepared for The Hogg Foundation for Mental Health of The University of Texas, 1961.

Crawford, F. R., Rollins, G. W., & Sutherland, R. L. Variations in the evaluation of the mentally ill: Part II—The viewpoint of the rural dweller. Journal of Health and Human Behavior, 1961, 2, 267–275.

Davis, J. T. The American Negro reference book. New York: Phelps-Stokes, 1966.

Freeman, H. E., & Kassebaum, G. C. Relations of Education and Knowledge to Opinions about Mental Illness. *Mental Hygiene,* 1960, 44, 1960, 43–47.

Gardner, E. A., and Associates. A Cumulative Register of Psychiatric Services in a Community. Paper presented at the American Public Health Association, October 1962.

Gorwitz, K. The demography of mental illness in Maryland. Paper presented at the Phipps Psychiatric Unit of the Johns Hopkins Hospital, November 1964.

Greenleigh Associates, Inc. *Diagnostic survey of tenant households in the West Side Urban Renewal Area of New York City,* New York, January 1965, pages 95–96.

Grossack, M. M. (Ed.) *Mental health and segregation.* New York: Springer Publishing Company, 1963.

Guptill, C. S. A study of the attitudes of Negro college students toward members of their race who have passed as white. Unpublished M.A. thesis, Emory University, 1950.

Howard, J. Race differences in hypertension mortality trends. *The Milbank Memorial Fund Quarterly,* 1965, *63*, 202–218.

Jaco, E. G. Attitudes toward, and incidence of, mental disorder: A research note. *Southwestern Social Science Quarterly,* 1957, **38**, 27–38.

Jaco, E. G. Mental health of the Spanish-American in Texas. In M. K. Opler (Ed.), *Culture and mental health.* New York: The Macmillan Company, 1959. Pp. 467–485.

Jaco, E. G. *The social epidemiology of mental disorders,* New York: Russell Sage Foundation, 1960.

Jeff, W. B. The relationship between certain socio-cultural factors, race and class, and programs in group-serving agencies. Unpublished thesis, Atlanta University, 1965.

Madsen, W. *Society and health.* Austin, Texas: The Hogg Foundation for Mental Health of The University of Texas, 1962.

McLean, H. V. The emotional health of Negroes. In M. M. Grossack (Ed.), *Mental health and segregation.* New York: Springer Publishing Company, 1963. Pp. 131–138.

Nunnally, J., Jr. *Tests and instruments.* New York: McGraw-Hill, 1959.

Pasamanick, B. A survey of mental disease in an urban population. In M. M. Grossack (Ed.), *Mental health and segregation.* New York: Springer Publishing Company, 1963. Pp. 150–157.

Plunkett, R. J., & Gordon, J. E. *Epidemiology and mental illness.* New York: Basic Books, 1960.

Smith, M. J. Some implications of lower class cultural traits for community organization in the urban slum neighborhood. Unpublished M.A. thesis, Atlanta University, 1962.

Srole, L. Opler, M. K., & Langner, T. *Mental health in the metropolis.* New York: McGraw-Hill, 1962.

The Negro family—The case for national action. Washington, D.C.: Office of Policy Planning and Research, United States Department of Labor, "For Official Use Only," 1965.

Wilson, D. C., & Lantz, E. M. Culture change and Negro state hospital admissions. In M. M. Grossack (Ed.), *Mental health and segregation*. New York: Springer Publishing Company, 1963. Pp. 139–149.

2.11   Orientation

Americans are imbued with the idea that this nation is composed of persons whose heritage lies in many different lands. What we sometimes forget is that these various subpopulations and ethnic groups have contributed differentially to our growth as a nation and to our social problems.

A case in point is the Japanese-Americans. Harry Kitano points out that they have lower rates of criminality (including juvenile delinquency), a lower incidence of psychological disorder of nearly all types, higher rates of advanced education, and generally exhibit a strong commitment to the positive values of the mainstream of American life. In building his case, Dr. Kitano presents a broad spectrum of research and statistics from Japan and the United States.

There are disquieting symptoms, however. As the Japanese-Americans become more acculturated, they are becoming more like other Americans and are giving evidence of rising pathology of many kinds. In reading this excellent article, one can only conclude that there is much that we might learn from the Japanese-Americans and there is much that they might learn about themselves. Otherwise, the potential benefits to be derived from this group will be lost in the formlessness of contemporary American social life.

2.11   Japanese-American Mental Illness[1]

Harry H. L. Kitano

In earlier days, the phrase "immigrants from Asia" might have called to mind seething masses, cheap labor, and the inevitable inscrutable faces. Hopefully the same phrase today is related to a more favorable, if not more realistic image. We say hopefully because the Chinese and Japanese still remain as relatively faceless and nameless populations,

[1] This research was supported by NIMH Grant M-11112.

even to social scientists, and as a consequence they are often viewed as exceptions to generalizations of human behavior. For example, in a study just completed on Japanese crime and delinquency in the United States (Kitano, 1962), reactions of professionals included such phrases as "Do they have any delinquency at all?" and "But how relevant are the findings to other groups?"

Reasons for these views are not too hard to find. The stereotype of an exotic culture and the mysterious East is difficult to discard when systematic knowledge about the Japanese is often lacking, and when scientific data are scarce. Further, scholars of Japanese ancestry have been hesitant to pursue studies of their own ethnic group, and Japanese residential concentration in the western part of the United States has excluded them from on-going studies of European immigrants. But perhaps most important, the Japanese do appear to be exceptions, especially to generalizations concerning "problem minorities." Poverty, discrimination, life in the ghetto, and nonwhite skin color are usually associated with such problem groups, and minorities often live up to this expectation by responding with high rates of crime, delinquency, and mental illness. It is generally believed that the Japanese (and to a similar extent the Chinese),[2] although saddled with handicaps such as discrimination and life in the ghetto, have somehow refused to respond to their negative environment with high rates of delinquency and mental illness. Therefore, the point of view that the Japanese are somehow different and perhaps not influenced in expected ways by environmental conditions is often reinforced.

Peculiarly, there has been little scientific interest in the Japanese-Americans until recently. As early as 1933, Hayner described the unique behavior of the Japanese. In studying crime in the Puget Sound area, Hayner noticed the high rates of crime in the ghetto area for all groups except for the Japanese, who had low rates. Up to the present time, this has remained as an interesting, but unexplored, finding, and Petersen in a current issue of the *New York Times* (January 6, 1966) has said:

The Japanese Americans, in short, ought to be a central focus of social studies. Their experience converts our best sociological generalizations into partial truths at best; this is a laboratory case of an exception to test a rule. Conceivably in such a more intensive analysis, we might find a means of isolating some of the element of this remarkable culture and grafting it on to plants that manifestly need the pride, the persistence and the success of our model minority.

[2] Although the Chinese and Japanese are completely different populations, census and other data often lump them together under the term Orientals. Such a category is useless for cross-cultural study.

Are the Japanese really so exceptional? An earlier study by the writer (Kitano, in progress) illustrates the extremely low rates of official crime and delinquency in the Japanese group. But, the reasons behind the behavior do not appear to be so mysterious. A group with a strong family system, living in a cohesive community, with high values on achievement and conformity, and with overall styles of life congruent with the American middle class should be characterized by low rates of official crime and delinquency.

What do we know about Japanese-American mental illness? How prevalent is *ki-chi-gai* ("crazy") behavior in this population? Are there empirical hypotheses that may be explored to understand mentally ill behavior? The primary purpose of this chapter is to attempt to answer these questions.

EPIDEMIOLOGY

The true incidence of mental illness and mental health in any population is probably impossible to assess except in the most general manner. All mental health statistics have one thing in common—they represent data that are related to the "funneling effect." The funneling effect as described by Cressey (1961) in criminological research, holds that the accuracy of criminal statistics is dependent upon distance from the bottom of the funnel. Therefore, in terms of official statistics, crimes known to the police are a more accurate index of incidence than statistics of those arrested. In turn, the arrest rate is a more efficient index than the conviction rate, which in turn is more accurate than imprisonment rates.

Although there are many differences between statistics on mental illness and crime, general rates of mental illness can also be related to the funneling effect. Therefore, a more accurate index of the true rates of mental illness can be determined from trained residents of a community who have intimate knowledge of its inhabitants, rather than from a random sample of a population drawn for diagnostic purposes. The random sample in turn is probably more accurate than statistics of those persons coming to a mental health facility, the diagnosis at a clinic is more relevant than statistics limited to persons accepted for treatment, and a consideration of the population under treatment is more efficient than an analysis of those patients residing in a mental hospital. There are interrelationships among the various levels, but the one most often used is the least efficient—the statistics on hospitalization. The error is similar to estimating the size of an iceberg by looking at the exposed portion.

The Bottom of the Iceberg—The Top of the Funnel

It is difficult to hide in a Japanese community, even in a sprawling area such as Los Angeles. That is, it is difficult to hide from other Japanese, and the number of residents renders the ethnic interaction comparable to life in a small hamlet in Vermont. Common friends, common institutions, common interests, and common past experiences provide fertile ground for communication and knowledge about each other. A further experience, probably unique among all ethnic groups, was the wartime evacuation and relocation which forced the majority of Japanese to live together under rather intimate conditions. Therefore, persons who have grown up in the Japanese community are in a strategic position to provide an assessment of mental health and mental illness.

Fortunately, there are a number of Japanese-American professionals who have grown up in the ethnic community and have acquired training in the mental health professions. We asked sixteen of them (two PhD psychologists, four psychiatrists, and ten MSW social workers) to complete a short check list concerning use and need of therapeutic resources by the Japanese in the United States. We followed up the check list with short interviews with selected respondents.

The Japanese have a convenient way of describing generations. The term Issei means first generation and refers to the immigrants from Japan, most of them arriving in the United States between 1900 and 1924. In general, Japanese currently over the age of 60 are probably Issei. The term Nisei means second generation and refers to the American-born children of the Issei immigrant. Their current estimated age range is 30–60; their modal age lies in the 40–45 category. The term Sansei means third generation and refers to the American-born children of Nisei-parents. They constitute the bulk of the adolescent and school-age population.

Mail responses to the check list were excellent. Of the sixteen contacts, fifteen responded within one week and are included in the coding. There was unanimous agreement (see Table 1) among the professionals that all three Japanese generations have seldom used the therapeutic resources of the larger community, including hospitalization. Most agreed that only the Issei used ethnic community services (that is, the social services provided by the Japanese community) at all.

Sharpest disagreement arose on Item 4, which refers to the need for therapy and mental health by Japanese generations. Sixty percent of the respondents indicated that all three of the Japanese generations were in need of services; the remaining proportion felt that the general mental

TABLE 1. Perceptions of Japanese Professionals Regarding
Three Generations of Japanese and Mental Health[a]

Generation	Have required hospitalization	Have used therapeutic resources of the community	Have used therapeutic resources of ethnic community	Have needed but not used therapeutic resources
Issei	No	No	A little	Yes
Nisei	No	No	No	Yes
Sansei	No	No	No	Yes

[a] $N = 15$.

health of the Japanese was quite good. There is, of course, a professional bias among mental health workers concerning the need for services for almost everybody. Nevertheless, it is interesting to note the discrepancy between "need" and "use" of services by the entire Japanese population.

Follow-up interviews were held with the professionals to gain more information about their perceptions of overall Japanese mental health. Most of them could recall very few signs of public "mentally ill behavior," either as they were growing up (including life in the wartime evacuation camps) or among their present ethnic acquaintances. However, all agreed upon the difficulty of assessing mental illness among a group where public "acting-out" behavior was kept under relatively formalized controls, and where the preferred modes of behavior encouraged formalism, politeness, and withdrawal.

However, the professionals who indicated a "need for therapy" among the Japanese referred primarily to current indications of conflict. The majority agreed that husband-wife roles and parent-child relationships were powerful sources of tension, but that the Japanese would not use professional services. As one psychiatrist commented,

Every time I give a public lecture (usually sponsored by a church or service club) on family problems, sexual information or child rearing, the place is packed and they ask all kinds of questions. Some of the questions are remarkably naive and others appear to indicate quite a bit of conflict but I'm sure the questioners will never go for professional advice.

Others corroborate these perceptions—high interest and possible signs of problems regarding parent-child relationships, high attendance at public lectures—but report virtually no follow-up for further professional help.

The Middle View

Statistics from social agencies, often thought of as providing preventive and therapeutic services, constitute our second-level view. These agencies (family service, child guidance clinics) can be divided into two types— those representing the minority group (the ethnic agency) and those serving the larger community.

The number of Japanese using the professional services of the larger community is extremely small. We attempted to obtain a sample of Japanese using the Family Service Agency and Child Guidance Clinic in Los Angeles for a proposed study (Archer, Staugas, & Hoffman, 1962) and found that even though over 80,000 Japanese were theoretically eligible for these services, less than five cases could be counted in any single year. The writer worked for two years in a Child Guidance Clinic which served the San Francisco Public Schools, and during this period there were no referred cases involving children of Japanese ancestry. Therefore, the perceptions of Japanese professionals concerning the nonuse of larger community services by the ethnic group is strongly supported.

Closer to true incidence, however, are data gathered from agencies serving the Japanese community. For many Japanese, especially for those who are less acculturated, the facilities of the ethnic community are more acceptable resources. A family service agency, developed by the Japanese community in 1962, served an average of thirty active counseling cases per month during its over two years of existence (Archer et al., 1962).

The most relevant source for analyzing mental health in the Japanese community on the agency level is the social service provided by the Japanese Chamber of Commerce of Los Angeles. An analysis of that caseload between the years 1962–1964 is presented in Table 2. Of the 604 cases, approximately 20 percent were classified "mentally ill." The majority of these cases were referred to County and State facilities.

Further analysis of the caseload shows an older male Issei population living on minimal income from lower status occupations and living in relatively isolated positions.

The most common diagnosis for mental illness was schizophrenia and a typical case might be illustrated by the following story. Mr. H., owner of a small hotel in the "Little Tokyo" area of Los Angeles, begins to notice gradual deterioration of Mr. Watanabe (fictitious name). Mr. Watanabe had moved into the hotel with two other bachelor Issei—although information was difficult to obtain, all three had come from the same *ken* ("state") and had worked as fruit pickers the majority of their lives. Now they were too old to continue, so they came to Los Angeles for retirement. The low rates at the hotel (average rent $45 a month) and a communal kitchen helped to stretch the dollar. The nearby Japanese community,

TABLE 2. DESCRIPTION OF CASELOAD OF SOCIAL WELFARE DEPARTMENT, JAPANESE CHAMBER OF COMMERCE, LOS ANGELES, 1962–1964

A. Generation	Percent[a]	B. Sex	Percent
Issei	83	Male	83
Nisei	7	Female	17
Sansei	10		
		D. Primary source of income	
C. Age		Public assistance,	85
55 or over	85	Social Security	
25–54	9	Nonpublic assistance	15
Under 24	5		
E. Primary occupations		F. Marital status	
Farm laborer	42	Widower-widow	36
Cook	15	Single, never married	30
Housewife	15	Married couple	15
Gardener	10	Divorced, never legally	15
Janitor	15	married	
Unknown	2	Under-age	5

[a] $N = 604$. Rounding errors lead to totals of less than 100 percent in some instances.

the recreation rooms at the Chamber of Commerce Building (*go, shogi, hana*—all Japanese games) filled up some space, but lack of money precluded gambling, once a favorite pastime. Savings were meager.

With the death of his two friends last year, Mr. Watanabe withdrew further and further from the outside world. He soon failed to get up from bed—problems of going to the bathroom, of getting up to eat and of cleanliness mounted. Eventually Mr. H. contacted the Japanese social worker, who in turn brought Mr. Watanabe to the County Hospital. The diagnosis was schizophrenia, and Mr. Watanabe was sent to a state hospital. There were no known relatives here in the United States.

The same story, with minor variations, describes much of the "mentally ill" caseload. One variation includes an elderly widowed Issei living with his married children—high conflict and lack of communication finally leads to his moving out to a cheap hotel. Eventually he experiences the loneliness, the absence of friends, the feeling that "no one cares," and similar symptoms (as had Mr. Watanabe), and eventually he is referred to the Japanese social worker.

Common behaviors indicating "mental illness" include "hearing voices" (of dead friends in Japanese), emotional weeping, heightened irritability, loss of toilet control and withdrawal.

The Top of the Iceberg—The Bottom of the Funnel

The data on hospitalization represent the least complete reflection of incidence, but it presents certain advantages. Hospitalization data are readily available and are quantifiable, so that instead of adjectives, precise ratios such as rates per 100,000 can be computed. Therefore, a comparison of hospitalization rates among Japanese in California, Hawaii, and Japan can be attempted, although such cross-cultural comparisons are quite deceptive. The problems of definition, diagnosis, availability of and access to the hospitals, and treatment objectives provide systematic differences which may invalidate all such comparisons.

The data on hospitalization are presented in terms of *admissions* and *hospitalization*. All statistics are computed in terms of rates per 100,000. Population figures by ethnic group are accurate for census years (for example, 1950, 1960); for in-between years, the closest census year figure is used as the denominator. Therefore, we are dealing with gross statistics and gross estimates, which will preclude the use of more sophisticated statistical techniques.

California State Department of Mental Hygiene admission rates for various groups are shown in Table 3. Longitudinal comparisons within groups remain remarkable consistent, especially if we take population increases into account. Perhaps the only group with rising rates of admissions is the Negro (190 in 1960, 280 in 1965), although even this increase may be related to population changes.

TABLE 3. Admissions of Patients by Ethnic Groups
California State Hospitals for the Mentally Ill, 1960–1965[a]

	Group (rates per 100,000[b])					
Year	Japanese	Caucasian	Mexican-American	Indian	Chinese	Negro
1960	40	150	40	150	70	190
1961	50	160	20	90	80	200
1962	50	170	30	140	90	210
1963	50	170	30	130	80	240
1964	60	170	40	170	90	250
1965	60	180	40	180	90	280

[a] Source: Adapted from *California State Department of Mental Hygiene*, Bureau of Biostatistics.

[b] Population base rates for each ethnic group are computed on 1960 population, United States Bureau of Census. Therefore, rates for the last several years are probably much lower for all groups.

TABLE 4. Admissions, Hawaii State Hospital for Mentally Ill
by Selected Ethnic Group, 1955 and 1960[a]

| Year | Group (rates per 100,000) | | |
	Japanese	Chinese	Caucasian
1954–1955	90	81	141
1959–1960	88	63	99

[a] Source: Adapted from *Hawaii State Hospital Psychology Report*, Volume III, December 1964, Appendix 2.

The more interesting comparisons are between groups. The group with the lowest rate of mental hospital admissions is the Mexican-American, followed very closely by the Japanese. Standing somewhere in the middle are the Chinese admission rates, followed by a cluster of relatively high rates for the Indian, Caucasian, and Negro.

Admission rate comparisons among the Japanese, Chinese and Caucasian in Hawaii are shown in Table 4. In general, admission rates are roughly similar for the Japanese in California and Hawaii; somewhat the same for the Chinese and much lower for the Caucasian in Hawaii when compared to California.

Hospitalization   Although rates of hospitalization provide the least effective method of measuring epidemiology, more complete data are

TABLE 5. Rates of Hospitalization for
Mental Illness for Six Prefectures
in Japan and Total, 1961[a]

Prefecture	Hospitalization Rate (per 100,000[b])
Hiroshima	117
Wakayama	122
Kumamoto	125
Fukuoka	153
Yamaguchi	115
Kagoshima	156
All Japan	130

[a] Source: Adapted from Masaaki Kato, *Annual Report on Mental Health*, 1962, National Institute of Mental Health, Japan, p. 12.
[b] Rates computed through population in prefecture.

TABLE 6. CALIFORNIA HOSPITAL RESIDENTS BY ETHNIC GROUP
FOR THE MENTALLY ILL FOR SELECTED YEARS[a]

| Year | Group (rates per 100,000[b]) | | | | | |
	Japanese	Caucasian	Mexican-American	Indian	Chinese	Negro
1950	216	300	188	356	535	364
1960	225	242	83	187	376	299
1964	198	213	74	174	361	296

[a] Source: Adapted from *California State Department of Mental Hygiene*, Bureau of Biostatistics.
[b] Rate for 1964 based on 1960 population.

usually available on hospital populations. For example, comparisons could be made on hospitalization rates among six prefectures in Japan (see Table 5), among six ethnic groups in California covering a span of 14 years (see Table 6), and among four ethnic groups using an age breakdown (see Table 7).

The six Japanese prefectures were chosen because they most closely represent the *ken* background of the Japanese populations in the United States (exception: a large number of Japanese immigrants in Hawaii are from Okinawa). There is relative uniformity in hospitalization rates among the prefectures in Japan and the overall Japanese totals.

TABLE 7. CALIFORNIA HOSPITAL RESIDENTS BY AGE-ETHNIC GROUP
FOR THE MENTALLY ILL, 1962[a]

| Ethnic Group | Ages (rates per 100,000[b]) | | |
	12–24	25–54	55 years or over
White	60	214[c]	649
Negro	47	142	222
Chinese	34	126	285
Japanese	12	80	218

[a] Source: Adapted from *Statistical Report of the Department of Mental Hygiene*, State of California, June 30, 1962, Table 12, p. 28.
[b] Population base rates for age-sex from estimates of population on 1960 U.S. Census.
[c] Ratios were computed and are to be read as follows: 12,188 whites of ages 25–54 in hospitals; estimated 5,698,000 whites of ages 25–54 in California; rate of 214 per 100,000 of whites, ages 25–54 in hospitals.

Hospitalization rates among various ethnic groups in California for 1950, 1960, and 1964 (Table 6) provide some interesting comparisons. The trend away from hospitalization in California mental institutions is seen in that all 1964 rates are lower than for 1950. The Chinese hospitalization rates are the highest of all groups; the Mexican figures present a relatively low hospitalized population. However, the proportionate drop in hospitalization rates is very low for the Japanese, and may indicate few alternative resources for a Japanese, once he gets to the stage of hospital referral.

Hospitalization rates of the Japanese in California are slightly higher than in Japan (Table 5), but these data are difficult to interpret.

Hospitalization rates computed on the basis of age distribution (Table 7) provide a firm generalization that the most vulnerable age for all population groups is the 55-or-over age categories. The year chosen for comparison was 1962 (because of the availability of data); therefore, there is a slight discrepancy between Tables 6 and 7. There appear to be many more white hospitalized residents of 55 years or older than for the Chinese, Negro, and the Japanese.

In general, the data supports a firm generalization that the Japanese contribute a very small proportion to the hospitalized, mentally ill population. However, it also appears that once he is hospitalized, he remains there longer. A hypothesis for further exploration include possible differences in the severity of the illness for the Japanese with the possibility that since their rates are so low, only the most severely disturbed end up at the hospital, and once there, they tend to remain.

CLASSIFICATION OF MENTAL ILLNESS

We have deliberately ignored some of the problems of definition, classification, and accessibility of mental health facilities in presenting the previous data. Terms such as mental health, mental illness, need of therapy, use of a social agency, admissions, and hospitalization are not consistent. Therefore, all generalizations are made with these limitations in mind.

An even more unreliable area is that of classification or diagnosis. What are some of the labels attached to Japanese once they arrive at diagnostic centers? The training of the professional, his techniques, his tools, and his insight determine to a large extent the "label" attached to the patient. Generally, the most common diagnostic category for hospitalized Japanese populations, whether in California, Hawaii, or Japan, was schizophrenia.

Enright and Jaeckle (1961) compared symptoms between Japanese and Filipino mental patients in Hawaii. The hospitalized Filipino tended to express feelings freely and directly, with frequent motor responses, while the Japanese mental patient tended to be more inhibited and restrained with ideational responses more frequent.

The other main difference was in the direction of behavior: The Filipino behaved outwardly, or alloplastically, so that attempts to resolve conflicts were through environmental manipulation and the expectation of changing the world. Conversely, the Japanese behaved inwardly or autoplastically, so that attempts to resolve conflicts were through internalization or modification of one's own behavior, rather than through changing external conditions.

A preliminary analysis of hospitalized Japanese, as well as interviews with our Japanese professionals corroborates the low degree of "acting-out" behavior among the Japanese mentally ill (as well as in the general ethnic population) and the high degree of withdrawal behavior.

1. At least as measured by official statistics, mental illness is not a major problem for the Japanese when compared to other groups.

2. The most vulnerable group for mental illness in the Japanese population is a single, old, lower-class male.

3. The rates of hospitalization, although subject to the most systematic biases, appear remarkably similar for the Japanese in Japan and in the United States.

4. The most common illness is schizophrenia, with withdrawal symptoms most common.

EXPLANATIONS: NONTHEORETICAL AND THEORETICAL

Nontheoretical hypotheses refer to explanations for Japanese-American mental illness that deal with technical factors such as data gathering, definitions, and research design. Therefore, possible explanations of mental illness may be through biased statistics, distortions in recording, unreliable classifications and other systematic "field" errors. All studies of "social problems" that are based in community settings (as opposed to the laboratory) are open to such criticisms, and the reliability and validity of our data can also be questioned.[3]

Our overall generalization that the Japanese are a *low group* in terms of official rates of mental illness appears to have validity because (1) there is consistency of data on all levels of the "funnel," (2) the data are

[3] We checked with one of the state hospitals to see how "ethnicity" is determined. There appears to be no systematic method of ascertaining the validity of the classification—in many instances a clerk who helps fill out the initial form checks whether in her judgment a person is Japanese or Negro or Indian. Some become quite skilled at this; there is a check at later stages when other personnel have time to become acquainted with the patient.

consistent with independent observations about the Japanese, and (3) the data fit logically with what we know about the Japanese. A replication of our study will undoubtedly yield the same results.

With the limitations of the data in mind, we turned to two broad theoretical hypotheses as possible explanations for the low rates of Japanese-American mental illness. The first hypothesis compares the Japanese with other ethnic groups in terms of over-all stress. It is what we would term a "compare the scars" technique, which assumes that those groups with the highest rates of mental illness are those who have faced the highest degree of "stress." Although this hypothesis is not a particularly fruitful one from our point of view, it does provide an opportunity to present a short background of the difficulties faced by this immigrant group to the United States.

PAST ATTITUDES TOWARD THE JAPANESE

Several quotations from leading Californians provide a flavor of the anti-Japanese campaigns which occurred frequently in the early half of the century. For example, McClatchy (1921), publisher of the *Sacramento Bee* in discussing the Japanese wrote:

The Japanese cannot, may not, and will not provide desirable material for our citizenship. 1. The Japanese cannot assimilate and make good citizens because of their racial characteristics, heredity and religion. 2. The Japanese may not assimilate and make good citizens because their government claims all Japanese, no matter where born, as its citizens. 3. The Japanese will not assimilate and make good citizens. In the mass, when opportunity offered, and even when born here, they have shown no disposition to do so . . . There can be no effective assimilation of Japanese without intermarriage. It is perhaps not desirable for the good of either race that there should be intermarriage between whites and Japanese . . . They cannot be transmuted into good American citizens.

Or, in the words of Marshall De Motte (1921), chairman of the State Board of Control of California,

It is utterly unthinkable that America or an American state should be other than white. Kipling did not say "East is East" of the United States, but if the star number 31 in Old Glory, California's star became yellow, West may become East. California has been loyal at all times to a flag that has honored her with the star of her own, so Californians, to a citizen, will see that the star of her glory shall not grow dim or yellow.

And finally, a citation from the Honorable James D. Phelan (1921), United States Senator from California:

Immigration and naturalization are domestic questions, and no people can come to the United States except upon our own terms. We must preserve the soil for the Caucasian race. The Japanese, by crowding out our population, produce disorder and Bolshevism among our own people who properly look to our government to protect them against this destructive competition. California, by acting in time, before the evil becomes even greater, expects to prevent conflict. . . .

We are willing to receive diplomats, scholars and travelers from Japan on terms of equality, but we do not want her laborers. We admire their industry and cleverness, but for that very reason, being a masterful people, they are more dangerous. They are not content to work for wages as do the Chinese, who are excluded, but are always seeking control of the farm and of the crop. . . .

The anti-Japanese feeling, which was most heavy in California, led to boycotts of Japanese-owned business, to anti-miscegenation laws, and to special discriminatory immigration and naturalization legislation. There was school segregation, restrictions on land ownership, and generally limited opportunity in the economic, political, and social spheres of the larger society. The "yellow peril" reached its peak with the 1942 wartime evacuation of all persons of Japanese ancestry, whether citizens or not, from the West Coast. If stress in the form of discrimination and limited opportunities is related in a simple, linear fashion to mental illness, we would expect to find large numbers of Japanese in mental institutions. It is obvious that a "compare the scars" approach is not an adequate explanation.

The second, and more fruitful, hypothesis conceptualizes stress in a more relative manner, so that a mere comparison of hardships faced by immigrant and ethnic groups is an insufficient explanation of behavior. From this perspective, the ability of an ethnic group to absorb stress and to provide alternative opportunities are important factors. Therefore, what may be considered heavy stress for one group might be handled without undue difficulty by another.

The ethnic community and family—their structure, their functions, their values, and their "culture"—are presented as the critical variables in understanding Japanese behavior. The strength of the culture was severely tested during the wartime evacuation of World War II, and the ability of the Japanese to rebound from this period may be cited as one example of the strength of the group.

The following areas will be analyzed: the ethnic community and family, their definitions and attitudes toward mental illness, and the possible relationship of mental illness to other behavior.

COMMUNITY ORGANIZATION

There are several generalizations concerning the Japanese community that are related to conformity and mental illness. In the most general sense, the Japanese community provides an "alternative legitimate opportunity structure"; that is, for most Japanese, an opportunity to satisfy economic, social, psychological, and political needs within the ethnic community when such opportunities are restricted in the larger society. Churches, mutual aid societies, small business firms, newspaper and radio networks, recreational, educational, vocational, social, health, and welfare organizations are developed and maintained by the Japanese community (Miyamoto, 1939). The existence of these pluralistic structures (especially during the early days when interaction with the American social system was much more limited) is probably a major factor in "absorbing" the stress of discrimination and prejudice.

The limited interaction between the Japanese community and the larger American system affected the use of larger societal institutions. One possible explanation for the low official rates of mental illness (and also of crime and delinquency) was the limited use of state and local facilities by the Japanese group. Instead, they "took care of their own." One positive consequence of the nonuse of public facilities was the avoidance of the institutionalization of a "mentally ill role," "public welfare role," or a "delinquent role." Therefore, the process of labelling, categorization, and reinforcement for developing and maintaining these dysfunctional roles was lacking in the Japanese system. An unfortunate consequence of some of our American health and welfare programming may be the reinforcement and subsequent continuance of certain dysfunctional role positions.

It is questionable whether the minority community could continue to handle its own problems if the number of "social problems" were large. Fortunately, a combination of its structure, its values, and its population kept problem behavior at a minimum. The population was a young one—the initial immigrant was a young male, in good health, vigorous and highly motivated toward work. There was a low initial probability of major health and welfare problems occurring in this type of population.

The most important single control in terms of mental illness, however, is the direction of preferred behavior prescribed by the Japanese. In general, reactions to stress and to frustration are directed "inward"— the concept of *"ga-man,"* which refers to "handling of pain and frustration without any outward signs," is typically Japanese. Therefore, in interpersonal relationships, the Japanese generally do not bother others, preferring instead to internalize problems. He might "eat his own heart out" and yet exhibit few overt signs of disturbance.

One other important option for handling problem behavior by the ethnic community was the use of the mother country. Immigration-emigration statistics indicate that from 1912 through 1941, the number of Japanese departing from the United States for Japan was larger than the number entering the country. There was also the "Kibei" custom, whereby an American-born child (Nisei) would be sent back to Japan to be reared by relatives in Japan. Although it is difficult to arrive at any precise figure, it is logical to assume that some families used both the Kibei system and the more permanent emigration to Japan as alternatives to handling problem behavior.

For example, one of our interviews in our study of crime (Kitano, in progress) is revealing:

I remember two brothers (Nisei) who were hard to handle. They would get drunk . . . were always fighting, always in trouble and were uncontrollable. Finally, their father came to talk to my father and other Japanese families in the neighborhood. . . . All agreed that these boys would hurt the reputation of the other Japanese and provide poor models for the younger boys. . . . So even though the brothers were already young adults and out of high school, they were sent back to Japan (1937). As far as I know, they never came back to the United States.

Several generalizations appear to be appropriate in describing the Japanese community:

1. The Japanese community is a cohesive, integrated body with many interdependent structures which play important roles in shaping desired behaviors. Desired behaviors include conformity and minimal "acting out."

2. The Japanese community provides a wide range of alternative opportunities (structural pluralism) that in many instances parallels the American system.

3. There is a strong group feeling which provides a "oneness" so that the behavior of one is a reflection on "all."

That the tightly knit ethnic community is a completely healthy development can be questioned. There is the risk of encapsulation, of a slowness of acculturation, of self-imposed isolation, restricted communication, and an overcontrol of adult supervision over the young.

Bradford Smith (1941) provides an apt summary to living in a Nihonmachi (Japanese town) before World War II:

The Issei liked it. They had created it . . . as a wall against prejudice and rejection, as a rebuilding of the life they had known at home, as a compensation for the return to Japan which they dreamed of . . . Nihonmachi was home. Most of these enclaves were small enough so that the environment could be rigidly controlled . . . They could be . . . bound into the community by many of their accustomed institutions—the temple, the school, the neighborhood group.

Etiquette, language, holidays—all were in the pattern of their upbringing . . . Those who failed to conform were soon brought about by the weapon of gossip and . . . economic sanctions could also be applied [p. 232].

Although there have been changes as years have passed, the Japanese community still today retains many of the aspects of small town life described by Smith.

THE FAMILY

The Japanese family is an intact (1.6 percent divorce rate, which remains constant by generation), cohesive unit. It is structured vertically, with father as the authority and with relatively clearly defined roles for mother and sibs. It retains social control through techniques of interdependence (Japanese children remain dependent upon their family much longer than American middle class children), shame, guilt, appeals to obligations, duty, and responsibility.

The Issei family was patterned to be self-sufficient; levels for help might include the extended family, then members of the same village or *"mura,"* then the "ken" or state, then other Japanese. As a consequence, problems were handled by family, friends, neighbors—then the ethnic community. Outside "experts" played a minimal role in such a process.

This type of family interaction appears to be somewhat typical of lower class immigrant groups, which helps to partially explain the low use of "professional" services by these populations.

The following generalizations can be made concerning the Japanese family:

1. The majority of Japanese families in the United States are intact. It is not unusual to find unmarried aunts and uncles as well as grandparents residing in the same household, even in urban areas.

2. Most families follow a vertical structure, that is, authority is primarily invested in the father and older males. Lines of social control and role functions are clearly defined. Duty and obligation are emphasized over love and motivation. Family complementarity may be more easily achieved under this model than one based on love and affection.

3. There remains a long family dependence on the part of Japanese children. It is still rare for children to strike out on their own at an early age. Marriage is delayed.

4. Good children and good family members are defined primarily in terms of obedient, conforming, and responsible behavior.

5. Parental techniques for obtaining conformity and control appear to be primarily nonverbal. Observations of Japanese families indicate

low verbosity, but a high degree of effectiveness in obtaining social control.

6. Voluntary interfamily social patterns are largely within the extended family, the ethnic group and the ethnic community. The relative homogeneity of interfamily and interethnic values strengthens social control functions.

7. The family is less apt to use outside "experts" and outside resources for the handling of social problems.

There have been changes by generations, but the Japanese family remains a tightly knit, cohesive group with a high degree of social control over its members.

Probably the most important role of the Japanese family in terms of mental illness is its protective function. The family name and the family identity might suffer if a member were mentally ill; therefore, most families would go to elaborate lengths to protect the public occurrence of such a catastrophe. Protection in this sense might include a high tolerance for "crazy behavior," a redefinition of family roles, and, finally, the use of external resources only if the effects of the deviant behavior caused major disruption in the family.

As a result of such ideas, Japanese families often view hospitalization as a final stage, with the point of view that once an individual is hospitalized, he is out of their hands. The concept of "cure" and "treatment" has to be discussed carefully, otherwise many Japanese families appear to be disinterested in their hospitalized member. This factor may be a further reason for the long hospitalization of Japanese patients.

Although we have discussed in general terms the community and the family, there are certain specific values and styles of life that may further help us understand Japanese behavior in the United States. We will present some of these changing values by Issei, Nisei, and Sansei generations.[4]

Ethnic Identity (Table 8)

Ethnic identity refers to the "degree of Japaneseness," as measured by self perceptions, identification, and participation in ethnic activities. This variable was a powerful predictor of delinquent and nondelinquent behavior (Kitano, 1969) —Japanese with a higher degree of ethnic

[4] The samples for comparison were drawn from available groups of Japanese in Los Angeles. The Caucasian group is a Psychology 1A class at UCLA. Test-retest reliability of the inventory was $r = .79$. Data are presented in percentage terms only.

identification were less delinquent than those with a low degree of ethnic identity. A behavioral consequence of ethnic identity would mean that in America one Japanese would be obligated to help another Japanese, even a total stranger, and that the success or failure of an individual Japanese would be a reflection on the entire group.

A knowledge of the degree of "Japaneseness" of an individual remains a powerful predictor of behavior today, even though the data show changes by generation. For example, predictions of marital choice, food habits, interaction with parents, attitudes toward education, and general styles of life might be comfortably made through knowledge of ethnic identity. On a higher level, the degree of an individual's identity (not necessarily ethnic) is believed to be highly important in understanding behavior.

Means-Ends (Table 8)

Traditional Japanese culture emphasizes both means (the process) and ends (the goals) as being of equal importance. Therefore, ethical behavior, or how one goes about a task, is as valuable as the outcomes or end results. The changes from means toward ends is illustrated by our data (Table 8), although all groups tested still placed relatively high emphasis on the importance of means. The way of playing the game is considered as important as winning.

Masculinity and Responsibility (Table 8)

Definitions of masculinity and responsibility are related to "acting-out" behavior. It is believed that the American culture provides less clarity for a male role, which may often result in behavior that attempts to validate masculinity.[5] Conversely, the more secure Japanese male role may restrain the impulsive "acting-out," which is thought of as more characteristically American. The inclusion of responsibility is also inherent in the Japanese definition of masculinity. The data indicate a trend by generation from the Japanese to the more American definition.

Individual-Group Orientation (Table 8)

Of special importance for group control and conformity are orientations and values emphasizing the individual and his relationship to the group. The American model of individualism, which is perhaps one key to

[5] A musician friend commented to us about the high quality of violin sections in Japan. It is not considered "feminine" for males to take up the violin; therefore there are probably many more males playing the violin in Japan than in the United States.

American behavior, is relatively alien to the Japanese. For example, at the time of Issei immigration, the Japanese constitution made no reference to "individual rights," but rather to individual obligations and duties to the state and to the family.

Consequently, there is less of an egoistic orientation (self-needs, self-enhancement) and more of an "alter" perspective. For example, one technique for treating criminals in Japan is through self-reflection, which emphasizes one's own responsibility in the criminal act and its consequences to others. Treatment success in these terms comes about when the criminal perceives and acknowledges his lack of responsibility, his lack of respect for others.

The change from the Japanese perspective to a more American point of view is reflected by the data.

Passivity (Table 8)

Passivity is related to a fatalistic orientation whereby an individual resigns himself to certain external conditions. It is also related to frustration tolerance—the Japanese phrase *shi-ka-ta-ga-nai* (usually accompanied by a shrug of the shoulders and meaning "it can't be helped" or "there's nothing you can do about it") illustrates this orientation. The wartime evacuation, business losses, natural disasters, and the like can all be covered by the phrase, and it is indicative of a style of life which counsels patience, tolerance, and repression. The changes in orientation from the Japanese to a more American perspective is illustrated by our data.

Realistic Expectations (Table 8)

Concepts such as frustration-aggression, anomie, and alienation are usually defined in terms of a discrepancy between expectations and reality. High expectations for success and blockage of legitimate opportunities for attaining goals provide background conditions for anomie, alienation, and illegitimate behavior (Cloward & Ohlin, 1961).

The Japanese as a group were an "underexpectancy" group—that is, aims for success were set so that goal attainment was not too difficult. A common practice was to settle for second best—rather than becoming a doctor, an individual might aim at a pharmacist level; rather than a Step III supervisory position, the Japanese-American might aim for Step I. The consequence is that many Japanese even today are over-trained for their level and perhaps even overproductive. Reaching for the stars is not a common practice, although changes by generation through acculturation are taking place. Probably both overexpectancy and underexpectancy are, in the long run, dysfunctional perceptions.

TABLE 8. GENERATIONAL RESPONSES (IN PERCENTAGES)
    TO TRUE-FALSE ATTITUDINAL ITEMS

Items	Issei $N = 18$	Nisei $N = 37$	Sansei $N = 48$	Caucasian $N = 82$
A. Ethnic identity				
1. Once a Japanese, Always a Japanese (T)	78	63	47	
2. I always look forward to going to prefectural (or family picnics) (T)	62	50	17	
3. I would prefer attending an all Japanese Church (T)	81	44	40	
4. I would prefer being treated by a Japanese doctor when sick (T)	69	50	26	
5. I prefer American movies to Japanese movies (F)	69	14	11	
B. Means-ends				
6. Even in a minor task a person should put all his energies into it (T)	95	86	86	78
C. Masculinity and responsibility				
7. It is only right for a man to marry a girl if he has gotten her into trouble (T)	79	80	48	36
8. My definition of a real man is one who adequately supports his wife and family under all conditions (T)	81	82	63	35
D. Individual-group orientation				
9. A person who raises too many questions interferes with the progress of a group (T)	88	43	19	40
10. One can never let himself down without letting the family down at the same time (T)	89	79	59	46
E. Passivity				
11. If someone tries to push you around, there is very little that you can do about it (T)	39	29	12	6
12. I would not shout or fight in public, even when provoked (T)	70	69	55	51
F. Realistic expectations				
13. I think I will be a success once I acquire a nice home, a new car and many modern appliances (T)	50	32	8	6

Other general styles of life that proved compatible to life in the United States included high achievement (high education), high savings, and a "future" orientation. The general influence of certain Japanese Meiji period values such as *shu-shin,* which emphasized duty, responsibility, and obligations was undoubtedly quite important in shaping Japanese-American behavior.

Possibly the most important point in presenting the values of the Japanese relates to their relatively fixed order, so that individual preferences are not given the same priority as within the American system. For example, the duties and obligation of the individual to the larger systems —the family, village, community, and nation—are relatively static, so that individual needs and preferences play a minor role in determining the significance of priorities.

One interesting facet of the Japanese styles of life emphasizing ritual, role-set, and formal behavior is the difficulty of separating normal and pathological behavior. A Japanese-American psychiatrist illustrates this point:

> Because of the relatively rigid, set ways for social interaction it's often difficult to diagnose where the role-set ends and possible psychiatric symptomology begins. The person who reacts to extreme stress with a pattern of unemotional and ritualistic behavior may be relatively easy to diagnose psychiatrically in another culture, but for the Japanese (especially the Issei), it's really hard to figure one way or the other.

The choice of occupations is also protective for many Japanese. The stereotyped Japanese gardener is an example of an occupation where the amount of social interaction can be held to a minimum and where *ki-chi-gai* or crazy behavior can be widely tolerated.

However, it is understandable that when a Japanese is referred to a mental institution, his behavior is usually described as rigid and compulsive. Schizophrenia is the most common classification.

The overall result of a tight, cohesive family and community system, with certain socialization procedures and emphasis upon certain values and styles of life, is a group with high conformity and low rates of overtly deviant behavior. Personality data show the Sansei male as more reserved, more humble, more conscientious, more shy, and more regulated by external realities than are Caucasian-American males. Conversely, Caucasian-American males are more outgoing, more assertive, more expedient, more venturesome, and more imaginative than are Japanese-American males (G. Meredith & C. Meredith, 1966).

Sansei females are more affected by feeling, more obedient, more suspicious and, more apprehensive than their Caucasian peers. On the other hand, Caucasian-American females are more emotionally stable, more independent, more trusting, and more self-assured than their Japanese-American counterparts (G. Meredith & C. Meredith, 1966).

Problems of leadership (Burma, 1953), of social backwardness (Kitans, 1962), and lack of creativity and overconformity may be a high price to pay for "good behavior."

JAPANESE ATTITUDES TOWARD MENTAL ILLNESS

There are several Japanese terms that describe mental illness. The word most commonly used by the Issei is *ki-chi-gai* ("crazy"); more professional and technical terms include *non-ro-seh* ("neurosis"), *sei-shin-byo* ("mental illness"), and *sei-shin-retsu-sho* ("schizophrenia").

Although there have been changes in both the conceptualization and treatment of the mentally ill in Japan (for example, introduction of group therapy, psychiatric social work, and psychiatric treatment), the main emphasis remains on physiological-neurological models. For example, on a recent trip to Japanese mental institutions, the writer noticed the widespread use of electro-shock therapy, of the measurement of GSR and ECG as more basic to the understanding and treatment of the mentally ill than interpersonal techniques.

General Japanese attitude toward the mentally ill, as well as other "gross deformities," has been that of fear, ostracism, and repression. The Issei brought to the United States many of these same attitudes, and the idea of an "hereditary taint" meant that families were hesitant to admit the existence of a *ki-chi-gai* person, since it might affect economic and social interaction (for example, chances for a job, for marriage).

THE LACK OF A "MENTALLY ILL ROLE"

A consequence of this perhaps unique combination of a young immigrant population, a strong family and community structure with its own resources, an emphasis on certain values and styles of life, a fear of and lack of sophistication regarding the origins and treatment of mental illness, and of limited use of psychiatric facilities was the lack of a clearly defined "mentally ill role." Although everybody could act *ki-chi-gai* at one time or another, there was no process by which his behavior could be diagnosed, labeled, treated, and the changed behavior reinforced. The term "tolerance for mental illness" may not be an entirely appropriate one since it connotes an understanding of the behavior in question—the tolerance is related more to the lack of "know-how," the form of the behavior, the lack of resources, and the lack of alternatives in handling the behavior.

For example, there is the case of an elderly Issei woman who died recently. During her lifetime she was rather widely known for her eccentric behavior—talking to animals, communicating with spirits, and displaying extremely erratic behavior in conducting her business. She was a widow left with running a small store; her absent-mindedness, her eccentric buying and spending habits and her extreme emotionality would have meant immediate failure for most stores. Instead, her loyal employees protected her, gradually taking over and handling her as they would a child. There was no thought of sending her for any psychiatric treatment (who could talk to her in Japanese?), no thought of hospitalization, and a rather amused tolerance for her odd and eccentric ways. She eventually retired, made periodic ritualistic visits to old friends, lived by herself on savings and social security, and at the time of her death had never been a statistic in any clinic or mental hospital.

The lack of a "mentally ill role" has both positive and negative consequences. It prevents an all too easy solution through quick hospitalization and the development of a mentally ill role as discussed by Szasz (1961), and it keeps the number of Japanese in mental hospitals extremely low.

However, it may hinder the use of appropriate resources (for example, clinics and "preventive services") when necessary, and leaves the ethnic community relatively helpless when its members do exhibit persistent symptoms of mental illness.[6] The rather large proportion of the aged with psychiatric symptoms has never been fully faced by the Japanese in the United States. Hospitalization of this old Issei group in state institutions where difficulties of language, dietary habits, and styles of life provide additional stress is not a pleasant prospect. Belatedly, the ethnic community is planning a nursing home and a facility for the aged. Third generation service groups are now showing an interest in the problems of its senior citizens.

RELATIONSHIPS AMONG MENTAL ILLNESS
AND OTHER FORMS OF DEVIANT BEHAVIOR

There are various ways of conceptualizing the relationship between mental illness and other forms of deviant behavior. For example, there is an oversimplified point of view that hypothesizes a homeostasis between internalization and "acting out," so that groups with low rates of mental illness are hypothesized as high in behavior such as delinquency, and

---

[6] For example, one possible reason for the low rates of Mexican-American mental illness may be the non-use of professional services. A medical doctor related to us that most Mexican-American children are literally "dying" by the time their parents bring them to the medical center.

vice-versa. It is obvious that the Japanese in the United States does not fit into such a model—he is low in mental illness and low in crime and delinquency (Kitano, in progress). Conversely, the Mexican American appears to provide a better fit—he is low in mental illness and high in delinquency. However, the reasons for this may be related to the type of data available on Mexican-American rates of mental illness.

Another point of view looks upon deviance as escape or release behavior, so that a certain amount is necessary for the health of any social system. From this perspective one might hypothesize a monstrous blow-up for the Japanese, since his rates of mental illness, of crime and of delinquency are so low. Furthermore, although rates of suicide in Japan are high, Iga (in progress) indicates no such abnormality of the Japanese rate in the United States. The Japanese population minimizes acting-out behavior.

However, we hypothesize other forms of acceptable "release" behavior within this ethnic group to absorb stress. These would be primarily in the form of "somatization," that is, with psychosomatic symptoms and an overconcern with bodily functioning. Although there was no formal testing of this hypothesis, impressionistic evidence, as well as research on the Japanese, lends support to the validity of this point of view. The extremely widespread use of potent drugs, the overconcern with high blood pressure, the hot baths, the masseurs, the practice of acupuncture, the concern with the stomach and other internal organs are characteristically Japanese, whether in Japan or in the United States.

Our overall explanation concerning Japanese-American mental illness and its relationship to other forms of deviant behavior emphasizes the relativity of stress and the cushioning effects of the family and community. From this perspective, certain groups of Japanese are "marginal," and it is this population that is more vulnerable to stress. Those with a weak ethnic identity—those from broken or conflict ridden homes—and those who have failed to integrate into either the Japanese or the larger social system will constitute the high-risk group in terms of mental illness, suicide, crime, and delinquency. Our empirical data strongly support this position.

For example, Japanese delinquents (Kitano, in progress) could be differentiated from a matched group of nondelinquents on many variables including broken homes, high conflict and lack of complementarity in the family life, less ethnic identity, and different values and styles of life. Our preliminary analysis of cases of suicides and of those hospitalized for mental illness[7] indicates surprising similarity.

A suicidal case is that of a 35-year-old man from Japan who had mini-

---

[7] A more comprehensive study under NIMH Grant OM-11112 is in progress.

mal job security and minimal income. He was not a member of either the the ethnic or the majority community, and he had no close relatives or close friends. His suicidal act arose from an unhappy love affair with a Caucasian divorcee.

A case of mental illness is that of a 40-year-old female, married to a non-Japanese. She was rejected by both families and had a psychotic break after the death of her husband. The stress of adapting to widowhood, including the rearing by herself of several young children was too much.

An analysis of Japanese-American hospitalized schizophrenics (Terashima, 1958) provides additional data. The lonely, isolated families and the lack of overall identity is common to the whole sample. The author in describing one of the cases says,

The patient, the youngest of 5 siblings, was not only rejected and neglected by his father who was domineering, irritable and seriously alcoholic, but he was also isolated from friends in his childhood. The entire family was shut off from social relationships . . . [p. 7].

We are confident that certain predictions can be made. We think it will be relatively easy to differentiate between "normal Japanese" and "abnormal Japanese" on a number of variables (most of these have been previously discussed). For example, we think that most clinicians analyzing interviews and case histories will be able to place samples into "normal" and "abnormal" categories with high accuracy. However, we also predict that there will be great difficulty in sorting the "abnormal" group into the correct dependent variables—suicide, mental illness, crime, and delinquency. The essential similarity of the case histories of the "abnormal" appears more than coincidental.

The interesting fact about the adaptation of the Japanese to life in the United States has been the ability of the ethnic system to provide a wide enough umbrella to control the development of a large "marginal group." There may be several reasons for this, including the essential congruence between American middle class and Japanese styles of life. Therefore, initially when interaction between the two systems was limited, the Japanese system played a major socializing role. At the current time, when the American system provides more ample opportunities, there is relative ease in moving over. It may be that other subcultures, less congruent to the American system (for example, possibly the Mexican-American) create special difficulties because integration into the ethnic or subgroup culture may mean a move away from the American system and therefore eventual conflict when interacting with American institutions (the public school system, for example).

Overall, we have attempted to provide a broad picture of a subcultural group and mental illness. We have assumed that behavior that can be labeled as "mental illness" arises from diverse sources. It may have biochemical, physiological, or genetic origins; it may arise from situational or constant stress; it may involve peculiarities of the individual or in his upbringing and family environment. Rather than concentrate on the "causal," we have described what happens within the ethnic community when such behavior occurs. Therefore, from this perspective the "form" of the behavior—how it affects others in terms of irritation and disturbance—is our important variable. The form ultimately affects the handling, the treatment, and the rates of mental illness.

In describing the Japanese system with their emphasis on a strong community and family, their values, their preferred modes of behavior, and their styles of life, we have presented a group where mental illness rates are low. Given the same system for whatever group—white, black, red, or yellow—we would expect the same low rates of mental illness. There appears to be little need to depend upon exotic or mysterious variables to explain the behavior of the Japanese in the United States.

THE FUTURE

There is a combination of factors that may be used for predictive purposes. Acculturation, changes in ethnicity and social class, the availability of trained mental health personnel (especially of the same ethnic background), and the nature of the population provide some clues for the future. It should be emphasized that on certain objective criteria of "success," such as education and income, the Japanese group in California have achieved a remarkable level. In both education and income, the Japanese rank higher than all other identifiable ethnic groups, as defined by the United States Census. Therefore on social class criteria, the Japanese are definitely upwardly mobile and will continue to be so, yet there are certain values and styles of life which remain ethnic. Most important for mental illness are attitudes and feelings that more clearly reflect older "Japanese traditions" than they do the sentiments of a highly educated, middle class population. The close family interaction model, with an emphasis on the extended family, friends, and neighbors for "assistance" on most matters limits the use of "experts" or professionals. This is gradually changing, both from pressures within (a breaking up of the ghettos, the extended family system) and from pressures without (in this case the most obvious being the large number of Japanese "professionals").

The pattern appears irreversible. The complexity of problems points to the need for the expert and the specialist. This means that the "wise old neighbor" whose main qualification might have been some knowledge of English (but who also provided a personalized service) or an older uncle, is no longer the most popular resource. The minimally trained Issei general practitioner, somewhat bumbling and with old-fashioned ideas about medicine, is being replaced by the young Nisei and Sansei specialist. A rising group of highly trained lawyers, social workers, psychologists, and psychiatrists is beginning to develop role positions modeled after appropriate middle and upper-middle class populations. The important part in this development is the training of ethnic personnel, so that they represent streams of acculturation arising from within the Japanese system rather than "experts" appointed from the outside by the American community. Therefore, hopefully, the changes in the Japanese social system will be through the incorporation of professionals in mutual interaction, rather than a dictation and one-way flow. Unfortunately, past experiences with professionals and experts has often been characterized by a one-way flow—the middle class professional to the lower class population. Phrases such as "imposing of values" and "taking clients where they are" are indications of this problem.

Finally, it is also of interest to note the changes in the handling of the mentally ill in the larger community. There have been swings to and from hospitalization, and the current American emphasis on "treatment in the home and the community" is congruent with the old Japanese-American way of handling mental illness, although the reasons may have been different. Ironically, the "cultural lag" phenomenon may mean that the earlier American influence of diagnosis and treatment is just catching up—for example, there is a cry for more hospitals and more hospital beds in Japan, and one proposed solution is to build "bigger and better institutions." The need for more personnel—psychiatrists, psychologists, and social workers employed in large institutions—may very well be the next step across the sea.

For the Japanese in the United States, the older ways of treatment through the family, extended family, and community will soon give way to the use of professionals, of experts, and of institutions. As more experts are produced, more Japanese will use their services, and community concern will rise since rates of mental illness will rise. Perhaps in due course, through acculturation and the passage of time, the rates of Japanese mental illness will then become more nearly equal to that of the majority group in the United States.

REFERENCES

Archer, M., Staugas, C., & Hoffman, N. A descriptive study of the services and of presenting problems, acculturation levels and social class positions of a Japanese-American social agency. Unpublished master's thesis, School of Social Welfare, University of California at Los Angles, 1962.

Arkoff, A. Need patterns in two generations of Japanese-Americans in Hawaii, *The Journal of Social Psychology*, 1959, **50**, 75–79.

Burma, J. Current leadership problems among Japanese-Americans. *Sociology and Social Research*, 1953, **37**, 157–163.

Cloward, R., & Ohlin, L. *Delinquency and Opportunity*. Glencoe, Ill.: The Free Press, 1961.

Cressey, D. Crime. In R. Merton & R. Nisbet (Eds.), *Contemporary Social Problems*. New York: Harcourt, Brace and World, 1961. Pp. 21–26.

De Motte, M. California . . . white or yellow? *The Annals*, 1921, **93**, 18–23.

Enright, J., & Jaeckle, W. R. Ethnic differences in psychopathology. Paper presented at the Pacific Science Congress, Honolulu, Hawaii, August, 1961.

Hayner, N. S. Delinquency areas in Puget Sound region. *American Journal of Sociology*, 1933, **39**, 314–328.

Iga, M., & Ohara, K. An interpretation of Durkheim's concept of anomie and suicide attempts of Japanese youth. Manuscript in progress, private copy.

Kitano, H. Changing achievement patterns of the Japanese in the United States. *The Journal of Social Psychology*, 1962, **58**, 257–264.

Kitano, H. Differential child rearing attitudes between first and second generation Japanese in the United States. *The Journal of Social Psychology*, 1961, **53**, 13–19.

Kitano, H. *Japanese-Americans: The evaluation of a subculture*. Englewood Cliffs, N.J.: Prentice-Hall, Inc., 1969.

McClatchy, V. Japanese in the melting pot: Can they assimilate and make good citizens? *The Annals*, 1921, **93**, 29–34.

Meredith, G., & Meredith, C. Acculturation and personality among Japanese-American college students in Hawaii. *The Journal of Social Psychology*, 1966, **68**, 175–182.

Miyamoto, F. *Social solidarity among the Japanese in Seattle*. Seattle, Wash.: University of Washington publications in Social Science, Vol. 11, No. 2, 1939, 57–130.

Phelan, J. Why California objects to the Japanese invasion. *The Annals*, 1921, **93**, 16–17.

Rotter, J. *Social learning and clinical psychology*. New York: Prentice-Hall, 1954.

Smith, B. *Americans from Japan*. Philadelphia: Lippincott, 1941.

Szasz, T. *The myth of mental illness*. New York: Hoeber-Harper, 1961.

Terashima, S. Cultural aspects of Japanese-American schizophrenic patients. Unpublished manuscript, University of California at Los Angeles Medical Center, 1958.

chapter three

Social Complexity

3.1 Introduction

In the previous section, we have taken a broad look at the influence of cultural systems on the development of psychopathology, and we have had the opportunity to examine closely the particular social pressures and their concomitant effects when an ethnic group resides within a "host" population.

Now it is time to turn our attention to those social forces that are more likely to be relevant to the daily lives of the readers of this volume—life in a complex, urban society. As nations become more industrialized and more populous, larger numbers of people must crowd into cities. Thus, the problems of urban living are gradually becoming the dominant problems of the world. When the separate colonies of America first declared their independence from England, only 13 percent of the people were able to support themselves in a manner other than in agriculture. Today, that ratio has been reversed, and less than 12 percent of our population is tied to the land to produce food for others. More importantly, more than 70 percent of the people live in cities or the larger metropolitan areas. Such rapid alterations in living patterns, combined with unpredictable technological changes, lead to unstable social environments and a potential for high incidence and prevalence rates of psychosis.

With such changes in the social structure, there are vital questions that impinge upon all of us if we are to develop a society that is livable. We are concerned with whether or not the ecology of cities in any way contributes to pathology (H. Warren Dunham). And, does the constant mobility of people from one location to another (one out of five families makes a significant change of residence each year) result in psychological burdens that are too great for many persons to cope with (Mildred Kantor)? A different kind of spatial mobility that has played an important part in the development of this nation is the immigration of persons from distant nations to take up new residence within our continental boundaries. Do immigrants face particular problems that are not common to their less mobile neighbors, and could such problems not only contribute to pathological behavior but also result in greater personal difficulties for their children (Benjamin Malzberg)?

As people live in cities, there is a greater probability that major value systems will come in conflict with each other and that these value systems will contribute differentially to the stability or pathology of their believers. The primary organizer of such values in most societies is religion. Thus, the relationship of kind of religious commitment and intensity of belief also becomes one of our topics for consideration (Leo Srole and Thomas Langner). Also, the protective life of contemporary society, as compared with the physical hardships encountered by earlier frontier Americans, and recent medical advances are resulting in an older population in the United States. What problems does this present for us? Are we likely to have more of our people who are unable to care for themselves, not because of the physiological infirmities of advancing age, but because they are no longer psychologically competent to run their own lives (Ivan Mensh)? And what about the problems presented by an achievement-oriented society, such as ours, where large numbers of persons are able to improve significantly their relative social and economic positions in life, while others correspondingly find that they are losing their personal battles to maintain status. Such rapid status position changes can result in the breakdown of behavior, and the question is how often and under what kinds of conditions this will occur (Kleiner and Parker).

All these are important and pragmatic questions which have consumed the interests of researchers in the social epidemiology of mental illness for many years. To put these questions in proper perspective, the section on social complexity and contemporary life opens with two papers addressed to theoretical problems that pervade the entire field of social psychiatry. First, we are concerned with whether or not our research efforts of the past century, or indeed even the past fifty years, are bearing fruit. Do we really understand the social epidemiological determinants of pathological behavior any better today than we did at the turn of the century? Are we really in a position to state emphatically that the uncounted millions thus far poured into social science research have been worthwhile? Some assessment of these questions must be made before we are free to deal with the more practical problems, and we must be made aware of how culture-bound we all have been in research attempts at viewing the limits of normalcy and pathology (Stanley C. Plog). Also, the concept of social class or socioeconomic status and its relationship to mental illness pervades the entire research field. Such findings are referred to in several chapters of this volume. However, questions about the adequacy of the concept and the way it has been used in research come immediately to mind. We must consider its utility and limitations and, ultimately, whether it has been beneficial or harmful to research (Raymond J. Murphy).

Such is the orientation of the next ten chapters. We are fortunate that we have experts who are competent to address themselves to these questions; their answers are not necessarily uniform, but many of the conclusions are new and startling. The reviews that are presented in this section serve the healthy purpose of periodic stock-taking and of informing us as to the probability that we can survive in the society of the future.

3.2 *Orientation*

In the following chapter, Stanley C. Plog presents a historical review of research on socioeconomic and demographic variables relevant to the study of disordered behavior during the period of time of important and relevant scientific literature—the last 125 years. In noting the changes in the areas of scientific interest in mental health problems and the analytic systems used to interpret the findings for the past century, the reader can only conclude that mental health researchers also are products of the social system that has produced them. Our current knowledge and understanding of individual pathology is limited by our ability to completely comprehend the social forces that have led to the development of mental health researchers.

However, Dr. Plog also points out those findings that have been more conclusive over a period of time and, therefore, seem to be less subject to those specific interpretations that are dependent upon the fads of each generation of researchers. Hopefully, our understanding of the causes of disordered behavior is increasing at an exponential rate, and we are developing more firm foundations for an imperfect science. History will judge our efforts. The question is how long we can wait for history's judgment.

3.2   Urbanization, Psychological Disorders, and The Heritage of Social Psychiatry

Stanley C. Plog

When we get piled upon one another in large cities, as in Europe, we shall become corrupt as in Europe, and go to eating one another as they do there. . . . In solving this question . . . we should allow just weight to the moral and physical preferences of the agricultural, over the manufacturing, man. (Thomas Jefferson, letter to John Madison, 1787)

The thought of a once beautiful America being spoiled by increasing urbanization and its citizens becoming degenerates because of the inherent evils of cities, has plagued politicians, citizens, and professionals from various disciplines since the nation was founded. Jefferson was not the first Colonial to warn against changes that were taking place in the social fabric, but he was often the most eloquent. His concerns have been frequently echoed across the nation since that time, and reflect not just the dangers of an America's losing its agricultural heritage, but also the constant fear that this nation would cease to exist unless it sought to preserve those special characteristics that made us free men and psychologically stable.

In essence, Jefferson was a social psychiatrist. He was concerned about the relationship of the social order to man's psychological health and, therefore, to his ability to govern himself. Similarly, hundreds of other public officials and popular writers have since voiced deep concern about the effect of uncontrollable social forces that could affect the "moral" nature of man and impair his psychological stability. Such concerns led the Congress of the United States to enact legislation requiring that the decennial census also include a survey of the number of institutionally hospitalized insane, beginning in 1840. With these statistics, it was easier to focus on important questions about the interrelationship of man and his social environment, and the use of census data has since become an accepted way of attempting answers to questions in the field of mental health and illness.

The focus of this chapter is to present a historical review of the published research of the nineteenth and early twentieth centuries related to the field of social psychiatry that is addressed to questions about the interrelationship of man and his social environment. Our review will carry us as far as the first quarter of the twentieth century, since the relevant research from that period to the present is adequately covered in several chapters in this volume (see Dunham, Kantor, Malzberg, Murphy, and Weakland).

There are those who suggest that the field of social psychiatry has developed since World War II in response to the increasing concerns of the nation and the world about man's ability to survive and maintain his stability in a social jungle. Studies have appeared that are addressed to almost every conceivable question, and it would seem that we are suddenly developing information in critical areas about man that previously had been neglected or overlooked.

To maintain such a viewpoint, however, it would be necessary to disregard a large body of historical literature that has been devoted to social psychiatric questions, but perhaps not so labeled. In fact, it would not be difficult to support the argument that the acceptance of Freudian ideas, with its emphasis on the examination of the single case or individual, delayed the development of social psychiatric research by at least fifty years. In spite of this, several hundred articles made prior to World War II are available, and they cover a variety of topics. The authors include physicians, neurologists, and early psychiatrists whose writings appear in professional and scientific journals. In reading these early articles, one experiences *deja vu* for almost any contemporary question in social psychiatry has been the subject of research 100 years ago or more. The primary difference is the development, in more recent years, of sophisticated statistical and research methodologies, and the correlated growth of a new social science vocabulary and jargon.

In reviewing the research of more than a century past, there are amazing similarities to current research in social psychiatry, similarities that cannot be passed over lightly. The major questions of that day cover most of the major questions raised in this volume. The primary sources of data are the same for these articles and deal with cross-cultural studies or are concerned with large populations of people, namely mental hospital admission rates and census statistics. Disagreements over questions that were thought to be important in previous periods and the meaning of the data are also readily apparent, and it is usually not too difficult to determine the biases of the individual researchers or authors. There is a considerable amount of moralism in many of the articles, a moralism which supported predetermined positions of the researchers. Though the language and tenor of contemporary social science research is more sophisticated, it also suffers from the fact that particular kinds of conclusions tend to come consistently from particular disciplines.

The more important similarity centers around the fact that the dominant questions about the influence of social factors on the determination or the course of mental illness are the same today as before, a fact that constitutes a serious indictment on the state of the art of social sciences. We have not progressed as rapidly as one would expect in developing answers to these century-old questions, nor does it appear that we have developed the methodology to provide sufficient answers or explanations in the near future.

The early reportings of mental health and illness data occurred in the early 1840s and were dependent upon the concurrent development of several things: (1) the inclusion of mental hospital data in the decennial United States Census (the first census was completed in 1790), (2) the acceptance of scientific methods in medicine as a legitimate procedure in the search for causes of disease, and (3) the establishment of journals devoted to "insanity" and "lunacy."

Two primary questions plagued the researchers of that period—whether or not mental illness was increasing over time and, if so, whether or not it was dependent upon "the rapid advance of civilization" (urbanization). The researchers were not unanimous on either of these questions, although some general conclusions could be derived from their work. A majority of these early pioneers in social psychiatry concluded, in fact, that mental illness was increasing and that this increase could be attributed to a variety of causes. Foremost among these causes was considered to be the rapid urbanization of the country and the attendant ills and hardships that are forced upon a population having to live in the cities. In eloquent rhetoric, in 1876, a Dr. Jamieson, physician to the Royal Asylum, Aberdeen, Northern Scotland, summarized "available" data for the three previous decades and concluded that,

I believe that the most remarkable medical phenomena in our time has been the alarming increase of insanity. Crime has been diminishing; prisons, here and there, have been shut up; but who hears of an asylum being shut down anywhere, or even of its numerous inmates decreasing? Are we but changing lawlessness for incapacity, cunning for weakness, and are we better because fools accumulate and thieves decay [Increase of Mental Disease, 1876, p. 139.]?

He goes on to report brief statistics about the number of inmates in public asylums in Aberdeen and an alarming increase in a variety of personality disorders for the period of 1844 to the time of the article and finally stated,

I believe that there is a great increase in diseased and half-invalided conditions; an increase in all diseases of the nervous system, or an increase of the nervous factor in all diseases; that there is an anemic physiognomy prevalent in all town inhabitants; a readiness to break down under trials; a tendency to be unduly influenced by slight causes; and a degeneration of physical character . . . a physical deterioration [which] is thought to be more observable in the male than the female section of the community [Increase of Mental Disease, 1876, p. 141].

A similar view was held by H. P. Stearns (1883), whose background and qualifications were not adequately identified. He stressed the fact that residents of cities do not have as much "fresh air" as those who are still engaged in agricultural pursuits and that "The thousands who are in the present immersed in the dense atmosphere of cities, large towns, manufacturing establishments and mines of various kinds, were accustomed in former times to live largely out-of-doors and were engaged in such pursuits as tended to develop and strengthen their whole system [p. 413]." Dr. R. Jones (1906), a resident physician and superintendent of the London County Asylum in Claybury, England, had a similar view in that, "With the progress of civilization, mental breakdown becomes more serious if not more frequent, and the varieties of insanity more chronic and less curable when life was simpler and men were more content [p. 632]."

The second major reason given by those who felt that rates of mental illness were increasing was that hereditary inbreeding by persons with congenital defects was leading to a predisposition for mental illness among large segments of the population. In summarizing inmate figures for the previous decade in England, H. C. Major in 1844 concluded that hereditary influences were the major factor out of twenty contributors to mental breakdown, contributing as much as 18.6 percent of the registered cases among males and 21.8 percent among females (Major, 1884). W. J. Corbet, a member of parliament from Wicklow County, Ireland, cried that he had been doing research on the topic for twenty years and there was an increase of 120 percent in the number of registered lunatics in the general population over that period of time, while the population increase was only 38 percent. No doubts were left that the major portion of this increase could be attributed to hereditary influences (Corbet, 1893). An intellectual giant of early psychiatry, William A. White, concluded similarly that insanity was increasing and that 70 percent of this increase came from "bad heredity." In his view, civilization furnished the environment that made bad heredity doubly dangerous, but hereditary factors were always primary. He warned ominously, "A bad heritage is always a source of danger and its possessor can never know when environmental conditions may appear which will make its latent activity kinetic [White, 1903, p. 278]." He finished his article with a stern warning that

No people in the world are freer than we are from the taints of vicious inheritance. Inhabitants of the most glorious country on earth, a country whose future for greatness, and power, and good, seems to have no limit, let us see that we make the best possible use of the bounties nature has showered upon us with so prodigal a hand.

But power and greatness are double-edged; they cut both ways, and already we are threatened with the dangers they have brought in their wake. The off-scourings of all Europe are hastening to our shores for that wealth they expect to find ready at hand, and today 50 percent of the nearly 25,000 insane of New York State are foreign born. The result of this great influx of defectives must of necessity have a constant leavening effect on the whole population. The danger from this source, however, is as nothing compared to that from war, the greatest curse that can afflict a nation.

In war it is not the defective that goes down to death, but the flower of a nation's manhood, and if modern theories of heredity are correct their place can never be filled—once gone they are gone forever, while the maimed, the diseased, the imbeciles and degenerates, unable to sustain the hardships of campaigning, stay at home and help populate the country with their ilk [pp. 278–279].

Occasionally an author would suggest that there had been an increase because of modern medical methods which afforded life protection for "incurable wrecks" and resulted in "interfering with the law of the survival of the fittest [Parker, 1906, p. 176]."

The similarity of most of these views about the presumed increase in insanity through urbanization or the hereditary inbreeding by social degenerates centered around a general belief that civilization was an unnatural state and that it forced conditions upon an individual or a population that were contrary to the fulfillment of normal needs or ways of interacting with a natural environment. This Rousseauian viewpoint suggested that the competitive jungle of modern life resulted in more breakdowns because of the maladaptability of a natural man to the rigors and competitions of a civilized society. These articles became more prevalent in the early 1880s, a time when ever-increasing industrialization and urbanization followed the Civil War, and the gradual closing of the American frontier became apparent to many social critics. Most of these professionals in the mental health field wrote in journalistic style, and their impassioned pleas were meant to wake up an America, which was in danger of losing the basic moral fiber that had contributed so much to its greatness. As early as 1844, C. D. Hayden, concluded that:

[It is our] free institutions which promote insanity . . . life in our republic has all the excitement of an Olympic contest. A wide arena is thrown open and all fearlessly join in the maddening rush for the laurel wreath, or golden chaplet which are the guerdons in that race which is to the swift, and rarely does any Hesperian fruit seduce the candidates from the contest. Are not the bitter rancor of partisans, the morbid excitement of politicians, the feverish anxiety of gambling speculators, the sickness of hope deferred, ambition maddened by defeat, avarice rendered desperate by failure, so many sources of insanity [Hayden, 1844, p. 178]?

In more tempered tone, J. P. Gray, the Superintendent of the State Lunatic Asylum, in Utica, New York, wrote more than 40 years later:

I will not give emphasis to the statement that insanity is a special disease of civilization because savages and uncivilized people show cases as well. But it is certainly fair to say that the duties and responsibilities, the toil and trials of civilization, far exceed those of savage life, and they are potent factors in the causation of insanity [Gray, 1885, pp. 13–14].

Before the turn of the century, the distinguished editor of the *American Journal of Insanity* sounded a warning that "either the average brain of today has become a more unstable structure than the average brain of our ancestors; or else the average stress of environmental forces brought to bear on the brains of our generation has become more severe than formerly" (Blumer, 1893, p. 310). He concludes that:

The struggle for mental supremacy is harder and harder. With the advance in general culture, there is less and less room in the ranks of mediocrity, more and more crowding even at the very top. Meanwhile the aspiration to be near the top has seized upon everyone. Not only do the classes elbow one another harder than ever before, that the masses are no longer content to remain the masses . . . the prizes are in view of all and none are debarred from striving for them; so an era of unrest, of vaulting ambition, has come upon our race. No man is satisfied . . . so success means an exaggerated, disproportionate success involving the failure of more and more competitors. The perpetual struggle thus involved in the attempt to reach an abnormal average of success imposes an environmental stress which is disproportionate to our present stage of evolution, and this is, in our opinion, the most potent factor in producing that disturbed equilibrium which manifests itself, among other ways, in an alarming increase of insanity [pp. 312–313].

However, in spite of this general alarm, there were those authors who did *not* feel that insanity was increasing, and their arguments against this increase usually were more unitary. In general, it can be said that these articles were more sophisticated in tone and content, and the authors demonstrated a greater awareness of the difficulties around problems of measurement. The majority of these articles appeared in the 1870s and 1880s, but summarized data of the previous 30 to 40 years. These authors universally accepted the fact that there had been an increase in the number of persons residing in asylums or mental hospitals, but they attributed this increase to factors not adequately considered by the other researchers, such as a general population increase, a more complete registration of "lunatics" as compared with former years because of more adequate census methods, a longer life span for the general population resulting in a longer risk-exposure period for the development of psychological problems, and the fact that improved medical facilities in asylums also resulted in a longer life span for patients (Alleged Increase of Insanity, 1872, 1894; Bucknill, 1862; Census, 1872; Dr. Dunglison's Statistics, 1860; General Board, 1884; Humphreys, 1890). At least one researcher, H. Rayner, suggested that even if there was a real increase, it would be reduced by the confinement of large numbers of insane to asylums, thereby resulting in a relative decrease in insanity because these persons could not reproduce themselves during the period of their confinement. By far the most sophisticated argument against any alleged increase in rates of psychosis was presented by E. H. Tuke (1886), who compared "the number of occurring cases of mental disorder in proportion to the population during the periods of time we desire to compare [p. 360]." This early attempt at developing age and sex standardized rates represents a practice now widely accepted among researchers. He investigated incidence figures, rather than just prevalence rates, tried to check out readmissions and eliminate transfer cases from one hospital to another, and finally took into account the increase in population from the period of 1859 to 1884 before suggesting that, "so far as statistics teach us anything, they fail to show the slightest increase in occurring insanity in this country since January 1, 1878, when we apply the only reliable test to the investigation of the problem under discussion [p. 360]." His approach and conclusions were amazingly similar to later work of Goldhamer and Marshal (1949).

Other major questions of social psychiatry also were the subject of study and concern during this period of time and are similar to contemporary discussions in social research. Various researchers wondered whether differences in rates of insanity could be related to patterns of immigration to a nation or migrations within that nation. The suggestions given varied as to whether the author represented a nation receiving immigrants or a nation sending emigrants from its shores. Authors writing in European journals, which were losing people to the United States, most often concluded that only the strong and healthy had the courage and the moral fortitude to want to leave, thus resulting in an accumulation of the unhealthy or mentally ill in the nation from which they had departed. As early as 1844, the suggestion was given by an unidentified mental hospital physician that "immigrants generally leave behind them the idiotic and insane, a state receiving immigration has less than its due proportion, and the parent state more [Hayden, 1844, p. 179]." Another unknown author concluded in 1883 that, "the decrease of the population by emigration, leaving the infirm, physically and mentally, to remain, causes the ratio of insane to the sane to be higher in the present generation than it otherwise would [Inspectors, 1884, p. 558]."

Likewise, H. P. Stearns (1883) concluded in England a year earlier that the extensive emigration of able-bodied men from Britain during the recent years left a proportion of the weak and insane that was much higher than otherwise would have been without a corresponding actual increase in insanity. On the same subject, W. A. White, who was then the first assistant physician of the Binghamton State Hospital in Binghamton, New York, suggested in 1903 that "the frontiersman who takes his family and goes West to open up new territory, engage in legitimate agricultural pursuits, and grow up with the country, is pretty apt to be of hardy stock and insanity, if it appears at all, comes in later generations [White, 1903, p. 267]."

Like many other authors, White uses mental hospital data to support his general conclusions that there is a decrease in mental illness as one moved from the East to the West of the United States.

The host countries for immigrants usually felt they were getting the better share of the lot, and very few articles can be found that are critical of immigration practices in the United States or elsewhere. Generally, it was concluded that a nation can best survive and grow with the healthiest of new blood coming from a variety of nations. The only critic of this general assumption who could be located in this review of the literature, was Dr. M. H. Ranney (1858), a resident physician at the New York City Lunatic Asylum, Blackwell's Island. He did not suggest that immigrants are a disturbed lot, but rather, that the pressures of life in the New World were often too much for even the hardiest of souls to maintain stability.

On landing in New York they soon learn that their hard expectations of prosperity, which had induced them to leave their native homes and sustained them on their voyage, were not to be realized, and awake to a consciousness of the wretchedness of their situation in finding themselves destitute in a strange land . . . The physical sufferings they have endured before leaving their homes, added to the privations of the sea voyage, the breaking up of attachments rooted in breast, their landing in a helpless and often destitute state on a strange shore, are causes well calculated to try the endurance of disciplined and strong minds. It is not astonishing, then, that those unaccustomed to self restraint, or without mental cultivation, should fall before such a combination of adverse moral and physical causes [p. 46].

Selected historical articles on the relationship of poverty to the production of mental illness also had variable conclusions, depending upon the kinds of data employed, the place where the author worked, and his philosophical predispositions. One of the earlier and more integrated theories was propounded by Dr. D. Yellowlees, Physician Superintendent of Glasgow Royal Asylum. He offered the hypothesis that poverty does not grant sufficient time or money for the individual to engage in activities that, by the nature of their immoral purpose, could lead to higher rates of mental illness. He used uncorrected statistics of the number of pauper patients in insane asylums to conclude that "adversity is favorable to mental stability and prosperity the reverse [Chapman, 1882, p. 189]." He offered some of his strongest arguments in reviewing the relationship of short term economic fluctuations to admissions rates of mental hospitals and wrote,

> The decreased production of insanity during the (labor) strikes seems mainly due to two causes—one fiscal, the other moral. There is no money to spend in drinking and there is no time to think of anything but the strike. This moral cause is more potent than might at first appear . . . the subject (of the strike) has the deepest personal interest for all, and so engrosses attention, that it gives stability and force to weak and wavering minds, just as a demented patient becomes reasonable and intelligent for a time when his attention is aroused and his scattered faculties concentrated by an illness or accident [Yellowlees, 1882, p. 472].

However, most authors of the day took strong exception with Yellowlees and their counter arguments are similar in tone and style to the major assumptions underlying current research on the effects of poverty and cultural deprivation on rates of mental illness. The strongest critic of Yellowlees's position was Dr. T. A. Chapman, Medical Superintendent of Hereford Asylum in England. Writing in the same year (Chapman, 1882), he tabulated the number of recoveries each year from 1870 to 1879 to suggest that, "Prosperity is a prophylactic of insanity," if not always, at least in most cases [p. 189]. Many more articles appeared near the turn of the century, usually with the similar conclusion that poverty had a debilitating effect on individuals in a variety of ways. W. A. White (1903), who has been quoted previously, also concluded very definitely that there is a relationship of "pauperism" to insanity, and he places blame on the individual who is poor, in that, "The individual who, unless absolutely incapacitated by physical disability, so far fails in the struggle for existence that he must be supported at the public expense, is certainly suffering from some form of mental defect [pp. 274–275]." Similarly, the Inspector of Lunatic Asylums in Ireland, Dr. W. R. Dawson (1911), used prevalence rates of the number of pauper insane in public institutions to suggest that agricultural counties with low wage rates and land values, also placed high on any ranking of the number of insane, and usually at the head of the list.

Many articles during the past 120 years also addressed themselves to the question of whether or not there were differences among Negroes and whites in rates of mental illness within the United States. These concerns and questions were prevalent before and immediately after the Civil War, and represented a further elaboration of many of the pro- and anti-slavery arguments. Even more than most of the topics previously discussed, the authors were guilty of holding strong biases and preconceived opinions which allowed them to choose statistics or research methods likely to be supportive of their basic positions. The great majority of these articles were by southern authors, and their conclusions were that slavery was beneficial to caste members and, therefore, a useful social institution for both whites and Negroes.

Using 1840 census data, which seemed to indicate an over-representation of free Negroes in the mental hospitals in New England states, C. D. Hayden (1844) concluded that:

The blacks are in a condition of social helotage, constituting the pauper caste and the heirs of all the ills which poverty entails upon its subjects. The Negro of the South on the contrary, cares not for the morrow, well-knowing that another will provide what he shall eat, what he shall drink, and wherewithal he shall be clothed; his simple mode of life secures him in health, and in the winter of life, he crowns a use of labor with an age of ease [p. 181].

Using the same census data, an unknown author presented an article in the *American Journal of Insanity* (Statistics, 1851) to point out in forceful language "amazing prevalence of insanity and idiocy among our free colored population over the whites and slaves [p. 150]." All available statistics of the day were summarized by another unknown author and a similar conclusion was reached that, "Insanity prevails to a greater extent among the white and free colored population than among the slaves. This is thought to be due to the freedom of the latter from care and anxiety, and from intemperance and other excesses."

The particular hardships of the transition from slavery to freedom among a population that was not used to freedom was a frequent subject of research by various authors during the period following the Civil War. Almost universally they arrived at the conclusion that slavery was a better form of existence for the Negro. A physician at the State Lunatic Asylum in Georgia in 1851 addressed a circular letter to the county officers in every county in the state requesting "reliable information" on the number of insane Negroes in their respective counties. When he finally reported his results (Insanity, 1874), the results of his "investigation" indicated that there were only forty insane Negroes in all of Georgia, which had a Negro population of over 400,000. However, he was "astonished" to find a very large number of insane colored people in mental institutions in the northern states when he later made a visit. His explanation was

When those people were in a state of slavery, they were taken care of and were not permitted to run into every possible excess, to remain up all night, to drink and to carouse, etc. When they were sick, they had proper medical attendance and nursing. They, as a class, were most assuredly not subject to such privations as were calculated to impair their health. Then the better class had no cares or anxieties about anything . . . now all this is reversed, and furnishes reasons, very satisfactory to my mind, for the manifest increase of insanity among the colored people [p. 155].

Only one article could be found in the nineteenth-century literature that developed the contrary conclusion (Jarvis, 1844). Again, the author had a preconceived and clearly specified bias; "to demonstrate that no reliance whatever can be placed on what purport to be facts, respecting the prevalence of insanity among the free Negroes, except for, in that fallacious self-condemning document, the 'Sixth Census of the United States' [p. 75]." In spite of the emotionally toned language, the author, Jarvis (Dorchester, Massachusetts), was more sophisticated in his approach to the problem. He compared the number of whites and Negroes in each town, city, and state to the number of listed white and colored "lunatics and idiots" in each respective district. The discrepancies he noticed in the census statistics included the fact that sometimes the number of insane in a town exceeded the total population listed for that area, that the northern states varied from having one in every fourteen Negroes insane (Maine) to one in every 297 (New Jersey), and that in some communities from one-tenth to two-thirds of the population were frequently listed as hospitalized psychotics. Thus, he argued that available census statistics were unreliable and could not be used to support any argument that suggested that slavery was a more proper form of existence for Negroes (Jarvis, 1844, p. 75).

We have presented an uncritical review of the important research conclusions of the past century that were addressed to major questions about the influences of social factors on incidence and prevalence rates of mental illness. It has been easy to see that the investigators allowed personal biases and predilections to influence the selection of their research focus, the kinds of data and statistics used, and the direction of the research results. In spite of the definitive claims of most of these authors, we can only conclude that we are not in the position to answer adequately most of the social psychiatric questions raised, and especially not the primary questions presented at the outset, that is, Is mental illness increasing? If so, what relationship does this increase have to the "advance of civilization" (urbanization)?

Not only have we not answered these questions, we do not seem to be close to any of the answers. The reasons for this are several: (1) the lack of comparative statistics over time, (2) the historical influence of Freudian psychology, and (3) the complexity of the questions being asked. Let us turn to each of these problems very briefly.

COMPARABILITY OF DATA

Most of the studies reported here have relied upon mental hospital statistics, especially when they were available from census data. Such statistics are notoriously unreliable, especially over a period of time, because of the lack of systematic record keeping systems in hospitals, the variability of admission practices at different hospitals, and the unreliability of diagnosis among psychiatrists responsible for the hospital admissions.

In the literature just reviewed, a variety of doubtful categories have frequently been included under the general rubric of "lunatic" or "insane." These marginal groups include the indigent poor, alcoholics, criminals, the aged and the infirm, and persons with chronic brain syndromes (especially those suffering from long-term effects of syphilitic infections). When the diagnostic categories are specified, the specific rates for each category are seldom given. Even today, there are no standardized ways of recording or reporting mental hospital data across the nation, though a few cities have developed some coordinated record keeping systems among their public institutions.

However, in spite of the inadequacies of this data, there is some merit to plotting the results of available studies on a graph to determine possible directional trends of hospitalization rates from 1840 to the present. The results are presented in Figures 1 and 2, which are summaries of available studies on incidence and prevalence rates over the past 125 years.[1]

[1] The graphs were developed by preparing available statistics into a uniform format (rates per 100,000 population), and by developing age and sex specific rates, where possible. When the reporting authors employed other methods for reporting their data, that is, the number of psychotics reported in a township or the percent of a population reported by professionals to be insane, attempts were made to determine the population of a township or other geographic area so that their rates could be converted to the format of the graphs. Wherever possible, the rates are mean averages for the average age of the population for that period of time. However, most statistics did not allow this kind of summary of the data. When information from the early studies was adequate, inappropriate categories of patients were eliminated in computing final totals, as paupers, alcoholics, and others who ended up in insane asylums because of their inability to care for themselves. Those articles that did not provide adequate information to develop specific statistics, were excluded from the compilation. The graphs, obviously, include many sources of error, since the per-

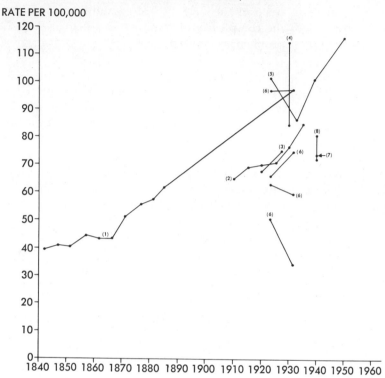

INCIDENCE OF MENTAL ILLNESS
(RATES PER 100,000)

FIGURE 1. This summary of research studies on the incidence of mental illness (1840–1960) is based on the references listed below. Corrections were made to standardize the data and to obtain patient figures per 100,000 population. As much as possible, inappropriate categories, such as criminal and pauper, and inappropriate medical disorders were excluded. It was impossible to standardize the rates for age and sex.

1. Goldhamer, H., & Marshal, A. W. *Psychosis and civilization.* Glencoe, Ill.: Free Press, 1949. Pp. 13, 76. [New York State in 1930 had 97 per 100,000 (p. 76).]
2. Malzberg, B. *Social and biological aspects of mental disease.* Utica, N.Y.: State Hospitals Press, 1940.
3. Malzberg, B. Mental disease among Jews: A second study with a note on the relative prevalence of mental defect and epilepsy. *Mental Hygiene,* 1931, *15,* 766–774.
4. Malzberg, B. New data relative to incidence of mental disease among Jews. *Mental Hygiene,* 1936, *20,* 280–291. [Rates represent averaged rates for males and females combined.]
5. Dunham, H. W. *Sociological theory and mental disorder.* Detroit: Wayne State University Press, 1959. P. 100.

Age-Specific Rates of First Admission for Psychosis by Sex and Year for the United States

Age	1923		1933		1939		1950	
	M	F	M	F	M	F	M	F
-19	15.4	12.0	13.4	10.1	16.4	13.3	19.9	18.0
20–29	78.3	53.1	60.3	43.2	66.9	53.3	65.0	68.9
30–39	100.8	83.8	71.2	56.2	89.9	74.8	71.5	90.7
40–49	106.2	96.7	84.0	67.8	106.0	83.4	85.2	98.7
50–59	110.7	97.2	100.1	75.4	110.3	94.6	90.3	102.5
60–69	145.4	106.8	130.4	90.2	140.6	106.8	142.2	125.4
70–	240.2	181.3	244.7	166.2	264.3	194.8	348.3	300.6

Since population totals in each age category are not known, an average rate for each year was considered to be the average of the 14 rates for the year. (For example, for 1923: (15.4 + 12.0 + 78.3 . . . 240.2 + 181.3) ÷ 14 = 102.0.) Averages obtained by this method are 1923: 102.0; 1933: 86.6; 1939: 101.1; and 1950: 116.2.

6. Jacob, J. S. A note on the alleged increase in insanity. *Journal of Abnormal and Social Psychology*, 1938, 33, 390–397.

	1923	1932
Georgia	50.3	34.7
Alabama	63.3	59.6
Illinois	97.2	97.9
United States	66.6	74.8

7. Lemert, E. M. An exploratory study of mental disorders in a rural problem area. *Rural Sociology*, 1948, 13, 48–64. [The upper peninsula of Michigan was combined with the southern industrial county rates.]

8. Stewart, D. D. A note on mental illness in rural Arkansas. *Journal of Social Problems*, 1953–1955, 1–2, 57–60. [For the year 1940: Arkansas State, 72.3 per 100,000; United States, 80.1 per 100,000.]

On the basis of the multiple problems in computing the data, it would be expected that no consistent picture would develop from plotting incidence and prevalence rates for the past 125 years. However, the surprising finding is the regularity of particular trends in the data. Except for a few studies with exceptional findings, Figures 1 and 2 suggest that there has been a constant, but gradual, rising trend in the *reported* incidence and prevalence rates of hospitalizations for psychosis since the

---

centage of ethnics or immigrants in each study is usually not identified, reports are included from differing ports of the nation or the world, and diagnostic categories are often not specified.

PREVALENCE OF MENTAL ILLNESS
(RATES PER 100,000)

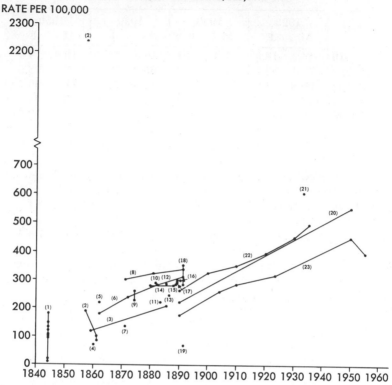

FIGURE 2. This summary of research studies on the prevalence of mental illness (1840–1960) is based on the references listed below. Corrections were made to standardize the data and to obtain patient figures per 100,000 population. As much as possible, inappropriate categories, such as criminal and pauper, and inappropriate medical disorders were excluded. It was impossible to standardize the rates for age and sex.

1. Ratio of the insane and idiotic to the population of different countries and great cities. *American Journal of Insanity*, 1844, *1*, 78.

    The following rates per 100,000 were developed from the ratios given:

Spain	10
Italy	20
Belgium	98
France	100
United States	102
England	120
Ireland	130
Scotland	146
Norway	180

302

2. Statistics of insanity in Europe. *American Journal of Insanity*, 1891, *17–18*, 348–349. [The following rates per 100,000 were developed: for 1861 in Germany, 83, and France (using the more conservative ratio of 1 in 1000), 100; for 1857 in England (averaging the figures for the agricultural and manufacturing counties), 2239; for 1857 in Scotland, 190.]

3. Tuke, D. H. The alleged increase of insanity. *Journal of Mental Science*, 1886, *32*, 360–376. [Per 100,000 in England and Wales, 1859: 117; 1885: 206.]

4. Dr. Dunglison's statistics of insanity in the United States. *American Journal of Insanity*, 1860, *17–18*, 111.

5. Arlidge, J. T. Lunacy reports and lunacy statistics. *Journal of Mental Science*, 1862, *8*, 417–429. [England and Wales, 1862: 220 per 100,000.]

6. Corbet, W. J. On the increase of insanity. *American Journal of Insanity*, 1893, *50*, 224–238. [Per 100,000 general population of England, Ireland, and Scotland, 1862: 181; 1872: 241; 1882: 284; 1891: 307.]

7. Deas, P. M. An illustration of local differences in the distribution of insanity. *Journal of Mental Science*, 1875, *21*, 61–67.

8. The alleged increase of insanity. *American Journal of Insanity*, 1894, *50*, 557–558. [Per 100,000 in England and Wales, 1871: 300; 1881: 325; 1891: 340.]

9. The lunacy blue books. *Journal of Mental Science*, 1874, *20*, 436–446. [For 1874, on the basis of the ratios given, the following rates per 100,000 were developed: England, 262; Scotland, 232.]

10. Thirty-seventh report of the commissioners in lunacy, March 31, 1883. *Journal of Mental Science*, 1884, *29*, 544–551. [The ratio of 1 per 346 produces 290 per 100,000 for the year 1882 in England.]

11. Twenty-fifth annual report of the general board of commissioners in lunacy for Scotland, for 1883. *Journal of Mental Science*, 1884, *29*, 552–558. [The ratio of pauper lunatics in asylums to the population is given as 185 to 188 per 100,111. Subtracting the 63 criminal lunatics from the 1883 figure of 10,510 insane leaves a total of 10,447 private and pauper patients. In 1883, 8793 patients were paupers.] The 1883 population was obtained as follows:

$$\frac{185}{100,000} \div \frac{8793}{X} = 4,752,973$$

Then

$$\frac{10,477}{4,752,973} = .0021+$$

And $(.0022)(100,000) = 220$ per 100,000.

12. Thirty-ninth report of the commissioners in lunacy (England), July, 1885. *Journal of Mental Science,* 1886, *31,* 518–529. [1 = .0029 = 290 per 100,000.]

13. Congress of psychiatry and neuropathology at Antwerp. *Journal of Mental Science,* 1886, *31,* 613–626. [Germany, 1886: 240 per 100,000.]

14. Thirty-seventh report of the inspectors on the district criminal and private asylums in Ireland, Dublin, 1888. *Journal of Mental Science,* 1889, *34,* 567–575. [Per 100,000 in England, 1880: 280; in Ireland, 1887: 280.]

15. Thirty-first annual report of the general board of commissioners in lunacy for Scotland, Edinburg, 1889. *Journal of Mental Science,* 1889, *35,* 412–417. [Per 100,000 in Scotland in 1888: 284; and in 1889: 289; in England in 1889: 291.]

16. Forty-fourth report of the commissioners in lunacy, 1st July, 1890. *Journal of Mental Science,* 1890, *36,* 540–544. [For England and Wales, 1890: 293 per 100,000.]

17. Forty-second report of the commissioners in lunacy, July, 1888. *Journal of Mental Science,* 1889, *34,* 555–561. [England, 1889: 1/346 = .0029 = 290 per 100,000.]

18. Ross, C. Statistics of insanity in New South Wales, considered with reference to the census of 1891. *American Journal of Insanity,* 1893, *50,* 11–20. [Per 100,000 in 1891, New South Wales: 277; Ireland: 346.]

19. Greenlees, T. D. A contribution to the statistics of insanty in Cape Colony. *American Journal of Insanity,* 1894, *50,* 519–529. [Cape Colony, 1891: 70 per 100,000.]

20. Pugh, T. F., & MacMahon, B. *Epidemiologic findings in United States mental hospital data.* Boston: Little, Brown, 1962.

21. Cohen, B. M., & Fairbank, R. Statistical contributions from the mental hygiene study of the eastern health district of Baltimore. *American Journal of Psychiatry,* 1938, *94,* 1153–1161.

22. Malzberg, B. *Social and biological aspects of mental disease.* Utica, N.Y.: State Hospitals Press, 1940.

23. Pugh, T. F., & MacMahon, B. *Epidemiologic findings in United States mental hospital data.* Boston: Little, Brown, 1962. [Although rates standardized for age and sex are available in this book, they have been combined and averaged to make them comparable with other rates used here.]

mid-nineteenth century. Impressive, too, is the relatively restricted range of variability for any particular time period on the graphs, and the very few studies that run counter to this trend. Thus, for whatever reasons, more and more persons have been hospitalized each decade over the past century for psychosis or related problems.

The reasons for the increasing use of mental hospitals are not clear from the data and do not necessarily reflect gradually increasing rates of mental illness due to urbanization or related factors. The possible explanations are many and are even the partial subject of several chapters in this volume. More mental hospitals have been built and are, therefore, more accessible to their potential users. Because of changing value systems of society, more persons are willing to seek professional psychiatric care during times of personal difficulty, and they are able to recognize the symptoms of severe personality disturbance more easily. Fewer older parents are living in homes with the families of one of their children, and the complexity and pressures of contemporary urban life have resulted in fewer families being willing to put up with extreme psychotic behavior on the part of one of their members. Thus, temporary hospitalization is more frequently thought of as an acceptable solution for close family members. Finally, modern medicine has resulted in more persons living to retirement age, increasing the general "risk exposure" period for senile psychosis, arteriosclerotic changes, and general physiological deterioration.

All of these explanations are meant only to suggest that the apparent increase in mental illness, on the basis of Figures 1 and 2 may not be real but our conclusions are subject to the inadequacy of previous and current methods of data collection and record keeping. Questions about causes of an *apparent* increase are unanswerable at the moment, and definitive conclusions cannot be given. However, it may also be, as Fried (1964) has suggested, that rates have been at least temporarily increasing and are the result of rapid and unstructured social change.

THE INFLUENCE OF FREUDIAN PSYCHOLOGY

Freud is rightfully given the credit for being the intellectual father of modern psychiatry, and he is responsible for major trends and developments that have become standard practices in the care and treatment of the mentally ill. However, his widespread acceptance also served to dampen interest in those problems that are now considered to be the purview of social psychiatry.

Freud's general theoretical system focused on individual treatment and an ontogenetic understanding of developmental trends within each individual. Largely excluded from consideration were the broad social factors that exert powerful influence on the development of personality, but which must be measured across large groups of people. Thus, by 1910, when Freudian thought was becoming popular, there was a significant decrease in the number of articles printed in the standard journals relevant to research on the social determinants of mental illness. For nearly a half-century, the subject matter of clinical psychiatry became the dominant focus of most of the professions dealing with mental illness. In contrast, superintendents of mental hospitals in the nineteenth century enjoyed great status and produced most of the research prevalent in the professional literature. With the rapid development of clinical psychiatry, prestige in psychiatry was no longer given to those who worked in state mental institutions, but to private practitioners, especially if they were psychoanalytically oriented. Hospital superintendents gradually became the least qualified professionals in the mental health field, and as a consequence, published very few articles which used social statistics in addressing research problems. Thus, Freudian psychology in some ways delayed the advance of one important area in the understanding of mental illness, and only a few researchers, some of whom are authors in this book (H. Warren Dunham and Benjamin Malzberg) continued to investigate their questions about mental illness which were sociocultural in nature. Without their continuing interest, it might have been even more difficult to pick up lost hypotheses and rediscover research methodologies relevant to the influence of social factors on mental illness.

COMPLEXITY OF THE QUESTIONS

Probably the most important reason that answers have not been forthcoming is that these questions, though simple in content, are exceedingly complex when put to a test. With present research methods and techniques, it is impossible to partial out the separate contributions of the multiple variables and factors that must be controlled in any study. The complete list of these factors is too long to include in this brief article, but any definitive study addressing itself to the question of the relationship of urbanization to whether or not mental illness is increasing must control for, at the very least:

Age and sex composition of the population
Ethnic composition of the population
Relevant subcultural or social class values held by subgroups, including beliefs about the causes of mental illness, willingness to accept professional treatment, and willingness to accept hospitalization
Socioeconomic status including affluence or poverty
Educational level
Type of occupation
Religious affiliation
Social and spatial mobility of the population
Geographic residence
Population density
Quality and type of housing

Size of family
Stability of family background
Availability of mental health treatment centers
Availability of recreational resources
Adequacy of medical care and attention
Rate of social change within the culture
Cultural stress (wars, hurricanes, epidemics, and so on)

In addition, any useful study would be dependent upon not only controlling for those factors listed above (and many more), but it would be assumed that an adequate psychiatric nosological system had been developed that measured up to acceptable standards of reliability and validity when utilized by practicing psychiatrists. This is not the case today, and there is very little possibility of significant improvements in psychiatric nomenclature or methods of diagnosis in the immediate future. Such a study would also be dependent upon the development of an appropriate epidemiological formula for measuring mental illness in a population and determining base line rates for computing changes over a period of time. Most studies rely on prevalence ratings for estimates of the degree of mental illness prevalent in a population, but a thorough review of the literature has convinced this author that a more accurate measure would be an index composed of

Mental illness in a population = Incidence of new cases

× Seriousness of each case

Thus, an index would be developed in which a psychotic episode was given a scale value larger (indicative of more serious impairment) than a mild anxiety attack, a delusional system was rated as a more severe personality disturbance than a fear of heights, a chronic and progressive brain syndrome was considered more debilitating than psychosomatically induced peptic ulcers, and so on. The advantage of using incidence rather than prevalence rates is that prevalence, by itself, does not provide an estimate of the number of new cases of mental illness developing each year, since no distinction is made between new and old cases. Prevalence rates are more readily affected by crude factors, such as the effectiveness of current treatment methods (psychotherapy or drugs), the chronicity of particular personality disorders, and their general distribution in the population. In contrast, incidence measures (which count the number of new cases) more immediately reflect changes in the social structure and their possible effect on mental health. These changes may be short-term (disasters, illness, family street, and so forth), or long-term changes (changes in society resulting from advancing technology, changing social mores, decline of religious belief, and so forth).

Obviously, it would be impossible to control for all of these factors in a single body. It may be that the conclusions will continue to be dependent upon the best guesses of contemporary researchers, or that there will gradually develop such a similarity of answers provided by the many separate studies about urbanization and mental illness that the final conclusion seems self obvious, if not statistically provable.

SUMMARY

We have reviewed, briefly, the social psychiatric research of the past 125 years and have concluded that

1. The kinds of questions asked today about the relationship of socio-cultural factors to mental illness are similar to those asked more than a century ago. Specifically, the continuing concern is with whether or not mental illness is increasing and, if so, whether or not it is related to the rapid advance of civilization (urbanization).

2. The kinds of research methodologies employed today are also quite similar to those of the previous century. Mental hospital admission rates and current cases under treatment constitute the primary sources of data, with an occasional attempt made to estimate prevalence in the community at large (the Midtown Manhattan Study, for example).

3. The conclusions developed from the research, which are often dependent upon the preconceived notions or biases of the researchers, are also similar over a period of time. The majority of the researchers from both periods feel that the complexity and pressures of modern living probably increase mental illness rates, that poverty and other factors of cultural deprivation have a deleterious effect on mental health, that minority group membership is disadvantageous to its members, that social upheaval causes problems for various members of society, and so on.

All of these similarities are true in spite of the development during recent years of more sophisticated statistical techniques and the utilization of a specialized jargon in the contemporary social sciences. We have not been able to answer the critically important questions about the effects of urban life on mental illness patterns, and contemporary research does not appear to be on the verge of important breakthrough.

These statements are not meant to present a pessimistic picture, but to re-evaluate, in a more honest light, the current "state of the art." It is only through increased research efforts and increased awareness of the magnitude of the problems involved that slow progress can be made. It can only be hoped that the period of complete dominance of Freudian thought in mental health research—to the exclusion of interest in the full range of variables affecting psychological stability—has passed, and that recent interdisciplinary efforts within social psychiatry will provide a model for cooperative and productive research. However, if any individual is hoping for dramatic achievements in the immediate future toward understanding the etiology of mental illness or in developing treatment methods and cures, he is, in all probability, going to be severely disappointed. Not many *enduring* professional reputations are likely to be made in the area of mental health research in the next generation, which, unfortunately, is likely to discourage some young and competent persons from entering the field. However, as social problems become more paramount in national affairs and politics, more of the nation's resources will be devoted to finding their solutions. Ultimately, we will discover the causes of psychological problems and effective methods for their treatment. Whether or not we will want to put those methods into practice is another question.

REFERENCES

The alleged increase of insanity. *Journal of Mental Science,* 1872, **18,** 229–231.

The alleged increase of insanity. *American Journal of Insanity,* 1894, **50,** 557–558.

Arlidge, J. T. Lunacy reports and lunacy statistics. *Journal of Mental Science,* 1862, **8,** 417–429.

Beach, F. Insanity in the coloured race in the United States, *Journal of Mental Science,* 1892, **38,** 145–146.

Blumer, G. A. The increase of insanity. *American Journal of Insanity,* 1893, **50,** 310–313.

Bockoven, J. S. *Moral treatment in American psychiatry.* New York: Springer Publishing Co., 1963.

Brigham, A. Millerism. *American Journal of Insanity,* 1845, **1,** 249–253.

Brown, M. English retrospect—Asylum reports for 1879. *Journal of Mental Science,* 1881, **27,** 17–18.

Bucknill, J. C. The statistics of insanity. *Journal of Mental Science,* 1862, **8,** 297–306.

The census. *Journal of Mental Science,* 1872, **18,** 120–122.

Chapman, T. A. On the effect of prosperity and adversity in the causation of insanity. *Journal of Mental Science,* 1882, **28,** 189–195.

Cohen, B. M., & Fairbank, R. Statistical contributions from the mental hygiene study of the eastern health district of Baltimore. *American Journal of Psychiatry,* 1938, **94,** 1153–1161.

Congress of psychiatry and neuropathology at Antwerp. *Journal of Mental Science,* 1886, **31,** 613–626.

Corbet, W. J. On the increase of insanity. *American Journal of Insanity,* 1893, **50,** 224–238.

Davidson, J. H. Observations on cannabis indica and syphilis as cause of mental alienation in Turkey, Asia Minor, and Morocco. *Journal of Mental Science,* 1883, **28**, 493–496.

Dawson, W. R. The presidential address on the relation between the geographical distribution of insanity and that of certain social and other conditions in Ireland. *Journal of Mental Science,* 1911, **57**, 571–597.

Deas, P. M. An illustration of local differences in the distribution of insanity. *Journal of Mental Science,* 1875, **21**, 61–67.

Dr. Dunglison's statistics of insanity in the United States. *American Journal of Insanity,* 1860, **111**, 17–18.

Dunham, H. W. *Sociological theory and mental disorder.* Detroit: Wayne State University Press, 1959.

Fried, M. Effects of Social Change on Mental Health. *American Journal of Orthopsychiatry,* 1964, **34**, 3–28.

General Board of Commissioners in Lunacy for Scotland. 25th annual report for 1883, 1884. *Journal of Mental Science,* 1884, **29**, 552–558.

General Board of Commissioners in Lunacy for Scotland. 31st annual report, 1889. *Journal of Mental Science,* 1889, **35**, 412–417.

General Board of Commissioners in Lunacy for Scotland. 37th annual report, 1883. *Journal of Mental Science,* 1884, **29**, 544–551.

General Board of Commissioners in Lunacy for Scotland. 39th annual report, 1885. *Journal of Mental Science,* 1886, **31**, 518–529.

General Board of Commissioners in Lunacy for Scotland. 42nd annual report, 1888. *Journal of Mental Science,* 1889, **34**, 555–561.

General Board of Commissioners in Lunacy for Scotland. 44th annual report, 1890. *Journal of Mental Science,* 1890, **36**, 540–544.

Goldhamer, H., & Marshal, A. W. *Psychosis and civilization.* Glencoe, Ill.: The Free Press, 1949.

Gray, J. P. Insanity: its frequency and some of its preventable causes. *American Journal of Insanity,* 1885, **42**, 1–45.

Greenlees, T. D. A contribution to the statistics of insanity in Cape Colony. *American Journal of Insanity,* 1894, **50**, 519–529.

Hayden, C. D. On the distribution of insanity in the United States. *3rd Literary Messenger,* 1844, **10**, 178–181.

Humphreys, N. A. Alleged increase of insanity. *Journal of Mental Science,* 1890, **36**, 236–239.

Hyslop, T. B. Occupation and environment as causative factors of insanity. *Journal of Mental Science,* 1906, **52**, 193.

The increase of mental disease. *Journal of Mental Science,* 1876, **22**, 138–141.

Influence of revolution in developing insanity in Paris. *American Journal of Insanity,* 1849, **5**, 281–285.

Insanity among Negroes. *Journal of Mental Science,* 1874, **20**, 154–156.

Inspectors of Irish Asylums. 32nd report, 1883. *Journal of Mental Science,* 1884, **29**, 558–564.

Inspectors on the District Criminal and Private Asylums in Ireland. 37th report, 1888. *Journal of Mental Science,* 1889, **34**, 567–575.

Jacob, J. S. A note on the alleged increase in insanity. *Journal of Abnormal and Social Psychology,* 1938, **33,** 390–397.

Jarvis, E. Insanity among the coloured population of the free states. *American Journal of Medical Science,* 1844, **7,** 71–83.

Jones, R. Medico-Psychological Association of Great Britain and Ireland: Presidential address on the evolution of insanity, delivered July 26, 1906. *Journal of Mental Science,* 1906, **52,** 629–661.

Leffingwell, A. Illegitimacy and the influence of seasons upon conduct. *Journal of Mental Science,* 1892, **38,** 428–432.

Lemert, E. M. An exploratory study of mental disorders in a rural problem area. *Rural Sociology,* 1948, **13,** 48–64.

The lunacy blue books. *Journal of Mental Science,* 1874, **20,** 436–446.

Major, H. C. Remarks on the results of the collective record of the causation of insanity. *Journal of Mental Science,* 1884, **30,** 1–7.

Malzberg, B. Mental disease among Jews: A second study with a note on the relative prevalence of mental defect and epilepsy. *Mental Hygiene,* 1931, **15,** 766–774.

Malzberg, B. New data relative to incidence of mental disease among Jews. *Mental Hygiene,* 1936, **20,** 280–291.

Malzberg, B. *Social and biological aspects of mental disease.* Utica, New York: State Hospitals Press, 1940.

Padover, S. K. (Ed.) *Thomas Jefferson on democracy.* New York: Pelican Books, 1946.

Parker, W. A. The increase of lunacy. *Journal of Mental Science,* 1906, **52,** 175–176.

Postell, W. D. Mental health among the slave population on southern plantations. *American Journal of Psychiatry,* 1953, **110,** 52–54.

Prange, A. J., & Vitols, M. M. Cultural aspects of the relatively low incidence of depression in southern Negroes. *International Journal of Social Psychiatry,* 1962, **8,** 104–112.

Public asylum reports for 1873. *Journal of Mental Science,* 1875, **20,** 634.

Pugh, T. F., & MacMahon, B. *Epidemiologic findings in United States mental hospitals data.* Boston: Little, Brown and Co., 1962.

Ranney, M. H. On insane foreigners. *American Journal of Insanity,* 1850, **7,** 45–53.

Ratio of the insane and idiotic to the population of different countries and great cities. *American Journal of Insanity,* 1844, **1,** 78.

Rayner, H. Presidential address, delivered at the annual meeting of the Medico-Psychological Association, held at the Royal College of Physicians, London, July 23, 1884. *Journal of Mental Science,* 1884, **30,** 337–353.

Rogers, T. L. The president's address. *Journal of Mental Science,* 1874, **20,** 327–351.

Rosen, G. Social stress and mental disease from the eighteenth century to the present: Some origins of social psychiatry. *Milbank Memorial Fund Quarterly,* 1959, **37,** 5–32.

Ross, C. Statistics of insanity in New South Wales considered with reference to the census of 1891. *American Journal of Insanity,* 1893, **50,** 11–20.

Startling facts from the census. *American Journal of Insanity,* 1851, **8,** pt. 1, 150–151.

Statistics of insanity in Europe. *American Journal of Insanity,* 1861, **17–18,** 348–349.

Stearns, H. P. Insanity: Its causes and prevention. *Journal of Mental Science,* 1883, **29,** 412–415.

Stewart, D. D. A note on mental illness in rural Arkansas. *Journal of Social Problems,* 1953–1955, **1–2,** 57–60.

Tietze, C., Lemkas, P., & Cooper, M. Schizophrenia, manic depressive psychosis and social-economic status. *American Journal of Sociology,* 1941–1942, **47,** 167–175.

Tuke, D. H. The alleged increase of insanity. *Journal of Mental Science,* 1886, **32,** 360–376.

Tuke, D. H. Does civilization favour the generation of mental disease? *Journal of Mental Science,* 1857, **4,** 94–110.

White, W. A. The geographical distribution of insanity in the United States. *Journal of Nervous and Mental Diseases,* 1903, **30,** 257–279.

Yellowlees, D. On the effect of prosperity and adversity in the causation of insanity. *Journal of Mental Science,* 1882, **28,** 472–473.

3.3 Orientation

Perhaps no other topic has served the proverbial purpose of "beating a dead horse" in medical sociology as much as studies on the relationship of social class to mental illness. The classics in the field, as the Chicago studies (Faris and Dunham), the New Haven studies (Hollingshead and Redlich), and the massive Midtown Manhattan investigation (Srole *et al.*), are now required reading in every good undergraduate program in sociology or social psychology throughout the country. And, any young researcher who wants to find an avenue for publication can reexamine the original data or replicate the studies, on a smaller scale, in another city or urban area.

It is refreshing to find a voice in the sea of acquiesing "Amens" in current research who calls for a reexamination of the assumptions underlying most of the research on class and psychological disorder. Raymond J. Murphy writes incisively and with clarity about those concepts of stratification research that are relevant to the study of psychological disorders. He raises such questions as, Is American stratification a system or systems? Does it constitute a class or a continuum? Are there many shared values among persons at similar class levels? What is the advantage of using subjective versus objective meanings of class levels?

Murphy points out how differing assumptions in class and stratification research can produce not only different research designs, but potentially differing results. The chapter is essential reading for anyone interested in the question of social class as related to mental illness.

3.3 Stratification and Mental Illness: Issues and Strategies for Research

Raymond J. Murphy

It has become increasingly evident that one of the most important trends in mental health research in the past decade is the growth of interdisciplinary efforts to understand the causes and treatment of mentally disturbed persons. Older parochial faiths have given way to a newly revitalized ecumenical spirit of collaboration among persons in the fields of anthropology, psychiatry, psychology, sociology, and social work. New graduate programs of training, such as community psychiatry, point the way to the creation of a new professional worker, skilled in the discipline of medicine and knowledgeable in the theories and methods of the behavioral scientist. It is also apparent from the results of such efforts that a key substantive area serving to interest and challenge persons from such diverse backgrounds is that of the relationship between stratification and mental illness. Such major efforts as those by A. B. Hollingshead and Redlich (1958), Miller and Swanson (1960), Srole, Langner, Michael, Opler, and Rennie (1962), and Parker and Kleiner (1966) testify to the attraction and utility of social stratification research for a multidisciplinary understanding of the causes and distribution of mental illness in the American community. The basic substantive findings of these studies, and others like them, are now becoming a part of our common understanding of the mentally ill.

The purpose of the present paper is to review some of the theoretical issues involved in stratification research and to suggest their possible implications for a better understanding of the mentally ill, and also to point out areas of further collaboration that would seem to be of value especially to the sociologist and psychiatrist. It is our feeling that a number of the issues raised by research into the structural factors related to mental illness point the way to a clearer understanding of, or empirical

support for, the working assumptions underlying each of these disciplines'
conception of human social behavior.

PROBLEMS AND ISSUES IN STRATIFICATION

Since most collaborative research tends to be focused specifically on a
substantive problem (rates of mental illness, for example), and since the
contributors to such studies are encouraged or pressured to seek a common working point of departure to facilitate their investigation, the
broader theoretical issues and problematics debated by their more endoga-
mous colleagues tend to be ignored or glossed over. Unresolved issues
concerning the most appropriate model or method for conceptualizing the
stratification system of the United States, for example, or the heuristic
value in alternative approaches to the problem of the genesis of neurotic
disturbances, tend not to enter extensively into the agenda of planning
operations. Such pragmatic concerns as budget, time, a prior agreement
to seek what is mutually acceptable to all research participants, plus the
inevitable impossibility of being a universal scholar, lead to a suspension
of problematics. It is our feeling that it may be useful to raise some of
these issues, both to inform the nonstratification specialist as to their
existence and also to indicate that buried in the academic disputes of
the specialist there seem to be potentially useful leads for continued
interdisciplinary research into the problem of mental illness and its treatment. Although, in fact, issues are seldom mutually exclusive in their
theoretical origins or implications, for the purpose of our present discussion we will briefly summarize four areas of debate among sociological
students of stratification.

American stratification: System or systems?   Given the size, industrial
complexity, and demographic heterogeneity of American society, one may
ask to what extent, and in what ways, it is possible to speak of *the* American stratification system. Most observers would agree that such ranking
criteria as occupational level, educational attainment, and amount of income are meaningful indicators of social position throughout the country.
A common language and national tradition with more or less general acceptance of a core of idealistic values (democratic representation, freedom
of thought and action, faith in the orderly process of change, and so on)
provide further bases for postulating a national system of rank. The
advent of the mass media made it even more likely that individuals would
come to share common values and aspirations, knowledge and fears. At
the same time, however, the forms and functions of stratification seem to
be affected by such factors as size of the population base, its demographic
composition, and regional traditions. Being in the upper class in Chicago

has different implications from being in the upper class in Rock Springs, Wyoming. In the small community, one can be identified and ranked on the basis of interpersonal relationships, personal tastes and idiosyncracies, and participation in a common set of institutions. In the large city, with its sea of anonymity, indirect measures of worth must be relied upon. The extremely complex division of labor in the metropolis, along with its physical size and the sheer numbers of people make it impossible for residents to gain an intimate understanding of strata differences or composition. In each community some form of stratification exists. However, it is not easy to compare these types meaningfully along the same dimension of rank. Bananas and pears are both types of fruit, yet none would argue that they are identical. For this reason, many sociologists cast doubtful eyes on such sweeping generalizations as that which implies that there are five or six classes in America. The number and types of strata may well vary with the community and the locale. The moral here seems to be that if one takes a technique developed to measure the stratification system of one community and mechanically applies it to other communities, different in size or composition, he may find that his data have little meaning, or more seriously, that they give him an erroneous understanding of the rank characteristics of the communities he studies.

In another sense, one may speak of *systems* of American stratification. Each of us represents a combination of statuses. We are graded in terms of the amount of formal education we have been able to complete, by the relative value of the work we do, by the life style we present, by the racial ancestry we have inherited, and so forth. Accordingly, we are participants in several different systems of stratification simultaneously. The worker or manager are incumbents of the stratification system of the factory as well as residents of separate neighborhoods which may be differentially ranked. This phenomenon of institutional stratification patterns further complicates the understanding of the significance of rank for behavior, and casts doubt on overly simplistic schemes for placing individuals into a single dimensional rank classification. It may be more accurate to construct measures of the relative position of an individual on each of several stratified dimensions in which he is involved, attempting to weight the contribution of each in a total assessment of that person's social standing. The work of Landecker, Lenski, and others in developing a measure of "status crystallization" illustrates this approach and suggests some useful leads for studying rates of mental illness, as we shall discuss presently (Landecker, 1960a, 1960b; Lenski, 1954).

The pattern of American racial and ethnic relations imposes another complication into the structure of social stratification. In the cities of the North and West, vast numbers of racial or ethnic group members live in largely self-contained ghetto communities. Such communities often contain highly developed institutional relationships and internal networks of exchange and authority. They tend to develop patterns of stratification that are known to the "insiders" but often only vaguely perceived by individuals outside the ghetto area. In such situations, the individual not only may be ranked with respect to the larger community or society, but has a status, too, within the segregated district he inhabits. Gordon (1964) has suggested that this fusing of socioeconomic position with ethnic status be called "ethclass." It follows that attempts to stratify members of urban subcommunities in terms of criteria or levels derived from the analysis of nonethnic groups are apt to be in serious error (Parker & Kleiner, 1966). This complication of status arrangements serves to remind us that a person's judgments of how well he is doing may depend upon which system of stratification he is using when he compares himself with others. A Negro who stands close to the top of his segregated community's socioeconomic structure may sense a feeling of accomplishment and self-satisfaction if he thinks about the ghetto, but he may feel frustrated and inadequate if he compares himself with those who inhabit upper-middle class white suburbs surrounding the city.

Finally, the historical importance on stratification of regional patterns of culture needs to be emphasized. In parts of New England and the South, for example, lineage is an important criterion for status. In the Midwest and West, one's ancestry appears to play a smaller role in the ranking of groups. The ranking of racial or ethnic groups differs somewhat according to regional tradition and to the proportions of such groups inhabiting a given area. We cannot assume universal social consensus concerning the worth or saliency of the criteria for ranking, nor that the saliency of any given criterion (race, age, style of life, and so on) will remain fixed over the passage of time. The high rate of population movement in the United States has altered traditional status relationships and created new patterns of stratification. It seems reasonable to conclude that innovations in transportation and mass communication have led to a breaking down of regional differences in the United States; yet the influence of tradition and regional history dies hard and meaningful differences can still be discerned.

In sum, we may conclude that the American stratification picture is a highly complex one involving variations induced by such factors as community size, ethnic composition, and regional tradition. Differences in the demographic characteristics of communities such as the labor force composition, age and sex distribution, and rate of migration further caution us against speaking of *the* system of American stratification. The multiple dimensions of status placement combined within the individual argue against a simplistic unitary scheme for ranking persons. Consequently, one must use care in specifying what aspects of stratification one is dealing with at what time and place, in the effort to predict rates of mental illness, or what dimensions of ranking are most crucial in our understanding of stress or other factors hypothesized to account for the development of symptoms of neurotic functioning. National stratification patterns may exist, but to ignore variations and complexities within the society can only invite oversimplification and distortion. Jonesville or New Haven are but two communities in the United States. We must ask not only what do they have in common with other communities in America, but also in what ways are they unique. How do the many complexities of ranking effect the etiology and frequency of mental disturbance?

The American scene: Class or continuum Another area of disagreement among sociological students of stratification centers about the most appropriate model for describing or conceptualizing the predominant patterns of ranked differentiation in the United States. Some argue for the concept of class as a useful and accurate description of the American scene. Others vigorously reject this formulation in favor of the idea of a continuum of status positions ranked from high to low, but without the natural breaks implied in the class idea. Both points of view offer plausible evidence as to their relevancy, yet our choice between them not only determines what method of study we will employ, but also, to a large extent, the findings we may anticipate at the conclusion of our efforts.

The concept of class owes its central meaning in stratification studies to the work of Karl Marx (1956). For Marx, classes were categories of persons sharing the same economic relationship to the ownership of the means of industrial production. As capitalism became fully developed, Marx argued, the stratification system would become transformed from one composed of land owners, merchants, craftsmen, peasants, unskilled workers, serfs, and so on, to a structure comprising two major classes: the owners of the means of production (the bourgeoisie) and those deprived of ownership, control, and the price of their own labor (the proletariat). This simplification of the structure would come about, he insisted, as the result of technological and social changes introduced by the owner class as a means of increasing efficiency and maximizing profits. Those unable to compete would sink down into the proletariat, swelling its ranks and adding to its leadership potential. For Marx, class relationships inevitably involved conflict—each class seeking to maximize the achievements of its goals at the expense of the other. The final downfall of the capitalist system would come about after a successful revolution by the proletariat had established itself in power. Without attempting to go into the matter of the accuracy of Marx's predictions for our society, or the application of many of his notions to an understanding of processes of stratification, it is important to realize that, by class, Marx meant far more than categories of persons in similar economic circumstances. Common economic situation, he posited, would, in time, lead to a shared sense of identity among those in a class. Class consciousness implies a sense of community, of common goals and aspirations, of an identification by the individual with others in the same economic situation, and an explicit rejection by him of other class interests or loyalties. Thus, the Marxian concept of class implies the qualities of a social group: awareness, interaction, shared loyalties and circumstances, and common ends. Classes to Marx were real entities, not abstractions convenient for research.

The ideas of a second German social scientist, Max Weber, have also been of great influence upon American specialists (Weber, 1947). While agreeing with Marx that classes involve persons in similar economic situations, Weber rejected the notion that classes inevitably took on the properties of groups. Rather, he treated them as categories of persons sharing a similar economic relationship to the market. Weber, furthermore, did not assume that relations among classes inevitably involved conflict. For him it was not inconceivable that harmonious and cooperative relations might exist among classes in society. Perhaps of greatest importance was Weber's assumption that modern industrial societies involve three major dimensions of stratification: classes, status groups, and parties. By status groups, Weber had in mind those strata formed on the basis of common educational attainment, occupational training, ancestry, and life styles, which gave rise to social interaction and a sense of social inclusion or exclusion. The concept of party involves differences in political power or influence in contemporary life. Weber argued that although each of these dimensions might well be correlated with the others, it was analytically useful to treat them as separate aspects of the stratification systems in modern society. The ward boss, for example, might be a person of considerable political power, but have little economic wealth or influence and stand low in the status groups in his community. Much of our present thinking about stratification derives from these ideas of Weber.

In contemporary usage, class has essentially one of two meanings. To some it means merely a statistical category comprising persons sharing roughly the same objective circumstances as measured by income, occupation, or educational attainment (Lenski, 1952). Few or no assumptions are made about class awareness, consciousness, identification or loyalty among those sharing similar objective characteristics. The presence or absence of such subjective states is left for empirical verification. Class, in this sense, represents a convenient and useful classification scheme for research. To others, however, class involves more than common socio-economic position. It may often imply, for example, shared values and life styles. To Warner and Hollingshead it indicates not only subcultural patterns in common, but also a sense of identification and awareness leading to predictable patterns of social interaction (Warner & Lunt, 1941; Hollingshead, 1949). In this latter usage, classes are treated as empirically locatable groups with determinate boundaries. It should be noted that both of the above researchers refer to *social* classes, implying more than economic factors as basic to class formation. In fact, Warner and Hollingshead seem to use the term class to refer essentially to that dimension of stratification called status group by Weber. These two investigators, like the majority of American stratification specialists see class relationships as basically harmonious, contributing to the functional integration of the community or society. Rather than regarding the members of higher classes as enemies worthy only of destruction, often those in lower levels are pictured as emulating and aspiring to positions above them.

Some sociologists would reject the idea of class entirely, arguing that while it may have been of great utility in understanding the stratification systems of European society, it finds little application in the American situation today. Nisbet (1959), for example, writes that:

The term social class is by now useful in historical sociology, in comparative or folk sociology, but . . . it is nearly valueless for the clarification of the data of wealth, power, and social status in the contemporary United States and much of Western society in general.

In his opinion, the conditions of contemporary life, especially the high rate of social mobility, the large number of functional associations, contemporary patterns in the consumption of economic goods, and the complex separation between property ownership and corporate control, have rendered useless the conception of class as a meaningful basis for stratification. Cuber and Kenkel (1954) argue that it is more accurate and useful to think of stratification in the United States as involving a continuum of positions and rewards conceived of by the individual as steps on a ladder of achievement. Instead of agreement among respondents as to the number of classes in a community, or the boundaries that demarked classes, these researchers report studies in which the majority of subjects could not identify such groups and instead seemed to regard their own positions, and others above and below theirs, as rungs on the competitive ladder. Similarly, other researchers have stressed that the majority of

Americans are so much concerned with their individual successes in competition that they fail to perceive of, or unite with, those with whom they objectively have much in common. In this view, the characteristic syndrome of the American is not class consciousness but rather individual status awareness (or anxiety). The stress on competition, territorial rather than economic political representation, geographical mobility, bureaucratic status arrangements, and widespread diffusion of material goods tend to blur class distinctions. A focus on racial, rather than economic differentiation, the historical commitment to democratic social relationships, and achieved rather than inherited privilege further prevent the perception of class identifications (Rosenberg, 1953). According to this view, the concept of class is of value only as a pragmatically useful way of statistically classifying persons sharing objective attributes in common, much as we might speak of persons of similar height or weight comprising a class. Sociologists are thus divided on the issue of the utility of the concept of class, on its empirical relevance in American life, and on its heuristic value in the formulation of research problems, especially those investigating causation. All agree that American society is stratified and that ranked differentiation has behavioral consequences. The question centers on which type of stratification best describes contemporary life and which offers the greater predictive power.

Values and social rank: Subculture or gradation? Closely related to the issues raised above is another area of contention: the question as to the linkage between stratum level and specific value orientations characteristic of those occupying this level. Those who prefer to regard social classes as identifiable groups in the society or community usually assume that each class contains specific patterns of values, mores, and traditions which serve to set the class culturally apart from other classes or groups in the structure and provide the individual with a set of meanings more or less unique to those sharing his class position. This notion of distinctive normative patterns associated with stratification levels is known as the treatment of "class-as-subculture" (Yinger, 1960). The concept of subculture derives from the work of anthropologists who have discovered and investigated population enclaves (often ethnic in composition) in the midst of large-scale industrial societies, set apart from other groups by a distinctive patterning of traditions, rituals, beliefs, and often language. The various immigrant communities in American cities, especially around the turn of the century, illustrate such subcultural groups. Those sociologists who see classes as discrete groups rather than statistical categories often argue for the cultural distinctiveness of classes (Gans, 1962). The early social ecologists frequently pointed out striking differences in behavior of those widely separated in social and economic space but residentially contiguous in the city (Zorbaugh, 1929). Warner and his associates have documented in detail the different paths of life associated with class level in the community (Warner and Associates, 1949). More recently, researchers have begun to detail the distinctive views and practices of those in the lower class (Miller & Reissman, 1961; Cohen & Hodges, 1963). The wealth of detail provided by Oscar Lewis in his attempts to portray "the culture of poverty" among Mexican laborers has encouraged similar efforts in this country (Lewis, 1959, 1961). Hypothetical models of the cultural patterns empirically linked to class levels have been developed (Kahl, 1957; Reissman, 1959). With all of this apparent support for the idea, the reader may well wonder why this is an issue. The answer involves both theoretical and empirical matters. As we have already suggested, many sociologists feel that classes as distinctive groups do not exist on the American scene. The vague notions about class, the relatively low level of class consciousness or identification, the absence of unique symbols of class membership, at least on a large scale, cast doubt, they feel, on the validity of the class model. If persons are not aware of themselves as a group, if they cannot state with certainty what they share in common with others at their level, if they disagree among themselves as to the criteria for status placement, and so forth, how can they perpetuate a self-conscious pattern of beliefs and practices marking them apart from others? Such researchers often point to the widespread diffusion of values in the society—the common aspirations for material success, the widespread commitment to political leaders, and high degree of consensus on issues as revealed by public opinion polls. According to this position, persons in varying socioeconomic positions differ not so much in kinds of belief or practice, but rather in the degree of adherence to values shared throughout the society and in their opportunities for achieving them. Such writers would argue that no sharp breaks in opinion or behavior exist of sufficient magnitude to justify the assumption of distinctive class subcultures. Rather, they posit a continuum of acceptance and participation in those cultural patterns widely disseminated by the characteristics of the mass society. Variations in practice or perspective are frequently attributed to differences in opportunity or resources among those in various socioeconomic levels. The poor differ from the rich not in preferences or ideals, but rather in the probability of realizing their desires or in the degree of sophistication with which they can articulate their goals and aspirations. Variations in child rearing, deferred gratification, thrift, long-range perspectives, and so on, they insist, are nearly as great *within* socioeconomic strata as *between* them. The idea of homogeneous clusters of distinctive values linked to stratum is thus rejected by those of this theoretical persuasion.

Another problem confounding the matter of class-linked cultural patterns is the fact that often the best examples of distinctively different patterns of behavior are found among groups who share not only a common economic position, but similar racial or ethnic ancestry as well. Gans's study of Italian working-class persons in Boston, for example, details a number of distinctive cultural traits, perceived and participated in by the residents of the neighborhood (Gans, 1962). The question may be asked, however, to what extent such patterns reflect common cultural ancestry, and to what extent they are reflective of an economic level shared by the majority of the residents. To determine this with accuracy, one would need a comparable case study of a group of working class persons, similar in economic position to the Italians but without their cultural ancestry. Unfortunately, such a directly comparable study does not exist. Hollingshead (1958), in his New Haven study of mental illness, notes that the community is structured vertically by racial, ethnic, and religious factors, and horizontally by a series of classes, yet he does not indicate to what extent his findings of class differences in rates of mental illness, types of treatment, attitudes about mental illness, or patterns of behavior, are confounded by shared traditions among the vertical groups in his sample. Studies have shown that certain variations in attitude and behavior are a function of differing occupational roles for those who occupy the same educational or income strata (Murphy & Morris, 1961). Such problems do not rule out the possibility that class-specific values exist. They do, however, indicate the necessity for more sophisticated techniques of analysis to isolate and define those elements of subculture that stem from common socioeconomic position.

The salience of stratification: Subjective and objective worlds   Our last example of intellectual disagreement among those who specialize in the study of social stratification is one that cuts across many of the issues we have examined. Basically, it concerns the significance of individual perceptions and subjective beliefs for an understanding of the stratification patterns of the society. All social scientists are committed to an understanding of the behavior of human beings as affected by membership in social systems. They vary in their utilization of subjective states and opinions as data in the quest for an understanding of human societies. It is possible, and often highly useful, to examine relationships and properties of social systems without reference to feelings or opinions of persons making up this system. The field of sociology has a long and noble history of such efforts. Durkheim (1951), for example, was able to account for differing rates of suicide in European societies without any consideration for the subjective moods, psychological predispositions, or personal motives of those who attempted this highly individual act. Much of the contemporary work in stratification consists in establishing relationships between socioeconomic levels and rates of group or individual phenomena. We are able to predict quite accurately, for example, how persons at a given level will vote in national elections, the religious denominations they will prefer, how much tolerance they will display to those of racial or ethnic origins differing from their own, the numbers of children they will indicate they want and the number they will have, the types of illness they will be most likely to develop and the kinds of treatment they will receive for their illnesses. Such information can be obtained without concerning ourselves about whether or not our respondents are aware of where they stand in the stratification hierarchy, whether they can enumerate classes in their communities, or whether they feel a sense of kinship with others in a similar economic level. Much of the valuable work in the effort to understand rates of mental illness is of this kind (Clark, 1948; Faris & Dunham, 1939; Jaco, 1959, 1960; Malzberg, 1940). Such studies have demonstrated that stratification and rates of mental illness are correlated: in general, the higher the socioeconomic position of the individual, the lower the rate of illness. Furthermore, among those receiving treatment for mental illness, the neuroses seem more characteristic among those higher in the structure than are the psychoses which tend to cluster in populations lower in the stratification system. The major value of such correlational work has been in establishing the existence of relationships among a variety of population samples over a period of time. They fail as do all correlational efforts, to provide us with evidence as to the dynamics of the process or processes by which persons come to develop, or escape developing, symptoms of mental disturbance. Specifically, what is the role of structural position in the etiology of mental disorder? How do the conditions of structure impinge upon the individual so as to cause him (or precipitate him) to develop clinical symptoms of disturbance? Leads that may be helpful in answering these questions have been hinted at above. If strata may be postulated to consist of distinctive subcultural patterns, it may be that certain of these patterns exert greater stresses on the individual than do others. Thus, by the logic of this approach, class differences in mental illness exist because normative expectations and pressures differ from one class to another. The ambiguity of strata, on the other hand, may make it difficult for the individual to judge where he is or how far he must go. In a highly competitive society, it may be argued, this is likely to produce considerable anxiety and concern. The point we wish to make here is that some knowledge of the person's perception, feelings, expectations, and aspirations, along with a detailing of his objective position, makes it possible to go beyond a descriptive portrait of the structural location of illness to the point where we can construct and test alternative hypotheses of dynamics and causation. How aware are individuals of their positions in the community or society? What difference does it make if some are highly aware and others, at the same level, can only with great difficulty speak about their place in the stratification scheme? How salient is position to the individual? Does he think and act in class terms, or are these meaningful only after the "expert" has pointed them out to him? Much of the work of sociologists has assumed that stratification position is known by and is important to the individual. The validity of these assumptions, however, needs constant empirical checking, especially if we seek to determine the causative significance of stratification for behavior.

Previous research has made it clear that not only do individuals differ in the ease with which they perceive their own positions or those of others in the community, but also that the view of the structure varies quite systematically as we move from top to bottom. Davis and the Gardners (1941) showed, for example, that persons near the bottom of a community's class structure saw greater differentiation in levels below the middle and that persons near the top were able to elaborate the subtle distinctions maintained by those above the middle of the structure. Both of these views describe the perception of reality as structure conditions it. The implications of systematic variation in perceptions of stratification have not, however, been drawn, insofar as they may bear on such matters as aspiration, reality testing, or sense of relative deprivation. Again, we may caution those concerned with mental illness that there is no one universal view of American stratification, whether we consider expert opinion or the opinions of the "naïve" participants in the social system. These discrepancies themselves are of significance. In a closed, fixed stratification system, one would expect little variation in descriptions as to what, and how many, levels exist. The fact of the existence in the United States of a considerable area for debate indicates that our system is flexible, changing, and sufficiently permeable to invite confusion. Logic and order may exist, but these qualities are more discernible in the models we construct than in the reality we study. Considerably more research will be needed to determine the relationship between objective and subjective meanings of stratification. Until we have such information, pragmatic necessities and the demands of our favorite hypotheses will determine the saliency of individual beliefs for understanding the correlates of stratification.

In this section of the paper we have briefly reviewed four major areas of intellectual disagreement among students of stratification: (1) whether there is *an* American stratification system, or whether it is more meaningful to speak of multiple systems within the community or nation; (2) the issue of class as an appropriate model for the description of American life (What are classes and do they exist in our society? Is it more appropriate to speak of a continuous gradation of statuses?); (3) the issue of the link between values and stratum (Do class subcultures exist? To what extent may one speak of classes as discrete social groups or communities?); and (4) the significance of subjective perceptions of stratification (How important is, and in what ways do, individual awareness of stratification figure in explanations of the link between stratum level and differential rates of mental disorder?). To these areas of contention, one could add many examples of dispute over appropriate methodological techniques for the measurement of the phenomena of stratification. Limitations of space preclude this here, although the matter is of obvious concern to those in the health sciences who may wish to use the indexes and scales that have been developed by the sociologist. Some of the more obvious implications of these theoretical issues for the continued interdisciplinary investigation of mental illness along with suggestions for future research will follow in the concluding section.

IMPLICATIONS OF THEORETICAL ISSUES
FOR MENTAL HEALTH RESEARCH

We have had several purposes in presenting this review of some of the problematics of stratification theory. In the first place, it is our hope that some understanding of intellectual issues, however brief and oversimplified, will lead workers in the mental health field to a somewhat greater appreciation of the complexities and subtleties of an area historically noted for its ideological and scientific debates. Sociologists have often been accused, with frequent justification, of vulgarizing the work of Freud and other theorists of the mind in their efforts to explain social sources of personal disorganization. A review of the literature produced by medically trained and behaviorally oriented psychiatric researchers often reveals the same lack of concern for, or knowledge of, stratification assumptions or approaches.

A second and related purpose of our effort is to caution researchers carefully to consider which of several points of theoretical departure makes the most sense to them in pointing the way to structural factors associated with clinical aspects of abnormality. Sensitivity to alternative formulations of American stratification may make collaborative work more productive, inasmuch as the theoretical orientation is selected by choice rather than out of the ignorance of variants. We suspect that there is a deceptive danger in the decision to utilize a simple, readily available measure of "class" unless one understands and is prepared to accept the underlying assumptions and implications of those who originally developed that measure. This procedure is somewhat analogous to the social scientist who uses the TAT without any appreciation of the theoretical assumptions contained in its use or of the intellectual arguments among clinicians centering on the parent theory of personality from which it was derived. It is unfortunate but true that genuine interdisciplinary work requires more than the knowledge that ready-made techniques of measurement exist in a neighboring discipline. Our hope is that eventually we will be able to develop better measures for variables with which we share an interest in common, through a sharing of intellectual concerns and understanding.

Perhaps the most important purpose to be served in a review of theoretical issues in stratification is that of suggesting the research implications and leads such issues provide. We feel that continuing research into the nature of American stratification will not only provide the sociologist with greater sophistication and predictive ability, but will make possible the testing of alternative assumptions concerning the nature of the link between rates and types of mental illness and socioeconomic position. Limitations of space preclude extended discussion of many potentially useful research questions; however, illustrative examples paralleling our discussion of issues will be provided.

System or systems? We have suggested that in the opinion of many sociologists the American social structure is composed of a number of stratification systems varying by size of community, population composition and density, region, and history. The implication here is that no one study of a given community can provide the basis for unqualified generalization to the rest of the society. Within a particular community, furthermore, there may be differing systems of rank affecting persons in varying ways. Potential links to mental health are thus likely to be highly complex. We might hypothesize, for example, that to the extent that status systems vary with population density or size of the community, it is plausible to assume that factors linking rates of illness with level may also vary. Kleiner and Parker (1963) provide some evidence that this is true. They show that high rates of mental disorder are associated with low status in large cities, but this relationship did not hold for smaller communities. They suggest that this may be due to the possibility that persons in low status positions in large cities have experienced greater downward mobility than have persons in equally low statuses in smaller communities. We would add that another potentially relevant factor would appear to be that the criteria for position vary with the size of the community. In the small town, family history, style of life, commitment to widely shared values, and the public display of morality appear to be major determinants of status. In the large city, the amount of education, type and level of occupation, and the ability to adjust to rapid change seem more crucial. It is possible that these somewhat different kinds of pressures may have differing effects on the mental health of individuals. Differences in the amount of pressure to achieve and the ease with which one may gain a "comfortable" self-identity may also be of significance.

If it is true that stratification systems differ by community size, one might well expect that persons who migrate from a small community to a large city would suffer greater status-linked emotional problems than would persons migrating from other large cities or persons who have lived their entire lives in a given city. The problem of fitting into a different system and of establishing a meaningful identity would appear to be important aspects of "culture shock" insofar as mental health is concerned. Parker and Kleiner (1966), in their study of Philadelphia Negroes, show, however, that persons who have lived all of their lives in Philadelphia have higher rates of mental illness than migrants from the South (predominantly rural). The authors argue that differences in the discrepancy between level of achievement and aspirations may account for this somewhat unanticipated finding. This study, in our opinion, illustrates the potential gains to be expected when sociological theory is coupled with psychological assumptions and techniques in an imaginative and flexible manner. It represents one of the most sophisticated investigative techniques yet developed and shows that a sensitivity to unresolved theoretical issues can greatly further analytical understanding of mental illness. The reader is urged to study the article by these authors in the present volume for an immediate example of the kind of collaborative research we have been urging.

The degree of consistency or inconsistency of statuses held by the individual is another potentially fruitful area for research. As we have already indicated, each person combines in his social self a number of ascribed and achieved status positions deriving from his participation in the familial, occupational, sex, racial, educational, and so on, institutions in society. Gerhard Lenski (1954) has argued that persons displaying inconsistent configurations of status (low crystallization) are likely to feel frustrated and will pressure for changes to more nearly equalize their status attributes. The Negro physician, for example, may take pride in his occupational accomplishment, but feel especially frustrated by the low rank accorded him by virtue of his race. According to this formulation, persons with relatively consistent status combinations (high status crystallization), whether such statuses are uniformly high or low, will evidence less psychological disturbance than will persons with inconsistent status configurations (low status crystallization). Nagi (1963), for example, hypothesizes that "the degree of anxiety generated in reaction to status threats is in part a function of the type of profile of the individual's status position." Some support for this notion is provided by Jackson (1962) in a study using national survey data. He reports that inconsistency due to higher racial-ethnic status as compared to occupational or educational rank is related to high stress symptoms. Other patterns of inconsistency did not reveal an association, however. Gibbs and Martin (1959) report inconclusive, but suggestive, evidence that the suicide rate in Ceylon varies inversely with the degree of status integration in the population. Findings such as these encourage further research into the problem of status marginality as a factor in mental illness. We would argue, however, that some measure of the degree to which persons perceive, and are concerned about, inconsistencies be included in such research. It is entirely possible that the various statuses held by a given individual are not of equal importance to him and thus that certain types of perceived inconsistency are more troublesome than others. The majority of studies thus far conducted on this topic seem to have ignored the question of saliency to the individual of inconsistent status combinations.

Finally, by way of example, we may mention another area in which the problem of the multidimensional aspects of stratification seems to have implications for the study of mental health. The fact that in our large cities, minority group members often reside in segregated communities, with their own internal status or class structures, means theoretically that the residents of such communities participate in the stratification structure of the ghetto as well as that of the surrounding metropolis and nation. Failure to take into account the criteria of rank in the ethnic community or to compare the relative position of the individual in each of these systems of stratification, may lead to errors of judgment. Hollingshead and his colleagues, for example, show that for the population of New Haven (predominantly white) there was a correlation of .72 between the level of education and occupation. Parker and Kleiner, studying the Negro ghetto of Philadelphia found, however, that these dimensions of stratification were much less highly correlated (.44). This confirms the observations of other researchers who have looked into the nature of stratification in the large urban Negro ghetto. Drake and Cayton (1945), for example, indicate that educational level was considerably more important than occupation in the subjective and objective placement of individuals and families in "Bronzeville," the Negro ghetto of Chicago. Visible characteristics associated with race, such as skin color and texture of hair, were also found to be criteria utilized in the ranking process in the community. The sources of status gratification or frustration, both within the community and in relation to the majority world must be considered in our efforts to understand the role of stratification in the creation or precipitation of mental illness among minority peoples. Here the concept of reference group would appear to have particularly valuable relevance. Further implications of possible subcultural patterns associated with minority communities will be discussed below.

Class or continuum   In essence, the debate about whether or not the American society contains classes centers on the heuristic utility of conceiving of discrete clusters of objective conditions and normative patterns as a means for predicting social behavior. Such utility can be demonstrated either by showing empirically that such discrete ranked categories exist as "natural" phenomena in the social world, or pragmatically by showing that a model consisting of arbitrarily constructed ranked groups has superior predictive power. Those who treat class as a statistical method of classification justify their categories by the ability to discriminate significant relationships in the population. Those who insist that classes exist as a part of the empirical order seek to demonstrate their claims through a detailed description of the multiple workings of class in everyday life. It is not our intention here either to reiterate or enter the debate as to the reality of class in American life. Rather, we wish to suggest some of the implications for research on mental health for those who opt for the existence of classes or contrastingly, those who are theoretically committed to the idea of a continuous gradation of ranked statuses. For many who prefer the class model, the idea of in-group identification and loyalty assumes importance. Whether interclass relationships are regarded as mutually cooperative or antagonistic, it is generally assumed that the members of any given class cooperate with each other and share common practices and views. Those who emphasize the status continuum model, however, view behavior as guided by the norms of competition and rivalry. Ties to the present or past are seen as weak, and loyalty to others in the same position is subordinate to an identification with those above in statuses regarded as desirable. The ideas of anticipatory socialization and status striving fit into this conception of stratification. Such a view seems to complement that of Karen Horney (1937) in her effort to link neurosis to competitive status aspirations. Uncertainty, status insecurity, and unfulfilled aspirations would thus seem to be major factors in accounting for mental illness. Partisans of the class model, however, while admitting that competition is a fact of American life, often seem to give priority to class differentials in patterns of child rearing, ego defense mechanisms, or normative expectations as significant factors in the etiology of mental disorder (Myers & Roberts, 1959; Miller & Swanson, 1960). The assumption here seems to be that certain types of illness, the neuroses most especially, are learned as a result of the normative requirements, expectations, and goals shared among the members of the class even though they may never be fully practiced or realized by all of its members. Differences in mental health may thus be related to discrepancies between expectation and accomplishment among the members of a given class and to normative differences that vary by class in the structure of the society. Lower class persons, it is argued, are exposed to differing expectations and requirements than are middle or upper class individuals, hence etiology may be class specific. In addition, such theorists are aware that resources and opportunities for accomplishment vary by class and that one source of frustration and anxiety may be that the representatives of middle class society (teachers, police, psychiatrists) demand adherence to norms and values which are either less attainable, or in contradistinction, to those in the lower class. In sum, the continuum notion implies that the majority of individuals share basic norms and values, but differ in their successes in accomplishment. Rather than sharp breaks in expectations or goals, differential opportunities or drive states are predicted. The class idea suggests differential norms and values as a product of variations in socialization. Factors in mental illness causation may thus be specific to class situation. These alternative formulations invite differing strategies of research and place differing explanations on the findings of stratificational relationships to illness.

Class as subculture A key to the most useful orientation to problems of the social etiology of mental illness will come from research into the structural distribution of values in the society. Surprising as it may seem, we lack detailed knowledge about the types and range of value commitment in the society. Much of the support for the idea of class specific values comes from child-rearing studies, themselves contradictory (Bronfenbrenner, 1958). We lack any inventories of belief that cover a wide spectrum of human interest. The clues we may get from various opinion polls and social surveys are limited, inasmuch as they have been collected from varying populations at separate points in time. It is plausible to assume that certain beliefs and practices are limited to a given socioeconomic level, yet others may be shared across the stratification structure. The location of class-specific values and those universal in the American culture remains a most crucial research need. Furthermore, we need also to determine which values are most significantly functional for mental health or illness. It is in research of this nature that those in the health research fields can be of greatest help to the sociologist. Values and normative beliefs play an important role in psychotherapy. An understanding of their structural origins seems necessary if greater successes are to be obtained by this technique of rehabilitation. The mutual exploration of value distributions would thus appear to be one of the most useful and promising areas for collaboration in the immediate future.

One of the great difficulties in determining the potential class location of values comes from the fact that often distinctive features of life that lend a communal air to behavior are a combination of socioeconomic and racial or ethnic patterns. Some of those "typical" values attributed to the lower class (for example, immediate gratification, short-range perspective, physical rather than verbal responses to aggression, authoritarian submission, and so on) may well reflect the perpetuation of traditional ethnic practices only partly explainable by economic position. We need, therefore, comparative investigations into groups at the same socioeconomic level, but differing in racial or ethnic background. In this way, we may be able to determine the relative significance of both ethnic and class values in the development of illness and response to it. Again, the research of Parker and Kleiner points the way into this complex problem. When we are able to point to those configurations of practice and belief that are unique to persons sharing the same stratum level, we will be closer to developing practical hypotheses about the function of stratification in determining rates of mental illness and effectiveness of various methods of treatment. Valuable community studies, such as those of Hollingshead and Warner, can be of even greater use if the researchers will give us some indication of ethnic variations in the patterns reported for the community classes as a whole. In a recent article, Dohrenwend (1966) suggests the importance of such information for the answer to an old, but important question: Does the relationship between social class and psychological disorder indicate social causation, with low status producing illness, or is the relationship evidence of social selection, with pre-existing disorder determining low social status? He indicates that "This substantive issue could turn on a simple question of fact: whether Negroes and Puerto Ricans in New York City have higher or lower rates of disorder than their class counterparts in more advantaged ethnic groups." Data adequate to answering this question do not exist, however, and Dohrenwend concludes that we must learn more about the cultural and situational factors that lead to different modes of expressing psychological symptoms and the conditions under which the symptomatic expression of psychological distress become evidence of underlying personality defect. Here would appear to be a "natural" area for productive collaboration between the sociologist and those in the health research areas.

Subjective and objective worlds   In our earlier discussion of this issue in this paper, we indicated some of the potential advantages of including subjective perceptions and feelings about stratification in our research formulations. If classes exist as viable groups in society, persons should be able to talk about them. If each class contains elements of cultural uniqueness, persons should be able to recognize them and verbalize their meanings for behavior. If class-linked stresses and frustrations exist, members of a class should be able to express their concerns or displeasures. If classes exist as communities, a sense of belonging and a sharing of loyalties should be demonstrable in the interviews with those who share common positions. Should we find considerable doubt in the minds of our respondents, or professed ignorance of such matters, our formulations about the nature of stratification may need revision. Lack of consensus on the part of those who share similar objective circumstances may indicate class structure in the process of formation, or it may simply mean that persons have learned the rhetoric of class stratification, but have difficulty in applying it to themselves. The point is that discrepancies between objective situation and subjective perceptions may tell us much about the nature of stratification in society and provide valuable clues to the connections between social structure and personality. Rogler and Hollingshead (1965), in their valuable study of familial factors relating to schizophrenia among the poor in Puerto Rico, point out that the persons interviewed (all at the same economic level) were unanimous about the existence of classes on the island but differed among themselves as to the number of classes that made up the system and as to the criteria that defined membership in a class. Some indicated that two classes existed, others suggested four or five, the majority said three. The authors suggest that "The number of classes a person perceives and how he labels them are not as important as the fact that he knows that there are classes in the society [p. 60]." Perhaps so, but this does not rule out the possibility that persons who share common objective socioeconomic status, yet have different perceptions of the structure, may also differ in clinically significant ways. One wonders if those who see themselves at the bottom of a structure with five classes may not sense greater frustration and despair than those who see only one group above them. In any case, it seems curious that Rogler and Hollingshead, while granting that variations in perception exist, and despite the finding that the model number of classes recognized was three, chose to analyze class relationships to schizophrenia in a framework of five classes similar to those utilized in the study of New Haven.

The considerable doubt about self-placement evidenced by respondents in the research of many investigators suggests another promising lead for research into mental illness. As we have suggested above, it has been argued by some social scientists and a number of social theorists that one of the consequences of living in a rigidly stratified society, such as a caste structure, is that the individual has a clear, unambiguous understanding of his place in society. He clearly knows his rights and privileges, his duties and opportunities. As a consequence, he may well have less anxiety about himself and others. To the extent to which this logic is accurate, we might hypothesize that the lack of clear-cut class boundaries or other status reference points, rather than a high development of class awareness, constitutes a major factor in inducing types of neurosis. Utilizing objective measures of class position, such as occupation, educational achievement, or residential dwelling area, as our only criteria for stratification placement obviates the opportunity to investigate such a notion and thus cannot tell us what significance the degree of subjective ambiguity about status may have for generating conflict or stress in the individual.

Finally, subjective ambiguity seems to be important in one other sense. Much research by psychologists and sociologists has shown that discrepancies between achievement and subjective aspirations are often linked to stress or other symptoms of potential illness. "Over-achievers" often seem to lack a realistic understanding of the system in which they are competing. Such lack of awareness, it may be argued, is functional in the sense that it is a defense against self-blame for failure, or on the other hand, it may be dysfunctional if it serves to drive the person into a contest for unattainable goals. Research is needed here to determine the conditions under which ambiguity or status self-delusions arise and the significance of such status confusion for the health of the individual. Again, subjective data on stratification seem crucial.

SUMMARY

In this paper, we have tried to suggest that the area of social stratification represents a wide-open field for research into social factors involved in mental illness. Despite more than thirty years of investigation into the structural correlates of illness, many questions remain unanswered, and in all probability the most important questions remain to be asked.

Research, like many other areas of human endeavor, often develops into well-worn paths of exploration. While the familiar avenues of investigation provide a sense of security and continuity, potentially greater yields may be expected if we let our creative imagination range over the whole spectrum of complexities involved in the etiology of mental illness. Robert Lynd long ago advised the sociologist that there is value in the outrageous hypothesis. We have been suggesting here that the theoretical issues in stratification are not closed; our knowledge is vastly incomplete, and contradictory hypotheses abound. This is not cause for despair or alarm. It is rather an invitation to participate in an exciting intellectual quest. The issues and debates among theorists of the mind are in a similar state of ferment. Here is the opportunity to assess some of our most cherished assumptions, not by parochial defense of established "truths," but by collaborative discovery of the empirical tenability of competing faiths.

REFERENCES

Bronfenbrenner, U. Socialization and social class through time and space. In E. E. Maccoby, T. M. Newcomb, & E. L. Hartley (Eds.), *Readings in social psychology*. New York: Henry Holt, 1958.

Cohen, A. K., & Hodges, H. M. Lower-blue-collar characteristics. *Social Problems,* 1963, **11,** 303–334.

Clark, R. E. The relationship of schizophrenia to occupational income and occupational prestige. *American Sociological Review,* 1948, **33,** 325–330.

Cuber, J. F., & Kenkel, W. F. *Social stratification in the United States*. New York: Appleton-Century-Crofts, 1954.

Davis, A. Gardner, B. B., & Gardner, M. R. *Deep South*. Chicago: University of Chicago Press, 1941.

Dohrenwend, B. P. Social status and psychological disorder: An issue of substance and an issue of method. *American Sociological Review,* 1966, **31,** 14–34.

Drake, St. C., & Cayton, H. *Black metropolis*. New York: Harcourt-Brace, 1945.

Durkheim, E. *Suicide* (Transl. by J. A. Spaulding and G. Simpson). Glencoe, Ill.: The Free Press, 1951.

Faris, R. E., & Dunham, H. W. *Mental disorders in urban areas*. Chicago: University of Chicago Press, 1939.

Gans, H. J. *The urban villagers: Group and class in the life of Italian Americans*. New York: The Free Press, 1962.

Gibbs, J. P., & Martin, W. T. Status integration and suicide in Ceylon. *American Journal of Sociology,* 1959, **64,** 585–591.

Gordon, M. M., *Assimilation in American life: The role of race, religion, and national origins*. New York: Oxford University Press, 1964.

Hollingshead, A. B., *Elmtown's youth*. New York: John Wiley & Sons, 1949.

Hollingshead, A. B., & Redlich, F. *Social class and Mental Illness*. New York: John Wiley & Sons, 1958.

Horney, K. *The neurotic personality of our time*. New York: W. W. Norton & Co., 1937.

Jackson, E. F. Status consistency and symptoms of stress. *American Sociological Review,* 1962, **27,** 469–480.

Jaco, E. G. Social stress and mental illness in the community. In M. B. Sussman, (Ed.), *Community structure and analysis*. New York: Thomas Y. Crowell & Co., 1959. Pp. 388–409.

Jaco, E. G. *The social epidemiology of mental disorder: A psychiatric survey of Texas*. New York: Russell Sage Foundation, 1960.

Kahl, J. *The American class structure*. New York: Rinehart, 1957.

Kleiner, R. J., & Parker, S. Goal-striving, social status, and mental disorder: A research review. *American Sociological Review,* 1963, **28,** April, 189–203.

Landecker, W. S. Class crystallization and its urban pattern. *Social Research,* 1960, **27,** 308–320. (a)

Landecker, W. S. Class boundaries. *American Sociological Review,* 1960, **25,** 868–877. (b)

Lenski, G. E. American social classes: Statistical strata or social groups? *American Journal of Sociology,* 1952, **58,** 139–144.

Lenski, G. E. Status crystallization: A non-vertical dimension of social status. *American Sociological Review,* 1954, **19,** 405–413.

Lewis, O. *Five families.* New York: Basic Books, 1959.

Lewis, O. *The children of Sanchez.* New York: Random House, 1961.

Malzberg, B. *Social and biological aspects of mental disease.* Utica, N.Y.: State Hospitals Press, 1940.

Marx, K. *Selected writings in sociology and social philosophy,* T. B. Bottomore & Maximilien Rubel, Eds., London: Watts & Co., 1956.

Miller, D. R., & Swanson, G. E. *Inner conflict and defense.* New York: Henry Holt & Co., 1960.

Miller, S. M., & Riessman, F. The working class subculture: A new view. *Social Problems,* 1961, **9,** 86–97.

Murphy, R. J., & Morris, R. T. Occupational situs, subjective class identification, and political affiliation. *American Sociological Review,* 1961, **26,** 383–392.

Myers, J. K., & Roberts, B. H. *Family and class dynamics in mental illness.* New York: John Wiley & Sons, 1959.

Nagi, S. Z. Status profile and reactions to status threats. *American Sociological Review,* 1963, **28,** 440–443.

Nisbet, R. A. The decline and fall of social class. *Pacific Sociological Review,* 1959, **2,** 11–17.

Parker, S., & Kleiner, R. J. *Mental illness in the urban Negro community.* New York: The Free Press, 1966.

Reissman, L. *Class in American society.* Glencoe Ill.: The Free Press, 1959.

Rogler, L. H., & Hollingshead, A. B. *Trapped: Families and schizophrenia.* New York: John Wiley & Sons, 1965.

Rosenberg, M. Perceptual obstacles to class consciousness. *Social Forces,* 1953, **32,** 22–27.

Srole, L., Langner, T. S., Michael, S. T., Opler, M. K., & Rennie, T. A. C. *Mental health in the metropolis.* New York: McGraw-Hill, 1962.

Warner, W. L., Meeker, M., & Eells, K. *Democracy in Jonesville.* New York: Harper & Brothers, 1949.

Warner, W. L., & Lunt, P. S. *The social life of a modern community.* New Haven: Yale University Press, 1941.

Weber, M. *From Max Weber: Essays in sociology* (Ed. & transl. by H. Gerth & C. W. Mills). New York: Oxford University Press, 1947.

Yinger, J. M. Contraculture and subculture. *American Sociological Review,* 1960, **25,** 625–635.

Zorbaugh, H. W. *The Gold Coast and the slum.* Chicago: University of Chicago Press, 1929.

ADDITIONAL BIBLIOGRAPHICAL REFERENCES

Bendix, R. & Lipset, S. M. *Class, status, and power.* New York: The Free Press, 1966.

Foote, N. N., Goldschmidt, W. R., Morris, R. T., Seeman, M. & Shister, J. Alternative assumptions in stratification research. In *Transactions of the Second World Congress of Sociology.* London: International Sociological Association, 1954. Pp. 378–390.

Gordon, M. *Social class in American sociology.* Durham, N.C.: Duke University Press, 1958.

Gursslin, O. R., Hunt, R. G., & Roach, J. L. Social class and the mental health movement. *Social Problems,* 1959–1960, **7**, 210–218.

Miller, D. R., & Swanson, G. E. *The changing American parent.* New York: John Wiley & Sons, 1958.

Murphy, R. J. Some recent trends in stratification theory and research. *The Annals of the American Academy of Political and Social Science,* 1964, **356**, 142–167.

Ossowski, S. *Class structure in the social consciousness.* New York: The Free Press, 1963.

Ranulf, S. *Moral indignation and middle class psychology.* New York: Schocken Books, 1964.

Turner, R. H. Life situation and subculture: A comparison of merited prestige judgments by three occupational classes in Britain. *British Journal of Sociology,* 1958, **9**, 299–320.

3.4   Orientation

Over thirty years ago, H. Warren Dunham was a partner in the monumental Chicago studies, which investigated the relationship of geographical areas of a city to the development of psychoses. The surprising finding that schizophrenia is in many ways a product of inner city life while the manic-depressive psychoses do not show such similar relationships has been the subject of many other community-oriented studies, even though the explanations for these differential rates has evoked a considerable amount of debate. It is nearly universally agreed, at least, that the social and ecological structure of cities have an impact on personality and ultimately can lead to the development of psychoses.

In this chapter, Dunham brings his research findings up to date by asking two questions:

1. Is there "evidence that distribution patterns of mental illness and specific psychoses within the city have shifted in form" since the time of the original Chicago studies?

2. "Are [there] valid differential rates between local area populations in a large city and [does] a population in one area produce more mental illness than a population in another area?"

Dr. Dunham suggests four reasons why we would expect the pattern of mental illness in cities to be changing, and he provides the results of his current research, to indicate not only the ways in which cities are changing, but also the resulting effect on the distribution patterns of mental illness.

3.4 City Core and Suburban Fringe: Distribution Patterns of Mental Illness

H. Warren Dunham

In this chapter I propose to examine the distribution patterns of mental illness in the city in order to assess them within the context of the social changes that have taken place in American cities over the past three decades. Further, I intend to inquire whether or not the changes in city life that have taken place have produced any radical shift in the types of community milieus where the different types of mental illness are to be found. These concerns are of fundamental significance for certain theoretical positions that have evolved from correlations between types of urban milieus and selected types of mental illness. However, in order to assess the distribution patterns of mental illness in relation to the social changes in American cities, it is necessary to compare contemporary distribution patterns with those of an earlier period (Faris & Dunham, 1939; Green, 1939).

Those studies that purported to examine the distribution of mental illness in the 1930s were quite definite in asserting that all types of mental illness, including most of the individual psychoses with the exception of the manic-depressive group, showed a concentration of high rates at the center of the city with rates declining in all directions toward the city's periphery. While there were certain variations in the distribution patterns of the individual psychoses, there seemed to be no doubt that all were highly concentrated in those local areas of the city that were marked by impoverishment, below-standard housing, ethnic conflicts, unstable families, and mobile populations, by virtue of which, for the most part, the people appeared to be isolated from the mainstream of American life. In fact, Schroeder (1942) asserted categorically, "There are insanity areas comparable to the delinquency areas of Chicago which Shaw discovered more than a decade ago."

These earlier findings point up two questions: What evidence can be gathered showing that the distribution patterns of mental illness and specific psychoses within the city have shifted in form, thus disturbing the older reported concentration of cases of mental disorder at the city's core? Can it still be demonstrated that Schroeder's earlier contention stands up today or, in other words, can it still be established that there are valid differential rates between local area populations in a large city, and that a population in one area produces more mental illness than a population of another area? In this paper these two basic questions will be examined.

ARE RATE PATTERNS CHANGING IN FORM?

The first issue is quite complicated, especially because of the variety of types among the mentally ill. However, there seems to be every reason to believe that the distribution patterns of mental illness will undergo sharp shifts because of the influence of certain factors that emerged during the past twenty-five years. These factors that have been at work and should bring about shifts in the distribution pattern of mental illness in large cities would include the following: (1) accelerated social change set in motion by automotive technology, urban renewal, new educational programs, and the civil rights movement; (2) the widening definition of mental illness; (3) changing attitudes in the cities toward the mentally ill; and (4) the multiplication of psychiatric facilities for care, treatment, rehabilitation, and research. I submit that these are the chief factors that are at work to bring about shifts in the distribution patterns of mental illness in the large cities of the country.

Social Change

Today, as never before in the history of mankind, the process of social change becomes increasingly evident to larger numbers of people everywhere. It has been commonplace for two or three decades among intellectuals to recognize the significance of urbanization and industrialization as twin stimuli for bringing about social change. In recent years these phenomena, discussed openly on editorial pages and via radio and television, have acquainted more and more people with the processes of change all over the world. Further, there is the increasing awareness of the role that the new technology is playing with respect to changing the character of manufacturing and transportation, and even of office work. In the world of a hundred years ago, in the technologically advanced countries, social change was hardly perceptible except over a generation. Today, social change is measured in decades and, in some cases, two- or three-year periods; sometimes it almost seems to take place before our very eyes. In fact, it comes so rapidly that man's patterns of thinking and behavior hardly catch up with the new change before further changes take place (Ogburn, 1950).

The consequences of change apply not only to the thought processes and behavior patterns of man, but also to the necessity to adapt our institutional structures. It has been only in the last decade that communities all across our land have awakened to the defects and inadequacies of our school systems. High school dropouts, for whatever reason, which were of little concern to communities thirty-five years ago because such dropouts would be absorbed into the work force, now become a problem of major proportions because they have none of the skills that are required to fit them into the work force. A recent conference in Michigan estimated that approximately two million young people had literally retired before the age of twenty because they could not find work. Such a group can and may still become a tremendous explosive force in the society unless some means is discovered, and discovered quickly, to locate these persons and incorporate them into various training programs that will equip them with new working skills appropriate to our changing economy (Foster, 1961; see also Fuhrman, 1960).

In another framework, the vast urban renewal program that has developed, as stimulated by the federal government during the past decade, has taken the bulldozer quickly through our urban slums in an unselective fashion, disrupting old stable neighborhoods and scattering the inhabitants to new neighborhoods within the city where old friends are lacking and old contacts lost (Gans, 1962). Within the cities this activity has been carried on by city planning groups which, while giving lip service to the psychic and social needs of people, in practice actually ignore these needs in their zest to erect new physical structures and build new bands of green belt near old city core (Jacobs, 1961; Wolf & Lebeaux, 1965). The development of high-rent apartments and expensive private houses near the city's core as in Detroit—the suburb at the center—will be a crucial factor in changing old ecological patterns.

The awakening of our Negro citizens to the possibility of achieving full citizenship as guaranteed by the Constitution, resulting in part from the Supreme Court's decision that segregated schools are unconstitutional, represents still another factor in bringing about changes in urban ecological organization. Their pressure, exerted on the schools, business organizations, the courts, and voting patterns, has been tremendous. Their pressure has not only activated the political right to oppose, but also activated large segments of lower and middle class society to support the civil rights movement. While there is marked dispute about some gains that have been achieved, there seems to be no doubt that in the white collar areas more and more positions have become open to Negroes, and business organizations that had never given a thought to the hiring of Negroes are hiring them today.

Thus, the new technology, the cultural lag in the schools, planned urban renewal, and the civil rights movement are the major forces that are changing the face of cities and their institutions in the United States. In a very definite sense it might be said that the current war on poverty, as outlined by the federal government, represents a realization of an age-old promise of science and technology. That is, through science and the new resulting technology it becomes really possible to eradicate those ancient scourges of mankind: war, disease, ignorance, and poverty.

The Widening Definition of Mental Disease

Perhaps our widening definition of mental illness more than any other is crucial in changing our perception of distribution patterns of mental illness. This factor highlights the perennial problem in psychiatric circles as to what constitutes a case (*Discussion*, 1953). This issue, while not settled, was much easier to cope with a quarter of a century ago, when practically the only available facilities for psychiatric help were the state and private mental hospitals. For, at that time, it was clear that for the most part the "violent and furious" were hospitalized and the minor disturbances were generally neglected. But with the mounting frustration over the treatment and cure of persons with major psychoses, particularly schizophrenia, there gradually resulted a turning away of psychiatric efforts from the real psychoses, toward persons with minor psychiatric symptoms who seemed to be the best risks for therapy. This widening definition of mental illness is not noticeable with respect to the hard core psychoses. But its impact is registered in the "minor" emotional disturbances as reflected in such concepts as neurotic tendencies, withdrawal symptoms, mild depressions, character disturbances, passive-aggressive personalities, and the like. The old saw that anybody who goes to a psychiatrist ought to have his head examined contains perhaps more than a grain of truth. For when the person does, the examining psychiatrist has literally a host of labels to apply, even though he may not force the patient into one of the diagnostic groups as listed and coded by the official psychiatric manual.

This state of affairs was well documented by two recent and carefully designed epidemiological studies of mental illness. Srole, Langner, Michael, Opler, and Rennie, in the Midtown Manhattan Study (1962), report that 80 percent of a sample population of 1660 were found to have some kind of psychiatric symptoms. Along the same line, Leighton and his associates (1963), in their epidemiological study in Sterling County, conclude from all their available information, ". . . that at least half of the adults in Sterling County are currently suffering from some psychiatric disorder defined in the APA Diagnostic and Statistical Manual." The significant question here, of course, is what percentage of cases found to be psychiatrically impaired in these two studies are actually impaired by minor emotional disturbances?

A comparison of the community epidemiological surveys of mental illness in the 1930s with comparable surveys in the 1950s supplies the same kind of evidence. In making this comparison, one is struck with the fact that four to five times more cases of all kinds of mental disorder are reported in the more recent surveys than in those of the 1930s (Plunkett & Gordon, 1960). The only thing that seemingly can account for such a discrepancy is the widening definition in recent years of what constitutes a case of mental disorder.

The net has also been widened by the recent attempt to place into the psychiatrically sick role all those persons who might be regarded as failures in social adaptation. Consequently, delinquents, sex offenders, alcoholics, drug addicts, homosexuals, prostitutes, beatniks, communists, and the racially prejudiced have all been, from time to time and in different clinical settings, fitted into one or another psychiatric diagnostic category, some of which have the APA official stamp and some of which do not. This is not to say that none of the persons found in these categories is mentally sick; indeed, some are. But any diagnostic category is likely to lose its significance unless carefully worked out criteria are rigidly applied. It also means that many of the persons whom we try to force into some psychiatric slot are likely to be regarded as normal and acceptable in their various subcultural milieus. In fact, much of their behavior also will be found acceptable in the more conventional areas of social life.

One other factor that has contributed to this widening definition has been the extensive and intensive education of psychiatrists in psychoanalytic theory and the use of psychoanalytic technique. This is not to say that psychoanalytic treatment should not be used with the clinically neurotic or the mild psychotic reaction types, but only that it is used and extended to those professionals in the community, excluding the psychiatrists in training, who are functioning at some acceptable level of adequacy in their occupations and families and at the same time are earning $10,000 to $25,000 per year. The problem becomes complicated when such persons are considered to be psychiatrically sick and in need of treatment. Thus, any epidemiological survey of all kinds of mental disorders, which includes cases seen by private psychiatrists, is likely to be weighted by such cases, producing a distorted picture of the incidence of valid psychiatric illness in the community.

All of these bits of evidence go to support my contention that what currently is defined as mental illness is a result of the widening definition of mental illness over the past two decades. This makes for tremendous difficulty in epidemiological studies, for, with respect to total mental illness, there is no basis for the comparison of contemporary rates with earlier rates. Epidemiological study of mental illness is also hampered by policy differences in the various clinics relative to those cases that will be accepted for treatment and those that will not. Consequently, it is almost impossible to have any basis for establishing a true count of mental illness in the community; the line that separates the sick from the well is a variable and confusing one.

Changing Attitudes toward the Mentally Ill

A certain amount of evidence has accumulated over the past two decades that would indicate a marked shift in the attitudes of our people toward the mentally ill in the various communities across the land. That is, while the stigma attached to mental illness still lingers on in certain quarters, the irrational fear of the mentally ill that used to be manifested is gradually disappearing. For example, Woodward (1951), in his survey of a sample of the Louisville population in 1950, showed that a great majority of the people who were questioned held a naturalistic view of the development of mental illness. Gurin's study in 1959 took much the same point of view and indicated a marked willingness of people to take their troubles voluntarily to those experts whom they thought might help them (Gurin, 1960). An attempt to tap the public opinion toward psychiatric home care (Crocetti & Lemkau, 1963) indicated a definite sympathetic and helpful attitude toward the mentally ill in over three-fourths of the persons in the sample. For example, to a statement, "The best way to handle people in mental hospitals is to keep them behind locked doors," 77 percent of 1737 persons gave a "no" response. To the statement, "Almost all persons who have a mental illness are dangerous," 74 percent gave a "no" response. It is responses of this character that serve to point to the new attitude about mental illness that has been developing among our people.

Then too, the bombardment of various communities over the past decade via radio and television concerning the problem of mental illness has helped to spread this sympathetic and more tolerant attitude. In fact, it has reached the point in some communities that it seems that the people have been promised more than psychiatrists can deliver. For they often come voluntarily now to the various outpatient clinics in the urban centers. This ground swell of persons who seem willing to be identified as psychiatric cases contributes, when they enter official counts, to the changing rate patterns of mental illness in the community.

Increase in Psychiatric Facilities

Since World War II, many developments have taken place that helped to do away with the apathy about mental illness that seemed prevalent during the first half of the century. The psychiatric experience accumulated in the war effort, the entrance of the federal government into the mental health field, the discovery of the new tranquilizing and energizing pharmaceuticals, the increase of foundation monies for mental health research, and the various sociological studies of mental health facilities all contributed to creating a climate of optimism relative to the care and treatment of the mentally ill. This new optimism was reflected in an increase in the number of psychiatrists,[1] the development of new treatment facilities, and new research efforts to evaluate psychiatric facilities and therapeutic results.

The frustrations over the older, more chronic cases, as we have seen, have been reflected in the widening definition of what constitutes mental illness, which, in turn, helped to contribute to the idea that much was being accomplished, even with respect to the chronic cases who often had been long-time residents of our mental hospitals. The application of the new drugs appeared to be moving them to some level of recovery, thus making it possible for more of them to return to their families in the community. This led to new projects geared toward rehabilitation and caring for any remissions occurring in their home settings. Thus, day hospitals, night hospitals, halfway houses, and convalescent homes began to put in their appearance, first in England and then in this country, as treatment centers that would encourage and support the mentally ill for living in the community. These new projects were further abetted by an increase in the number of public and private outpatient clinics in order, again, to keep the patient out of the hospital as long as possible.

The changed attitudes on the part of the people toward mental illness discussed above have helped to encourage two new developments. If people who are sick in their minds are to be regarded and acted toward in

[1] From 1940 to 1965 the number of psychiatrists in this country increased by 477 percent, or from 2,403 in 1940 to 13,880 in 1965. (Source: American Psychiatric Association.)

much the same way as are persons who are physically ill, then it also follows that such persons should have access to the general hospitals. This produced the development of psychiatric wards in general hospitals, often made possible because of the inclusion of provisions for mental illness in various health insurance plans. While it is true that most plans only cover approximately a month's illness, nevertheless, it was enough to help encourage the general hospitals to include facilities for the mentally ill. As a further development along this line, it was interesting to note that the new auto contracts signed in Detroit in 1964 carry certain provisions for the treatment of any mental illness that may arise among the workers.

The second development has been in terms of the techniques aimed at the rehabilitation of the person who has been mentally ill. The empirical experience that developed after World War II in connection with the rehabilitation of handicapped veterans obviously precipitated the notion that such procedures might work also with persons who are apparently recovering from their mental illnesses. These techniques are, of course, directed toward creating a more satisfactory self-image and equipping the person with skills that enable him to function in the community, if not at his previous level, at least at a level where he feels necessary and accepted. Rehabilitation is behind such therapeutic facilities as day hospitals, convalescent homes, halfway houses, and the like, which are used both to prevent prolonged hospitalization and to help fit back into the community those people who are recovering from a mental illness.

The latest development in this increasing number of psychiatric facilities has been the proposal for community mental health centers throughout the country. The purpose of these centers is to bring together the total psychiatric facilities of the community in one location so that treatment potentialities can be maximized. It is visualized that these centers would serve populations from 50,000 to 200,000 persons and would combine in one location all of the facilities necessary for diagnosis, treatment, prevention, and research, thus insuring continuity of care.

Some Evidence of Changing Rate Patterns

In the account above, we have attempted to make a logical analysis of those factors observable in cities in the past two decades that should contribute significantly to changing the rate patterns of mental illness that have been reported for urban communities in the United States. In the earlier Faris and Dunham (1939) study, I was often struck by the fact that the great bulk of the subcommunities in Chicago had, for the most part, rates for total mental disorder that were relatively low, while only about ten or twelve subcommunities had rates that might be regarded

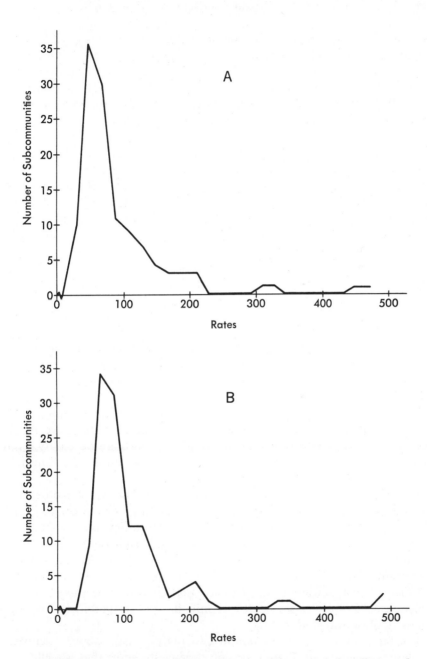

FIGURE 1. Frequency polygons of first admission rates for all mental disorders in Chicago, 1922–1934: A, state hospitals; B, state and private hospitals. Subcommunities $N = 120$. All rates per 100,000 population, 15–64 years of age.

as high. The frequency distribution of the subcommunities in Chicago by size of rates for total mental disorders are shown in Figure 1. One notes in this distribution the small number of subcommunities with high rates.

Now, if our analysis of the factors at work in the urban community has any validity, we would expect distributions of such rates for Chicago at the present time to approach a more normal distribution. That is, there would be a few communities with low rates and a few with high rates, and the bulk of the communities would fluctuate around the average. Unfortunately, we do not have these data for Chicago, but we do have a comparison for the patterns formed by the schizophrenic rates in Detroit for 1936–1938 as contrasted with the patterns for 1956–1958. These distributions are shown in Figure 2. One notes immediately the greater spread of the subcommunities for the more recent period in contrast to the distribution of schizophrenic rates for the earlier period. While the distribution for 1956–1958 does not quite fit a normal curve, it should be noted that in this period seventeen subcommunities have rates larger than 100, as compared to six in the earlier period.

This same difference also stands out when the distribution of schizophrenic rates in Detroit in these two time periods are broken down by sex. In the distribution of male first admission schizophrenic rates in the 1936–1938 period one notes that only seven subcommunities have rates above 100 but in the 1956–1958 period nineteen subcommunities had rates above 100, indicating that schizophrenia is distributed throughout the city much more widely in the recent period. The pattern formed by the female rates almost approaches a normal curve in the more recent period. Again, one notes that for the earlier period there were only seven subcommunities with rates above 100. These distributions are shown in Figure 3.

This evidence, scanty as it may be, serves to document our contention that the rate patterns of mental illness in our large urban communities are changing. These changing patterns appear to follow both population and income shifts. That is, the city core has been continually losing population, some pushing out to the suburbs and others settling in those subcommunities beyond the city's core. In a like manner, the tendency of the income distribution to approach a normal curve for those incomes under $10,000 is associated with this shift in the rate patterns of mental illness (Goldsmith et al., 1954).

The factors that we have attempted to analyze in the above discussion can be regarded as social pressures of varying strengths that are effective in changing the distribution patterns of rates for total mental disorder as well as specific psychoses in our cities. Thus, it can be predicted that future studies that attempt to examine the distribution of mental dis-

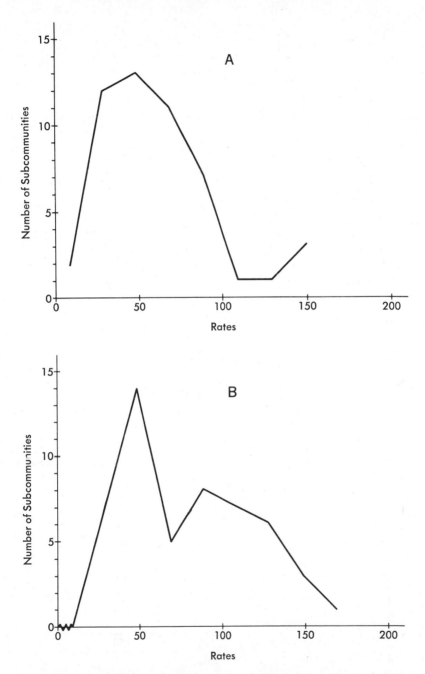

FIGURE 2. Frequency polygons of first admission rates for schizophrenic cases, Detroit: A, 1936–1938; B, 1956–1958. Subcommunities $N = 51$. All rates per 100,000 population, 15–64 years of age.

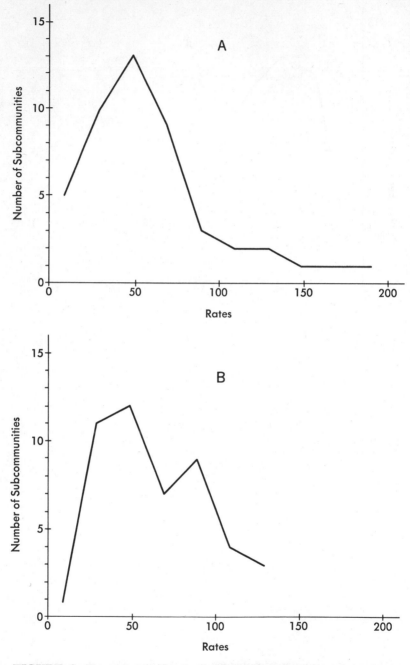

FIGURE 3. Frequency polygons of first admission rates for schizophrenic cases, Detroit: A, male, 1936–1938; B, female, 1936–1938;

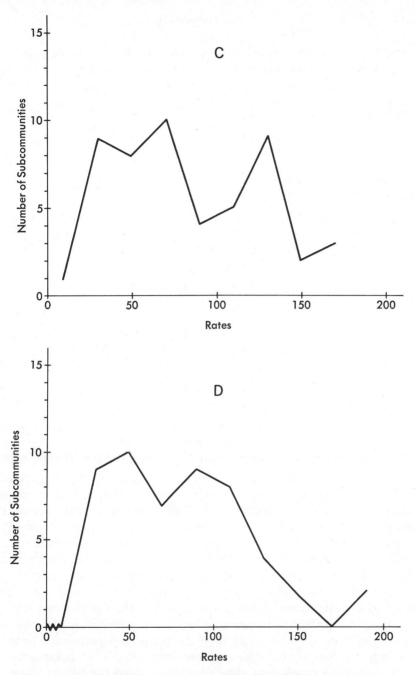

C, male, 1956–1958; D, female, 1956–1958. Subcommunities $N =$ 51. All rates per 100,000 population, 15–64 years of age.

orders in our large metropolitan centers may come up with rate patterns which, while still pointing to differential areal rates, will tend to show concentration of medium high rates in certain areas beyond the city's core. Further, as our cities attain a more marked social and economic equilibrium, it would be expected that rates by local areas for total mental disorders, and especially for schizophrenia, would approximate a normal curve.

DO DIFFERENTIAL RATES OF MENTAL ILLNESS
MEAN WHAT THEY SEEM TO MEAN?

We turn now to an examination of the second question, where we want to determine if significant differential rates between local areas of the city signify that the population in one area actually breeds more of one type of mental disorder than does the population in another area.

In order to effect such an analysis, we propose to examine the following questions: (1) To what extent do the original findings of the Faris and Dunham study stand up today? (2) What has been the character of the criticism of the Faris and Dunham study? (3) To what extent did the findings of recent studies support those of Faris and Dunham? (4) What is the most plausible explanation of differential rate patterns of mental disorders and, particularly, schizophrenia within the city?

Previous Epidemiological Mental Disease Findings

In any attempt to examine differences or similarities that exist between city core and suburban fringe, it is appropriate to recall the issues raised by the Faris and Dunham (1939) findings concerning the distribution of different psychoses in Chicago. The central finding of that study established that the high rates of schizophrenia were concentrated at the center of the city, with the rates declining in all directions toward the periphery, while the distribution of manic-depressive rates appeared to be randomly scattered throughout the city. This difference in the distribution rate pattern of these two psychoses in the city did not receive much attention in subsequent discussions of the study, for the critics concentrated on the schizophrenic distributions to discover if they really meant what they seemed to indicate, namely, that one kind of an urban population seemed to produce a significantly larger number of schizophrenics than another type of population. Yet, the failure of the manic-depressive rates to form a pattern similar to the schizophrenic rates might be interpreted as meaning that the manic-depressive reaction enabled the person to relate to his immediate environment in a much more effective fashion than could the person who developed schizophrenia. In contrast, the schizophrenic reaction was of the type that prevented a meaningful relationship with family and peer group members and so the person withdrew from these relationships and selected an environment where he would more likely be left alone and so did not have to become involved in close interpersonal relationships.

In this earlier study of the various distributions of schizophrenic rates, while the ratio between the high- and low-rate areas was approximately 3.5:1, a difference which was statistically significant, the problem of the interpretation of this difference was constantly present. Myerson (1941) sounded the alarm when he reviewed the study and pointed to the drift hypothesis as explaining the concentration of cases that made up the high-rate areas. A decade or so later, Gerard and Houston (1953) tried to explain the concentration of schizophrenic cases at the center of the city by showing that they were to be accounted for primarily by schizophrenics living alone, and that if one looked at the distribution of schizophrenics coming from a family base, the differences between high and low-rate areas tended to disappear. Clausen and Kohn (1959), in a study of the distribution of first admission schizophrenic rates in Hagerstown, Maryland, showed a complete absence of rate differences among the different socioeconomic areas of the city. Even before this study, Hare (1956) in Bristol, England, attempted to determine whether the "attractor" or the "breeder" hypothesis best explained schizophrenic rate differentials in the city and was forced to conclude that, while the issue was not resolved completely, the evidence did seem to favor the "attractor" hypothesis. And the most impressive and monumental study of Leighton et al. (1959) showed that as far as the psychoses were concerned there appeared to be no difference in the rate between disorganized and organized communities.

The Epidemiology of Schizophrenia in Detroit

These recent findings have thus failed to support the implication of the Faris and Dunham study that one type of urban population produced more schizophrenics than did another type. It was exactly this point that I wished to test for an urban population when I designed an epidemiological study of schizophrenia for the city of Detroit (Dunham, 1965).

Here, my intent was to select two subcommunities that presented a demographic similarity with respect to age, sex, and race, but differed markedly with respect to the quality of their cultural life. Another qualification was that these two subcommunities should differ significantly with respect to the size of their incidence rates of schizophrenia, based upon first admissions to state hospitals. We were able to obtain a fair similarity on age and sex, but by 1958 it was extremely difficult to secure comparability with respect to race. However, the ratio of schizophrenic

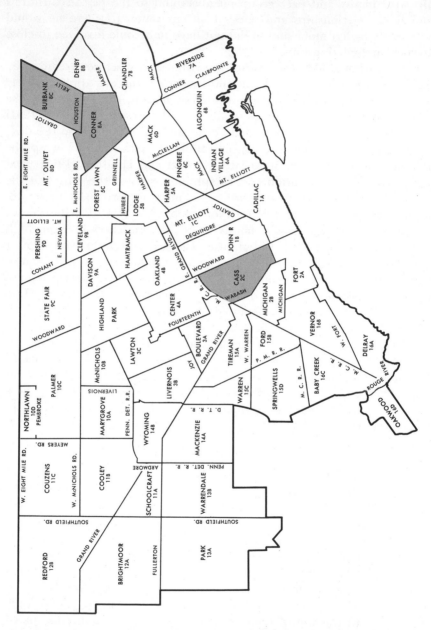

FIGURE 4. Location of research subcommunities in Detroit. United Community Services of Metropolitan Detroit Research Department, 1952.

cases for the two subcommunities, based upon first admissions to state hospitals, was in the expected range of 4:1. We finally selected these two subcommunities after comparing them on the basis of certain population characteristics with seven other high-rate and six other low-rate subcommunities. On the above criteria we selected Cass, located at the city's core and Conner-Burbank, located at the extreme outskirts of the city, as shown in Figure 4. They differed from one another with respect to economic level and cultural organization. The intent then was to search diligently through the records of all psychiatric facilities, both inpatient and outpatient clinics and public and private hospitals, as well as private psychiatrists, to find those schizophrenic cases that had been admitted to or had been seen by a psychiatric facility for the first time during 1958.

TABLE 1. Number and Incidence Rates[a] for Three Diagnostic Groupings[b] Resulting from Intensive Screening[c] in Two Subcommunities, Detroit, 1958

Diagnostic Grouping	Cass			Conner-Burbank				Ratios	
	No.	Rate	r_1	No.	Rate	r_2	$r_1 - r_2$	C/C-B	C/C-B[d]
Schizophrenic	46	1.24	.18	24	.45	.09	.20	2.8:1	2.7:1
Nonschizophrenic	63	1.69	.21	48	.90	.13	.25	1.9:1	1.9:1
Additional	238	6.39	.41	35	.65	.11	.43	9.8:1	9.8:1
Total	347			107					

[a] All rates per 1000 estimated population, 15 years and over, 1958.

[b] The diagnostic groups used in this survey were three in number: (a) schizophrenic—any case that was ever given a diagnosis of schizophrenia at any psychiatric facility; (b) nonschizophrenic—this category includes primarily cyclothymic, involutional, psychoneurotic, and schizoid personality cases; (c) additional psychiatric cases—this category includes most of the psychopathies, some addiction cases, and cases admitted to psychiatric facilities but not given any diagnosis.

[c] By intensive screening we refer to the fact that every one of our cases in the initial schizophrenic group and two-thirds of our cases in the nonschizophrenic group were examined by a psychiatrist plus the fact that there was a careful check on each case in the three diagnostic groups to determine whether or not there had been a previous psychiatric hospital admission or any contact whatever with a psychiatric facility. This means that if a case had been admitted to a psychiatric facility in 1959 and after a careful study of the history of this case, by the record, the project psychiatrist, and a sociological interview, it was discovered that the case had first been admitted in 1958, such a case was added to the number of cases in the base year, 1958. This, of course, applied to cases first picked up in 1958 and when subsequent admissions were discovered in a previous year, such cases were dropped from the base year.

[d] Ratio based on rates from estimated total population, 1958.

Comparable data were gathered for the two subcommunities for the years 1956 and 1957.

By this procedure we attempted to test a null hypothesis that the incidence rates of schizophrenia will not vary significantly between the two subcommunities. The data used to test this hypothesis initially are presented in Table 1. It should be noted immediately that the ratio for schizophrenics between high- and low-rate subcommunities is still approximately 3:1, which is in line not only with our original study but with several other studies that have reported areal rates for large cities (Dunham, 1965). The nonschizophrenic ratio is approximately 2:1 which is a considerable reduction from the earlier study, while the additional group presents a ratio of almost 10:1 between high- and low-rate areas.

It is perhaps interesting to note that when the rates were computed for these three diagnostic groups for 1956, 1957, and 1958 without intensive screening, the ratios are almost identical to the 1958 data with intensive screening. The one ratio which apparently is out of line is the ratio for nonschizophrenics in 1956. These are shown in Table 2.

However, this is not the final note, for it was necessary to turn to the data and ask, "To what extent are the cases that make up our rates indigenous to these two culturally contrasting subcommunities?" This question touches on geographical mobility and points to the necessity for

TABLE 2. NUMBER AND INCIDENCE RATES FOR THREE DIAGNOSTIC GROUPINGS WITHOUT INTENSIVE SCREENING FOR 1956, 1957, 1958 IN TWO SUBCOMMUNITIES, DETROIT[a]

| | 1965 | | | | | | 1957 | | | | |
| | Cass | | | Conner-Burbank | | | Cass | | | Conner-Burbank | |
Diagnostic Grouping	No.	Rate	r_1	No.	Rate	r_2	No.	Rate	r_1	No.	Rate	r_2
Schizophrenics	33	.81	.14	18	.34	.08	41	1.05	.16	20	.38	.08
Nonschizophrenics	55	1.35	.18	24	.45	.09	58	1.49	.20	44	.83	.13
Additional	353	8.64	.46	62	1.16	.15	321	8.22	.46	76	1.42	.16
Total	441			104			420			140		

| | 1958 | | | | | | | | |
| | Cass | | | Conner-Burbank | | | Ratios: Cass/Conner-Burbank | | |
Diagnostic Grouping	No.	Rate	r_1	No.	Rate	r_2	1956	1957	1958
Schizophrenics	30	.81	.15	16	.30	.08	2.5:1	2.7:1	2.7:1
Nonschizophrenics	56	1.50	.20	43	.80	.12	3.0:1	1.8:1	1.9:1
Additional	269	7.22	.44	51	.95	.13	7.4:1	5.8:1	7.6:1
Total	355			110					

[a] Population 15 years old and over.

examining the evidence on the length of time that these cases were residents of the two subcommunities. It must be borne in mind that our first concern was to determine if the ratio of the rates between the two subcommunities would change significantly when geographical mobility was taken into account. To provide some basis for a judgment in this matter, we divided the cases in the two subcommunities into two groups: those under and those over five years in residence. We then calculated rates for both categories in each of the diagnostic groupings in the two subcommunities. The results of this analysis are shown in Table 3.

It is immediately noticeable that when cases are counted that have been

TABLE 3. NUMBER AND RATES BY LENGTH OF RESIDENCE AND DIAGNOSTIC GROUPING IN TWO SUBCOMMUNITIES, DETROIT, 1958[a]

	Cass							
	Schizophrenic		Non-schizophrenic		Additional		Total	
Length of Residence	No.	Rate	No.	Rate	No.	Rate	No.	Rate
Under 5 years	28	.75	27	.73	20	.54	75	2.01
Over 5 years	8	.22	15	.40	15	.40	38	1.02
Total	36	.97	42	1.13	35	.94	113	3.03
Unknown	3	.08	6	.16	4	.10	13	.35
Total	39	1.05	48	1.29	39	1.04	126	3.38

	Conner-Burbank							
	Schizophrenic		Non-schizophrenic		Additional		Total	
Length of Residence	No.	Rate	No.	Rate	No.	Rate	No.	Rate
Under 5 years	13	.24	11	.21	6	.11	30	.06
Over 5 years	11	.21	33	.62	24	.45	68	1.02
Total	24	.45	44	.83	30	.56	98	1.08
Unknown	0	.00	2	.03	1	.02	3	.00
Total	24	.45	46	.86	31	.58	101	1.08

[a] Based on estimated population for 1958, 15 years and over: Cass, 37,229; Conner-Burbank, 53,504.

resident in the subcommunity for at least five years, the rates for schizophrenia prove to be identical, while the rates in the other two diagnostic
groups actually are higher in Conner-Burbank, the more homogeneous
subcommunity. It is also worth noting that for those schizophrenic cases
that had been in the subcommunity for five years or less, the ratio comparing the two subcommunities remains at the original level of 3:1. In
the nonschizophrenic group for those in the subcommunity for less than
five years, the ratio increased to approximately 3.5:1, while in the addi-

TABLE 4. NUMBER AND RATES BY LENGTH OF RESIDENCE
AND DIAGNOSTIC GROUPING IN TWO SUBCOMMUNITIES,
DETROIT, 1958[a]

	Cass							
	Schizophrenic		Non-schizophrenic		Additional		Total	
Length of Residence	No.	Rate	No.	Rate	No.	Rate	No.	Rate
Under 5 years	28	1.00	27	.95	20	.71	75	2.65
Over 5 years	8	.63	15	1.18	15	1.18	38	2.99
Total	36	.87	42	1.02	35	.85	113	2.76
Unknown	3	.07	6	.14	4	.10	13	.32
Total	39	.94	48	1.16	39	.95	126	3.08
	Conner-Burbank							
	Schizophrenic		Non-schizophrenic		Additional		Total	
Length of Residence	No.	Rate	No.	Rate	No.	Rate	No.	Rate
Under 5 years	13	.63	11	.53	6	.39	30	1.45
Over 5 years	11	.25	33	.73	24	.54	68	1.52
Total	24	.37	44	.67	30	.46	98	1.50
Unknown	0	.00	2	.03	1	.01	3	.04
Total	24	.37	46	.70	31	.47	101	1.54

[a] Based on population in residence 5 years and under, 1960: Cass, 28,316; Conner-
Burbank, 20,739. Based on population in residence 5 years and over, 1960: Cass, 12,696;
Conner-Burbank, 44,762.

tional diagnostic group the ratio was reduced slightly to approximately 5:1. These ratios are to be contrasted with the ratios obtained by intensive screening as shown in Table 2.

It must be noted that these rates have been computed on the basis of the estimated population 15 years old and over in 1958. However, one might argue from this procedure that even though two-thirds of the population of Cass is a mobile one, the total population formed the demographic and cultural environments for those schizophrenic cases that had been in the subcommunity for more than and less than five years. Thus, the use of the total population to compute the rates is warranted. However, it is also argued that the more correct procedure would base these rates upon the population that was in the community for at least as long as the two groups of patients composing the three diagnostic groupings. In line with this argument, further rates were computed based on the population that had been in residence in each of the two subcommunities for under and over five years. These data are shown in Table 4.

This analysis shows for those in residence five years or more that the ratios between the two subcommunities for the three diagnostic groupings are considerably reduced but tend to favor the more disorganized community in each instance. The ratios for those in residence over five years are 2.5:1, 1.5:1, and 2.2:1 respectively. The ratios for those in residence under five years are 1.6:1, 1.8:1, and 2.4:1 respectively. Thus, the picture is reversed as compared to the previous table where the rates were based on the total population in each of the two subcommunities.

Further, it should be noted that while the differences in the rates between the two subcommunities for those who have been there five years or longer for schizophrenics and nonschizophrenics are not significant because of the reduction in the case base, the ratios between the two subcommunities, although reduced slightly, are still in the same direction for both categories of residence, as was true when the cases were combined. Here, it is perhaps appropriate to call attention to the trend of the rates rather than to the absence of a statistically significant difference between them. Only in the additional diagnostic group does the rate difference between the two subcommunities stand up with a critical ratio of 4.5.

As a final step, we examined those few cases that have been residents of our two subcommunities practically from birth onward. We found three cases that were residents in Cass for twenty years or more and five cases that were residents in Conner-Burbank for the same length of time. With one exception, these eight cases spent their childhood years in one or the other of these two subcommunities. If one computed rates for these cases, the two subcommunities would emerge with almost identical rates in terms of their nearly lifetime residents who broke down with schizophrenia.

These data lead to the following conclusions: (1) With a complete coverage of cases admitted to all psychiatric facilities in an area and with careful intensive screening of such cases to establish diagnosis and exact year of first admission, the ratio of schizophrenic patients between two widely separated and culturally contrasting subcommunities in a large urban center remains approximately 3:1. (2) When the factor of length of residence is taken into account, the ratio for the schizophrenic patients and for the other two diagnostic groups between the two subcommunities are reduced to a nonsignificant level. (3) When lifetime residence is counted in the two subcommunities, there appears to be little difference in the proportion of schizophrenics that come out of contrasting types of population. These conclusions imply that the 3:1 ratio of schizophrenic cases between different types of communities in a city is a function of the mobility of the cases and certain undetermined selective processes. They further imply that the true incidence of schizophrenia in culturally contrasting communities is approximately at a parity.

One other finding with respect to the mobility of our cases was brought to light when we examined the areas of the city from which the cases came before taking up residence in one or the other of the two subcommunities. These data, shown in Table 5, were distributed according to the following procedure: First, rates for the subcommunities were grouped into quartiles on the basis of a distribution from all first admission schizophrenic cases that had entered state hospitals from Detroit. The first two quartiles represented the inner city, and the third and fourth

TABLE 5. Number and Percentage of First Contact Psychiatric Cases by Diagnostic Grouping and Location of Previous Residence from Two Subcommunities, Detroit, 1958

	Cass						Conner-Burbank					
Location of previous residence	Schizo-phrenic		Nonschizo-phrenic		Additional		Schizo-phrenic		Nonschizo-phrenic		Additional	
	No.	%	No.	%	No.	%	No.	%	No.	%	No.	%
Inner city	25	78.1	23	74.2	21	60.0	15	62.5	14	35.9	12	44.4
Outer city	2	6.3	2	7.4	5	14.3	5	20.8	17	43.6	10	37.0
Other U.S. & foreign	5	15.6	6	19.4	9	25.7	4	16.7	8	20.5	5	18.6
Total	32	100.0	31	100.0	35	100.0	24	100.0	39	100.0	27	100.0
Unknown	7		17		4		0		7		4	
Total	39		48		39		24		46		31	

quartiles plus the suburbs represented the outer city. Other parts of the United States and foreign countries represented a third category. Second, the cases were distributed in these categories according to their previous residences. This table shows that in the schizophrenic grouping, 78.1 percent of the cases recorded for Cass came from the inner city, while at the same time 62.5 percent of our cases recorded for Conner-Burbank came from the inner city. The assumption that the cases came from the same universe is supported by accepting the null hypothesis of no difference on the basis of a critical ratio of 1.3. In the nonschizophrenic group, the difference between the two subcommunities is significant as shown by a critical ratio of 3.6. Thus, we rejected the null hypothesis for this grouping and inferred that the origin of our nonschizophrenic cases in Conner-Burbank were quite different from those casees in Cass. However, in the additional group we accepted the null hypothesis on the basis of a critical ratio of 1.2. These findings point to the fact that both the schizophrenic and additional cases have been extremely mobile as compared to the nonschizophrenic cases.

Although we present these findings for our three diagnostic groups, our attention was always centered on the schizophrenic group. Perhaps we have not been able to demonstrate conclusively that one type of urban population produces no more schizophrenics than another type of urban population, but we think we have cast considerable doubt on the proposition that communities in an urban complex that have been shown to be marked by extreme disorganizing conditions are likely to produce more schizophrenics than such communities in an urban complex that are not so marked. If the validity of such a proposition can be accepted, then it is necessary to look for factors other than general life conditions and styles that may be conducive to bringing about differential rates of schizophrenia among subcommunities in a large urban center. The singular points of origin of the majority of the schizophrenic cases found in both Cass and Conner-Burbank suggests the following question: In what specific ways did those families that produced schizophrenics and moved out of the inner city differ from those families who produced schizophrenics and stayed in the inner city?

The question is crucial, and we have tried to develop an interpretation that seemed most valid in terms of our data. We have been struck by the fact that a certain number of schizophrenics are found in every subcommunity of the city and that the ratio between high and low rate areas tends to stay at about 3:1, which is in line with the ratios found in all similar studies. We have further noted that this ratio is reduced when we take account of the residential mobility of our cases. We have further noted that all of our cases, with the exception of one, who were living alone at the time of their first psychiatric contact were in Cass. This fact suggests that when the young person who is destined for a schizophrenic breakdown leaves the nuclear family to seek work in the city, he invariably meets many disappointments and ends up in an anonymous social situation which characterizes Cass. Further, we have recognized the significance of the observation made in a recent study (Freeman, Simmons, & Berger, 1960) that "Families containing schizophrenic patients move for the same reasons as do other families in the community." In the light of these facts, we hypothesized that rate differences for schizophrenia found within the confines of a large, urban, industrial city are to be explained by differing initial life chances present in families that produce schizophrenics. In other words, when a person who later is to develop this disorder is born into a family where the life chances are better than average, he will reap certain benefits with respect to education, health, income, and residence, provided he stays with the family. Thus, families with good life chances are more likely to change their residence, and when such families contain potential schizophrenics they will be moving when the family moves. If this hypothesis stands up, we would conclude that significant rate variations in the incidence of schizophrenia in the different areas of a given geopolitical unit in the United States is caused by a social-selective process that functions to maintain a balance between the needs of schizophrenic persons and the characteristics of the social organization of the diverse areas of that unit.

This analysis of the study has been concerned primarily with the attempt to determine if there are any differences in the size of the schizophrenic rates between the core and the periphery of the city. However, there is the pattern of rates formed by some of the other psychotic groups that Faris and I did examine in our earlier study. These other psychoses, namely, manic-depressive, general paresis, alcoholic psychoses, and the old-age group, have not received much attention in recent epidemiological studies, which, while they often contain diagnostic distinctions, concentrate primarily on the schizophrenic disorders, the total psychoses group, and in some instances, the psychoneuroses and character disturbances. We have already commented on the contrast between the manic-depressive distribution and the schizophrenic distribution in the earlier study and noted that the manic-depressive cases gave evidence of less residential mobility than did the schizophrenic cases. This is also supported by my recent study (see Table 5).

In referring to the distribution patterns of alcoholic psychoses and drug addiction in the earlier study we noted that the concentration of cases seemed to be largely explained by the tendency of these cases to select the more anonymous areas in the urban community where they

TABLE 6. Number and Percentage[a] of General Paresis and CNS Syphilis First Admissions to All Facilities[b] by Sex, 1923–1962[c]

Year	Males		Females		Total	
	No.	%	No.	%	No.	%
1922	5678	8.10	1474	2.10	7152	10.20
1938	6092	5.85	2125	2.04	8217	7.89
1948	3565	2.56	1499	1.08	5064	3.64
1962	312	.19	127	.08	439	.27

[a] Refers to a percentage of total first admissions.

[b] Includes all state, city and county, and private facilities, excluding Veterans' hospitals.

[c] Source: U.S. Department of Health, Education, and Welfare Publications, *Patients in Mental Institutions*, 1923, 1938, 1948, 1960, and 1962.

might escape surveillance. Again, in the earlier study the correlation of the general paretic rates with vice areas and syphilitic case rates, while they did not explain the rate patterns, did suggest, by implication, that proximity to sources of infection might account for the high rates in certain areas of the city. The gradual control of syphilis has reduced cases of general paresis to almost a disappearing point and this may account for the absence of new epidemiological work with this psychosis. Some evidence on this point is shown in Table 6.

The early association that we found between the old-age psychosis and the areas of poverty merely suggested that the families in poverty-stricken areas tended more easily to place their older members in psychiatric hospitals. However, we are discovering that, with the aging of our population, these psychoses of old age have no relationship to any particular population but rather are likely to be related to the number of older people in the population and numerically are possibly on the increase owing to the increasing age of the population. As the current population of older people, those long-time residents of the city core, die out and are not replaced, there will be a real increase in the geriatric disorders in the peripheral and suburban areas, especially in the oldest areas.

SUMMARY AND PREDICTIONS

This analysis of the pattern of mental illness in our large cities has pointed up two positive findings. First, I have attempted to show that certain forces are at work in the American city that are making obsolete the traditional ecological organization which seemed to characterize American cities from their initial beginnings up to World War II. Thus, it is not unexpected that rate patterns for various social problems will also be subject to change. I have pointed out that this seems to be true for patterns of mental illness. Thus, when the current set of forces have worked themselves out, a new ecological organization of the city will emerge. In its ideal form, it should provide a greater equilibrium in its organization. This means that with respect to the various subcommunities of the large urban centers, population, income, and family size will tend toward a more normal distribution. Of course, the rate patterns for all kinds of social deviancy, including mental illness, will also shift toward this new equilibrium. Thus, we predict that, with respect to mental illness, when the new ecological organization of the city is completed, only a few of the subcommunities will have high rates and a few will have low rates, but the bulk of the subcommunities will converge toward an average rate. If this trend continues, and I confidently expect it will, there will be a grave question concerning the attaching of any significance to the living conditions and cultural organization in its subcommunities for explaining the high rates of the psychoses, particularly schizophrenia.

In answering the second question, we have presented certain evidence to show how a high schizophrenic rate in a subcommunity of the city has developed. The analysis pointed to mobility as the chief factor to account for the spread of schizophrenia cases in the urban community. The analysis also questioned that any schizophrenic rate in a subcommunity of the city can be regarded as a product of an indigenous population. This means, of course, that schizophrenic rate differentials can hardly be explained by the cultural climate in a subcommunity, but are more likely to be accounted for by a social selection process, aided and abetted by the actions of schizophrenics themselves in selecting areas of residence where their chances of survival in the free community would appear to them to be enhanced.

This analysis suggests a greater caution in using differential rate distributions of various forms of pathological behavior to infer a connection between the behavior in question and the surrounding social conditions. It seems most likely that differential rate patterns in cities for various types of social deviancy may be significant as a means for studying the organization of the city, rather than as a device for dredging up the etiological factors to account for the deviancy in question.

REFERENCES

Clausen, J. A., & Kohn, M. L. Relation of schizophrenia to the social structure of a small city. In B. Pasamanick (Ed.), *Epidemiology of mental disorders.* Washington, D.C.: American Association for the Advancement of Science, 1959.

Crocetti, G. M., & Lemkau, P. V. Public opinion of psychiatric home care in an urban area. *American Journal of Public Health*, 1963, **53**, 409–414.

Discussion of "Definition of a case for purposes of research in social psychiatry." In *Interrelations between the social environment and psychiatric disorders*. New York: Milbank Memorial Fund, 1953.

Dunham, H. W. *Community and schizophrenia: An epidemiological analysis*. Detroit: Wayne State University Press, 1965.

Faris, R. E. L., & Dunham, H. W. *Mental disorders in urban areas: An ecological study of schizophrenia and other psychoses*. Chicago: University of Chicago Press, 1939.

Foster, I. Some facts about the labor market in the sixties. *The American Child*, 1961, **43** (3), 5–8.

Freeman, H. E., Simmons, O. G., & Bergen, B. J. Residential mobility inclinations among families of mental patients. *Social Forces*, 1960, **38**, 320–324.

Fuhrman, M. School dropouts and juvenile delinquency. *Federal Probation*, 1960, **24** (3), 34–37.

Gans, H. *Urban villagers*. New York: Free Press, 1962.

Gerard, D. L., & Houston, L. A. Family setting and the social ecology of schizophrenia. *Psychiatric Quarterly*, 1953, **27**, 90–101.

Goldsmith, S., Jaszi, D., Kaitz, H., & Liebenberg, M. Size distribution of income since the mid-thirties. *The Review of Economics and Statistics*, 1954, **36**, 1–32.

Green, H. W. *Persons admitted to the Cleveland State Hospital, 1928–1938*. Cleveland: Cleveland Health Council, 1939.

Gurin, G., Veroff, J., & Feld, S. *Americans view their mental health*. New York: Basic Books, 1960.

Jacobs, J. *The death and life of great American cities*. New York: Random House, 1961.

Leighton, D., Harding, J., Macklin, D., Macmillan, A., & Leighton, A. *The character of danger*. New York: Basic Books, 1959.

Myerson, A. Review of *Mental disorders in urban areas*. *American Journal of Psychiatry*, 1941, **96**, 995–997.

Ogburn, W. F. *Social change with respect to culture and original nature*. New York: Viking Press, 1950.

Plunkett, R. J., & Gordon, J. E. *Epidemiology and mental illness*. New York: Basic Books, 1960.

Schroeder, C. W. Mental disorders in cities. *American Journal of Sociology*, 1942, **47**, 40–47.

Srole, L., Langner, T., Michael, S., Opler, M., & Rennie, T. A. C. *Mental health in the metropolis: The midtown Manhattan study*. New York, McGraw-Hill, 1962.

Wolf, E., & Lebeaux, C. *Studies in change and renewal in an urban community*. Unpublished manuscript, Wayne State University, 1965.

Woodward, J. L. Changing ideas on mental illness and its treatment. *American Sociological Review*, 1951, **16**, 443–454.

3.5　*Orientation*

America is a highly mobile nation. About 20 percent of the population change their places of residence each year. Such mobility is facilitated by a complex system of coast to coast highways, and an interlocking network of competing routes for airlines, trains, and buses.

For more than a century, researchers have investigated the effects of immigration on recipient nations and emigration on those nations that face a net outflow of people. However, it is only recently that attention has been given to the migration that occurs within nations, perhaps because general population mobility within any nation is a rather recent phenomenon.

Mildred Kantor summarizes the research in this important topical area and indicates the difficulty of the problem. As she points out, the relationship between migration and mental illness is complex and varies with the social characteristics of the migrants, the social psychological aspects of the situation surrounding migration, and the social characteristics of the sending and receiving communities. She distinguishes between those facts about migration that are relatively well established, and those that require further investigation. Also, she suggests that a reliance on the old concepts used in social mobility research may not be sufficient for an adequate understanding of the problem, and it is necessary to study the discrepancy between aspirations and achievements in migrant and nonmigrant populations for a complete understanding of the problem.

3.5　Internal Migration and Mental Illness[1]

Mildred B. Kantor

"Migration causes adjustment problems that precipitate mental illness." "Migration is a way of adapting to problems and results in improved adjustment in the new setting." "There is no relationship between migration and mental illness." "There is an association between migration and mental illness, but the association varies under different conditions."

[1] The author is indebted to John C. Glidewell, PhD, for critical comments and review of various drafts of this paper; to Mary Elizabeth Thompson for research assistance; and to Jeanne Medalie for typing drafts of the manuscript.

These are commonly voiced statements concerning the relationship of migration to mental illness, and one might find some research support for each statement. How does one resolve the dilemma posed by apparently inconsistent research findings?

The purpose of this paper is to look for resolutions of the dilemma of apparently inconsistent and contradictory research findings concerning the relationship of internal migration in the United States to mental illness. No attempt is made to present an exhaustive survey of all relevant work; only those references directly pertinent to an argument are cited.

The position taken in this paper is that migration, in and of itself, does not precipitate the development of mental illness. Migration, however, does involve changes in environment which imply adjustments on the part of the migrant. These adjustments may be reflected in improved or worsened mental health. There are conditions, nevertheless, under which there is an increased risk of the development of emotional disturbance among migrant groups. These conditions can be specified in terms of characteristics of the sending and receiving communities, characteristics of the migrants, and circumstances under which the migration occurs. These conditions will be examined in the following sections of this paper.

INITIAL CONSIDERATIONS

Some clarification of the concepts "migration" and "mental illness" will be helpful in interpreting the available evidence.

Let us first consider "migration," or intercommunity residential change. What is the extent of migration? Personal observation and statistical evidence indicate that our society is a highly mobile one. According to official reports (Shryock, 1964; Taeuber & Taeuber, 1958), approximately twenty percent of the population of the United States changes residence each year. This proportion has been relatively stable since 1947; however, the number of such movers has increased because of population growth. Shryock noted that there were about thirty-five million such movers in 1960.

All changes in residence are not considered to be migration, however. Demographers generally classify residential changes from one part of a community to another as local moving, and reserve the term "migration" for residential changes from one community to another. Accordingly, Shryock noted that approximately twelve million of the residential changes that occurred in 1960 could be classified as migration and approximately twenty-four million as local moving. Although the emphasis in this paper is upon migration, references will be made to those studies of local moving that are relevant to the presentation.

The distinction between migration and local moving is contingent upon the definition of community. In 1948 Hollingshead reviewed the field of community research and concluded that the community has been "assumed to be an organized structural and functional entity with spatial, temporal, and sociological dimensions." In a later article, Hillery (1955) analyzed ninety-four definitions of community from the period 1901 to 1950. He found that a majority of the definitions included area, common ties, and social interaction as elements of community. In 1956 Blackwell defined community as "a locus for a set of basic, interacting institutions through the functioning of which a majority of the residents find it possible to meet their needs and have developed something of a sense of togetherness, with a consequent potential ability to act together as an entity." Blackwell noted further that not all local areas exhibit the characteristics of community, that specific localities may be designated as conforming more or less to the concept of community. In all of these definitions there are spatial and social elements. Accordingly, distance of the residential move, and amount of change in the social environment of the mover are apparently involved in the distinction between migration and local moving. Theoretically, intercommunity residential change involves greater distances and more environmental change than intracommunity residential change.

Operationalization of the distinction between migration and local moving involves the establishment of appropriate cutting-points. County and state lines are spatial cutting-points used by many demographers and sociologists (see, for example, studies by Bogue, 1959; Shryock, 1964; Snipes, 1965; Kleiner & Parker, 1959; Jaco, 1960; Lee, 1958, 1963). The term "migration" is reserved for the movements across the lines. Although the use of this type of boundary as a cutting-point facilitates data collection and tabulation, it presents problems because the conceptualization is not clear. The theoretical basis for the operational definition is spatial distance, the larger movements being those across the boundary lines. However, some movements across county or state lines may be very small with respect to the distance covered and, conversely, some intracounty and intrastate movements may cover large distances.

To pursue this problem further, let us examine the relationship between distance of residential move and amount of change in the environment of the migrant. In theory, a move that covers a great distance involves more environmental change than a move that spans a small distance. In actuality, the situation may be quite the reverse. A move that spans a great distance may involve less environmental change than a move that spans a small distance. An example of such a situation is the relocation of an entire self-contained army base from one section of the country to another. The environment of the ordinary soldier changes very little as a result of the relocation; however, a great distance is spanned. This would suggest that distance and environmental change ought to be considered separately in relation to the consequences of migration for the individual migrant.

Environmental change implies the severance of old relationships and the establishment of new ones. In addition to the change in living quarters, migration may involve changes in occupation, school, church, and social ties for the migrant and members of his family. The minimum change required is change in residence. Local moving may also involve some or all of these changes; here, too, the minimum change required is change in residence. Theoretically, the amount of change differentiates migration from local moving. Operationalization of this distinction is not a simple task. To resolve this problem many researchers select populations for study in such a way that the change in environment for the group classified as migrant is a gross environmental change. Rural sociologists, for example, have generally classified as migrants all persons who move away from farms (Burchinal, 1963; Leybourne, 1937; Omari, 1956). Such a move usually involves a complete change in the way of life of the migrants as well as a change in area of residence.

Also relevant to the amount of change involved in a residential move are characteristics of the sending and receiving communities, characteristics of the migrants, and the circumstances under which the move occurs. The greater the similarity between the receiving and sending communities, the less environmental change there is. What are some of the conditions that contribute to similarity between the sending and receiving communities? When the distance of the residential move is small, and when change of residence is the only change that occurs, there is a high degree of similarity between sending and receiving communities. With the addition of simultaneous changes in occupation, school, church, and social ties, and with an increase in the distance between sending and receiving communities, the degree of similarity decreases. More old relationships are severed and new ones must be established.

The size of the group that moves also contributes to the similarity between sending and receiving communities. When a large group moves, it is possible for the migrants to establish in the receiving community the way of life that they had in the sending community, and they are more likely to do so than a small group. At the very least, there are familiar faces with whom the migrant can interact and persons who might help orient him to the new surroundings. Striking examples of settlement patterns in relation to the size of the migrating group are found in the movement and relocation of ethnic and racial groups, and of migrants from rural to urban areas (Gans, 1962; Wirth, 1928; Kiser, 1932; Rose & Warshay, 1957).

The amount of change that occurs as a result of any residential move is not the same for all migrants. Characteristics such as age, social status, and preparedness affect the amount of change experienced by the individual. For example, a short-distance move may imply a complete change in environment for a child, owing to the fact that he cannot get around by himself, although there is little or no change involved for the parents. Fenichel (1945) proposes, in fact, that for a child a change in residence is analogous to a change in a parent. Persons of high social status may experience less environmental change than persons of low social status (Burchinal & Bauder, 1963). An involuntary move for a person who is not prepared to move may involve more environmental change than a voluntary one for a person who is prepared to move (Fried, 1965).

Finally, it is important to note that changes in family structure and gross social changes such as war and economic depression are often related to the occurrence of a residential move. For example, the birth of a child often results in a residential move to a dwelling unit with more space. Moves that occur under such circumstances are likely to involve more environmental change than moves that occur in the absence of such circumstances.

In summary, we may say that migration is not a simple concept. It has a number of aspects, and each of these aspects may have implications for mental illness. Migration has been defined as change of residence from one community to another, in contradistinction to local moving, which has been defined as change of residence within a community. Distance of the move is fundamental to this distinction. Amount of change in the social environment is another important element, and this is influenced by characteristics of the sending and receiving communities, characteristics of the migrants, and the circumstances under which the move occurs. This multiplicity of variables involved in the definition of migration suggests the potential utility of a matrix of types of migration based upon spatial and social elements. One could then define specific residential changes in terms of both distance and changes in the social environment.

Now let us consider the concept "mental illness." This also is not a simple concept. An understanding of its many aspects is relevant to our review of research. The definition of it influences the type of data that is reviewed and interpretations of the data. Since problems of definition of mental illness have already been discussed in the article by Theodore Sarbin, there is no need for further consideration of them here. Let us merely note several points that have particular pertinence for this paper.

The first point is that the term "mental illness" includes a variety of types of mental disorder that are due to different causes. Conceivably, each type of disorder could have a different relationship with migration. Some researchers work with the general concept "mental illness"; others select particular types of mental disorder for study, for example, schizophrenia, manic depressive psychoses. The adequacy of working with types of mental disorder in this case is dependent upon the accuracy with which one type of disorder can be distinguished from another type of disorder. However, the research based upon the total concept must assume that the whole is representative of the parts, that the relationship of migration to mental illness is similar to the relationships of migration to particular types of mental disorder.

The second point concerns the definition of a case of mental illness. Incidence and prevalence figures for mental illness are usually based upon diagnosis of symptomatic behavior by a psychiatrist or upon hospitalization due to diagnosis of mental illness by a psychiatrist. These figures are an underestimation of the true incidence and prevalence figures, since cases that do not come to the attention of a psychiatrist are not included. The underenumeration is due in part to difficulties in identifying or screening cases of mental illness. The problem involves more than the assessment of attributes, however; it is related to the referral process and to the acceptance of a patient for treatment. Whether or not an individual comes to the attention of a psychiatrist is a function not only of his behavior, but also of the norms of the community in which he lives and of the tolerance of the community for his behavior.

A wide range of operational indexes of mental illness has been used in research studies. Faris and Dunham (1939), Tietze, Lemkau, and Cooper (1941), Hollingshead and Redlich (1958), Clausen and Kohn (1959), Jaco (1960), and Lee (1963), for example, used data based upon diagnosis of symptomatic behavior by a psychiatrist or upon hospitalization due to diagnosis of mental illness by a psychiatrist. Pasamanick, Roberts, Lemkau, and Krueger (1959) used data based upon examinations by non-psychiatric physicians and a diagnosis arrived at by clinical evaluation procedures. Questionnaire methods designed to obtain information on psychosomatic and other psychopathological symptoms were used by Srole, Langner, Michael, Opler, and Rennie (1962) and Sewell and Haller (1959). If the criterion for definition of mental illness is related to migration, choice of a particular index may affect the findings. For example, there may be a relationship between patient status and migration, but there may be no relationship between reported symptoms and migration. In an attempt to clarify the findings concerning the relationships between indexes of mental illness and migration, data relevant to a sample of different indexes will be reviewed separately in the following sections of this paper.

In summary, we may say that neither migration nor mental illness is a simple concept. Each has a number of aspects that might affect the relationship between them. Researchers have not been uniform in their operationalization of either concept. This has been a source of confusion in the collation and interpretation of research findings. In this review of the literature, an attempt will be made to clarify research findings with respect to some of the aspects of migration and mental illness that have been noted above.

PATIENT STATUS DATA

In this section of the article, aspects of migration will be examined in relation to patient status, which is defined as diagnosis of symptomatic behavior by a psychiatrist and hospitalization due to diagnosis of mental illness by a psychiatrist.

Malzberg's early work (1936a, 1936b) directed attention to the possible existence of associations between interstate migration in the United States and hospitalization for mental illness. In separate analysis of white and Negro population groups, he found higher rates of mental hospitalization for migrants into New York State, from other states of which they were natives, than for nonmigrant natives of New York State.

In later work with Lee (Malzberg & Lee, 1956), Malzberg found continued support for these early findings. Further, he was able to control for color, sex, and age, which are among important factors affecting comparisons of rates of mental illness in different groups. In addition, separate comparisons were made for total psychoses, schizophrenia, manic-depressive psychoses, and psychoses other than these two types, and recency of migration was examined as a possible important factor. For total psychoses and for the three groups of psychoses that were examined separately, rates of admission to hospitals in New York State were found to be much higher for in-migrants than for nonmigrants, even when age, sex, color, and time of migration were controlled. In addition, this study revealed much higher rates for migrants who had come into the state within the preceding five years than for migrants who had been in the state more than five years.

For New York State, it appeared that rates of admission to mental hospitals were higher for in-migrants than for the nonmigrant natives. Why this was true could not be ascertained from the available data. Malzberg and Lee speculated that such differentials might arise in three different ways: "from selection in the place of origin, from stresses of migration or adjustment to the new environment, or from differentials in prevailing rates of mental disease in the originating and the New York State populations" (p. 123). They were inclined to favor a combination of the first two possibilities and to discount the third. As they indicated, the higher rates of mental hospitalization among recent migrants than among those who had migrated earlier point to selection in the place of origin of persons who already had some degree of mental illness. Further, this finding suggests that New York State might be atypical in attracting unstable individuals who are either hopeful of using its psychiatric facilities or of finding an anonymous place for themselves in New York City.

Later studies lent further credence to the Malzberg and Lee findings and helped to dispel the impression that the New York State data were unique. The work of Locke, Kramer, and Pasamanick (1960) produced findings similar to those of Malzberg and Lee for migrant and native-born populations of Ohio. Specifically, "white and non-white males and females born in Ohio were found to have lower rates" of admission to mental hospitals "than their counterparts who were born elsewhere in the United States and subsequently migrated to Ohio."

Lazarus, Locke, and Thomas (1963) collated the Locke data for Ohio on migration status by age, sex, and race with similar data for New York and California. They found the same pattern of higher rates of mental hospitalization for in-migrants than for nonmigrants in all three states. The magnitude of the differentials, however, varied by diagnosis, race, sex, and state. For schizophrenia there appeared to be no differences in hospitalization rates of white[2] in-migrants and nonmigrants in Ohio and California. In New York State, however, higher rates for schizophrenia were found for white in-migrants than for nonmigrants.

With respect to race, the magnitude of the migrant-nonmigrant differentials (for all disorders) was greater for nonwhites than for whites. In addition, there were variations in these differentials by state. For whites, the highest migrant-nonmigrant differentials were found in New York State, the next highest in Ohio, and the lowest in California. For nonwhites, the highest differentials were found in California, the next highest in New York, and the lowest in Ohio. Further, within each racial classification, the magnitude of the migrant-nonmigrant differentials varied by sex. For the white population, the magnitude of the differentials between migrants and nonmigrants was greater for females than for males.

[2] Data were not available for nonwhite first admissions with a diagnosis of schizophrenia. For nonwhites, only data for a general category of "all disorders" were available.

The reverse situation was found for the nonwhites. There the magnitude of the differentials was greater for males than for females.

An additional difference among the states appeared in the pattern of variations in magnitude of the migrant-nonmigrant differentials by sex within each racial category. Ohio, for some reason, was an exception to the findings stated in the previous paragraph. In Ohio, for the white population, there was no difference in the migrant-nonmigrant rates for schizophrenia, and, for all disorders, the magnitude of the differentials was greater for males than for females. The reverse situation was found for the nonwhite population. There, for all disorders, the magnitude of the differentials was greater for females than for males.

The variations in the magnitude of the differentials among the states appear to indicate either selective migration into different areas of the United States or diverse consequences of living in different areas of the United States for in-migrant and nonmigrant populations. The variations in the magnitude of the differentials by race, sex, and diagnosis point to the necessity for continued exploration for the potential influence of additional factors.

Divergent findings from the work of Kleiner and Parker (1959) also point to the involvement of other factors in the association between inter-state migration and patient status. Further, their data support the suggestion that there might be diverse consequences of living in different parts of the United States for migrant and nonmigrant groups. Kleiner and Parker studied interstate migrant and nonmigrant Negroes in Pennsylvania. They compared a sample of 2013 first admissions to Pennsylvania state psychiatric hospitals during the period from 1951 to 1956 with the census population by nativity and age. Their findings indicated that the southern Negro migrant population was under-represented and both northern migrants and natives were over-represented in the statistics on first admissions.

Pursuing this finding in a later study, Kleiner and Parker (1965) suggested that intervening social-psychological variables such as social status, status consistency, and the discrepancy between one's achievement and level of aspiration might explain the data. They compared a sample of 1423 persons admitted to selected psychiatric agencies on an inpatient or outpatient basis in 1960–1961 with a representative sample of 1489 from the Philadelphia Negro community. In this study, a "migrant" was defined as an individual who spent the majority of his first seventeen years of life outside of Philadelphia, and a "native" as an individual who spent the majority of this period in Philadelphia. Classification as a "southern" or "northern" migrant was determined on the basis of where he lived during those seventeen years. With age and sex controlled, the incidence of mental illness among the native-born was significantly higher than among the southern migrants.[2] Neither social status nor status consistency could account for the observed differences in illness between the migrant and the nonmigrant groups. However, the discrepancy between aspiration and achievement was significantly higher for the native-born than for the migrants. This finding is consistent with other research showing larger discrepancy scores for psychotic, neurotic, and maladjusted individuals than for healthier individuals (Kleiner & Parker, 1963), and it is especially important because it directs attention to social psychological aspects of demographic phenomena.

Jaco (1960) also produced findings divergent from those of Malzberg and Lee (1956), Locke et al. (1960), and Lazarus et al. (1963). In part, the differences may be due to methodological differences. Jaco adjusted his rates on a different basis than did the other researchers, and he also used a different definition of migration. In part, there may be actual differences in the selection of migrants in their community of origin and in Texas as a receiving environment. In either case, a closer look at Jaco's work will contribute to an understanding of the relationship between migration and patient status.

Jaco studied 11,298 Texas residents who were diagnosed psychotic and sought treatment for the first time in their lives during 1951 and 1952. In compiling cases for his migrant group, Jaco made a distinction between "transients" and "migrants" and used data only for "migrants." Transients, defined as people who had changed place of residence frequently or who had lived in the state for a very short time without showing any intent of establishing residence there, were eliminated from the study. Also, he included in his migrant group not only interstate migrants but also migrants from outside the United States, predominantly from Mexico. The majority of the foreign-born migrants, however, could be isolated in analyses by subculture, because they were Mexican-American. The findings indicated that rates of mental illness were not significantly higher for migrants to Texas than for natives of Texas. The Mexican-American group, however, showed higher rates for migrants than for the native-born. This was especially true with respect to the incidence of schizophrenia among migrant Mexican-American females. This finding could have been due to difficulty in acculturation to a new environment or to selection of an illness-prone migrant group. The finding for the native Americans could have been due to the distinction between "migrants" and "transients."

---

[2] Northern migrants were not considered in this study because they constituted a relatively small proportion of the migrant population.

A different approach to the investigation of the relationship between migration and mental illness was taken by Faris and Dunham (1939) and by Freedman (1950). Their studies of Chicago utilized areal distributions of indices of migration and of mental illness. Specifically, they directed attention to the possible existence of associations between mobility characteristics of areas of a city and rates of mental illness of the population living in these areas. Faris and Dunham (1939) used percent of home ownership and percent of hotel and lodging-house residents as indexes of areal stability. They found a negative association between percent of home ownership and rates of schizophrenia, a positive association between percent of hotel and lodging-house residents and rates of schizophrenia, and similar, but less strong, associations for the manic-depressive psychoses. In addition, they defined areas of the city in terms of indexes of social disorganization, including mobility characteristics, and found a steady decline in rates of schizophrenia from the center of the city to the periphery accompanying a decline in the rates of the indices of social disorganization. No such regular pattern was found for the manic-depressive psychoses.

Freedman (1950) analyzed data from the 1940 census, in which migrants were defined as those persons who lived in different counties (or quasi-counties[3]) in 1940 and 1935. On an areal basis he found a high positive correlation of this index of migration status with admission rates for manic-depressive psychoses, but not for schizophrenia. Further, the correlations among various indexes of social disorganization and the migrant rates were not found to be consistent, and in almost every case the correlations with intracity mobility rates were greater than with intercity migration rates.

The findings of both the Faris and Dunham and the Freedman studies were important for several reasons: (1) they pointed to diagnosis as a factor in the relationship between migration and mental illness and suggested that specific types of mental illness might be related to specific types of population movements; (2) they indicated associations between types of mental illness and characteristics of areas of a city; and (3) they led to interpretations which stimulated further research.

Among the possible explanations for their findings, Faris and Dunham noted "that persons who are mentally abnormal fail in their economic life and consequently drift down into slum areas because they are not able to compete satisfactorily with others" (p. 163). An alternative explanation also discussed was that the mode of life in particular areas of the city is

[3] In this classification a city with 100,000 or more inhabitants is treated as a quasi-county, and the remainder of its county as another.

conducive to the development of mental illness. On the basis of his findings, Freedman advanced the hypothesis that it is not the amount of mobility alone that distinguishes disorganized from normal urban areas, but also the extent to which the population is accustomed to mobility. Later investigators contributed to the clarification of some of these relationships.

The work of Tietze et al. (1942) provided support for Freedman's finding of differences between intracity and intercity mobility with respect to rates of mental illness. They examined data collected in a survey of the Eastern Health District of Baltimore in 1936. Information concerning mental deviants (including psychotics, adult neurotics, psychopathic personalities and adult behavior deviates, and children with behavior disorder) was obtained from case records of hospitals, clinics, courts, and social agencies, and analyzed in relation to two indexes of spatial mobility (length of residence within a given house and length of residence within the city of Baltimore). Tietze et al. found higher rates of mental deviation among persons who changed residence within the city than among nonmobile persons, but could find no such relationship for length of residence in the city. They concluded that intracity mobility rather than intercommunity migration is important in relation to mental deviation. In addition, they noted that possible interpretations of these findings are that "mobile families are on the move for reasons not associated with their mental makeup and that adjustment difficulties and personality disorders of every kind are the results of this moving around" and that "families with a tendency to mental deviation may not adjust well wherever they find themselves and therefore change their residence oftener than do more stable people" (p. 39). As they observe, their data favor the constitutional factor; equally high rates would be anticipated in both groups of migrants if change in environment were the major factor.

The findings of these early ecological studies led to a consideration of the possible existence of associations between social mobility and mental illness. A detailed review of relationships between social mobility and mental illness is beyond the scope of this paper; however, those aspects of the relationships with particular relevance to spatial mobility will be examined here.

One interpretation of the concentration of people with mental disorders in the poorer areas of the city is that the disorders are so handicapping that afflicted individuals inevitably become downward mobile. Another interpretation is that downward mobility produces so much stress for the individual that mental disorder is a highly probable outcome. The studies of Gerard and Houston (1953), Lystad (1957), Jaco (1959), Hollingshead and Redlich (1954, 1955, 1958), Lapouse, Monk, and

Terris (1956), and Clausen and Kohn (1959) provide information concerning these issues.

Gerard and Houston (1953) studied 305 first admission male schizophrenics in Worcester, Massachusetts. They found a clustering of cases in the lower socioeconomic areas of the city. These cases were predominantly single, separated, or divorced men who were living alone. There was an absence of such a concentration for schizophrenics who lived with their families. These findings led them to suggest "that the overall central concentration of male schizophrenics is due to the 'drifting' or instability of the single and divorced men, who have moved away from their family settings into the central, deteriorated areas of the city which offer them residential facilities."

In both the Lystad and Jaco studies, the presence of mental illness was found to be associated with downward mobility, but not necessarily a consequence of the downward mobility. It is important to note, however, that geographic mobility was not consistently found to accompany the downward social mobility. Examination of these studies in greater detail will provide further clarification of the relationships among geographic and social mobility and mental illness.

Lystad (1957) studied social mobility and geographic mobility in relation to the occurrence of schizophrenia among ninety-four first admissions for the years 1953 and 1954 and ninety-four nonschizophrenics obtained from the outpatient clinics of a semiprivate hospital in New Orleans. She initially intended to study foreign migration as well as internal migration; however, only three controls were from another country, so this was not feasible, and the study became one of internal migration. The measure of mobility used was length of time lived in the city. Lystad found that schizophrenic patients showed less upward mobility and less geographic mobility than the matched group of mentally well persons.

Jaco (1959) also did not find a relationship between spatial mobility and mental illness, but did find one between downward occupational mobility and mental illness. In this study, he designated high- and low-rate areas for psychoses in Austin, Texas, by classifying according to census tract all first admissions of diagnosed functional psychoses to the local state hospital from 1940 to 1952. Within these areas, a random sample of residents was selected for interview concerning interaction patterns and social conditions within the area. The measures of spatial mobility examined were the number of persons renting or owning their places of residence (assuming that renting indicates potentially higher mobility on the part of the occupants), the number of times moved within the city, number of places lived before migrating into the city, and length of residence in present abodes. Occupants of areas in which there were high rates of psychoses rented their homes significantly more than those in areas with low rates of psychoses, but there were no differences in the number of moves they made within the city. In addition, he found that occupants of high-rate areas had lived in significantly fewer places before migrating into the city and had a significantly greater length of residence in their present abodes than those living in low-rate areas. On the basis of these findings, Jaco concluded that amount of home ownership is not a good index of spatial mobility, and that there was no association between spatial mobility and the prevalence of mental illness in the community.

Among the studies that do not support the "drift" hypothesis are those of Hollingshead and Redlich (1954, 1955, 1958), Lapouse et al. (1956), and Clausen and Kohn (1959). Hollingshead and Redlich (1955) studied the social mobility of twenty-five psychoneurotics, twenty-five schizophrenics, and sixty control subjects. Contrary to the "drift" hypothesis, they found that neurotic and schizophrenic patients were more upwardly mobile than the control subjects. With respect to geographic mobility, they found (Hollingshead & Redlich, 1958) no relationship between patient status and migration to the New Haven community from elsewhere in the United States, nor was there a relationship between onset of schizophrenia and movement to slum areas.

The findings of Lapouse et al. (1956) were similar to those of Hollingshead and Redlich. Their sample comprised all patients (there were 587) with a diagnosis of schizophrenia on first admission from a Buffalo, New York, address to the two state hospitals in the Buffalo area between January 1, 1949, and December 31, 1951. Tracing residential moves back to 1925 for a subsample of 114 patients and a matched control group, they could find no evidence of downward drift. There was an inverse relationship between the areal distribution of the schizophrenic patients and the socioeconomic status of the areas. However, Lapouse et al. demonstrated that the high rates of schizophrenia in low-income areas were neither the result of downward mobility nor of recent migration into these areas of mobile men who live alone.

Clausen and Kohn (1959), while essentially supporting the findings of Hollingshead and Redlich and of Lapouse et al. direct attention to the importance of occupational and residential change that occurs on the same status level. They found that Hagerstown schizophrenics had changed their places of residence and their jobs more frequently than normals of comparable background. However, they could find no evidence of unusual upward or downward mobility in either the occupational shifts or the residential histories.

Discussion

Patient status data are generally obtained from case records of psychiatrists and from records of agency and hospital admissions. Thus, they designate a population that has some degree of mental illness at the time of admission as a patient. The majority of the studies that utilize this type of data attempt to relate the fact of mental illness to social variables recorded on the case record. Studies of rates of mental illness of migrant and nonmigrant populations are generally of this nature. Some of the studies examine data for matched groups of patients and non-patients. In either type of study, it is possible for the researcher to collect additional data. However, it is not possible to assess the psychological characteristics of the patients and the controls prior to diagnosis. Therefore, the question of whether the mental illness occurred prior to, concomitant with, or as a result of migration cannot be answered directly. Valuable information is provided by these studies nonetheless, and their particular contributions should be cited.

The studies reviewed indicate the existence of a positive association between interstate migration and patient status. Interstate migrants generally were found to have higher rates of mental illness than non-migrants. Studies in which this was not so point to the amount of migration or transiency (Jaco, 1960) and to social-psychological factors (Kleiner & Parker, 1965) as intervening variables. It appears that there might be a positive association between frequency of migration and incidence of mental illness. It also appears that there may be social psychological factors, such as discrepancy between aspiration and achievement, that might be differentially associated with the occurrence of mental illness in migrant and nonmigrant groups.

Variations among the states in the comparative rates of mental illness for migrants and nonmigrants point to the possible influence of characteristics of the place of destination, selection at the place of origin, and social characteristics of the migrant and nonmigrant populations. Characteristics of areas of destination and selection of migrants at places of origin have not been studied in relation to patient status. Selected social characteristics of migrant and nonmigrant populations have been included in studies of patient status; however, they have been treated mainly as control variables in order that the relationship between migration and mental illness might be more systematically examined. This has been done because of the possibility that differences in rates of patient status might be associated with differences in the social characteristics of migrant and nonmigrant populations rather than with the migration process itself. The studies reviewed indicate that race and sex are two social characteristics that may be associated with differential occurrence of mental illness in migrant and nonmigrant groups. Further exploration of the relationships between migration and mental illness is needed for population groups that vary in these and other social characteristics in relation to characteristics of areas of origin and destination and in relation to the circumstances under which the migration occurs.

The studies reviewed also indicate an association between rates of mental illness and mobility characteristics of urban areas. This association, however, varies with diagnosis and type of mobility. Indexes of mobility that have been used most frequently include length of residence in a city (a measure of intercity migration), length of residence in a house (a measure of intracity mobility), and home ownership (a measure of areal stability and social organization). Diagnoses most frequently studied include schizophrenia, manic-depressive psychosis, mental deviation, and the psychoses. There is a considerable range in the specificity of these.

Home ownership appears to have an inverse relationship with rates of schizophrenia, manic-depressive psychosis, and the psychoses in general. However, there is some question concerning the validity of home ownership as an index of spatial mobility. In at least one study (Jaco, 1959), a negative association was found between home ownership and both number of moves within the city and length of residence in a particular house.

A distinction between migration into a city and mobility within a city appears to be important in clarifying the relationship between mobility characteristics of urban areas and mental illness. In most of the studies, high rates of mental illness were associated with high rates of intracity mobility. The correlations of rates of mental illness with rates of migration into the city were lower by comparison, and in some cases no relationship was found. For schizophrenia, the findings were consistent in all of the studies reviewed; a positive association was found between schizophrenia and intracity mobility, but no association was found between schizophrenia and migration into the city. Other diagnoses led to contradictory findings in some of the studies. In part, the conflicting findings may be due to the fact that some of the studies utilized areal distributions of indexes of mental illness and mobility, while others correlated information concerning mobility and mental illness for individuals in sample populations. In part, variations in findings may be due to the possibility that specific types of mental illness might be related to specific types of mobility.

In general, the findings for mobility characteristics of urban areas in relation to mental illness are consistent with those reported above for interstate migration in relation to mental illness. To the extent that intracity mobility is an index of transiency, these data also indicate that there may be a positive association between amount of mobility and mental illness. Further, the finding that schizophrenia appears to have different relationships with various types of mobility and migration than do other diagnostic categories of mental illness is also consistent with the findings from the other studies.

Several studies found concentrations of admissions to mental hospitals in lower socioeconomic areas of cities. Efforts to explain these concentrations led to the "drift" hypothesis, namely, that persons who are mentally ill fail in their economic life and, consequently, drift into deteriorated urban areas. Other studies found an association between downward social mobility and mental illness, but no association between geographic mobility and mental illness for the same populations. Additional studies demonstrated associations between mental illness and upward and horizontal mobility, in some cases accompanied by geographic mobility, in some cases without it. Therefore, it appears that these concentrations are not due to the drifting into these areas of persons who are already ill. Nor are persons who are hospitalized for mental illness necessarily on the downgrade economically. Other explanations besides the "drift" hypothesis are obviously needed. It does appear, nevertheless, that occupational change is positively related to rates of mental illness regardless of the direction of the change.

In summary, patient status data have given us important information concerning the relationship between migration and mental illness. Now let us see what contributions data from other sources can make to further understanding of this relationship.

ADJUSTMENT DATA

In this section, aspects of migration will be examined in relation to various nonpsychiatric indices of adjustment. These include indexes of psychological adjustment such as diagnoses by nonpsychiatric clinical methods, reports of psychosomatic and psychopathological symptoms elicited by interview and questionnaire methods, and indexes of social adjustment such as assimilation into the receiving community and community satisfaction. Studies utilizing these types of data have generally focused upon populations involved in particular kinds of movement such as rural-urban migration, forced relocation, and classroom mobility. These studies have disclosed a variety of information concerning characteristics of sending and receiving communities, characteristics of migrants, and circumstances surrounding migration in relation to adjustment. The scope of this paper does not permit a complete review. Let us, however, examine the results of selected studies relevant to each of these aspects of migration with respect to their implications for the patient status data presented above.

Sending and Receiving Communities

Amount of change in the environment includes change in physical and social aspects of the surroundings of the individual. One way of examining consequences for adjustment of amount of change in the surroundings of the migrant is to compare the adjustment of migrants from sending communities with varying degrees of similarity to selected receiving communities.

Among the first to study this type of problem were the rural sociologists who directed attention to the adjustment of migrants from farms into urban areas, a movement between two dissimilar types of communities, generally involving a change in the way of life of the migrant as well as a change in the area of residence.

Leybourne (1937) studied a group of 653 "hillbilly" white migrant families from the western plateaus of the Southern Appalachians. These migrants came to Cincinnati with no industrial experience and had to take low-paid unskilled jobs; in comparison with 434 white Cincinnati families, their position in industry and education was found to be unfavorable. Leybourne found that the Cincinnati residents held many mistaken ideas and attitudes concerning the migrants and were hostile toward them, making it difficult for the migrants to become an integral part of the community. Cincinnati residents felt, for example, that the migrants had come to the city to take advantage of welfare programs, while in reality the migrants were unable to obtain positions that paid enough to keep them off the welfare rolls. Leybourne attributed these misapprehensions to social isolation of the migrants resulting in part from lack of knowledge concerning the way of life of the migrants and in part to a tendency of the migrants to associate with members of their own group and to maintain habits of life appropriate to isolated rural areas.

Later studies by Rose and Warshay (1957), Tilly (1965), Omari (1956), and Burchinal (1963) supported these early findings and pointed to other relevant aspects of migration. Rose and Warshay (1957) studied the efficiency of problem-solving (finding a home, joining organizations, using city facilities) of 110 migrants to Minneapolis from other areas in the United States outside a 40-mile radius of the city. They found that migrants with already existing primary group contacts in the new community were more likely to remain isolated from the rest of the community than migrants without such contacts. Further, these "isolated" migrants were more likely than the others to feel disheartened or pessimistic about their life accomplishments, and they were more likely to be frustrated in contacts outside the primary group because they did not share sufficient meanings and values with the greater society.

In an effort to examine more closely the relationship between characteristics of receiving and sending communities and adjustment of migrants, Rose and Warshay compared the adjustment of urban-urban migrants with the adjustment of rural-urban migrants. They found that migrants from one urban area to another were likely to act more "efficiently" in solving the adjustment problems than were those from a rural area to an urban area. In addition, they found that the rural-urban migrants were more likely to rely upon the primary group contacts in getting settled.

Tilly (1965) also found that the least assimilated of a group of 244 rural and urban migrants to Wilmington, Delaware, were those with kin and friendship contacts in the new community. Further examination of the characteristics of the migrants in relation to assimilation status indicated that the migrants who came to Wilmington through contacts with kin and friends were more likely to be lower socioeconomic status than higher socioeconomic status migrants and more likely to be rural-reared than urban-reared. The data, in fact, indicated an interaction between socioeconomic status and migration from rural and urban areas; the higher the social status of the migrant, the more urban experience he was likely to have had. In the comparisons with respect to assimilation, however, the rural-urban differences were found to be much weaker than the socioeconomic status differences. As Tilly noted, this might be interpreted to mean that rural or urban origin made a difference only for low socioeconomic status migrants, that high socioeconomic status aids assimilation in exposing the individual to urban ways of life regardless of where his residence happens to be.

These studies indicate that social isolation of migrants in a new community is negatively associated with assimilation and with socioeconomic status. Low socioeconomic status migrants with kin and friendship contacts in the new community are less likely to be assimilated than high status migrants who do not have already established social contacts. Length of residence as a mediating factor in these relationships was noted by Tilly (1965) and by Omari (1956). Tilly found his indicators of assimilation to be positively associated with length of residence in the new community, while Omari found positive associations between socioeconomic status and length of residence and between community satisfaction and length of residence for 200 male Negro migrants to Beloit, Wisconsin.

Further confirmation of the importance of length of residence as a mediating factor in assimilation to a new community comes from Burchinal's (1963) study of 208 rural migrant, 391 urban migrant, and 582 nonmigrant adolescents in Cedar Rapids, Iowa. Comparisons among these three groups of children showed that they were much alike in personality characteristics, participation in activities and clubs at school, relations with school friends and teachers, intelligence scores, scholastic achievement, absenteeism, and emotional relationships between parents and children. To Burchinal these results suggested that after several years of residence in a new community migrant children become indistinguishable in many characteristics from children who have always lived there.

In summary, these data point to the importance for adjustment of the mode of orientation into the new community, length of residence in it, and socioeconomic status of the migrant, rather than to the degree of similarity between sending and receiving communities. Migrants who rely upon kin and friendship groups for orientation into a new community are less likely to be assimilated than those who are without such contacts. Reliance upon primary groups for orientation into a new community appears to be associated with low socioeconomic status. Low socioeconomic status migrants are less readily assimilated into a new community than are high socioeconomic status migrants. Length of residence in the community is a mediating factor, however. The longer migrants reside in a community, the more likely are they to become assimilated into it and to be satisfied with it.

Characteristics of Migrants

Migrants may be described in terms of physical, social, and psychological characteristics. These characteristics may affect the amount of change experienced by the individual and the adjustment of the individual to change. Comparison of groups that vary in physical, social, and psychological characteristics is one way of approaching an understanding of their consequences for adjustment.

One group of studies that give us information concerning a wide range of characteristics of migrants in relation to adjustment is that which focuses upon the academic, social, and emotional adjustment of the child. These studies generally use the classroom as the basis for the selection of samples for study. Since the particular focus of these studies is the child, it is important to note several unique features of the position of the child with respect to residential mobility. First, although concern for his welfare may be expressed by the parents, the child has little or no voice in the decision about mobility. His move is generally involuntary; he must accompany his parents in a residential move. Second, the meaning of a move is different for the child than for the parents. A short-distance move, for example, may imply a complete change in environment for the child, owing to the fact that he cannot get around by himself, although there is virtually little or no change involved for the parents.[4]

Studies by Joy (1933), Sackett (1935), Tetreau and Fuller (1942), Gilliland (1958), and Snipes (1965) indicate that mobility enhances the academic position of some children in the classroom. Children from the upper social classes profited more from their experiences in moving than did those from the lower social classes; children with high intelligence profited more than children with low intelligence. Because of the relationships between social class and intelligence, it is not possible to ascertain how much of the effect is attributable to social class and how much to intelligence. None of the investigators examined the effects of either of these variables while the other was held constant.

In addition, although the evidence is not consistent, there may be some optimal number of moves or amount of experience with changing schools, beyond which achievement gains no longer occur. Tetreau and Fuller (1942) found, for example, that transient children who had been in not more than two schools previously fared better in the achievement area than those who had moved more often, while Gilliland (1958) found that the superiority of the transients in mean achievement increased as the number of schools attended increased, and Snipes (1965) found that the greater the number of changes of residence, the greater the likelihood of retention in a grade in school.

The Snipes study also points to the relevance for adjustment of the grade level of the child at the time when the move occurs and of the distance of the move. Pupils who moved during the later grades tended to be retained more than either the nonmovers or the pupils who had moved during Grades 1, 2, and 3. Pupils who had not moved since entering school, or who had moved to the present school from outside the state, were more likely to be promoted than retained. More pupils were retained after having moved within the state than could be expected by chance. These findings are positively correlated with socioeconomic status. Because of the relationships between social class and these aspects of migration, it is not possible to ascertain how much of the effect is due to social class and how much to each aspect of migration.

With respect to the emotional acceptance dimension of classroom social structure, the findings have been markedly different. Kerr (1945), Downie (1953), and Liddle (1955) all found that newcomers to classrooms were

[4] Fenichel (1945, p. 97) indicates, in fact, that for the child a change in residence is analogous to a change in a parent.

significantly underchosen in sociometric studies of acceptance. Downie (1953) also found that one or two previous moves, or having been in the school from one to three years after having moved, produced greater than average acceptance by the other pupils. The implications of Downie's work were that emotional acceptance increases, generally, with the time the child has been in the school and with some mobility experience. In reviewing his results, Liddle also saw some trends in improved acceptance with time in the smaller classroom unit.

The question may be raised as to whether these effects are brought about by moving or whether they are associated with moving for other reasons. The relevant evidence is not clear-cut. Smith and Demming (1958) found no significant differences between late and early entrants on either teacher ratings or the California Test of Personality, although, like the other studies, they found the late entrants lower in social status (but making progress through the year). Smith, in a later study (1959), also found that late entrants scored higher on achievement tests than early entrants but nevertheless had lower social acceptance. These findings suggest that the low social status was a function of newness per se rather than personality traits that characterize children who move or their academic standing.

However, it has been noted by many others that the very highly mobile children are often older than their classmates, and, in several studies (Bedoian, 1954; Elkins, 1958), it has been found that the older children in a classroom were most likely to be rejected and the younger, most accepted. Thus, this would suggest that the age of the migrants relative to their classmates may be a factor contributing to their acceptance or rejection.

Kantor (1958, 1965) has contributed enormously to the question of cause and effect by getting measures of the migrant children before they moved. Her subjects were third graders in St. Louis County. She found that the children who moved were more emotionally maladjusted, as measured by teacher ratings, than those who remained in the classroom. Further, she followed the children who moved within the St. Louis metropolitan area and studied the increase or decrease in behavior symptoms reported by their mothers. Changes in residence without change of social context appeared to have no effect upon the number of symptoms reported. A family move, however, is often accompanied by a change in the father's job (Andrews, 1945; Dewey, 1948; Myers, 1950). Kantor found that when the move was accompanied by the father's change to a more highly regarded occupation, the child retained more old symptoms or developed more new ones than did the children of the nonmobile families. This would suggest that the emotional maladjustment of the migrants relative to their classmates may be a factor contributing to their rejection.

With respect to the process of assimilation in the classroom, Liddle (1955) found that new children are more often cautious than aggressive in their approach and are often seen as withdrawn. They do, however, make approaches to the group, particularly to the most obviously respected child or teacher. Early approaches often seem to be some form of imitating the behavior of the children seen by the newcomer as most highly regarded (Phillips, Shenker, & Revitz, 1951).[5] Early influence attempts are probably often unsuccessful, but, after a period of conformity or imitation and learning the group's frames of reference, the new child's influence attempts become more successful (Merei, 1949). The initial period of conformity or imitation was observed by Merei even when the child was assigned a leadership role. While social class and intelligence factors set limits on the child's assimilation, the acceptance and power of the new child increases to these limits over time. The time required to reach a stable position was not indicated by the research findings reviewed.

In summary, the data indicate that residential mobility has different consequences for different indexes of adjustment in children. Residential mobility appears to enhance the academic adjustment of upper social class children and of children with high intelligence. However, residential mobility appears, at least at first, to interfere with the social adjustment of the child. The data indicate also that in both instances there are mediating factors. With respect to academic adjustment, it appears that there may be an optimum amount of mobility beyond which achievement gains no longer occur. With respect to social adjustment, length of time in the classroom, some mobility experience, age of child, and emotional adjustment of the child at the time of entry into the classroom appear to be influential. The social position of the child improves with length of time in the classroom and some mobility experience, but worsens with increasing disparity in age between the child and his peers and with the presence of emotional disturbance in the child.

Circumstances Surrounding Migration

Migration can occur under a wide variety of circumstances. These circumstances may affect the amount of change experienced by the indi-

---

[5] Phillips, Shenker and Revitz (1951) and Merei (1949) studied groups outside of the classroom context, but their research is relevant to the assimilation of the newcomer into the classroom. Phillips, Shenker and Revitz (1951) studied groups composed of children from neighborhood houses and nearby public schools; Merei (1949) studied children from two Hungarian day nurseries.

vidual and the adjustment of the individual to the change. Examination of the adjustment of individuals who migrate under varying conditions is one way of learning about the consequences of migration for adjustment.

Studies of forced relocation give us information concerning the adjustment of individuals who move under a particular set of circumstances, specifically, a situation where the decision to move is made by someone other than the migrants. In many instances it is difficult to distinguish between forced and voluntary migration. Consequently, studies of forced relocation have generally focused upon dramatic movements, such as displacement from a leveled slum area or relocation due to job reassignment. Several such studies will be reviewed here.

Fried (1963, 1965) studied the impact of forced relocation in the West End of Boston, an ethnic working-class community with approximately 12,000 residents. He found that, for the majority of those who were displaced, leaving their residential area involved a moderate or extreme sense of loss and an accompanying affective reaction of grief (Fried, 1963). This grief reaction was manifested in feelings of painful loss, continued longing, general depressive tone, frequent symptoms of psychological or social or somatic distress, active work required in adapting to the altered situation, sense of helplessness, occasional expressions of direct and displaced anger, and tendencies to idealize the lost place. As in other situations of loss, however, Fried found that most people manifested remarkable powers of recuperation despite their experience of grief. Readiness for social change was noted (Fried, 1965) as the critical mediating factor in adaptation, and a willingness to cut the strong social ties within the community was noted as a primary indicator of readiness for change. The forces that most directly facilitated assimilation and cultural preparedness for leaving the community were those that promoted social mobility and readiness for transitions in social roles. Further, these evidences of preparedness for change tended to minimize the importance of conditions in the receiving community. Fried did find that objective experiences of improvement with relocation can partly counteract the effects of lack of preparedness for the change. However, objective improvements, whether in residential status, household density, or other living conditions, occurred more frequently for those who were ready to use the relocation situation as an opportunity for maximizing their achievement of goals.

Support for Fried's finding concerning the importance of readiness for change in relation to adjustment is provided by Pedersen and Sullivan's study (1963) of the movement of army families. They examined the effects of geographical mobility and personality factors on emotional disorders in a group of twenty-seven male disturbed and thirty normal male children of regular army officers. They found that, although the groups could not be distinguished with respect to incidence of mobility, parent attitudes relevant to mobility were highly significant. The mothers of normal children scored significantly higher than mothers of disturbed children on the acceptance of mobility scale. No difference was observed for fathers on this scale. In addition, on the identification-satisfaction with military role scale, both mothers and fathers of the normal children scored significantly higher than the corresponding parent in the disturbed group. These data suggest that definable parent attitudes relevant to mobility may serve to mediate stress effects to children.

When a change in residence is not voluntary, the attitude toward the move apparently becomes very important with respect to the adjustment of the migrants or movers. Those who are prepared to move and those who have favorable attitudes toward moving adjust better than those who are not prepared to move and those who are dissatisfied with mobility.

Discussion

In this section of the paper, aspects of migration have been examined in relation to nonpsychiatric indexes of psychological and social adjustment. Some individuals designated maladjusted by these criteria might have been diagnosed mentally ill, had psychiatric evaluations been possible. For the most part, however, the types of disturbance designated by these indexes are less serious. Nevertheless, to the extent that the development of difficulties in psychological and social adjustment is related to the development of mental illness, an understanding of the relationship between migration and adjustment is significant for an understanding of the relationship between migration and mental illness.

With respect to characteristics of sending and receiving communities in relation to the adjustment of migrants, the findings indicate that the mode of orientation into the new community and the length of residence in it are more important than similarity between the two communities. Migrants who rely upon primary groups for their orientation to the new community are more likely to become socially isolated and less likely to be assimilated than those who do not have already established contacts. Length of time in the community, however, is a mediating factor. The longer migrants remain in a community, the more likely they are to become assimilated into it and to be satisfied with it. It is important to note, nevertheless, that there are specific groups for whom similarity between sending and receiving communities is important. The data indicate, for example, that urban-reared, lower socioeconomic status migrants become assimilated into urban areas more readily than rural-reared, lower socioeconomic status migrants.

Comparison with the patient status data reported earlier points to an interesting similarity. The finding that length of residence is negatively associated with social maladjustment is consistent with the negative association reported for length of residence and diagnosed mental illness. There is apparently some initial maladjustment on the part of migrants upon their entrance into the new community. Selection at the point of origin or maladjustment as a result of the migration are possible explanations of these data. With the passage of time, alleviation of the maladjustment occurs. On the one hand, some of the maladjusted and mentally ill may be hospitalized and treated upon their arrival. Some of the maladjusted, on the other hand, may become adjusted with a growing familiarity with the new environment.

With respect to the characteristics of migrants in relation to adjustment, the findings indicate the importance of socioeconomic status, mobility experience, and age. Upper socioeconomic status migrants adjust better than lower socioeconomic status migrants. A moderate amount of mobility appears to aid adjustment, while transiency or high mobility hampers it. The closer the age of migrant children is to the age of the children in the receiving community, the more likely are they to make a good adjustment.

For socioeconomic status and mobility experience, related data concerning patient status are available. Several studies found concentrations of admissions to mental hospitals in lower socioeconomic areas of cities; data concerning characteristics of individuals were unavailable in these studies, however, and it could not be determined what the relationship was for individuals. The present overview indicates that the areal relationship holds for individuals as well, and that there is an inverse relationship between socioeconomic status and maladjustment and mental illness. With respect to amount of mobility, the data concerning migration and adjustment confirm the findings concerning migration and mental illness, that is, that a high amount of mobility is associated with high likelihood of disturbance.

With respect to the circumstances surrounding migration in relation to the adjustment of the migrants, the attitudes of the migrants toward the move appear to be crucial factors. Those migrants who have favorable attitudes toward the move make a better adjustment than those migrants who are not prepared for the move. Similar findings from disparate situations, such as displacement from a leveled slum area and job reassignment, give us some indication of the generality of the importance of attitudes in relation to adjustment to spatial movement. No directly comparable patient status data were available. Nevertheless, it behooves us to note that the attitude findings are in line with the Kleiner and Parker (1965) finding that social psychological factors are significant for an understanding of the consequences of migration for the individual.

SUMMARY

This article reviews and organizes selected research findings and observations concerning internal migration in the United States in relation to mental illness. Studies of various nonpsychiatric indexes of adjustment have been reviewed in addition to studies of psychiatric diagnoses of mental illness. This was done to provide a broader base for an understanding of the relationship between migration and mental illness and to stimulate consideration of many factors that might otherwise be overlooked.

Clearly, there is a relationship between migration and mental illness. The relationship is not a simple one, however. It varies with social characteristics of the migrants, social psychological aspects of the situation surrounding the migration, and characteristics of the sending and receiving communities. In addition, the relationship differs for different indexes of mental illness.

With respect to social characteristics of migrants, the findings of patient status studies indicate that race and sex may be associated with differential occurrence of mental illness in migrant and nonmigrant groups. Studies of various nonpsychiatric indexes of adjustment indicate in addition the importance of socioeconomic status, mobility experience, and age.

With respect to circumstances under which the migration occurs, the patient status studies indicate that social psychological factors such as discrepancy between aspiration and achievement might be differentially associated with the occurrence of mental illness in migrant and nonmigrant groups. Studies of nonpsychiatric indexes of adjustment point in addition to the importance of the attitudes of migrants toward the move.

With respect to characteristics of receiving and sending communities, the patient status studies show variations among the states in the comparative rates of mental illness for migrants and nonmigrants that point to the possible influences of characteristics of places of destination and selection at places of origin. Actual characteristics of areas of destination and selection of migrants at places of origin, however, have not been studied in relation to patient status. Studies of nonpsychiatric indexes of adjustment indicate that the mode of orientation into the new community and the length of residence in it are more important than similarity between the two communities. There are, however, specific groups, lower socioeconomic status migrants for example, for whom similarity between sending and receiving communities is an aid to assimilation and adjustment.

REFERENCES

Andrews, R. B. Urban fringe studies of two Wisconsin cities: A summary. *Journal of Land and Public Utilities Economics,* 1945, **21**, 375–382.

Bedoian, U. H. Social acceptability and social rejection of the under-age, at-age, and over-age pupils in the 6th grade. *Journal of Educational Research,* 1954, **47**, 513–520.

Blackwell, G. W. *The nature of community and methods of community analysis.* Paper prepared for Conference, Study of the Community, Northwestern University, March 1956.

Bogue, D. J. *The population of the United States.* New York: Free Press, 1959.

Burchinal, L. G. How do farm families adjust to city life? *Iowa Farm Science,* 1963, **17**, 6–8.

Burchinal, L. G., & Bauder, W. W. "Adjustments to the new institutional environment. Paper presented at the Conference on Family Mobility in Our Dynamic Society, Iowa State University, October, 1963.

Clausen, J. A., & Kohn, M. Relation of schizophrenia to the social structure of a small city. In B. Pasamanick (Ed.), *Epidemiology of mental disorder.* Washington, D.C.: American Association for Advancement of Science, 1959. Pp. 69–94.

Dewey, R. Peripheral expansion in Milwaukee County. *American Journal of Sociology,* 1948, **54**, 118–125.

Downie, N. M. A comparison between children who have moved from school to school with those who have been in continuous residence on various factors of adjustment. *Journal of Educational Psychology,* 1953, **44**, 50–53.

Elkins, Deborah. Some factors related to choice-status of 90 eighth-grade children in a school society. *Genetic Psychology Monographs,* 1958, **58**, 207–272.

Faris, R. E. L., & Dunham, H. W. *Mental disorders in urban areas.* Chicago: University of Chicago Press, 1939.

Fenichel, O. *The psychoanalytic theory of neurosis.* New York: W. W. Norton & Co., 1945.

Freedman, R. *Recent migration to Chicago.* Chicago: University of Chicago Press, 1950.

Fried, M. Adaptation to social change: Displacement and restitution. Research Memorandum 20, Center for Community Studies, West End Research Project, February, 1963.

Fried, M. Transitional functions of working-class communities: Implications for forced relocation. In M. B. Kantor (Ed.), *Mobility and mental health.* Springfield, Ill.: Charles C Thomas, 1965.

Gans, H. *The urban villagers*. Glencoe, Ill.: The Free Press, 1962.

Gerard, D. L., & Houston, L. G. Family setting and the social ecology of schizophrenia. *Psychiatric Quarterly*, January, 1953, **27**, 90–101.

Gilliland, C. H. *The relationship of pupil mobility to achievement in the elementary school*. Abstract of Research Study No. 1–1958. Ann Arbor, Mich.: University Microfilms, 1959.

Hillery, G. A., Jr. Definitions of community: Areas of agreements. *Rural Sociology*, 1955, **20**, 111–123.

Hollingshead, A. B. Community research: Development and present condition. *American Sociological Review*, 1948, **13**, 136–146.

Hollingshead, A. B., & Redlich, F. C. Schizophrenia and social structure. *American Journal of Psychiatry*, 1954, **110**, 695–701.

Hollingshead, A. B., & Redlich, F. C. Social mobility and mental illness. *American Journal of Psychiatry*, 1955, **112**, 179–186.

Hollingshead, A. B., & Redlich, F. C., *Social class and mental illness*. New York: John Wiley & Sons, 1958.

Jaco, E. G. Social stress and mental illness in the community. In M. B. Sussman (Ed.), *Community structure and analysis*. New York: Thomas Y. Crowell Co., 1959. Pp. 388–409.

Jaco, E. G. *The social epidemiology of mental disorders*. New York: Russell Sage Foundation, 1960.

Joy, G. E., *Some aspects of a moving population—A comparative study of transient children in the Panama Canal Zone schools*. Unpublished M.A. thesis, University of Michigan, 1933.

Kantor, M. B. Some consequences of residential and social mobility for the adjustment of children. In M. B. Kantor (Ed.), *Mobility and mental health*. Springfield, Ill.: Charles C Thomas, 1965.

Kantor, M. B., & Gall, H. S. *A study of some consequences of physical and social mobility for the adjustment of children*. Research proposal, St. Louis County Health Department, Clayton, Mo., 1958.

Kerr, M. A study of social acceptability. *Elementary School Journal*, 1944–1945, **45**, 257–265.

Kiser, C. V. *Sea island to city*. New York: Columbia University Press, 1932.

Kleiner, R., & Parker, S. Migration and mental illness: A new look. *American Sociological Review*, 1959, **24**, 687–690.

Kleiner, R. J., & Parker, S. Goal-striving, social status, and mental disorder: A research review. *American Sociological Review*, 1963, **28**, 189-203.

Kleiner, R. J., & Parker, S. Goal-striving and psychosomatic symptoms in a migrant and non-migrant population. In M. B. Kantor (Ed.), *Mobility and mental health*. Springfield, Ill.: Charles C Thomas, 1965.

Lapouse, R., Monk, M., & Terris, M. The drift hypothesis and socio-economic differentials in schizophrenia. *American Journal of Public Health*, 1956, **46**, 978–986.

Lazarus, J., Locke, B. Z., & Thomas, D. S. Migration differentials in mental disease. *Milbank Memorial Fund Quarterly*, 1963, **41**, 25–42.

Lee, E. S. Migration and mental disease: New York State, 1949–1951. In *Selected Studies of Migration Since World War II*. New York: Milbank Memorial Fund, 1958. Pp. 141–152.

Lee, E. S. Socio-economic and migration differentials in mental disease, New York State, 1949–1961. *Milbank Memorial Fund Quarterly*, 1963, 41, 249–268.

Leybourne, G. Urban adjustment of migrants from the Southern Appalachian Plateaus. *Social Forces*, 1937, 16, 238–246.

Liddle, G. P. *An analysis of the sociometric scores of newcomers*. Unpublished manuscript, Quincy Youth Development Project, Quincy, Ill., 1955.

Locke, B. Z., Kramer, M., & Pasamanick, B. Immigration and insanity. *Public Health Reports*, 1960, 75, 301–306.

Lystad, M. H. Social mobility among selected groups of schizophrenic patients. *American Sociological Review*, 1957, 22, 288–292.

Malzberg, B. Migration and mental disease among Negroes in New York State. *American Journal of Physical Anthropology*, 1936, 21, 107–113.

Malzberg, B. Rates of mental disease among certain population groups in New York State. *Journal of the American Statistical Association*, 1936, 31, 545–548.

Malzberg, B., & Lee, E. *Migration and mental disease*. New York: Social Science Research Council, 1956.

Myers, J. K. Assimilation to the ecological and social systems of a community. *American Sociological Review*, 1950, 15, 367–372.

Omari, T. P. Factors associated with urban adjustment of rural southern migrants. *Social Forces*, 1956, 35, 47–53.

Pasamanick, B., Roberts, D. W., Lemkau, P. W., Krueger, D. B. A survey of mental disease in an urban population: Prevalence by race and income. In B. Pasamanick (Ed.), *Epidemiology of mental disorder*. Washington, D.C.: *American Assn. for Advancement of Science*, 1959, 183–201.

Pedersen, Captain F. A., & Sullivan, Captain E. J. *Effects of geographical mobility and parent personality factors on emotional disorders in children*. Paper read at the 40th annual meeting of the American Orthopsychiatry Association, Washington, D.C., June 1963.

Phillips, E. L., Shenker, S., & Revitz, P. The assimilation of the new child into the group. *Psychiatry*, 1951, 14, 319–325.

Rose, A. M., & Warshay, L. The adjustment of migrants to cities. *Social Forces*, 1957, 36, 72–76.

Sackett, E. B. The effect of moving on educational status of child. *Elementary School Journal*, 1935, 35, 517–526.

Sewell, W. H., & Haller, A. O. Factors in the relationship between social status and the personality adjustment of the child. *American Sociological Review*, 1959, 24, 511–520.

Shryock, H. S. *Population mobility within the United States*. Chicago: Community and Family Study Center, University of Chicago, 1964.

Smith, W. D. *Late school entrance, social acceptance, and children's school achievement*. Unpublished manuscript, Florida State University, 1959.

Smith, W. D. & Demming, J. S. *Pupil mobility and adjustment.* Unpublished manuscript, Florida State University, 1958.

Snipes, W. T. Promotion and moving. *Elementary School Journal,* 1965, 65, 429–433.

Srole, L., Langner, T., Michael, S., Stanley, T., Opler, M. K., & Rennie, T. A. C. *Mental health in the metropolis: The midtown Manhattan study.* New York: McGraw-Hill Book Co., 1962.

Taeuber, C., & Taeuber, I. *The changing population of the U.S.* New York: John Wiley & Sons, 1958.

Tetreau, E. D., & Fuller, V. Some factors associated with the school achievement of children in migrant families. *Elementary School Journal,* 1942, 42, 423–431.

Tietze, C., Lemkau, P., & Cooper, M. Schizophrenia, manic-depressive psychosis, and social-economic status. *American Journal of Sociology,* 1941, 47, 167–175.

Tietze, C., Lemkau, P., & Cooper, M. Personality disorder and spatial mobility. *American Journal of Sociology,* 1942, 48, 29–39.

Tilly, C. Migration to an American city. Agricultural Experiment Station & Division of Urban Affairs, University of Delaware, in cooperation with Farm Population Branch, Economic Research Service, United States Department of Agriculture, 1965.

Wirth, L. *The ghetto.* Chicago: University of Chicago Press, 1928.

3.6   Orientation

As was pointed out by Stanley C. Plog, research in the mental health fields in the United States was completely dominated during the second quarter of this century by Freudian concepts of the individual basis of pathology. A few voices cried out in the wilderness about the necessity of looking at social, cultural, and ethnic determinants of rates of psychosis and styles of pathological behavior, but their cries went largely unnoticed.

One such lonely voice was Benjamin Malzberg. At a time when one risked research oblivion by utilizing concepts of pathology other than those of Freud, Malzberg recognized the opportunity that existed to observe the impact of culture contact and ethnic patterns of living on rates of mental illness in the United States. He patiently sifted through the data on recent and long-term immigrants to the United States, especially persons of European Jewish origin, to determine the effect of a variety of cultural and ethnic independent variables.

The present article represents a summary and some of the conclusions of Malzberg's current work. While relying on new data, the chapter largely confirms his earlier findings. The flavor and excitement of his early discoveries are present as we see how social systems of complex societies have an effect on society's participants. Thus, the possibility of an individual's experiencing a psychotic episode is dependent not only upon the combination of societal pressures and strains impinging upon him, but also the psychological strengths and weaknesses he has developed as a result of having been reared within a particular ethnic or subcultural group.

3.6   Are Immigrants Psychologically Disturbed?

Benjamin Malzberg

ALL FIRST ADMISSIONS

It is generally held that migrant populations have a higher incidence of mental illness than nonmigrants, whether migration be of external or internal origin (Malzberg & Lee, 1956). Internal migrants differ from immigrants by being more homogeneous. They are usually of the same race and national origin; they speak the same language; and they share a common overall culture. Yet there are stresses to which immigrants are subjected that are similar in many respects to those experienced by internal migrants. We know, for example, that in Canada those of French-Canadian origin have, in general, lower incidence rates of mental illness than Canadians of British origin. They have a lower incidence than the British in Quebec, yet their incidence is higher in Ontario. Among themselves, French-Canadians have a lower incidence in Quebec than in Ontario. Similarly, the British have a lower incidence in Ontario than in Quebec (Malzberg, 1964). It is apparent that where migrants are a minority, they tend to have higher rates of mental illness than in their places of origin. If, then, this is characteristic of native-born internal migrants, it must also be true of foreign-born. It is not surprising therefore that immigrants were usually reported as having higher rates of mental illness than indigenous populations.

There were no large-scale investigations of the relative frequency of mental illness among native and foreign-born in the United States prior to the report of the Bureau of the Census that dealt with "insane" in hospitals on December 31, 1903, and admissions during 1904 (*Insane*, 1906). Previous studies, based upon limited coverage, all reported higher rates for the foreign-born, but made no corrections for the obvious differences with respect to the age distributions of the two populations. Since the mentally ill were almost all aged 10 years or over, the census report of 1904 presented comparisons based upon the white population of the United States aged 10 and over in 1900. On this basis, the native-born, who included 80.5 percent of the white population, represented only 70.2 percent of the total admissions. The foreign-born, however, represented 29.8 percent of the admissions, but only 19.5 percent of the total population. It was concluded, therefore, that the "insane" were more numerous among the foreign-born whites than among the native-born.

But such a comparison could hardly be considered conclusive, since it disregarded completely the difference in age distribution above the lower limit of 10 years. This was corrected in the next report of the Bureau of the Census, dealing with total admissions to all hospitals for mental disease in the United States during 1910 (*Insane,* 1914). It was shown that native whites had an admission rate of 57.9 per 100,000, compared with 116.3 for foreign-born whites, the latter being in excess by 100 percent. But when the rate for foreign-born was recomputed on the basis of the age distribution of the native white population in 1910, the rate for the former was reduced to 70 per 100,000, compared with 57.9 for the native white, an excess of only 21 percent, compared with 100 percent on the basis of crude rates (*Insane,* 1914).

But the report recognized that there were other factors related to the relative differences in rates. Some of these were demographic, such as the difference in sex distribution, in geographic distribution, and in degree of concentration in cities. Other differences were social and psychological. "The change of environment which the immigrants experience in coming to the United States must have an important influence. Without doubt the strain to which they are subjected in the effort to adjust themselves to new physical, economic and social conditions in a strange land tends to increase insanity, but the influence of this factor cannot be segregated or measured on the basis of available statistics" (*Insane,* 1914, p. 27).

This report formed the basis of the discussion of immigration and mental illness in Vol. II of the Report of the United States Immigration Commission (*Reports,* 1913). No new data were added, so that the statistical conclusions remained as before.

In 1922, the Committee on Immigration and Naturalization of the House of Representatives, sixty-seventh Congress, received a statement by Harry H. Laughlin, which was published as "Analysis of America's Modern Melting Pot" (Hearings, 1923). In effect, this report ended with the conclusion that after all possible allowances for shocks or strains associated with immigration, the newer generation of immigrants had higher incidence rates of mental illness than the native-born.

It is not necessary to indicate the numerous fallacies in this investigation. They are discussed in detail elsewhere (Malzberg, 1940). But it must be made clear that such a comparison based upon admissions to selected mental hospitals spread throughout the United States introduced a bias against foreign-born which could not be corrected statistically.

In seeking a better and more legitimate basis for such comparisons, we shall utilize data of first admissions to hospitals for mental illness both public and private, in New York State. The great advantage of New York for such a comparison lies in the large population from which such data are derived, uniformly, completely, and without selective bias. It is true that such statistics do not include the growing number of community clinics, nor do they include the mentally ill who are treated privately. One might go further and point to the unknown total of mentally ill who receive no treatment at all. It is suggested, therefore, that the incidence of hospitalized cases is not necessarily a correct picture of the relative distribution of mental disease among the components of the general population.

But far from clarifying the issue, the introduction of statistics of non-hospitalized cases would introduce errors of measurement that cannot be determined accurately, and cannot be submitted to correction. For example, the comparative incidence of the psychoneuroses cannot be measured on the basis of admissions to clinics, because ethnic groups differ widely in the importance they attach to such disorders and in their willingness to apply for treatment.

There is a range of mental illness from the least to the most disabling. The lower part of the range differs in social consequences from the severely disabling disorders at the other end of the range. The latter, which require hospitalization, are the more immediate concern of society. In effect, therefore, comparisons of relative incidence of mental illness are most fruitful when they are based upon admissions to hospitals for long-term treatment of mental disease in states with liberal policies affecting admission to, and discharge from, such hospitals.

In basing incidence upon first admissions to hospitals, public and private, we are studying those conditions of mental illness that are of the deepest concern to society. We are in agreement, therefore, with Greenwood and Yule, when they state "We do not see why objections which no sensible man would allow to influence him in the ordinary affairs of life should suddenly acquire scientific importance when the question is one of interpreting statistics."

In 1910, native-born constituted 69.8 percent of the population of New York State, but only 52.6 percent of first admissions to the civil state hospitals for mental disease. Thus, native-born reached only 75 percent of their expected quota of first admissions. But the foreign-born included 30.2 percent of the general population and 47.4 percent of the first admissions, and therefore exceeded their quota by 57 percent. Thereafter, due primarily to changes in the immigration laws, the native-born constituted a growing proportion of the total population of New York State, and the foreign-born decreased steadily. In 1960, the percentages were 86.4 and 13.6 for native and foreign-born, respectively. Throughout this period, foreign-born included an excess number of first admissions to mental hospitals, in comparison with the expected quotas. The native-born showed a deficiency of such admissions. It appeared, therefore, that foreign-born had a relatively greater frequency of first admissions than native-born throughout the period from 1910 to 1960. It should be noted, however, that whereas the relative excess by foreign-born, as thus measured, held constant at approximately 60 percent, native-born first admissions increased relatively throughout the period, growing from 75 percent of the expected total in 1910 to 91 percent in 1960.

However, these trends, though suggestive of relative differences, are not given in sufficient detail to afford conclusive evidence. The first detailed analysis of such data for New York State was based upon first admissions to all mental hospitals, public and private during the fiscal years 1929 to 1931, inclusive (Malzberg, 1940). During this period, native-born whites had an average annual rate of 58.7 first admissions per 100,000 population. Foreign-born whites had a rate of 115.1, an excess over native whites of 96 percent; standardized with respect to age and sex, the excess was reduced to 19 percent. However, the statistics of the private hospitals included only the committed cases. The great majority of such admissions were on a voluntary basis, and represented 70 percent of the total. The voluntary admissions were almost all native-born. Hence, if the native-born first admissions were adjusted to include the voluntary admissions to private hospitals, the addition of such admissions would raise the standardized rate for native-born by approximately 10 percent, and thus reduce the relative excess of the foreign-born rate to only 8 percent. That this revision is reasonable may be verified by considering the differences between native and foreign-born during 1939–1941 (Mental Disease, 1955).

During 1941, the statistical reporting system of the New York State Department of Mental Hygiene was improved by requiring the inclusion of all first admissions to the licensed private hospitals, whether voluntary or involuntary. By adjusting the totals for 1939 and 1940 in accordance with the experience of 1941, it was possible to obtain complete totals of first admissions to all mental hospitals, public and private. During 1939–1941, there were 27,530 native white and 15,033 foreign-born white first admissions. The average annual rates of first admissions per 100,000 population were 91.8 and 175.1 for native and foreign-born, respectively, an excess by the latter of 91 percent. However, when standardized with respect to age and sex, the relative difference was reduced to 14 percent. A further correction was made by standardizing with respect to the urban-rural distribution of the two populations, in addition to holding the factors of age and sex constant. This reduced the relative excess of the rate of foreign-born to only 2 percent.

A similar comparison was made for 1949–1951 (Mental Disease, 1964). During this period, the average annual rates of first admissions to all hospitals for mental illness were 103.9 and 213.8 per 100,000 for native and foreign-born whites, respectively. The latter was in excess by 106 percent. But when standardized for age and sex, the excess by foreign-born fell to 18 percent. Because the additional data were not available, it was not possible to adjust for the urban-rural ratios during this period. However, an approximation was made by limiting the comparison to New York City. This resulted in reducing the excess to only 9 percent. Thus, between 1930 and 1950, the incidence of mental illness in New York was higher for foreign-born than for native-born, but the relative differences were so low as to be of only limited statistical significance.

The experience of Canada lends support to the conclusions derived from the data for New York State (Mental Disease, 1963). For the period 1950–1952, inclusive, the average annual crude rate of the foreign-born exceeded that for native-born by 75 percent. When the rates were adjusted for age and sex proportions, the excess was reduced to 23 percent. But the two populations were not distributed uniformly throughout Canada, and this affected the rate for foreign-born adversely, because they were concentrated largely in the more urbanized, eastern provinces. Hence, the analysis was restricted to the province of Ontario. It is significant therefore that the excess of the crude rate of the foreign-born over that for native-born was reduced to 46 percent, and when standardized, as for all Canada, the excess was reduced to 10 percent. But even within Ontario, the comparison was vitiated because of the relative excess of foreign-born in Toronto. Limiting the comparisons to this city, we found the "crude" rate of the foreign-born in excess by 29 percent. And when standardized, the excess fell to only 4 percent. This is not a statistically significant difference, and we are justified in concluding that the native and foreign-born populations did not differ significantly with respect to the relative incidence of mental disease.

These comparisons for New York State and Canada may be completed by the following detailed analysis of first admissions during 1960–1961 to all hospitals for mental disease in New York State. During these two fiscal years, there were 40,221 white first admissions to all hospitals for mental disease in New York State, of whom 31,239, or 77.7 percent, were native-born and 8,982, or 22.3 percent, were foreign-born. The percentages for the corresponding general populations were 85.7 and 14.3, respectively. This implies a relative excess of first admissions by foreign-born amounting to 56 percent, whereas the native-born had a deficiency of 9.4 percent. The average annual rates per 100,000 were 119.2 for native-born, and 205.8 for foreign-born. The latter was in excess by 73 percent.

But examination of the age distributions of the two populations shows that the excess was closely associated with the more advanced ages of the foreign-born. The median ages were 29.3 and 57.3 for native and foreign-born, respectively. Those under age 15 included only 3.5 percent of the foreign-born, but 31.2 percent of the native-born. At all ages under 45, the native-born population was in relative excess, where as the foreign-born were in significantly higher proportions at all higher ages. Since the rates of first admissions have relatively little significance at ages under 15, but are highest at advanced ages, it is obvious that the crude rates were weighted favorably for the native-born.

Actually, beginning with ages 15 to 19, the age-specific rates of the native-born were higher up to age 70. Beyond the latter age, the difference was not significant (see Table 1). The comparison held for each sex, but, in general, the relative excess of the native-born was higher among males.

The relative differences between the sexes varied significantly according to nativity (see Table 2). Excluding the age interval from 30 to 49,

TABLE 1. White First Admissions to All Hospitals for Mental Illness in New York State, 1960–1961, Classified According to Nativity

Age (years)	Native-born					Foreign-born				
	Males	Females	Total No.	Total %	Average annual rate per 100,000	Males	Females	Total No.	Total %	Average annual rate per 100,000
Under 15	684	219	903	2.9	11.1	17	10	27	0.3	17.6
15–19	1,187	876	2,063	6.6	106.4	40	30	70	0.8	99.6
20–24	1,357	1,110	2,467	7.9	160.7	69	63	132	1.4	117.1
25–29	1,290	1,323	2,613	8.4	156.9	88	121	209	2.3	146.2
30–34	1,308	1,504	2,812	9.0	149.3	104	143	247	2.8	130.0
35–39	1,290	1,462	2,752	8.8	141.9	137	161	298	3.3	124.0
40–44	1,226	1,396	2,622	8.4	139.8	104	127	231	2.6	114.7
45–49	1,104	1,232	2,336	7.4	134.6	131	211	342	3.8	107.1
50–54	1,003	1,054	2,057	6.6	138.1	225	288	513	5.7	114.7
55–59	945	922	1,867	6.0	154.7	272	331	603	6.7	107.6
60–64	797	765	1,562	5.0	162.9	362	399	761	8.4	134.4
65–69	760	809	1,569	5.0	211.6	455	504	959	10.7	181.1
70–74	674	841	1,515	4.8	297.9	679	589	1,268	14.1	302.1
75 and over	1,592	2,509	4,101	13.1	721.0	1,509	1,813	3,322	37.0	809.8
Total	15,217	16,022	31,239	100.0	119.2	4,192	4,790	8,982	100.0	205.8

TABLE 2. AVERAGE ANNUAL RATES OF WHITE FIRST ADMISSIONS TO ALL HOSPITALS FOR MENTAL ILLNESS IN NEW YORK STATE, 1960–1961, PER 100,000 POPULATION, CLASSIFIED ACCORDING TO AGE AND NATIVITY

Age (years)	Males			Females		
	Native-born	Foreign-born	Ratio	Native-born	Foreign-born	Ratio
Under 15	16.4	21.9	0.74	5.4	13.2	0.41
15–19	124.8	122.7	1.02	88.7	79.7	1.11
20–24	187.0	146.1	1.28	137.1	96.2	1.43
25–29	157.6	137.7	1.14	156.3	153.2	1.02
30–34	142.3	119.0	1.20	156.1	139.3	1.12
35–39	137.5	121.2	1.13	146.0	126.5	1.15
40–44	136.9	110.4	1.24	142.4	118.4	1.20
45–49	132.0	88.9	1.48	137.0	122.8	1.12
50–54	138.9	105.0	1.32	137.4	123.7	1.11
55–59	163.3	96.7	1.69	146.8	118.5	1.24
60–64	178.9	131.2	1.36	149.1	137.6	1.08
65–69	234.2	175.4	1.34	193.9	186.6	1.04
70–74	321.3	325.0	0.99	281.7	279.3	1.01
75 and over	754.3	785.3	0.96	701.3	831.4	0.84
Total	119.4	200.0	0.60	119.0	211.2	0.56

native-born males had significantly higher rates of first admissions than native-born females. But among the foreign-born, females had higher rates than males at all ages beyond 24. This agrees with the long-held opinion that *immigration introduces a more difficult process of adjustment for females.*

In view of the differences between native- and foreign-born with respect to age and sex proportions, the rates were standardized. These became 179.4 and 160.8 per 100,000 for native and foreign-born, respectively. The former was in excess by 12 percent. Thus, an excess of 73 percent by foreign-born on the basis of crude rates was revised, after adjustments for age and sex proportions, to produce an excess by native-born.

Native-born males had a higher rate than foreign-born in the ratio of 1.19 to 1 (see Table 3). The corresponding ratio among females was 1.07 to 1. We may again note the difference according to sex in each nativity group. Thus, the standardized rate for native males exceeded that for native females by 8 percent. Among foreign-born, on the contrary, the rate for females was in excess by 3 percent.

TABLE 3. Average Annual Standardized[a] Rates of White First Admissions
to All Hospitals for Mental Illness in New York State, 1960–1961,
per 100,000 Population, Classified According to Nativity

	Native-born	Foreign-born	Ratio
Males	182.4	153.7	1.19
Females	169.2	158.2	1.07
Total	179.4	160.8	1.12

[a] White population of New York State, aged 15 years and over on April 1, 1960 (in
intervals of 5 years), taken as standard.

The incidence of mental illness is affected by the distribution of the
population with respect to urban-rural distribution. In general, the rate
is significantly higher for the urban population. The urban population
was defined by the Bureau of Census in 1960 as comprising all persons
living in places of 2500 or more incorporated in cities, boroughs, and
villages, and the densely settled urban fringe, whether incorporated or
unincorporated, of such urbanized areas (United States, 1961). On this
basis, 94.1 percent of the foreign-born population lived in urban areas,
compared with 82.6 percent of the native-born. Furthermore, of the urban
populations, only 47.8 percent of the native-born, lived in New York City,

TABLE 4. White Urban First Admissions to All Hospitals
for Mental Illness in New York State, 1960–1961,
Classified According to Nativity

Age (years)	Native-born					Foreign-born				
			Total		Average annual rate per 100,000			Total		Average annual rate per 100,000
	Males	Females	No.	%		Males	Females	No.	%	
Under 15	638	204	842	3.1	12.8	17	10	27	0.3	19.0
15–19	1,057	749	1,806	6.7	112.9	36	29	65	0.8	98.9
20–24	1,200	969	2,169	8.0	161.7	68	57	125	1.5	115.6
25–29	1,145	1,134	2,279	8.4	163.0	85	112	197	2.4	145.4
30–34	1,158	1,306	2,464	9.1	157.1	100	128	228	2.7	127.6
35–39	1,090	1,274	2,364	8.7	145.8	133	151	284	3.4	125.9
40–44	1,046	1,199	2,245	8.3	141.7	98	122	220	2.6	116.1
45–49	949	1,079	2,028	7.4	138.2	124	197	321	3.8	106.4
50–54	872	935	1,807	6.7	143.6	215	273	488	5.8	115.8
55–59	832	813	1,645	6.1	162.0	253	308	561	6.7	105.7
60–64	678	675	1,353	5.0	170.3	345	370	715	8.5	133.4
65–69	642	710	1,352	5.0	224.7	423	475	898	10.7	179.9
70–74	572	729	1,301	4.8	322.1	628	541	1,169	14.0	297.0
75 and over	1,275	2,151	3,426	12.7	782.6	1,413	1,657	3,070	36.7	807.0
Total	13,154	13,927	27,081	100.0	125.0	3,938	4,430	8,368	100.0	203.7

TABLE 5. Average Annual Rates of Urban First Admissions to All Hospitals
for Mental Illness in New York State, 1960–1961, per 100,000
Population, Classified According to Age and Nativity

Age (years)	Males			Females		
	Native-born	Foreign-born	Ratio	Native-born	Foreign-born	Ratio
Under 15	19.0	23.7	0.80	6.3	14.2	0.44
15–19	136.3	118.4	1.15	90.6	82.1	1.10
20–24	196.3	149.6	1.31	139.6	90.9	1.54
25–29	166.3	138.9	1.20	159.7	150.8	1.06
30–34	151.8	120.7	1.26	162.1	133.6	1.21
35–39	140.0	124.7	1.12	151.0	126.9	1.19
40–44	140.0	110.4	1.27	143.3	121.2	1.18
45–49	135.7	89.2	1.52	140.3	121.3	1.16
50–54	144.6	106.7	1.36	142.7	124.0	1.15
55–59	173.4	95.2	1.82	151.8	116.2	1.31
60–64	177.2	132.3	1.34	156.2	134.4	1.16
65–69	251.0	173.8	1.44	205.2	185.7	1.11
70–74	357.6	322.3	1.11	298.8	272.1	1.10
75 and over	829.7	795.5	1.04	757.1	817.0	0.93
Total	126.0	199.9	0.63	124.1	207.2	0.60

compared with 71.3 percent of the foreign-born. It is evident, therefore, that if greater concentration of population affects the incidence of mental illness adversely, the effect will be greater in the case of foreign-born.

During 1960–1961, there were 35,449 urban first admissions to all mental hospitals, of whom 76.4 percent were native and 23.6 percent

TABLE 6. Average Annual Standardized[a] Urban Rates
of White First Admissions to All Hospitals for Mental Illness
in New York State, 1960–1961, per 100,000 Population,
Classified According to Nativity

	Native-born	Foreign-born	Ratio
Males	193.3	154.5	1.25
Females	175.7	155.1	1.13
Total	188.1	159.9	1.18

[a] White population of New York State, aged 15 years and over on April 1, 1960 (in intervals of 5 years), taken as standard.

were foreign-born (see Table 4). The percentages for the corresponding general populations were 84.1 and 15.9, respectively, implying an excess of foreign-born first admissions of 44 percent. The corresponding excess for the entire state was 60 percent. The average annual urban rates per 100,000 were 203.7 and 125.0 for foreign- and native-born, respectively, an excess of 63 percent for the foreign-born. The relative excess for the entire state was 73 percent. But again we must consider the differences among the native and foreign-born populations with respect to age and sex differences. Comparable age-specific rates were significantly higher for the native-born (see Table 5). Standardized rates are therefore summarized in Table 6.

Because of the heavy concentration of foreign-born in urban areas, their standardized rate did not differ significantly from that for the entire state. But the urban rates for the native-born were markedly higher. Therefore, a relative excess of 12 percent by the native-born increased to 18 percent, when the comparisons were limited to the urbanized sections of the general populations. Comparison by sex showed similar relative excess by the native-born.

We proceed next to a comparison of the rural populations. Following the definitions of the Bureau of Census, we exclude the urbanized areas, and consider the remainder as rural. During 1960–1961 there were 4772 rural first admissions to all mental hospitals, of whom 4158, or 87.1 per-

TABLE 7. White Rural First Admissions to All Hospitals
for Mental Illness in New York State, 1960–1961,
Classified According to Nativity

Age (years)	Native-born					Foreign-born				
			Total		Average annual rate per 100,000			Total		Average annual rate per 100,000
	Males	Females	No.	%		Males	Females	No.	%	
Under 15	46	15	61	1.5	3.9	—	—	—	—	—
15–19	130	127	257	6.2	76.5	4	1	5	0.8	109.7
20–24	157	141	298	7.2	129.5	1	6	7	1.1	152.4
25–29	145	189	334	8.0	125.2	3	9	12	2.0	161.1
30–34	150	198	348	8.4	110.7	4	15	19	3.1	168.0
35–39	200	188	388	9.3	122.2	4	10	14	2.3	95.1
40–44	180	197	377	9.1	129.3	6	5	11	1.8	91.9
45–49	155	153	308	7.4	115.2	7	14	21	3.4	118.1
50–54	131	119	250	6.0	108.1	10	15	25	4.1	97.4
55–59	113	109	222	5.3	116.2	19	23	42	6.8	140.4
60–64	119	90	209	5.0	127.3	17	29	46	7.5	152.9
65–69	118	99	217	5.2	155.1	32	29	61	9.9	201.4
70–74	102	112	214	5.1	204.7	51	48	99	16.1	379.6
75 and over	317	358	675	16.2	515.1	96	156	252	41.0	845.8
Total	2,063	2,095	4,158	100.0	91.3	254	360	614	100.0	240.1

TABLE 8. Average Annual Rates of White Rural First Admissions
to All Hospitals for Mental Illness in New York State, 1960–1961,
per 100,000 Population, Classified According to Age and Nativity

Age (years)	Males			Females		
	Native-born	Foreign-born	Ratio	Native-born	Foreign-born	Ratio
Under 15	5.7	—	—	2.0	—	—
15–19	74.0	181.8	0.41	79.2	42.4	1.87
20–24	137.1	56.0	2.44	122.0	213.8	0.57
25–29	111.4	111.1	1.00	138.3	187.6	0.74
30–34	95.9	88.7	1.08	125.4	220.7	0.57
35–39	125.2	62.2	2.01	119.3	120.7	0.99
40–44	121.5	110.6	1.10	137.4	76.4	1.80
45–49	113.1	84.3	1.34	117.3	147.7	0.79
50–54	109.8	77.7	1.41	106.3	117.3	0.91
55–59	114.5	121.1	0.94	117.9	161.6	0.73
60–64	143.0	111.4	1.28	111.2	195.6	0.57
65–69	171.7	200.4	0.86	139.1	202.5	0.69
70–74	204.6	363.3	0.56	204.8	298.6	0.69
75 and over	552.3	660.4	0.84	486.2	1,022.3	0.48
Total	89.5	201.8	0.44	93.1	277.1	0.34

cent, were native, and 614, or 12.9 percent, were foreign-born (see Table 7). Of the corresponding general rural population, 94.7 percent were native and 5.3 percent were foreign-born. Thus, the latter exceeded their quota by 143 percent, whereas the native-born reached only 92 percent of their quota. The average annual rates per 100,000 were 240.1 and 91.3 for foreign- and native-born, respectively, the former being in excess by 163 percent. Unlike the urban population, the rural foreign-born population had a higher rate than the native-born. When we compare age-specific rates (see Table 7), we may observe that native-born have generally lower rates throughout the age range. But this was due primarily to the contrast between females (see Table 8). With two exceptions, native-born females had significantly lower rates. Among males, the trend varied with age. Thus, below age 55, native males had higher rates than the foreign-born. They had lower rates at ages 55 and over.

If we standardize the rates, we find no significant difference among males with respect to nativity (see Table 9). But the rate for foreign-born females was in excess by 43 percent. Although there was no significant sex difference among native-born, the rate for foreign-born females ex-

TABLE 9. AVERAGE ANNUAL STANDARDIZED[a] RATES
OF WHITE RURAL FIRST ADMISSIONS TO ALL HOSPITALS
FOR MENTAL ILLNESS IN NEW YORK STATE, 1960–1961,
PER 100,000 POPULATION, CLASSIFIED ACCORDING TO NATIVITY

	Native-born	Foreign-born	Ratio
Males	136.8	137.8	0.99
Females	135.9	194.7	0.70
Total	139.2	173.7	0.80

[a] White population of New York State, aged 15 years and over on April 1, 1960 (in intervals of 5 years), taken as standard.

ceeded that for males by 41 percent. Clearly, rural life in New York State was a severe experience for foreign-born females. Because of their high rate, the total standardized rate for foreign-born, exceeded that for native-born by 24 percent, in contrast to a higher rate for urban native-born.

We now make a final comparison of rates of first admissions, by standardizing simultaneously for age, sex, and urban-rural proportions. The results are summarized in Table 10. Despite the high rate for the rural females of foreign birth, the native-born had a higher standardized rate than foreign-born. The rates were 179.4 and 161.7, respectively, an excess of 11 percent by the native-born. The excess was especially marked among males. But even among females, the rate for native-born was in excess by 4 percent.

Another factor of importance in relation to the incidence of mental illness is the distribution of the population with respect to social status. A decisive factor appears to be position on the economic ladder. Admis-

TABLE 10. AVERAGE ANNUAL STANDARDIZED[a] RATES OF WHITE FIRST ADMISSIONS
TO ALL HOSPITALS FOR MENTAL ILLNESS IN NEW YORK STATE,
1960–1961, PER 100,000 POPULATION,
CLASSIFIED ACCORDING TO NATIVITY

	Native-born	Foreign-born	Ratio
Males	183.6	152.1	1.21
Females	168.8	161.8	1.04
Total	179.4	161.7	1.11

[a] White population of New York State, aged 15 years and over, classified according to urban-rural distribution on April 1, 1960 (in intervals of 5 years), taken as standard.

sions to mental hospitals have been classified in broad economic categories as being in dependent, marginal, or comfortable circumstances (New York State,1943). "Dependent" is defined as lacking in the necessities of life or receiving aid from public funds or persons outside the immediate family. By "comfortable" is meant having accumulated resources sufficient to maintain self and family for at least four months. "Marginal" constitutes the remaining population, which fluctuates between self-support and dependency. It has been shown that the dependent class has the highest rate of first admissions to mental hospitals and that the rate is lowest in the comfortable class (Malzberg, 1963a). It is therefore significant that of foreign-born white first admissions in New York State during 1949–1951, 31.1 percent were in dependent economic circumstances, compared with 20.7 percent of native-born white first admissions. The percentages in the comfortable class varied in the reverse order, being 21.7 and 15.6 for native- and foreign-born respectively. Hence, we may infer that an additional standardization of rates of first admissions on the basis of economic status would result in a further reduction of the rate for foreign-born and an increase for native-born. Unfortunately, the statistical data permitting such an adjustment are not available. But comparisons of populations in limited areas (New Haven, Connecticut, for example) confirms this conclusion (Hollingshead & Redlich, 1958).

Comparisons of native- and foreign-born have considered the latter as an entity. But in so doing, we have arrived at an average result. The foreign-born are of varied origins, and their incidence of mental illness varies accordingly.

Comparative data are available for 1950 (see Table 11). In that year,

TABLE 11. Average Annual Standardized[a] Rates of White First Admissions to All Hospitals for Mental Illness in New York State, 1949–1951, per 100,000 Population, Classified According to Nativity and Parentage

	Foreign-born			Native-born of foreign parentage			Ratio		
	Males	Females	Total	Males	Females	Total	Males	Females	Total
England	138.8	137.2	140.7	158.9	142.3	157.3	0.87	0.96	0.89
Ireland	240.7	216.9	231.7	228.4	194.3	220.2	1.05	1.12	1.05
Germany	157.3	175.5	169.4	144.2	147.2	152.4	1.09	1.19	1.11
Poland	167.3	207.6	191.3	151.9	146.1	155.5	1.10	1.42	1.23
Russia	169.8	153.0	164.1	160.2	146.9	157.1	1.06	1.04	1.04
Italy	146.2	130.4	141.3	139.2	102.8	114.6	1.05	1.27	1.23
All foreign-born	168.2	180.5	178.7	190.8	160.4	178.4	0.88	1.13	1.00

[a] White population of New York State, aged 15 years and over on April 1, 1950 (in intervals of 5 years), taken as standard.

the foreign-born white population of New York State totaled 2,500,429. The largest total, 503,175, came from Italy. Russia followed with 353,835. The nationalities next in order were Germany, 270,661; Poland, 254,065; Ireland (Eire), 182,581; England and Wales, 104,875. Together these nationalities included 1,669,192, or 67 percent of the total of foreign-born in New York State in 1950.

During 1949–1951, the average annual standardized rate of foreign-born white first admissions to all hospitals for mental illness in New York State was 178.7 per 100,000. But the rates varied from 140.7 for those born in England and 141.3 for those born in Italy to a maximum of 231.7 for those born in Ireland. There is a consistency in these comparisons, for the English and Italians have always had low rates of admissions, as shown by census reports, and the Irish have always shown the highest incidence (*Insane*, 1914, p. 31). There is a further confirmation of the distribution of rates for English and Italian born, as similar results occurred in Canada during 1950–1952 (Malzberg, unpublished manuscript). It is noteworthy that the English, who represent the older type of immigration from western Europe, and the Italians, who represent the newer immigration, both had lower rates than the average of 152.0 for all native-born whites in New York State during 1949–1951. Natives of Poland had the high rate of 191.3. Immigrants from Poland consisted of two different ethnic streams, Slavic and Jewish. It is known that the average rate of first admissions for Jews is less than the average for the entire white population of New York State (Malzberg, 1960, 1963b). We therefore infer that the high rate for immigrants from Poland must be attributed to the Slavic element. Similarly, the rate for Russia, 164.1, is less than the average for all foreign-born in New York State. But as with Poland, this must be attributed to the relatively low rate for Jews, who constitute the majority of Russian-born immigrants.

There is no evidence, therefore, for the establishing of invidious comparisons between immigrants from western and those from eastern and southern Europe in relation to the incidence of mental disease. Rates may be high, as for the Irish or Slavs, or they may be low, as for English, Italian, and Jews. Germans, with a relatively low rate of 169.4, were in the middle of the range between high and low.

Thus, the fact of ethnic origin does not explain the varying distribution of the incidence of mental illness in New York State. This conclusion is supported by the comparison of annual rates of first admissions among native-born of foreign parentage. The average rate for all native-born of foreign parentage was 178.4 per 100,000. But the lowest rate, 114.6, occurred among native-born of Italian parentage. The highest, 220.2, occurred among native-born of Irish parentage. The native-born of Polish and Russian parentage, predominantly Jews, also had rates well below the average.

We may also note that with the exception of English, the native-born of foreign parentage all had lower rates than the parental generations. Since the ethnic factor is presumably constant, it must be inferred that the variations between the two generations are due to external factors of environmental origin.

SCHIZOPHRENIA

It has been shown that over a long period (1930 to 1950), the over-all rates of first admissions to all mental hospitals in New York State did not differ significantly as between native- and foreign-born. In 1960–1961, in fact, the foreign-born had a lower rate. Detailed investigations for 1949–1951, showed that some foreign-born groups had lower standardized rates for mental disorders of organic origin. But there is a marked difference with respect to so-called functional disorders, especially schizophrenia (dementia praecox).

During 1929–1931, the average annual rates of first admissions for schizophrenia to all public and licensed private hospitals for mental illness in New York State were 15.2 and 30.2 per 100,000 for native and foreign-born whites, respectively, the latter being in excess in the ratio of 2 to 1. When standardized, however, the relative excess was reduced to 48 percent. In considering all first admissions, we adjusted for the omission of voluntary first admissions to private mental hospitals, which resulted in reducing the relative excess of the foreign-born to approximately 8 percent. A similar correction may be made with respect to schizophrenia, which reduced the excess to 38 percent.

A better comparison was possible during 1939–1941, because of better reporting by the private mental hospitals. During these years, the average annual rates of first admissions for schizophrenia were 24.9 and 30.7 per 100,000 for native- and foreign-born, respectively, an excess by the latter of 23 percent. When standardized with respect to age and sex, the excess increased to 39 percent. Introduction of a correction for the urban-rural ratios reduced the relative excess to 27 percent.

During 1949–1951, the crude rate of first admissions for schizophrenia among the native-born exceeded that of the foreign-born by 20 percent. But when the correction was made for age and sex differentials, this was reversed and the foreign-born rate was in excess by 28 percent.

The corresponding experience of Canada agrees closely with that of New York State. During 1950–1952, inclusive, the crude rate of first admissions for schizophrenia in Canada among foreign-born exceeded that of native-born by 58 percent. When standardized with respect to age and sex, the excess increased to 77 percent. Some attention was given to the question of degree of urbanization, by limiting the comparison to the province of Ontario. The excess of the standardized rate for foreign-born was reduced to 40 percent. By limiting the comparison still further to Toronto, the excess was reduced to 24 percent (Malzberg, 1963a).

Thus, it appears that foreign-born had significantly higher rates than native-born with respect to the frequency of schizophrenia. Subsequent data for New York State also show a higher incidence for foreign-born, but the relative difference in comparison with native-born was reduced.

Schizophrenia constituted the largest group of admissions to hospitals for mental illness in New York State. Such first admissions in 1960–1961 represented 25.6 percent of the total white first admissions. But this varied with nativity, being higher for native than for foreign-born, largely because of the age factor. There were 10,355 white first admissions for schizophrenia during 1960–1961, of whom 9182, or 88.7 percent, were native-born, and 1173, or 11.3 percent, were foreign-born. The percentages for the corresponding general populations were 85.8 and 14.3, respectively. In contrast to all first admissions, the foreign-born had less than their expected quota for schizophrenia, whereas the native-born were in excess. The average annual rates per 100,000 were 35.0 for native-born and 26.9 for foreign-born.

But, whereas the age distribution of the foreign-born raised their

TABLE 12. White First Admissions for Schizophrenia to All Hospitals for Mental Illness in New York State, 1960–1961, Classified According to Nativity

Age (years)	Native-born					Foreign-born				
	Males	Females	Total No.	%	Average annual rate per 100,000	Males	Females	Total No.	%	Average annual rate per 100,000
Under 15	243	91	334	3.6	4.1	8	3	11	0.9	7.2
15–19	488	396	884	9.6	45.6	21	20	41	3.5	58.3
20–24	779	627	1,406	15.3	91.6	53	44	97	8.3	86.0
25–29	681	769	1,450	15.8	87.1	69	79	148	12.6	103.6
30–34	646	811	1,457	15.9	77.4	79	82	161	13.7	84.7
35–39	535	707	1,242	13.5	64.0	86	89	175	14.9	72.8
40–44	426	590	1,016	11.1	54.2	54	61	115	9.8	57.1
45–49	280	354	634	6.9	36.5	49	65	114	9.7	35.7
50–54	151	189	340	3.7	22.8	45	64	109	9.3	24.4
55–59	104	120	224	2.4	18.6	24	50	74	6.3	13.2
60–64	45	65	110	1.2	11.4	25	29	54	4.6	9.5
65–69	15	44	59	0.6	8.0	17	25	42	3.6	7.9
70–74	5	9	14	0.2	2.8	12	8	20	1.7	4.8
75 and over	4	8	12	0.1	2.1	5	7	12	1.0	2.9
Total	4,402	4,780	9,182	100.0	35.0	547	626	1,173	100.0	26.9

average "crude" rate for total first admissions, it reduced the rate for schizophrenia. The reverse was true of native-born. The age range for schizophrenia may be placed between 15 and 44. Only a fifth of such first admissions are outside this range. Forty percent of the general native white population were within this age range in 1960, compared with only 22 percent of the white foreign-born. On the contrary, three-fourths of the foreign-born were aged 45 and over, compared with only a fourth of the native-born. Clearly, the low "crude" rate of the foreign-born resulted from the high proportion of foreign-born at those ages with low age-specific rates, whereas the native-born were concentrated at ages where the rates are high.

If we compare age-specific rates (see Table 12), we find that they were generally higher for foreign-born. If we compare the sexes, it becomes evident that native-born males had lower rates than foreign-born males, excluding ages 55 to 64. But among females the ratios of corresponding rates varied irregularly, the rates being generally lower for native-born at the youngest ages and at advanced age, but higher between ages 20 to 44 (see Table 13).

TABLE 13. Average Annual Rates of White First Admissions for Schizophrenia to All Hospitals for Mental Illness in New York State, 1960–1961, per 100,000 Population, Classified According to Age and Nativity

Age (years)	Males			Females		
	Native-born	Foreign-born	Ratio	Native-born	Foreign-born	Ratio
Under 15	5.8	10.3	0.56	2.3	4.0	0.58
15–19	51.3	64.4	0.80	40.1	53.1	0.76
20–24	107.3	112.2	0.96	77.4	67.2	1.15
25–29	83.2	108.0	0.77	90.8	100.0	0.91
30–34	70.3	90.4	0.78	84.2	79.9	1.05
35–39	57.0	76.1	0.74	70.6	70.0	1.01
40–44	47.6	57.3	0.83	60.2	56.9	1.06
45–49	33.4	33.3	1.00	39.4	37.8	1.04
50–54	20.9	21.0	1.00	24.6	27.4	0.90
55–59	18.0	8.5	2.12	19.1	17.0	1.12
60–64	10.1	9.1	1.11	12.7	10.0	1.27
65–69	4.6	6.6	0.70	10.6	9.3	1.14
70–74	2.4	5.7	0.42	3.0	3.8	0.79
75 and over	1.9	2.6	0.73	2.2	3.2	0.69
Total	34.5	26.1	1.32	35.4	27.6	1.28

TABLE 14. Average Annual Standardized[a] Rates of White First Admissions
for Schizophrenia to All Hospitals for Mental Illness
in New York State, 1960–1961, per 100,000 Population,
Classified According to Nativity

	Native-born	Foreign-born	Ratio
Males	43.7	51.4	0.85
Females	46.6	46.8	1.00
Total	44.8	48.5	0.92

[a] White population of New York State, aged 15 years and over, on April 1, 1960 (in
intervals of 5 years), taken as standard.

When standardized, the average annual rates per 100,000 were 44.8 for
native-born and 48.5 for foreign-born, the latter being in excess by 8
percent (see Table 14). The rate for foreign-born males was in excess by
18 percent. But there was no significant difference in rates between
females. The latter remained true, even when the age range was limited to
15 to 44.

The importance of the urban-rural distribution of population with
respect to the incidence of mental disease was emphasized in connection
with the over-all rates of first admissions. It is known that schizophrenia
is affected strongly by the degree of urban concentration. We may there-

TABLE 15. White Urban First Admissions for Schizophrenia
to All Hospitals for Mental Illness in New York State,
1960–1961, Classified According to Nativity

Age (years)	Native-born					Foreign-born				
	Males	Females	Total No.	Total %	Average annual rate per 100,000	Males	Females	Total No.	Total %	Average annual rate per 100,000
Under 15	228	86	314	3.8	4.8	8	3	11	1.0	7.7
15–19	449	361	810	9.7	50.5	19	19	38	3.4	57.8
20–24	727	572	1,299	15.6	99.5	52	42	94	8.4	86.9
25–29	634	689	1,323	15.9	94.6	68	73	141	12.6	104.1
30–34	598	727	1,325	15.9	84.4	77	73	150	13.4	83.9
35–39	480	639	1,119	13.4	69.0	83	84	167	14.9	74.0
40–44	377	528	905	10.9	57.1	53	59	112	10.0	59.1
45–49	246	315	561	6.7	38.2	47	61	108	9.7	35.3
50–54	137	172	309	3.7	24.6	44	62	106	9.4	25.1
55–59	89	110	199	2.4	19.6	24	45	69	6.2	13.0
60–64	42	52	94	1.1	11.8	25	26	51	4.6	9.5
65–69	13	34	47	0.6	7.8	16	25	41	3.7	8.2
70–74	5	9	14	0.2	3.4	10	8	18	1.6	4.6
75 and over	4	7	11	0.1	2.5	5	7	12	1.1	3.2
Total	4,029	4,301	8,330	100.0	38.4	531	587	1,118	100.0	27.2

fore evaluate the incidence of mental illness among native and foreign-born whites when the urban-rural ratio is held constant.

There were 9448 first admissions for schizophrenia during 1960–1961 from urban areas of New York State. Of this total, 8330, or 88.2 percent, were native-born and 1118, or 11.8 percent, were foreign-born. The percentages for the corresponding general populations were 84.1 and 15.9, respectively. Thus, the native-born exceeded their expected quota of first admissions, and the foreign-born had a deficiency. The average annual rates per 100,000 were 38.4 and 27.2, respectively.

Comparisons based upon the total populations of New York State showed that the comparison of crude rates was spurious, owing to the age differences between native and foreign-born. This holds also when the urban populations are compared. If we consider corresponding age-specific rates (see Table 15), it appears that the native-born urban population had, in general, lower rates of first admissions with schizophrenia than the foreign-born. Foreign-born males had generally higher rates than native-born, except between ages 45 and 64. Among females, however, the rates were generally higher for native-born (see Table 16).

TABLE 16. Average Annual Rates of White First Admissions
          for Schizophrenia to All Hospitals for Mental Illness
          in New York State, 1960–1961, per 100,000 Population,
          Classified According to Age and Nativity

Age (years)	Males			Females		
	Native-born	Foreign-born	Ratio	Native-born	Foreign-born	Ratio
Under 15	6.8	11.2	0.61	2.7	4.3	0.63
15–19	57.9	62.5	0.93	43.7	53.8	0.81
20–24	118.9	114.4	1.04	82.4	67.0	1.23
25–29	92.1	111.1	0.83	97.0	98.3	0.99
30–34	78.4	92.9	0.84	90.2	76.2	1.18
35–39	61.7	77.8	0.79	75.8	70.6	1.07
40–44	50.2	59.7	0.84	63.1	58.6	1.08
45–49	35.2	33.8	1.04	41.0	37.6	1.09
50–54	22.7	21.8	1.04	26.2	28.2	0.93
55–59	18.5	9.0	2.06	20.5	17.0	1.21
60–64	11.6	9.6	1.21	12.0	9.4	1.28
65–69	5.1	6.6	0.77	9.8	9.8	1.00
70–74	3.1	5.1	0.61	3.7	4.0	0.93
75 and over	2.6	2.8	0.93	2.4	3.4	0.71
Total	38.6	27.0	1.43	38.3	27.4	1.40

TABLE 17. Average Annual Standardized[a] Rates of White Urban First Admissions for Schizophrenia to All Hospitals for Mental Illness in New York State, 1960–1961, per 100,000 Population, Classified According to Nativity

	Native-born	Foreign-born	Ratio
Males	47.9	52.6	0.91
Females	49.3	46.6	1.06
Total	48.2	48.9	0.99

[a] White population of New York State, aged 15 years and over on April 1, 1960 (in intervals of 5 years), taken as standard.

When the rates were standardized, they became 52.6 and 47.9 per 100,000 for foreign-born and native-born males, respectively, an excess of 10 percent by the former (see Table 17). Among females, however, the rate for native-born was in excess by 6 percent. The total rates balanced each other, being 48.2 for native and 48.9 for foreign-born.

We may consider next the differences in rates of first admissions among the rural populations. Of the total rural white population, 94.7 percent were native and 5.3 percent were foreign-born. Of the rural first admissions, 93.9 percent were native and 6.1 percent were foreign-born. Hence,

TABLE 18. White Rural First Admissions for Schizophrenia to All Hospitals for Mental Illness in New York State, 1960–1961, Classified According to Nativity

Age (years)	Native-born					Foreign-born				
			Total		Average annual rate per 100,000			Total		Average annual rate per 100,000
	Males	Females	No.	%		Males	Females	No.	%	
Under 15	15	5	20	2.3	1.3					
15–19	39	35	74	8.7	22.0	2	1	3	5.5	65.8
20–24	52	55	107	12.6	46.5	1	2	3	5.5	65.8
25–29	47	80	127	14.9	47.6	1	6	7	12.7	94.0
30–34	48	84	132	15.5	42.0	2	9	11	20.0	97.3
35–39	55	68	123	14.4	38.7	3	5	8	14.5	54.4
40–44	49	62	111	13.0	38.1	1	2	3	5.5	25.1
45–49	34	39	73	8.6	27.3	2	4	6	10.9	33.7
50–54	14	17	31	3.6	13.4	1	2	3	5.5	11.4
55–59	15	10	25	2.9	13.1		5	5	9.1	16.7
60–64	3	13	16	1.9	9.7		3	3	5.4	10.0
65–69	2	10	12	1.4	8.6	1	1	1	1.8	3.2
70–74						2		2	3.6	7.7
75 and over		1	1	0.1	0.8					
Total	373	479	852	100.0	18.7	16	39	55	100.0	21.5

TABLE 19. Average Annual Rates of White Rural First Admissions for Schizophrenia to All Hospitals for Mental Illness in New York State, 1960–1961, per 100,000 Population, Classified According to Age and Nativity

Age (years)	Males			Females		
	Native-born	Foreign-born	Ratio	Native-born	Foreign-born	Ratio
Under 15	1.9			0.7		
15–19	22.2	90.9	0.24	21.8	42.4	0.51
20–24	45.4	56.0	0.81	47.6	71.2	0.67
25–29	36.1	37.0	0.98	58.5	126.4	0.46
30–34	30.7	44.3	0.69	53.2	132.4	0.40
35–39	34.4	46.6	0.74	43.1	60.3	0.71
40–44	33.1	18.4	1.80	43.2	30.6	1.41
45–49	24.8	24.1	1.03	29.9	42.2	0.71
50–54	11.7	7.8	1.50	15.1	15.6	0.97
55–59	15.2			10.8	35.1	0.31
60–64	3.6			16.1	20.2	0.80
65–69	2.9	6.3	0.46	14.1		
70–74		14.2				
75 and over				1.4		
Total	16.2	12.7	1.28	21.3	30.0	0.71

contrary to the urban populations, rural native-born had less than their expected quota of first admissions for schizophrenia, and the foreign-born were in excess. The average annual rates per 100,000 were 18.7 for native and 21.5 for foreign-born.

TABLE 20. Average Annual Standardized[a] Rates of Rural White First Admissions for Schizophrenia to All Hospitals for Mental Illness in New York State, 1960–1961, per 100,000 Population, Classified According to Nativity

	Native-born	Foreign-born	Ratio
Males	22.7	30.1	0.75
Females	30.6	50.6	0.60
Total	27.6	40.1	0.69

[a] White population of New York State aged 15 years and over on April 1, 1960 (in intervals of 5 years), taken as standard.

In general, native-born had lower age-specific rates than foreign-born (see Table 18). This was clearly evident among females. Among males, the native-born had lower rates at ages under 40, the crucial age periods for this disorder (see Table 19).

Hence, when standardized, the rates per 100,000 became 27.6 for native and 40.1 for foreign-born, the latter being in excess by 45 percent (see Table 20). Foreign-born males and females both had higher standardized rates than native-born. Among males, the excess amounted to 33 percent. Among females, it amounted to 65 percent.

We now conclude the comparisons by standardizing simultaneously for age, sex, and urban-rural differences (see Table 21). The average annual rate of first admissions for schizophrenia per 100,000 then became 44.0 for native and 47.8 for foreign-born, an excess of 9 percent. The excess was higher among males, the foreign-born rate being higher by 12 percent. Although foreign-born females had a higher rate than native-born, the excess was not significant, amounting to only 2 percent.

Thus we began with an excess of 30 percent by native-born on the basis of crude rates. When standardized by age and sex, however, the foreign-born had a rate of 48.5, which exceeded that for native-born by 8 percent. The relative excess remained at 9 percent, when we added an adjustment due to the urban-rural ratio of populations.

It has been shown that the distribution with respect to economic status influences the relative difference in incidence of mental illness. There are such differences in connection with schizophrenia, and they favor the native-born. The percentage classified as in comfortable economic circumstances is small. Nevertheless, 19.4 percent of the native-born first admissions during 1949–1951 were in this category, compared with 16.9 percent of the foreign-born. The percentages of those classified as dependent were 14.2 for native and 18.0 for foreign-born. Hence, we

TABLE 21. Average Annual Standardized[a] Rates of White First Admissions for Schizophrenia to All Hospitals for Mental Illness in New York State, 1960–1961, per 100,000 Population, Classified According to Nativity

	Native-born	Foreign-born	Ratio
Males	44.1	49.3	0.89
Females	46.4	47.5	0.98
Total	44.0	47.8	0.92

[a] White population of New York State, aged 15 years and over, classified according to urban-rural distribution, on April 1, 1960 (in intervals of 5 years), taken as standard.

may infer that a correction for economic status would reduce further the relative differences in rates of first admissions between native- and foreign-born. However, the relative distributions of economic status differ only slightly among native- and foreign-born in this diagnostic category, and therefore are not likely to affect the difference in incidence significantly.

Rates of first admissions for schizophrenia vary with respect to nativity and ethnic origin. The average standardized rate for all foreign-born whites during 1949–1951 was 52.7 per 100,000. But this varied from a low of 26.6 among English-born to a maximum of 73.1 and 65.4 among those born in Poland and Russia, respectively. Jews constitute high proportions of immigrants from these countries. As it has been shown that the annual rate of first admissions for schizophrenia among Jews does not exceed the average for the white population of New York State (Malzberg, 1960, 1963b), it follows that the high rates for Poland and Russia must be due to the Slavic element in these populations. Irish-born had a high rate of 60.2. Italian-born had a low rate of 48.4. Hence, as with total first admissions, high and low rates occurred among immigrant populations from Europe without reference to their geographic origin (see Table 22).

When we examine the distribution for the second generation of foreign white stock in New York State in 1950, we find the lowest rate, 36.3, among natives of Italian-born parentage; and the highest, 59.0, among natives of Irish-born parentage. Native-born of Polish and Russian-born parentage had relatively low rates, which again must be attributed to the high proportion of Jews among them.

If we compare the native-born of foreign parentage with the corresponding parental generations, we find that, with the exception of Eng-

TABLE 22. Average Annual Standardized[a] Rates of White First Admissions for Schizophrenia to All Hospitals for Mental Illness in New York State, 1949–1951, per 100,000 Population, Classified According to Nativity and Parentage

	Foreign-born			Native-born of foreign parentage			Ratio		
	Males	Females	Total	Males	Females	Total	Males	Females	Total
England	27.3	26.3	26.6	45.5	41.4	44.6	0.60	0.64	0.60
Ireland	71.2	50.1	60.2	63.0	52.1	59.0	1.13	0.96	1.02
Germany	58.0	58.3	58.2	40.1	41.8	42.0	1.44	1.39	1.39
Poland	66.7	78.3	73.1	56.4	52.0	55.7	1.18	1.51	1.31
Russia	90.9	41.1	65.4	41.8	47.4	46.0	2.17	0.87	1.42
Italy	56.9	40.2	48.4	35.0	35.6	36.3	1.63	1.13	1.33
All foreign-born	57.2	50.3	52.7	51.6	46.7	49.1	1.11	1.08	1.07

[a] White population of New York State, aged 15 years and over on April 1, 1950 (in intervals of 5 years), taken as standard.

land, the native-born all had lower rates of first admissions for schizo-phrenia.

This is in accord with an environmental explanation of the distribu-tion of mental disease. The ethnic factor is constant, but the second generation benefits from a superior social status with respect to educa-tion and occupation, both of which are correlated inversely with the incidence of mental illness (Malzberg, 1963a).

With respect to England, we noted previously that English-born had a lower rate than native-born, but that native-born of English parentage had a higher rate than all natives of native parentage. The second gen-eration of English also had a higher rate than English-born. This is true also with respect to schizophrenia, the English-born having a lower rate than all native-born and native-born of English parentage. The latter also had a higher rate than all natives of native parentage. Data with respect to nativity are available for Canada, and they show agreement with the experience of New York State. Those born in England had a lower rate than all native-born in Canada.

"It is possible that the English-born underwent a favorable selection before emigrating. This might have been self-selection, the healthier and more vigorous being more likely to emigrate. Selection may also have been exercised by American authorities at place of origin of the migrating stream" (Malzberg, 1964, p. 54).

SUMMARY

Foreign-born were uniformly reported as having higher rates of first admissions to mental hospitals than the native-born populations of the host countries. Investigators who reported such results seemed to imply that the differences were due to the unfavorable characteristics of the immigrant populations. Yet, when the important factors of varying age and sex proportions were considered, the relative differences were reduced significantly. The equally important factor of urban-rural distribution has been generally neglected. Yet, when this factor is added to age and sex differentials, the rates of first admissions to mental hospitals were almost equivalent for native- and foreign-born. In fact, during 1960–1961, the average annual rate of first admissions, standardized for age, sex and urban-rural ratios, was higher for native than for foreign-born. If the factor of social status, as measured by degree of education, occupa-tion, and income, could also be considered, it would undoubtedly strengthen the conclusion that differences in "crude" rates can only be explained by facts of demographic and social origin that operate inde-pendently of the hypothetical racial and ethnic qualities of the migrat-ing populations.

It has been shown that rates of first admissions among foreign-born vary with the duration of residence in the host country (Mental Disease, 1964). Thus, for constant age, that part of the foreign-born population with the longest residence has the lowest rate of first admissions, and the most recent has the highest rate. This has been demonstrated for New York State on the basis of a five-year dichotomy with respect to internal migration (Malzberg & Lee, 1956, Ch. 5), but it has been proven in greater detail on the basis of Canadian experience. For the years 1950–1952, the lowest average annual rates of first admissions, when age was held constant, occurred among the immigrants who had the longest residence in Canada, and the highest occurred among the most recent years. It is not unreasonable to conclude that the phenomena of anomie, present in the early stages of immigration, disappear with or are modified by the passage of years. There may be some selection among an immigrant population, whereby the more vigorous do not develop a mental illness, live longer, and therefore constitute an increasing proportion of the immigrant population with the passage of time. It is also true, however, that the processes of adaptation are difficult for immigrants during the early years. For most foreign-born, there is the necessity of learning a new and difficult language. There must be economic stabilization, following the acquisition of a new occupation, one with which he had had no previous familiarity. He must throw off as quickly as possible those outward traits that mark him as different from the native-born and tend to separate him from the generally accepted community norms. In the course of time, these indications of difference tend to disappear. Thus, it follows that an immigrant aged 40 years, for example, who has been a resident for twenty years, is less likely to develop mental illness than an immigrant of the same age, who has been resident only a year or less. It is probable, because of the restrictive immigration laws, that the foreign-born with periods of long residence in the United States now represent a growing proportion of the total foreign-born population.

The foreign-born are not a homogeneous population, and the ethnic and national components were therefore considered. In 1950, the leading groups of foreign nativity in New York State were from Italy, Russia, Germany, Poland, Ireland and England. Of these, there were two, England and Italy, that had lower standardized rates than the native-born, their rates being 140.7 and 141.3, respectively. The highest rate, 231.7, occurred among the Irish-born. German-born had a relatively high rate, but Russian-born, who were primarily Jews, had a low rate. Hence, it is evident that high and low rates of first admissions occurred among emigrants from both northwest and southeast Europe, disproving the invidious judgments by earlier investigators.

When comparisons are made between native-born of specific foreign parentage and those of native parentage, the results parallel closely those for the foreign-born. The important fact is, however, that, with the exception of the English, the foreign-born had higher rates than the second generations. Since the ethnic origins were the same for both generations, it follows that the relative differences in rates of first admission must be ascribed to environmental factors, such as education, which are more favorable for the native-born.

We have considered rates that are an average for the native- and foreign-born. But the rates vary in accordance with specific mental disorders. The alcoholic psychoses are generally less frequent among the foreign-born. But the difference is most marked with respect to schizophrenia. Contrary to the comparison with respect to total first admissions, foreign-born have higher rates of schizophrenia than native-born. The relative excess has decreased since 1930, but the difference remains significant. It is generally believed that constitutional factors have etiological relations to schizophrenia, and that these factors appear disproportionally among migrants (Odegaard, 1932).

But the average incidence of schizophrenia varies among the foreign-born populations. The English-born had a rate of 26.6, compared with 41.3 for native-born and 52.7 for all foreign-born. Italians had a rate of 48.4, higher than for native-born but lower than the average for all foreign-born. The highest rates occurred among Polish and Russian-born. But Jews, who formed high proportions of these populations, had rates of first admissions for schizophrenia that did not exceed the average for New York State (Malzberg, 1960, 1963b). Hence, the high rates for Polish- and Russian-born must be attributed to the Slavic element among them. Irish-born had a rate of 60.2, significantly higher than the rates for all foreign-born.

In general, native-born of foreign parentage had lower rates of schizophrenia than the corresponding generations of foreign-born. But this was reversed in the case of the English, the foreign-born having a significantly lower rate. The difference between the two generations of Irish was not significant. But among Germans, Italians, Polish, and Russians, the rates for the foreign-born exceeded the corresponding rates for the second generation by 30 to 40 percent.

REFERENCES

Greenwood, M. & Yule, G. *Udney Proceedings of Royal Society of Medicine,* 1915 (Section of Epedemiology and State Medicine), p. 137.

Hearings before the Committee on Immigration and Naturalization. House of Representatives, Sixty-second Congress. Third Session, November 21, 1923. Serial 7-C. Washington, D.C.: Government Printing Office, 1923.

Hollingshead, A. B., & Redlich, F. C. *Social class and mental illness.* New York: John Wiley & Sons, 1958.

Insane and feebleminded in hospitals and institutions, 1904. Bureau of Census. Washington, D.C.: Government Printing Office, 1906.

Insane and feebleminded in institutions, 1910. Bureau of Census. Washington, D.C.: Government Printing Office, 1914.

Malzberg, B. *Social and biological aspects of mental disease.* Utica, N.Y.: State Hospitals Press, 1940.

Malzberg, B., & Lee, E. S. *Migration and mental disease: A study of first admissions to hospitals for mental disease, New York, 1939–1941.* New York: Social Science Research Council, 1956.

Malzberg, B. *Mental disease among Jews in New York State.* New York: Intercontinental Medical Book Corporation, 1960.

Malzberg, B. Mental disorders in the United States. In *Encyclopedia of mental health,* Vol. III, pp. 1051–1066. New York: Encyclopedia of Mental Health (Franklin Watts, Inc.), 1963. (a)

Malzberg, B. *Mental health of Jews in New York State.* Albany, N.Y.: Research Foundation for Mental Hygiene, 1963. (b)

Malzberg, B. Mental disease among English-born and native-whites of English parentage in New York State, 1949–1951. *Mental Hygiene,* 1964, **48**, 54. (a)

Malzberg, B. *Mental disease in Canada, 1950–1952: A study of comparative incidence of mental disease among those of British and French origin.* Albany, N.Y.: 1964. (b)

Malzberg, B. *Migration in relation to mental disease.* Albany, N.Y.: Research Foundation for Mental Hygiene, Inc., 1968.

Mental disease among native and foreign-born white populations of New York State, 1939–1941. *Mental Hygiene,* 1955, **39**, 545–567.

Mental disease among native and foreign-born in Canada, 1950–1952. Albany, N.Y.: 1963.

Mental disease among foreign-born in Canada, 1950–1952, in Relation to Period of Immigration. *American Journal of Psychiatry,* 1964, **120**, 971–973. (a)

Mental disease among native and foreign-born whites in New York State, 1949–1951. *Mental Hygiene,* 1964, **48**, 478–499. (b)

New York State Department of Mental Hygiene. *Statistical guide.* (12th ed.) Utica, N.Y.: State Hospitals Press, 1943. P. 52.

Odegaard, O. Emigration and insanity. *Acta Psychiatrica et Neurologica,* Supplement 4, 1932.

Reports of Immigration Commission, 61st Congress, 3d Session. Vol. II, Immigration and Insanity. Washington, D.C.: Government Printing Office, 1913.

United States Bureau of Census. *United States census of population, 1960. General population characteristics.* New York. Final Report PC (1)-34B, p. VI. Washington, D.C.: United States Government Printing Office. 1961.

3.7 *Orientation*

The social forces of city life are often hypersegmented and cen-
trifugal, and their impact on the lives of urban dwellers can be
divisive and pathological. It is commonly assumed that one of the
social structures that provides a stabilizing influence against such
destructive forces in the lives of many people is the common bond
shared by persons of similar religious belief.

The article by Leo Srole and Thomas Langner examines the significance of America's three great religious communions, Protestantism, Catholicism, and Judaism, on the mental health of urban
dwellers. The report is an outgrowth of the important midtown
Manhattan study, and has been specially adapted for the current
volume. Unlike most other investigators, Srole and Langner possess
the research sophistication to control age, social class, and degree
of religiosity of the parents for the respondents in their study sample. Thus, we are presented with convincing evidence to support
more informative conclusions.

3.7   Protestant, Catholic, and Jew: Comparative Psychopathology[1]

Leo Srole and Thomas S. Langner

In the antiphony of voices that express American society, Protestantism,
Catholicism, and Judaism stand out as the nation's three great religious
communions. The significance for mental health of personal roots in
these different religious traditions is the complicated and difficult question that shall engage us in this article.

In the early 1950s, a large-scale, intensive study of the Midtown Manhattan area of New York City was initiated by the Cornell University
Medical School to determine the prevalence of mental illness and psychological disorder among persons living in a large and densely populated urban area. The complete description of the study and the research methods utilized is available in the two volumes published since

[1] The major portion of this chapter is reprinted, with permission of the authors
and publisher, from Chapter 16 of *Mental Health in the Metropolis: The Midtown Manhattan Study,* New York: McGraw-Hill, 1962.

1962 (Srole, Langner, Michael, Opler, & Rennie, 1962; Langner & Michael, 1963). For the purposes of this article, it is only necessary to summarize, very briefly, the research methods and procedures employed in the study.

A sample of 1911 individuals was selected for study from an area of 175,000 persons of diverse socioeconomic status, nationalities, religious beliefs, urban and rural backgrounds, and length of residence in New York City. The sample was drawn randomly, first selecting city blocks, then dwelling units, and finally specific persons from ages 20 through 59, within the dwelling units. A total of 1660 interviews were completed, representing 87 percent of the original random sample.

The method used to estimate the level of mental health was a personal interview, averaging two hours in length, and covering a wide variety of demographic and sociocultural variables. Questions related to the mental health of the respondent focused on (1) recent mental pathology, (2) somatic illnesses that often have a psychological origin, (3) psychophysiologic manifestations of emotional illness, (4) memory difficulties, and (5) current interpersonal functioning within social settings of family, work, and peer groups.

Working from the questionnaires and the additional detailed notes provided by the interviewers, two psychiatrists made independent ratings of the degree of symptom formation of each respondent. Final classifications were on a six-point scale varying from "well" to "incapacitated."

In the Midtown study, as many as fifteen separate questions were asked about each person's religious orientation, identification, and behaviors, past and present. Obviously, the individual's religious identification can change between childhood and adulthood, and such changes may be the result of personality processes that also work themselves out in forms subsumed under the concept of mental health. Thus, adults' replies to the interview question, "To what religious faith do you *now* belong?" must be considered in the nature of a concurrent, reciprocal, and etiologically ambiguous variable relative to their mental health. On the other hand, in replies to questions on the faith that each parent grew up in, we have the individual's religious origin, potentially standing as an antecedent and independent variable to the dependent variable of his current mental health.

We shall presently consider changes in religious identification between parents and their adult offspring. But here we first want to classify the sample adults by religious origin and to examine the mental health distribution in each of the four religious categories shown in Table 1.

We know that among the religious groups in the sample there are differences in age composition and socioeconomic origin. We have previously found that these two demographic factors are independently related

TABLE 1. Home Survey Sample (Age 20–59), Respondents' Distributions
on Mental Health Classification by Religious Origin
(in Percentages)

Mental health categories	Religious origin			
	Catholic	Protestant	Jewish	Others[a]
Well	16.1	22.6	16.0	22.6
Mild symptom formation	35.4	36.1	41.7	30.1
Moderate symptom formation	22.2	19.8	25.8	20.8
Impaired	26.3	21.5	16.5	26.5
Marked symptom formation	13.9	12.5	11.3	17.0
Severe symptom formation	9.0	6.9	3.8	5.7
Incapacitated	3.4	2.1	1.4	3.8
$N = 100\%$	(832)	(562)	(213)	(53)

[a] Almost two-thirds of these respondents had parents who were identified as Christians
of the Eastern (Greek or Russian) Orthodox Church. The remaining parents were either
members of non-Western religious cults or were reported as having grown up in no
known religious faith. These respondents are too diverse in religious backgrounds and
too few in number to be brought into subsequent analyses in this chapter.

to respondent mental health. Thus, if interesting differences appear in
Table 1, there is a decided chance that these differences are not real, but
rather are spurious results of intergroup variations in age and SES origin.
In Table 2, we present the mental health distributions that could be
expected were the three religious-origin groups identical in these latter
respects.[2]

This standardization almost completely levels the Protestant-Catholic
differences seen in Table 1. The impairment differences observed between Jews and the other two groups in the table remain statistically
significant, however. Reference to Table 1 locates the Jewish difference
specifically in smaller Severe and Incapacitated frequencies, i.e., at the
end of the impairment range rather than in the Marked category.

On the other hand, in Table 2, Jews are also seen with the lowest
prevalence of Wells at a not insignificant distance from the Protestants'
Well frequency. With the lowest rates both of the Well and the Impaired,
Jews of course are found more heavily concentrated than Protestants or
Catholics in the subclinical range in between, above all in the most pop-
ulated mental health category, namely, Mild symptom formation.

[2] This is accomplished by the technique of standardization. In this method,
the less-populated mental health categories in the Impaired range cannot be
separately sustained. Accordingly, they are merged in Table 2.

TABLE 2. Home Survey Sample (Age 20–59), Respondents' Distributions on Mental Health Classification by Religious Origin as Standardized for Age and SES Origin (in Percentages)

Mental health categories	Religious origin		
	Catholic	Protestant	Jewish
Well	17.4	20.2	14.5
Mild symptom formation	34.5	36.4	43.2
Moderate symptom formation	23.4	19.9	25.1
Impaired	24.7[a]	23.5	17.2[a]
$N = 100\%$	(832)	(562)	(213)

[a] $t = 2.6$ (.01 level of confidence).

We might follow the matter one step further. Suppose we look at the religious-origin groups within each of the three SES-origin strata, retaining standardization for age differences. We then find in all three strata the essential mental health picture discerned in Table 2. However, there are differences of degree—the most suggestive appearing in the lower stratum (E–F) of SES origin. Here respondents of Protestant, Catholic, and Jewish origin have almost identical Well frequencies, but their Impaired rates are 32.0, 30.5, and 19.4%, respectively.

If Jews convey the most favorable group picture of mental health in the SES stratum having the highest concentration of mental morbidity, then one possible hypothesis that can be suggested for future testing is this: Midtown respondents of Jewish parentage tend to reflect some kind of impairment-limiting mechanism that operates to counteract, or in some degree contain, the more extreme pathogenic life stresses during childhood. This hypothesis appears to be consistent with the repeatedly confirmed relative immunity of Jews to such self-impairing types of reactions as alcoholism (Snyder, 1955) and suicide.

If such a "this-far-and-no-farther" control mechanism exists, its source is a question that here can only be a subject of speculation. One factor often hypothesized by psychiatrists as potentially pathogenic is the strong Jewish family structure. However, this factor may conceivably be eugenic on balance, in the specific sense that powerful homeostatic supports are brought into play at danger points of crisis and stress that in other groups may be unbalancing for the family and impairing for the individual.

If subsequent investigation should lend support to this inference, the mechanism involved may have historical, broadly psychosocial roots, of a kind defined by the following hypothesis: A group that for thousands of years has been beleagured by chronic environmental threats of destruction survives by developing internal processes of resistance, deep within the dynamics of the family itself, that counteract in some measure the more extreme kinds of exogenous crises and check the more extreme forms of pathological reaction.

Also potentially relevant, although stemming from another framework is the inference Janis (1958, p. 352) draws from his classic study of surgery patients:

> Arousal of some degree of anticipatory fear may be one of the necessary conditions for developing inner defenses of the type that can function effectively when the external danger materializes. . . . If a person is given appropriate preparatory communications before being exposed to potentially traumatizing stimuli, his chances of behaving in a disorganized way . . . may be greatly decreased. Thus, from the standpoint of preventive psychiatry, it is of considerable importance to determine how preparatory communications can be made to serve an effective prophylactic function.

To translate this formulation for the present discussion, mobilization of anxiety about the instability of the Jewish exilic environment may historically have been established as a conditioning pattern of the Jewish family structure. In one direction, such anxiety, subsequently magnified in the adult by extrafamily life conditions, may be reflected in our finding of an unusually large concentration of Midtown Jews in the subclinical Mild category of symptom formation. On the other hand, this large component of historically realistic anxiety, as generated in the Jewish family, may function prophylactically to immunize its children against the potentially disabling sequelae of the more severe pressures and traumas of existence.[3] Later in this chapter we may see other expressions of this process.

Also to be emphasized is that, like earlier studies of patients, the Midtown Home Survey shows a somewhat higher over-all frequency of mental morbidity in the Catholic group than in the Protestant group. However,

---

[3] Here may also be the seedbed of the Jewish community's proverbial gift, through its long history, for rising from adversity and for converting a handicap into an asset. Alexander King points to another possible consequence: "Jewish humor, as I learned at one of its very sources, was a racial anti-biotic, whose original cultures the children of Israel had carried out of Egypt, more than two thousand years ago, and whose health-preserving properties had been nurtured through the centuries in all the ghettoes and outposts of persecuted Judaism." A. King, *Mine Enemy Grows Older*, 1958, p. 171.

this difference was found to be a wholly spurious consequence of the fact that Protestants in the aggregate are younger and of considerably higher socioeconomic antecedents than are Catholics.

HOME SURVEY SAMPLE: MENTAL HEALTH
AND PARENTAL RELIGIOSITY

In the section preceding we have been concerned with the respondent's religious origin as based on the faith in which his parents had grown up. This is a formal, demographic kind of classification, but it tells us nothing about the degree of parental commitment to the doctrines, commandments, and practices enjoined by their religious institution.

Seen in historical perspective, this dimension of individual commitment to the tenets of the faith—or "religiosity"—is extremely sensitive to changes in the environing society. The Protestant Reformation is an excellent case in point. The period in which our respondents' parents had been born roughly spanned the half century from 1864 to 1914. These, of course, were years that saw vast scientific, technological, and economic changes which made themselves felt along the entire broad front of Western institutions. Not the least of these impacts registered on the church and on the individual's anchoring ties to it.

We can hypothesize that this factor of relative religious anchorage or commitment had direct effects on parents' roles and on the home atmosphere, with radiating consequences for the development of the child as observed when he himself had grown into adulthood.

Interviewing each respondent, we asked this key question as a short-cut approach to his parents' religious orientation:[4] "How important would you say religion (belief in religion) was to your parents? For example, would you say it was: Very important? Somewhat important? Or not important at all?"[5]

We were of course aware that a reply to this question is essentially the respondent's judgment applied to his recall of observed words and

[4] Originally also asked for this purpose was a question on parents' frequency of church (or synagogue) attendance—"when you were growing up." Subsequently, we recognized more fully that as a universal index of religiosity, frequency of church attendance had a number of serious deficiencies. Accordingly, it is not being employed here for this purpose.

[5] If respondent indicated that father and mother differed in this respect, the interviewer recorded the specific nature of the difference. Later, with an eye on the parent likely to have had the larger influence on the home's religious atmosphere, we classified such cases according to importance of religion reported for the mother.

deeds as they reflected parental attitude toward religious tradition.[6] We could assume that the judgment hinged in part on a norm or image of the "faithful" man that is specific to each church system and, in part, on the respondent's recall of reality modifications in this ideal among the parents' local contemporaries.

Within the Study's taxonomy of test factors (Srole *et al.*, 1962, Ch. 2), parental religiosity certainly stands to the dependent variable of respondent mental health as a chronologically antecedent factor. But we deal with the respondent's *judgment* of such religiosity, and this "filter" is potentially open to influence from psychological processes related to the dependent variable. However, parental religiosity qualifies as an independent, as well as antecedent, test factor to the extent that the respondent's judgment took its measure from long and relatively close observations of parental behavior. We can produce no evidence to illuminate this issue. As a matter of the investigators' opinion, however, until shown otherwise we will assume that respondents' reports of parental religiosity provide a reasonable approximation of independence from the dependent variable.

A final preparatory point must now be clarified. Earlier in this chapter, the respondent's religious origin was used, as determined by the criterion of descent through the religion of parents' upbringing (much as had nationality origin in the preceding chapter). This criterion was appropriate to our purposes of inclusive demographic classification at that point. With religiosity now the factor of central interest, we must gear this factor to identification of religious groupings based on a more refined criterion. That is, instead of religious origin or descent of parents, we refer to this criterion as parents' *religious-group identification,* as ascertained from respondent replies to the interview question: "What religious faith did *you* grow up in?"

Of course, the religion a parent had experienced during his own childhood tells us nothing with certainty about his religious identification during adulthood. However, we can be confident that the religious tradition which enveloped the child is a fairly reliable indicator of the religious-group identification conveyed, however minimally, by his parents. This criterion, of a specific religious identification *conveyed* to one's

---

[6] Whether this reply would have coincided with the judgments of the parents themselves, their clergyman, or their friends at the time, is information beyond access to us. Even if accessible, these judgments would not necessarily be of transcending relevance compared to the respondent's judgment from his personal vantage point.

children, is the basis for our present classification of respondents' parents by religious group.

With a locus in any given religious system, individuals vary in degree of acceptance of its disciplining claims upon their thought and behavior. In this perspective, parents who had stood with the "faithful," by the light of locally modified standards of the church at large, would likely be seen by the child as having given their religion very important weight in their lives. On the other hand, parents deviating considerably from the faithful model, while remaining more or less anchored in the church, would probably be judged as holding their religion no more than "somewhat important." Finally, parents remaining formally identified as in the fold of the church but whose behavior suggested that its religious tenets were to them "not important at all" were probably at best peripheral, nominal members of the institution.

Let us first record how the sample respondents' parents are distributed on this gross scale of reported religiosity:[7]

Very important (rVI)	52%
Somewhat important (SI)	37%
Not important at all (NIAA)	11%

Table 3 shows next how respondents' parents located within *each group fold* are distributed by religiosity as reported to us. We need not pause to speculate on the explanations for the differences that appear in Table 3.[8] However, they are consistent with general observations that

[7] If personal importance of religion is seen as a continuum ranging (1) from complete submission to the expectations of one's church to (2) more or less complete independence of one's church, it is clear that in this distribution about half of the parents stand at the VI range of the continuum. With benefit of hindsight, were we to test this factor again, we would enlarge the number of categories in the scale, perhaps to four, in order to sort out religiosity differences within the present VI category and to produce a closer approximation to a normal distribution curve.

In this direction, Fichter has applied the following fourfold classification of Catholics: [a] *"Nuclear,* who are the most active participants and the most faithful believers. [b] *Modal,* who are the normal, practicing Catholics easily identifiable as parishioners. [c] *Marginal,* who are conforming to a bare arbitrary minimum of the patterns expected in the religious institution [d] *Dormant,* who have 'given up' Catholicism but have not joined another denomination." J. H. Father, S.J., "The Marginal Catholic: An Institutional Approach," *Social Forces,* vol. 32, no. 2, pp. 167–172, December, 1953.

[8] It might be added that parents' religiosity also varies inversely with their

TABLE 3. Home Survey Sample (Age 20–59), Distributions of
Respondents' Parents on Religiosity Classification
by Parental Religious-group Identification (in Percentages)

	Parents' religious-group identification		
Parents' religiosity	Catholic	Protestant	Jewish
Very important (VI)	67.4	40.0	31.1
Somewhat important (SI)	28.1	45.8	48.4
Not important at all (NIAA)	4.5	14.2	20.5
$N = 100\%$	(805)	(541)	(190)

close conformity to the normative expectations of one's religious institution characterizes more adherents of the Catholic church than Protestants
or Jews.

Furthermore, if we could assume that at some not-too-distant period
in the past almost all adherents of each religious faith were in the top
level of religiosity, it seems apparent that this was far from the case
among the respondents' parents a generation ago. Even within the relatively stable Catholic group, one in every three parents in the eyes of
their offspring stood at less than a very important level of religious commitment. Thus, the erosions of traditional religious anchorages among
adults of a generation ago can seemingly be discerned from the data
presented in Table 7.3.

Our primary concern here is addressed to this question: What are the
detectable consequences of parental differences in religiosity for the
mental health of the children they raised to adulthood? Let us first direct
this question to the Midtown sample respondents of Jewish-identified
parents. In Table 4 they are distributed on a threefold classification of
the mental health continuum.

---

socioeconomic status. That is, the higher the SES level, the lower, on the average,
is the religiosity reported. However, when both the SES and religious-group
factors are analyzed simultaneously, religiosity varies more among religious groups
within any given SES stratum than among SES strata within any given religious
group.

More accurately stated, in all parental-SES strata such analytical control tends
to eliminate the differences in religiosity distributions between Protestants and
Jews seen in Table 3 and tends to magnify the distribution differences between
each of the latter two groups and the Catholics. For example, in the parental
lower-SES stratum the "very important" frequencies of Catholic, Protestant, and
Jewish parents are 74.0, 39.8, and 37.5%, respectively.

TABLE 4. Home Survey Sample (Age 20–59), Distributions of Respondents with Jewish-identified Parents on Mental Health Classification by Parental Religiosity (in Percentages)

	Parental religiosity		
Mental health categories	VI	SI	NIAA
Well	8.5	18.5	15.4
Mild–Moderate	76.2	63.0	64.1
Impaired	15.3	18.5	20.5
$N = 100\%$	(59)	(92)	(39)

Among offspring of the several religiosity categories of Jewish parents, no significant difference in mental health composition is to be seen. In the light of the relatively small number of cases in the two extreme columns of Table 4, we must consider our evidence from the Jewish segment of the Midtown sample as statistically inconclusive.

The difficulty of insufficient sample numbers is not encountered to the same degree among respondents of Protestant-identified parentage. In fact, this group is sufficiently numerous to be examined on our present test variable as subdivided by our three-way stratification of parental socioeconomic status. In Table 5 we present the mental health distributions only for the respondents who are of upper-SES descent (A–B).

Mental health composition is almost identical in the three religiosity categories of Table 5. However, when we similarly categorize respondents of Protestant-identified parents who had been in our middle or lower strata of socioeconomic status, we find a rather different pattern of mental

TABLE 5. Home Survey Sample (Age 20–59), Distributions of Respondents from Upper SES-origin and Protestant-identified Parents on Mental Health Classification by Parental Religiosity (in Percentages)

	Parental religiosity		
Mental health categories	VI	SI	NIAA
Well	26.7	25.7	27.0
Mild-moderate	56.5	55.0	56.8
Impaired	16.8	19.3	16.2
$N = 100\%$	(101)	(109)	(37)

TABLE 6. HOME SURVEY SAMPLE (AGE 20–59), DISTRIBUTIONS OF RESPONDENTS
OF LOWER AND MIDDLE SES-ORIGIN AND PROTESTANT-IDENTIFIED
PARENTS ON MENTAL HEALTH CLASSIFICATION BY PARENTAL RELIGIOSITY
(IN PERCENTAGES)

	Parental religiosity		
Mental health categories	VI	SI	NIAA
Well	20.9	22.3	12.5
Mild-moderate	51.3	60.4	50.0
Impaired	27.8[a]	17.3[b]	37.5[a,b]
$N = 100\%$	(115)	(139)	(40)

[a] $t = 2.1$ (.05 level of confidence).
[b] $t = 2.9$ (.01 level of confidence).

health composition. Since the pattern is quite similar in these parental
strata, and the number of cases is relatively small in the lower of the two,
Table 6 combines the respondents of these two SES-origin groups (C–D
and E–F).

If the VI- and SI-reared respondents are alike in their Well frequencies,
the latter are better off in having a significantly lower Impaired rate,
accompanied by a correspondingly higher frequency in the subclinical
(Mild-Moderate) range of the continuum. Relative to these two groups,
moreover, the NIAA-sired respondents have the largest impairment rate
and the smallest Well representation.

In short, we discern the most favorable mental health picture in the
SI religiosity column and the least favorable in the NIAA segment, with
the VI category standing more or less intermediate. On the yardstick of
impairment rates, therefore, the pattern of relationship between parental
religiosity and respondent mental health can be described as being of
the general J-curve type.

Of course, the generality of this pattern remains in question when we
consider that it does not seem to appear among Jewish-bred respondents
or among Protestant-reared people of high SES origin. However, respondents of Catholic-identified parents have not yet been examined in
this respect. Analysis reveals the presence of this distribution pattern
among such Catholics on *all* three SES-origin strata. However, because
the number of respondents with NIAA parents is so small in each of
these strata, we can best delineate the pattern by viewing, in Table 7,
the entire Catholic-identified group as differentiated in terms of parental
religiosity.

TABLE 7. Home Survey Sample (Age 20–59), Distributions of Respondents with Catholic-identified Parents on Mental Health Classification by Parental Religiosity (in Percentages)

Mental health categories	Parental religiosity		
	VI	SI	NIAA
Well	17.1	15.0	5.5
Mild-moderate	56.0	63.3	58.4
Impaired	26.9	21.7	36.1
$N = 100\%$	(543)	(226)	(36)

Although the intra-Catholic differences in Table 7 do not achieve firm statistical significance, we again see the lowest Well frequency and highest Impaired rate in the NIAA column. Moreover, the SI category again emerges with the smallest prevalence of impairment; the VI respondents in turn stand intermediate in this respect.

All in all, therefore, the J-curve pattern observed among Protestant-sired respondents of lower and middle SES origins seems to be paralleled among Catholic offspring of all SES-origin strata. We can thereby infer, first, that this is a key pattern for respondents from both Protestant and Catholic childhood homes that were of lower or middle socioeconomic position. Jews of such SES origin do not seem to fit this pattern, but because of their small numbers in these strata, we lack confidence that this negative finding in their case is statistically conclusive.

Second, we can infer that a finding of no relationship between parental religiosity and respondent mental health seems to characterize both Protestants and Jews of upper socioeconomic descent. Here, Catholics of like SES origin seem to deviate, presenting instead the J shaped curve. However, their number in this stratum is relatively small, and we cannot be sure that this positive finding in their instance is statistically stable.

Accordingly, we are left with the residual inference that in lower- and middle-class homes, parental religiosity tends to be related to childrens' adult mental health—at least if the home had been Protestant or Catholic identified.

To be sure, the affinity uncovered in these parental-SES strata is not strikingly strong. On the other hand, this relationship has come through a measure of religiosity that rests on the narrow base of a single interview question and offers only a crude trichotomous classification. Accordingly, it is a plausible expectation that with a broader base of information and more refined classification of parental religiosity the relationship may well emerge in clearer form and enlarged magnitude.

Suggestive evidence lending support to the link between parental religious behavior and offsprings' mental health comes from a study of King and Funkenstein (1957), who report:

. . . there is a constellation of psychological and sociological factors which are associated with the cardiovascular reactions of healthy subjects [male college students] in acute stress. The constellation includes the immediate emotional reaction of the subject, his attitudes in the area of religious values, his perception of parental behavior in discipline, and the *church-going behavior of his parents* [italics added]. . . . We leave it to further research to spell out the manifold implications of these associations. We do suggest that they are of sufficient strength to encourage further inter-disciplinary research among the fields of physiology, psychology and sociology.

From another context, a leading mental hospital chaplain has observed: "We have found that, with the mentally ill, religion and its faith and practices have sometimes been used as a means of control, domination or manipulation with marked and serious emotional consequences" (Bruder, 1958, p. 3).

The relationship seemingly discerned in the Midtown sample poses a series of questions that cannot be answered at this time. First, why is this relationship apparently specific to the lower two-thirds of the parental-SES range and seemingly nonoperative among respondents from the upper third of that SES range? What specific elements can explain why the VI type of home in the susceptible SES strata seems to be more eugenic for offsprings' mental health than the NIAA home, and why does the SI home tend to be the most eugenic type of all? Under the secularizing pressures of industrial, urban society, are different modes of religiosity chosen by parents of broadly different types of personalities? If so, the apparent consequences of parental religiosity for offsprings' mental health may partially dissolve themselves into consequences of more comprehensive aspects of parents' characters.

On the other hand, assume broad personality similarities in a group of parents who diverge in religiosity: What consequences of the latter variable alone would flow into the intrafamily processes, e.g., into performances of parental roles, and thereby into the psychological conditioning of their offspring? What effects do variations in parental religiosity have upon family stability under crisis? For children, especially in adolescence, what are the intrafamily consequences when they veer away from the religious orientation of parents under pressure of peers and larger social influences?

By the inroads made into the religious anchorages of a large segment of the population, we see one cutting edge of the vast sociocultural changes of the past century. In particular we have seen the impacts of

TABLE 8. Home Survey Sample (Age 20–59), Distribution of Respondents' Current Religious Group by Their Religious Origin (in Percentages)

Current religious group	Religious origin		
	Catholic	Protestant	Jewish
Catholic	90.0	4.1	1.9
Protestant	2.5	78.6	1.9
Jewish	0.0	0.4	75.6
None	5.8	14.2	16.9
Other	1.7	2.7	3.7
$N = 100\%$	(832)	(562)	(213)

these historical forces on the religious moorings in the generation parental to our sample adults, and we can glimpse possible residue of such forces in the mental health of these respondents.

MENTAL HEALTH AND RELIGIOUS MOBILITY

We have been concerned about presumptive changes in religiosity among parents who had been identified with a specific religious group. Here we focus on direct evidence of a more drastic kind of change— among respondents in this instance, namely, a change in religious-group *identification* itself, or what we shall call *religious mobility*.

For respondents' religious-group lineage we shall take their religious origin, and we shall compare this with their replies to the interview question: "To what religious faith do you *now* belong?" In Table 8 we can ascertain the relative prevalence of religious mobility in the Midtown sample population.

This table clearly shows that respondents of Protestant or Jewish origin have total religious mobility rates (21.4 and 24.4%) more than twice that of Catholic-derived people (10%). However, in all three origin groups most of the movement has been not into another group, but into the disidentified no faith or "unchurched" ranks.

Of particular relevance to us here is the mental health composition of the several subgroup segments that have sufficient numbers of cases. Given the number of these segments, perhaps the most summary indication of such composition might be in terms of the Impaired-Well ratio[9] as presented in Table 9.

[9] It may be remembered that this expresses the number of Impaired cases per 100 Well respondents in a given group.

TABLE 9. HOME SURVEY SAMPLE (AGE 20–59), IMPAIRED-WELL RATIO
    OF SAMPLE RESPONDENTS BY RELIGIOUS ORIGIN
    AND CURRENT RELIGIOUS GROUP

| | Religious origin | | |
Current religious group	Catholic	Protestant	Jewish
Catholic	163	57	...
N^a =	(747)	(23)	(4)
Protestant	25	87	...
N =	(21)	(442)	(4)
Jewish	...	...	92
N =	(0)	(2)	(161)
None	200	170	120
N =	(48)	(80)	(36)

[a] N is the total number of respondents in the specific cell to which the Impaired-Well ratio value refers.

As we have just seen, Protestants who changed to Catholicism and Catholics who shifted to Protestantism are small in numbers. But to judge from the Impaired-Well ratios as derived from so few cases, such church-to-church changers appear in a somewhat more favorable mental health condition than do the stable Protestants and Catholics. Compared to the latter and the nonmobile Jews, however, the currently unchurched *respondents* from all three religious-origin groups uniformly present a less favorable mental health picture.

Since religious mobility is in the realm of voluntary behavior, it seems likely in large part to be psychologically determined. Hence, Table 9 probably tells us more about the kinds of people who change their religious group identification than it reveals about the mental health consequences of such change.

A potential programmatic utility of the data is to highlight to metropolitan religious organizations the mental health weighting of adherents they are losing to the unchurched, unreachable condition.

HELP-NEED, THE PATIENT-HISTORY VARIABLE,
AND PROFESSIONAL ORIENTATION

We turn finally to the patient-history factor as applied exclusively to the population at help-need, namely, the sample respondents who are in the Impaired category of mental health. Because religious origin is the

TABLE 10. HOME SURVEY SAMPLE (AGE 20–59), DISTRIBUTIONS OF
IMPAIRED RESPONDENTS ON PATIENT-HISTORY CLASSIFICATION
BY RELIGIOUS ORIGIN (IN PERCENTAGES)

| | Religious origin | | |
Patient history	Catholic	Protestant	Jewish
Current outpatients	1.8	8.3	20.0
Ex-patients	19.7	24.0	20.0
Never-patients	78.5	67.7	60.0
$N = 100\%$	(219)	(121)	(35)

most comprehensive criterion for classification by religious grouping, it is used with the Impaired segment of the sample in Table 10.

Of course, the ex-patients shown in the table include people who had been hospitalized, as well as those who had used ambulatory facilities. Accordingly, if the ex-patient rates are quite similar in the three columns of the table, we can be sure—from our Treatment Census data earlier reviewed—that the exhospitalized representation in the "mix" is quite different in the three religious groups.

More clear-cut are the current out-patient frequencies. We discern that among those now in a state of help-need, Jews have a current out-patient rate more than twice that of Protestants and approximately ten times that of Catholics. This illuminates the finding earlier drawn from the New Haven Study and our Treatment Census analysis that Jews emerge with higher ambulatory treatment rates than either Protestants or Catholics (see Srole et al., 1962, p. 303).

From our Home Survey sample we have already seen (Table 1) that Jews have a lower impairment rate than either of the other two religious groups. This seemed to be at direct variance with the Treatment Census finding that Jews were the highest of the three groups in Total Patients rates. The seeming paradox is set aright by the finding that between two groups of like size a low mental morbidity rate and a strong tendency to seek therapy can bring more Impaired people to a treatment facility than a high morbidity rate and a relatively weak tendency to seek therapy.

This statement stands irrespective of the fact that determinants other than mental morbidity enter into the varying motivations that lead one to treatment—especially of the voluntary out-patient type. One of these determinants is certainly the Impaired respondent's socioeconomic status. When the latter factor among the Impaired is controlled, the interreligious differences in current out-patient rates are narrowed but by no means eliminated. In most previous studies of patient populations sorted by religious groupings, lack of control for the SES variable has obscured its contribution to the large interreligious differences in patient rates.

However, that more than socioeconomic status is involved in patient rate differences may be gathered from questions put to the Midtown sample adults bearing on a dimension that we designate *professional orientation*. This was derived from our Midtown respondents through open-ended questions that posed certain psychiatric problems in a hypothetical family. One question was: "Let's suppose some friends of yours have a serious problem with their child. I mean a problem with the child's behavior, or difficulty getting along with others. The parents ask your advice what to do. What would you probably tell them to do about it?" A similar query was phrased in terms of an advice-seeking friend with a problem spouse.

Respondents were first sorted into those who in either or both situations would recommend consulting a psychotherapist of some kind. Sorted next were all the remaining respondents who would advise seeing a physician. In the third category were placed those who at most would refer such friends to some other kind of professional person, principally a clergyman or member of a social agency staff. The residue contained all respondents whose replies to both questions contain no suggestion of professional help of any kind.

Since professional orientation is strongly related to socioeconomic status of respondents, in Table 11 distributions on the former variable appear standardized for respondents' own SES. The criterion of classification by religion is again religious origin.

TABLE 11. Home Survey Sample (Age 20–59), Respondents' Distributions on Professional Orientation Scale by Religious Origin as Standardized for Own-SES Differences (in Percentages)

Respondent recommendation	Religious origin		
	Catholic	Protestant	Jewish
Psychotherapist	23.8	31.4	49.2
Physician	13.3	12.5	7.9
Other professional	13.0	7.5	3.1
Nonprofessional	49.9	48.6	39.8
$N = 100\%$	(832)	(562)	(213)

Catholics and Protestants are alike in that within each group about half could perceive no professional help as relevant for either of the stipulated problem families, and about one in eight would refer such problems to a physician. They differ in that fewer Catholics than Protestants would recommend a psychotherapist, and correspondingly more Catholics would advise other kinds of professionals, principally clergymen.

Jewish respondents, to a degree well beyond the other groups, see psychotherapists as the most appropriate source of help for the disturbed individuals outlined to them. In fact, they are the only group where this response is more frequent than the "no professional" recommendation.

SUMMARY

Home interviews were conducted with 1660 representative adults of the Midtown Manhattan area, which were later classified by two psychiatrists according to the degree of psychological impairment of the persons interviewed. On the chronologically antecedent criterion of parental religion, the sample's groups of Jewish, Protestant, and Catholic derivation had impairment rates of 16.5, 21.5, and 26.3 percent respectively.

Standardization for intergroup differences in age and SES origin reduced the Protestant and Catholic groups to near identity in mental health distributions. Respondents of Jewish origin retained a significantly lower Impaired rate—one wholly explained by smaller numbers in the Severe and Incapacitated subcategories of impairment. However, they were relatively underrepresented in the Well category and overrepresented in the Mild to Moderate range of symptom formation.

Analysis further revealed that the more favorable impairment rate of the Jewish-origin group was principally characteristic of its low SES-origin members. A number of hypotheses and speculations were advanced as possible explanations of these findings.

Within each religious-origin group we differentiated respondent parents on a threefold gradient of religiosity, that is, commitment to and anchorage in their faith. Reflected in the data were substantial erosions in religious moorings among adults of a generation ago. The Midtown evidence further suggested a J-curve type of relationship between parental religiosity and offspring mental health in Protestant and Catholic families belonging to the lower two-thirds of the SES-origin range. Seemingly discernible here were the echoes in contemporary adults of the reverberating sociocultural upheavals generated during the nineteenth century.

REFERENCES

Bruder, E. E. *Administrative concerns in a public mental hospital chaplain program.* Academy of Religion and Mental Health, N.Y., 1958.

Janis, I. *Psychological stress.* New York: J. W. Levy & Sons, 1958.

King, S. H., & Funkenstein, D. Religious practice and cardiovascular reactions during stress. *Journal of Abnormal Social Psychology,* 1957, **55,** 135–137.

Langner, T. S., & Michael, S. T. *Life stress and mental health.* Glencoe, Ill.: The Free Press, 1963.

Snyder, C. R. Culture and Jewish sobriety. *Quarterly Journal of Studies in Alcohol,* 1955, **16,** 700–742.

Srole, L., Langner, T. S., Michael, S. T., Opler, M. K., & Rennie, T. A. C. *Mental health in the metropolis: The midtown Manhattan study.* New York: McGraw-Hill, 1962.

3.8 Orientation

Although America is often viewed as a culture addicted to youth, the number and proportion of our aged citizens is rapidly increasing. They are playing an increasingly important role in our political life, and it remains to be seen what kind of influence they will have in determining the directions of American social life and mores.

Ivan N. Mensh is an authority on the many problems of the aged, especially the state of their psychological health. He summarizes statistics to point out that aging populations have special social, economic, and psychological problems, over and above the physiological problems associated with growing older. Among the institutionalized aged, at least, symptomatologies of physical health and psychological health are often confused, and there is an enormous number of older psychiatric patients whose ranks may have been artificially swelled by improper diagnosis and confusion of medical and psychological symptoms. Basic information is lacking in many areas, and much remains to be learned about the influences of aging on attitudes, motivation, and personality. We also need to learn much more about the influence and effect of economic, environmental, and psychological interventions into the lives of aging persons, in addition to the effect of standard medical care. Mensh approaches all these topics, and more, in this significant contribution toward understanding the impact of aging populations.

3.8 The Aging Population and Mental Health

Ivan N. Mensh

In 1961 there appeared a summary of population data on the older in-dividuals in the United States (Staff Reports, 1961). The report indicated the significance of the basic data as "part of the background . . . [for] the growing recognition of the American aged population as a new and quite different phenomenon in our history" (p. 1). Although all of the data reported are important to a consideration of mental health among the aged, certain of the findings are especially relevant. For example, since the turn of the century there has been an 80 percent increase in the proportion of persons 65 years of age and older, from 5 to 9 percent; and during just the 1950–1960 decade alone the increase was 35 percent, whereas the general population increased only by 19 percent during the same period. In absolute numbers, there were 3.1 million persons aged 65 and older in 1900, and 16.6 million by 1960.

In addition to mental health and other health considerations of the aged, these figures imply important political possibilities, some potential, others already functioning. Of the voting age population in 1920, 8.1 percent were past 65, and barely more than a generation later this pro-portion had nearly doubled, 15.4 percent by 1960. The Medicare national program for the elderly, passed after several years of defeat and delay, suggests not only the direct political effect of the aged but also their indirect political power in legislative decisions.

Other characteristics deserve special mention because of their relation-ships with mental health. These are sex and marital status; rural farm and nonfarm, and urban distributions; and employment of the elderly in the work force. These variables are not independent, as we shall see. Although the ratio of aged women to aged men is 121:100 nationally, on farms this ratio is 84:100. Sex differences also are prominent in labor force statistics, with a decline for men past 65 during the period 1900–1960 from 64.9 percent of this population to 33.6 percent; and a shift for women past 65 from 9.3 to 11.2 percent. Finally, there are the important data on marital status, indicating the great sex difference in this charac-teristic and all of the personal, social, and economic implications of this difference for mental health. Among men past 65, 70 percent are married, more than twice the proportion of aged women who are married (one-third). Nearly half of all of the aged are widowed, single, or divorced.

The increase by about 16 years in life expectancy, from 54 in 1920 to 70 in 1960, also has to be examined in light of the increase in numbers of aged at each of the later decades. From 1920 to 1960, the increases (1960 over 1920) were 236 percent for those 65 and older, 279 percent for those 75 and older, and 920 percent for those 85 and older. In other terms, for those 75 and older, there was an increase from 30 to 34 percent, and for those 85 and older, an increase from 1.8 to 5.6 percent, about a three-fold increase in proportion. In projections of our national population growth, there is the estimate that by the year 2000 there will be over 32 million persons aged 65 or older, or more than the total United States population in 1860. In evaluating this population projection, the differing sex ratio should again be considered, for the gap in longevity between men and women in the United States has widened. At the beginning of the twentieth century, a man who had lived to age 65 had an expectation of 11.5 years of life, and by 1950 this expectation had increased to 12.8 years; but in the next dozen years there was but slight change in life expectancy for men aged 65. During the period 1900–1950, women's expectancy increased for those at age 65 from 12.2 to 15.0 years, and by 1962 to 16.0 years. Current expectations are that 20 percent of men at age 65 will attain 20 more years, while about a third of women at age 65 will survive to age 85.

Increased longevity generally is attributed to progress in public health, nutrition, and living standards. Further increases may come with methods for reducing deaths from cardiovascular-renal diseases and from cancer. Because of the improvement in public health, nutrition, and general living standards, there already has been a significant reduction in mortality from tuberculosis, pneumonia, and other infectious diseases, as well as from accidents. Decreases from these major causes of death in later life therefore would not have the effect on longevity that may occur with advances leading to the reduction of mortality from the cardiovascular-renal diseases and cancer.

The economic, social, psychological, and medical consequences of longevity are not always favorable, unfortunately. The first of these has been attacked by such programs for retirement income as the national Social Security system and private pension plans (today there are over 25,000 plans covering 23 million workers), and the last by private health insurance programs and federal legislation of the Medicare program. By the end of 1962, about 9 million aged, slightly more than half of the total number of the aged in the United States, had some form of prepaid insurance against medical expenses. The others had no health insurance of any kind. The social and psychological consequences of aging should be seen in the contexts of an economic society and the physical and psychological changes that may develop in aging individuals

(Planning Committee, 1960; President's Council, 1963; Special Staff, 1961).

The physical, psychological, and social characteristics of older individuals must be evaluated within the economic and political environments of their societies. Among the many factors to be considered is the ratio of the older population, retired for the most part (depending upon the criteria of retirement, 64–87 percent of men and 87–97 percent of women), to the population in the productive years (18–64), that is, still in the labor force. The former have been increasing at a higher rate than the rest of the population, as previously noted, owing to increased longevity and, in the United States, to larger number of births in the 1875–1925 period and the heavy immigration from Europe. There has been, however, a leveling off in the ratio of older people, because of the increase in number of children born over the past quarter-century, with a more rapid increase of children than of older people since 1950. These changing curves are relevant to data on the population dependent upon the individuals in the productive ages—for 1960 there were 63 million in the population under age 18 and 16 million 65 years old and over, constituting 44 percent of the total population and a ratio of 77 dependents to each 100 persons in the productive age range. Despite the numbers of older and retired persons in today's population, the dependency ratio is considerably smaller than that about 1900; and, even if the ratio rises to 93, a probable forecast for the year 2000, there will remain larger numbers in the productive age range than in the pre-work and retirement age groups.

The changing numbers at various parts of the age curve have other significance as well. The United States was a young nation in its chronology and in its population characteristics until relatively recently; prior to 1900 only 4 percent of the population was over age 65. This proportion has nearly tripled since then, so that an older person in today's society is more likely to meet other older individuals and to influence and be influenced by them. These older individuals increasingly represent an important political and economic group, and a more active one. Unfortunately, there are many older people with inadequate incomes. The 17 million aged 65 and over in 1961 had a total income of $35 billion, of which $11 billion came from earnings. Median money income for two-person families was $5315 and $2530 for head of household under 65 and head aged 65 or over, respectively; and for persons living alone the amounts were $2570 and $1055. In view of complaints and grumblings about governmental intervention and a "socialized state," it is important to observe that in 1950 about half of all money paid to the aged under government programs was public assistance, and in 1961 this proportion had dropped to one-eighth. Through increases in pension rates, social security benefits and the numbers of people eligible for retirement benefits, purchasing power of this group past 65 has been rapidly increasing, at a rate about as rapid as that for any other age group. This development has brought with it financial advantages and related political power for the older population. However, as with other age groups, there has not been as yet any significant political effort by the elderly. Advantages have come instead indirectly from health and social changes that have affected other age groups as well in varying degree.

In spite of the benefits of social, psychological, medical, and economic gains in recent years, there remain for the older person the difficult adjustments to retirement, to physical changes, and to the increasing losses among friends and family, a loss no longer made up by others as the circle of family and friends steadily diminishes during the later years. The relative plateau in work, leisure, and other personal and social activities that has developed during the middle years of 40–65 moves into a decline at a far slower rate than generally is reported for the biological functioning of individuals past 65. Physical and psychological performance is maintained, and effective social behavior continues because the individual has learned to work efficiently and to respond to his culture's emphasis upon efficiency and physical and psychological vigor. For example, in this country, many women during these middle years return to activity other than the home, or move into these other social spheres and continue these involvements into the later years. But for both men and women, there comes a time when their activities are reduced by personal or social changes, and a new readjustment becomes necessary. Thus, the cycle of preparation continues—preparation in youth and early adulthood for a career, the career period of adulthood and middle years, the beginning adjustments away from full-time career involvement in the 60s, and the final preparation for an indefinite period of changed activity and social interaction. Within these generalities there exists a wide range of diversity, varying as a function of the individual and his personal, social, and economic circumstances. It is this range of variation that tempers the findings and conclusions of investigators seriously engaged in systematic studies of older individuals.

Other population changes also function in any evaluation of the significance of the older part of our population. Beginning about age 50, women outnumber men, and this difference widens with increasing years. Present predictions suggest that by 1980 the ratio of men to women will have dropped from 82:100 (in 1960) to 72:100. Another continuing change is in the proportions of older white, foreign born, and nonwhite populations. Changes in immigration have markedly reduced the foreign-born numbers and will be even more significant as the effects of restrictions cumulate. Changes in mortality rates for nonwhites are slowly reducing the differences in proportions of white-nonwhite individuals, and these changes, too, will increase more and more in coming years to reduce the differences in the proportions.

A changing third characteristic of the older population contributes further to social change—educational level. Fifteen years ago, only about 25 percent of persons 65 and older had more than eighth grade schooling, and about one in six had completed high school, proportions just about half those for the entire population aged 25 years and older. This is not surprising, in light of the proportion of foreign-born among older individuals, and the low urban-rural ratio during the earlier years of our older citizens. These factors, together with early school-leaving and early age of beginning work, produced the differences in educational level between those past 65 and those in the 25–65-year age range. With the decade-by-decade increase in educational level in the United States, however, the wide discrepancy in educational level between the older population and the younger age groups will be lessened, with attendant other changes related to education in our society in terms of retirement planning and activities during later years, and to cultural values and expectations.

Urban-rural pattern changes were observed above as one of the variables in the change in educational level. The urbanization of America, and suburbanization in large metroplitan areas, has drawn younger people from the farm and rural areas and, interestingly enough, also attracted older women. The net result is a marked shift in the population and the related ratio of economic producers to nonproducers or dependents (those under 18 and 65 or older). More older men and older women live in rural areas (129:100), in contrast to the ratio (80:100) in urban areas. For older Americans of both sexes there is an inverse relationship between their proportion in the population and size of community, with the proportion in newer suburban areas as low as 1 percent. There are, especially in the Southwest and South, increases in the population of older residents ranging from 50 to 90 percent.

Other chronological and time relationships are relevant to psychological, social, and economic adjustments of the older population. In this country, the median age of men at time of first marriage is 23, age at birth of last child is 29, marriage of last child 50, death of spouse 64, and his death 72 years. For his wife, the ages are, respectively, 20, 26, 48, 61, and 77. For both, there must be adjustments in many spheres to no longer having children at home, after half of the parents' lives have been

involved in child rearing; and widowhood or widowerhood after 50 years
or more of marriage and partnerhood. Here again, there are the greater
numbers of widows than widowers, because women are younger at first
marriage than men, and fewer women than men remarry because of the
disparate numbers in the "marriageable pool." These data mean that
about two-thirds of older men but only one-third of older women will
still be married after age 65.

Household arrangements constitute another socially and economically
relevant variable. Most couples prefer to live in their own household,
and about 80 percent of those past 65 are able to continue this living
arrangement. In successive decades after age 60, the proportions of independently living older individuals and couples drop significantly until,
in those past 85, about two-thirds of the aged live in households headed
by other people. But housing for older persons must be evaluated with
their lower incomes and special medical and health needs, as contrasted
with housing needs for younger people. The 1960 United States Census
of Housing included studies of housing of senior citizens. For 26 percent
of owner-occupied dwellings where the household head was 65 and over,
the housing was deficient (dilapidated, deteriorated, or sound, but lacking
some or all plumbing facilties); and for renter-occupied housing the
proportion was 40 percent.

Three more areas round out the range of significant variables for the
aged. These hold as well for the younger population but, as indicated
above, with different impact. The areas are the related ones of employment, income, and urbanization. Estimates today indicate that the aggregate income before federal, state, and local income and other taxes for
the United States population 65 years of age and over is $35 billion,
from which come $5 or more billion in taxes. Various public income-
maintenance programs (OASDI, railroad retirement, other public retirement systems, and public assistance) comprise 35 percent of the income,
10 percent comes from private pension plans and other private sources,
43 percent from earnings and other income (10 percent from earned income only), and the balance from such other sources as dividends, interests, rents, annuities, and so on, with 4 percent with money income. With
from one-fifth to one-third of all older people living in households with
adult children, there is, no doubt, a significant amount of support from
these and other relatives in the forms of housing, food, gifts, other contributions, and medical care costs. Although the aggregate cash income
of the population past 65 is about 10 percent of the total national income
and 6–7 percent of the gross national product (the total value of all goods
and services produced), estimates indicate that the majority of older

people, especially the retired, have less income than is necessary to provide a minimum adequate budget.

Income does not derive only from employment, since among the older population only 10 percent have income only from earnings. Employment represents more than income, however, because of its personal and social rewards and interactions. Thus, as with marital status, living and household arrangements, ethnic origin, and education, employment has relevance significantly related to the psychological, social, economic, and political characteristics of the aged and the larger society in which they live. For example, the economic, physical, social, and psychological situations of single, older persons more often are poorer than those of the aged still married. Similarly, these areas of interaction varied as a function of ethnic origin when neighborhoods in cosmopolitan centers represented concentrations of specific ethnic or national groups. Today there still remain such concentrations in some major cities, but their composition is much changed from the peak period of European immigration (1880–1920). These generalizations also apply to urbanization, a major development with far-reaching consequences for the aged and for the younger population, and one that represents a nearly universal characteristic of societies, states, and nations in most parts of the world. For example, in the United States, one-third of the total population lived on farms in 1910. In the following half-century the ratio dropped to 7 percent, about one-fifth of the proportion in 1910, and since World War II more people have left farms than there now are living on farms. Among the aged, 8 percent live on farms and nearly 25 percent in nonfarm rural areas, totalling one-third in rural areas, an 8 percent decrease from the number a decade earlier in spite of an increase of a million aged in the rural population. These changes in urban-rural proportions still reflect the important observation, among others, that more than 5 million aged Americans live in rural areas, where there are far fewer health care facilities, personnel, and community programs than exist in urban regions, yet the health and other needs of these older individuals are greater than for the population under age 65. Although the incidence and prevalence of poor health may not be greater in rural than in urban areas, facilities, personnel, and health programs are far less available.

One study (Youmans, 1963) does suggest certain differences between the aged in a rural area and those in an urban area. This empirical research provided many details about the aged in a rural, agrarian county in an economically depressed region of the southern Appalachians, and the aged in the metropolitan community of Lexington, both in Kentucky. Although there are geographical and other sampling variations limiting the generalizability of the study, the data deserve review, for both methodological and substantive reasons. Four areas of living conditions were examined—economic and health status, leisure-time activities, and the perceived problems and advantages of aging. The study was conducted in 1959 and consisted of home interviews of 627 respondents aged 60 or older in an area-probability sample of households in a rural county and 609 in an urban area. The samples were drawn from populations of 14,000 and 112,000, respectively. Economic status variables related to work and retirement, income, housing, property and equipment, economic losses with age, economic attitudes, and the widowed woman. Health status variables were ailments, role impairments and health services, needs, and costs. Family relationships, community activities, hobbies and pastimes, attitudes, and needs were studied in the area of leisure time. To gauge status of the respondents, data were obtained on age, sex, education, occupation, color, marital status, religion, housing area, type of community, and socioeconomic condition.

The responses and their tabulation suggest the associations between socioenvironmental variables and living conditions, and attitudinal and other behaviors of these older individuals. In the area of economic status, the urban male respondents had incomes triple those of the rural men, even though more of the latter were in the labor force. Also, the property owned by the urban-living older males were double that of the rural men, with more of the latter owning homes, but these were in poorer condition than the homes of the urban dwellers. Men past 75, compared to those in the 60–64 age range, were less often in the labor force, had smaller incomes and estates, fewer owned homes, and these homes were in poorer condition. However, the younger respondents, ages 60–64, reported stronger feelings of economic deprivation. These feelings of deprivation were equally often reported by men and widowed women, interestingly enough, although the economic status of the widow was much lower than that for married men and their wives. A quarter of men and widows disliked their living arrangements, a third judged their financial state at present worse than at age 50, and 50 percent said they did without things because of lack of money.

In the area of health, more than two-thirds reported symptoms of poor health consistently or intermittently, with more ills voiced by rural persons and by those of low socioeconomic status. There was not an increase in reports of poor health with older age groups nor were there sex, mental status, or role differences in the number of illnesses reported. However, role impairments and fewer activities for both men and women were reported significantly more often with increasing age. Related to reports of ailments were reports of many serious problems with more than 60 percent of all respondents reporting such problems. Further, more than half saw no advantages to aging, over 40 percent were pessimistic in their outlook on life, and health problems were of much greater concern than financial problems.

In the area of medical care, about half of all respondents had seen a physician during the preceding five years, one-third had been in hospital, and one-fifth had a nurse or friend in to the home to help them. One-fifth said they needed additional health care, and about a third had health insurance coverage.

In leisure periods, church-going was the commonest activity and, for most, the only community participation. There were not urban-rural differences, although relationships with friends and neighbors were more often reported by rural than urban dwellers. In the close relationships of families, 80 percent had children living and, of these, 44 percent lived in the households of children. Family visits were directly related to geographical distances between homes of siblings and children. Hobbies occupied leisure time for many, with these activities usually sedentary, as, for example, listening to the radio, watching television, and reading. There were but slight urban-rural differences. About one-fourth desired more activities and, for many, free time appeared to be a burden.

Urban dwellers were decidedly less pessimistic than rural aged, reported fewer serious problems, were less concerned about health, and saw more advantages in aging. Although age and work status were not associated with a pessimistic outlook, there were significant associations of this attitude with low socioeconomic status, sex (men more pessimistic), race (nonwhites reporting more pessimism), and marital status, with less pessimism among older persons who had never married.

Reference to the older woman has been made several times in this discussion. In the specific field of mental health, it is this sample of the population of older individuals that represents special problems, both for themselves and for the society of which they are part. Whereas in both Britain and the United States there was a population increase in the decade of the 1950s, there was a decrease in the number of beds for mental patients, from 584,000 to 543,000 in the United States and from 143,000 to 140,000 in Britain. Resident rates have been going down steadily, and admission rates have as steadily risen. However, resident rates for patients 65 and older have been rising, and admission rates are highest for this group and for the 35–44 age group. For example, in Britain, admissions of patients 75 years and older increased nearly 80 percent from 1951 to 1959. Among Britain's mental patients in hospital, older women occupy 46 percent of the total days' stay and 30 percent of the total time in hospital for all psychiatric patients, rates far higher even

than the traditional long-stay women schizophrenic patients, for whom
the figures are 16 and 17 percent, respectively. For males, the rates for
schizophrenics are 30 and 27 percent, and for aged males the rates are
21 and 16 percent.

Mental hospital discharge data reflect a high probability of discharge
in the early months of hospitalization, with a sharp drop after six months
and one year, with two years clearly tending as the period after which
chronic hospitalization is highly likely. For men in the 15–64 year range
the percentage remaining in hospital two years or more after admission
is 9–10 percent, and over 11 percent for those 65 or older. For women
patients the percentages are 6–9 percent for those under 64, and nearly
21 percent for the older mentally ill women, proportions two or three
times greater than for the younger women, and about twice that for male
patients. These resident rates for older patients arise from the 20 percent
of all mental hospital admissions in Britain who are past 65 years of age.
Among these geriatric patients, the fortunate ones who were able to leave
hospital were discharged on the average about six weeks after admission.
Of the remainder, the mean interval between admission and death was
only twenty weeks for men and forty-eight weeks for women. In the
United States, long-term studies indicate only 16 percent of older patients were discharged by release or transfer, 19 percent died within a
month following admission, and 57 percent died within the first year of
hospitalization. It is of further importance that these rates appear to
have varied only slightly during the past 30 years and are representative
of data reported in such major population areas as those contained in
Ohio, Maryland, New York, and California (Mensh, 1963; Whittier &
Williams, 1956).

It is important also to observe that the already enormous population
of older psychiatric patients may, in error, be swelled by "the confusion
and confounding of age with physical and psychological health" (Mensh,
1959). The importance of such diagnostic discrimination has been reported by Kidd (1962) and Mensh (1959) in the physical-psychological
dimension, and for prognosis by Kay, Roth and their associates (Kay &
Roth, 1955; Kay, Norris, & Post, 1956; Roth & Kay, 1956); Weiss, Gildea,
Davis, and Mensh (1958); Davis, Weiss, Gildea, and Mensh (1959); and
Mensh, Weiss, David, and Gildea (1959). Mensh (1959, p. 517) concluded
that "medical or administrative decisions may confuse psychologic and
physical illness in patients in later life." Kidd's (1962) study of patients
evaluated as mental, mental-physical (mental symptoms predominant),
physical-mental (physical symptoms predominant), or physical, indicated
that 24 percent of the patients aged 60 or older in the mental hospital
wards, and 34 percent of older patients in a general hospital geriatric

unit were "misplaced and ought to have been in the other type of hospital." Age, social class, economic status, and marital status were associated with misplacement, with more frequent errors of placement among patients past 75, in lower social classes and lower economic status, single and widowed, and those referred from either welfare institutions or lodgings. Symptoms of restlessness, disorientation, and impaired ability to communicate were more frequent among the misplaced patients.

There are two groups of hospitalized mental patients among the aged which must be separately examined, but this discrimination seldom is made. There are those patients who are 60, 65, or older on admission, and those who are admitted at earlier ages and whose chronic illness necessitates continued hospitalization. Thus, in a 15 percent random sample of a California state hospital with a high proportion of elderly patients (Palmer, 1962; Scott & Devereaux, 1963), 89 percent of the patients in hospital for two or more years were admitted prior to their becoming 65 years old—"Obviously, at any given date a new group of yesterday's chronic, middle-aged patients become today's geriatric patients. . . ." In this study, the authors suggest that many chronic patients in the 40–64-year range, and "most" chronic patients past 65 may be able to be cared for in community facilities other than psychiatric hospitals, freeing these state hospitals for treatment of younger patients and acute conditions. The data thus far (Booth & Swain, 1963) are not sufficiently complete to warrant more than a continued experiment to make such placements for middle-aged and older chronic patients, pending follow-up of the course of these patients when placed in other than state psychiatric hospitals. On those who remain in hospital, there are such observations as those summarized in previous pages, relative to longevity and associated variables, and measures of disability and consequent medical and nursing care. Meer and Krag (1964), for example, recommend their empirical scale of disability for measuring the degree of dependence on others to meet basic physical needs. Their study of the total geriatric population in a state hospital numbering 1340 patients indicated that "(1) female patients were significantly more disabled than male patients; (2) patients with organic mental diseases were significantly more disabled than patients with functional mental diseases; (3) disability increased significantly with age; and (4) disability was significantly associated with the type of patient movement during the year following the survey" (p. 445).

Age and sex differences also have been observed among patients coming to an outpatient clinic. These may sooner or later be found in state mental hospitals, but because many are able to maintain themselves in the community, they represent an important sample to observe. For example, Weiss, Rommel and Schaie (1959) studied the presenting problems of sixty-seven women and forty-five men in a city hospital psychiatric clinic, all above age 45 and drawn from a total population of about 600 patients seen during two years of clinic operation. Half of the patient sample were 65 and older.

The patients reported three or four complaints each, on the average, with a mean of five for women and three for men. In general, the complaints were related by the men to economic or occupational stresses; while the women reported somatic and reality-disturbance symptoms, displayed a greater variety of symptoms, and complained more about their symptoms. There were not age differences in the kinds of complaints, although patients aged 65 and older (65–78) generally complained less and had less variety in their complaints than those 45–64.

Weiss, Chatham, and Schaie (1961) reported statistically significant age-related problem areas for the patients coming to their outpatient psychiatric clinic in the city hospital under study. Patients in the younger age groups (in their late 40s) expressed most concern about somatic symptoms, changes in thinking, and their psychological state of mind or feelings of well-being. In the patients in late middle age, the problems related primarily to economic or to occupational situations. Among those in the older age groups (60s and 70s) most concern was voiced about problems that appeared to represent gross distortions of reality. All of the age groups seeking help in this metropolitan clinic desired situational aid for their problems and concerns, which were mostly about changes in emotional state and their overt anxiety. Thus, these latter variables were not age-related.

Finally, as investigators review the studies of older individuals, their own research and that of colleagues, there is general agreement that basic information on mental health and illness among these older persons is lacking in many significant areas. At least, there have evolved recommendations about the areas in need of study, but the studies themselves are only slowly coming into being, and thus reports of the designs and findings remain unfortunately few. For example, much needs to be learned about both cross-sectional and longitudinal samples of aging individuals as attitudes, motivations, intellectual and other personality characteristics change over a period of time. In some individuals the physical changes may overshadow the psychological changes, and in others the reverse may be observed. We already have seen how frequently physical and mental illness are confused when these conditions exist with old age as one of the variables under review. There is the further need to learn how specific interventions may affect the developing aging process in older persons. Such interventions may be economic and financial, medical and physical, environmental (in both physical and social categories), or psychological. The last may include forms of behavioral conditioning on the premise that older individuals are less "psychologically minded" and therefore the "talk of psychotherapy" may be less effective than specific behavioral conditioning methods. Many reports exist extolling the merits of group therapy for oldsters, on the criterion of efficiency and effectiveness, but few serious investigators are satisfied with the experimental controls reported in these studies. These primarily clinical studies reflect enthusiasm and willingness to try to help older persons with psychological disorders, but rarely are the research designs compatible with the findings and conclusions summarizing the experiences.

Other gaps in information exist in our knowledge of developing changes in behavior, normal or abnormal, throughout the life span of the human organism, that may predict the rate or other characteristics of aging in such a way that intervention may be other than empirical. The personal ecology of older individuals and their total social patterns as they affect the aged, and are affected by them, remain largely unknown, especially in the field of mental health and illness. This is not to deny the planning, concern, and beginning efforts which within the next decades may produce yields that presently are almost infinitesmal. It is important to observe the extensive literature in gerontology as well as the widespread interest among the general public and among many biological (Shock, 1962), social (Tibbits & Donahue, 1962), clinical (Blumenthal, 1962; Hoch & Zubin, 1961), welfare (Kaplan & Aldridge, 1962), and psychological (Planning Committee, 1960) investigators. Here lies the promise of the answers to questions on aging, questions which we only recently have been able to formulate so that there may be systematic studies of the many variables and their interactions in the human organism as it develops and ages. The lack of adequate sampling, data-gathering, methodology, and often even of hypotheses is far more apparent to today's investigators than it was a decade or more ago. This in itself represents a gain, in the development of more specific hypotheses and more effective methods for testing them, in mental health and illness, as in other areas of aging.

What are the implications of the data that do exist on the aging population and mental health? With increasing federal, state, and local support for mental health programs at the community level and increasing awareness of the mental health needs of older citizens, there also will be greater demand placed upon programs. Further, as better understanding of the preventive and treatment aspects of psychological care develops in this segment of our population, through health education and other media, it is anticipated that negative attitudes toward mental health care will be modified toward an acceptance of such programs. The increasing educational level of the aged in our society, and programs developed specifically for lower income and social groups (described above) make for greater acceptance of mental health programs.

Another development relates to recent concepts and efforts to reduce the number of aged in institutions, primarily in state mental hospitals, by appropriate placement in the community, especially in foster homes. These programs for maintaining older patients in the community, and returning them as rapidly as possible from institutional care, where this care has been necessary because of some acute condition, may prevent the isolation and alienation of older patients which, unfortunately, is so usual today.

There also are changes in the economic condition of the aged that will affect the psychologic adjustment of many. Reactions to situational stress because of financial deprivation frequently have been reported among the precipitating causes for seeking help, especially among older individuals who are single or widowed. The governmental and private health care and retirement programs which include more and more of the older population will provide relief from economic stress and also reduce the numbers of individuals who have been forced to live in substandard housing. Housing programs designed for the aged also will affect positively the economic and living situation of the elderly in ways that may reduce personal and social stresses on these individuals. For example, the research on housing by such investigators as Wilner (UCLA) in Los Angeles and Rosow (Western Reserve University) in Cleveland and their associates will for the first time provide reliable data on housing conditions among the aged and their reactions to the varied situations in which they live. Such basic data have been lacking, and many programs have been based therefore upon anecdotal or otherwise unsystematic information. Psychological adjustments related to the economics, physical environment, and personal and social environments now may be assessed where previously no systematic studies were available upon which to develop housing programs whose psychological and social impact upon the aged and other age groups may be significantly positive or negative. The mental health of nursing home residents, senior citizens' housing, and other living arrangements, other than studies of the number of family or other units and quality of housing, now will be more reliably evaluated and programs can be designed for varying degrees of adjustment and maladjustment in communities of older persons and in the general community in which so many aged still live.

It is obvious then that policies and plans for social action programs in our society must recognize (1) the increasing proportions and great absolute numbers of older individuals in our society; (2) the mental health needs of these citizens, especially the enormous numbers of older women with mental disorders; (3) the need for maintaining older people in the community except during periods of acute illness; (4) the distinction between physical illness and psychological disorder in the aged; (5) the impact of social changes—political, economic, legal, and other forms of social change—upon the aged as well as upon younger age groups; and (6) the need to maintain the perspective of developmental progression from infancy through adolescence and adulthood to the later years of maturity, rather than examining aging changes only from the period of age 60 and older.

REFERENCES

Blumenthal, H. T. (Ed.) *Medical and clinical aspects of aging.* New York: Columbia University Press, 1962.

Booth, R. S., & Swain, J. M. Mental disorders of the aged: The role of the state hospital in the treatment; Report of a pilot study. *Calif. Med.,* 1963, **98,** 320–324.

Davis, D., Weiss, J. M. A., Gildea, E. F., & Mensh, I. N. Psychiatric problems of later life. II. Clinical syndromes. *Amer. Pract. Dig. Treatment,* 1959, **10,** 61–65.

Hoch, P. H., & Zubin, J. (Eds.) *Psychotherapy of aging.* New York: Grune & Stratton, 1961.

Kaplan, J., & Aldridge, G. J. (Eds.) *Social Welfare of the aging.* New York: Columbia University Press, 1962.

Kay, D. W., Norris, V., & Post, F. Prognosis in psychiatric disorders of the elderly. An attempt to derive indicators of early death and early recovery. *J. ment. Sci.,* 1956, **102,** 129–140.

Kay, D. W., & Roth, M. Physical accompaniments of mental disorder in old age. *Lancet,* 1955, **269,** 740–745.

Kidd, C. B. Criteria for the admission of the elderly to geriatric and psychiatric units. *J. ment. Sci.,* 1962, **108,** 68–74.

Meer, B., and Krag, C. L. Correlates of disability in a population of hospitalized geriatric patients. *Journal of Gerontology,* 1964, **19,** 440–446.

Mensh, I. N. Psychiatric diagnosis in the institutionalized aged. *Geriatrics,* 1959, **14,** 511–517.

Mensh, I. N. Studies of older psychiatric patients. *Gerontologist,* 1963, **3,** 100–104.

Mensh, I. N., Weiss, J. M. A., Davis, D., & Gildea, E. F. Psychiatric problems of later life. III. Treatment and rehabilitation. *Amer. Pract. Dig. Treat.,* 1959, **10,** 225–228.

Palmer, J. T. Older patients in California state hospitals for general psychiatry: 1961. Sacramento, Calif.: State Department of Mental Hygiene, Research Division; *Biostat. Sect. Bull.* No. 20, 1962.

Planning Committee on Population Trends, Social and Economic Implications. *Background paper on population trends, social and economic implications.* Washington, D.C.: White House Conference on Aging, 1960. (Conference held in January 1961.)

Planning Committee on Research in Gerontology: Psychological and Social Sciences. *Background paper on research in gerontology: Psychological and social sciences.* Washington, D.C.: White House Conference on Aging, 1960. (Conference held in January 1961.)

President's Council on Aging. *The older American.* Washington, D.C.: United States Government Printing Office, 1963.

Roth, M., & Kay, D. W. Affective disorders arising in the senium. 2. Physical disability as an etiological factor. *J. ment. Sci.,* 1956, **102**, 141–150.

Scott, T., & Devereaux, C. P. Perpetuation of geriatric problems in California state mental hospitals. *American Journal of Psychiatry,* 1963, **120**, 155–159.

Shock, N. W. (Ed.) *Biological aspects of aging.* New York: Columbia University Press, 1962.

Special Staff on Aging. *The nation and its older people: Report of the White House Conference on Aging.* Washington, D.C.: United States Department of Health, Education, and Welfare, 1961.

Staff Report to the Special Committee on Aging, United States Senate. *New population facts on older Americans, 1960.* Washington, D.C.: United States Government Printing Office, 1961.

Tibbitts, C., & Donahue, W. (Eds.) *Social and psychological aspects of aging.* New York: Columbia University Press, 1962.

Weiss, J. M. A., Chatham, L. R., & Schaie, K. W. Symptom formation associated with age. *Arch. gen. Psychiat.,* 1961, 4, 22–29.

Weiss, J. M. A., Gildea, E. F., Davis, D., & Mensh, I. N. Psychiatric problems of later life. I. Nature and scope. *Amer. Pract. Dig. Treatment,* 1958, **9**, 1955–1959.

Weiss, J. M. A., Rommel, L. A., & Schaie, K. W. The presenting problems of older patients referred to a psychiatric clinic. *Journal of Gerontology,* 1959, **14**, 477–481.

Whittier, J. R. & Williams, D. The coincidence and constancy of mortality figures for aged psychotic patients admitted to state hospitals. *J. nerv. ment. Dis.,* 1956, **124**, 618–620.

Youmans, E. G. *Aging patterns in a rural and an urban area of Kentucky.* Lexington, Ky.: University of Kentucky Agricultural Experimental Station, Bulletin 681, 1963.

3.9   Orientation

The sociologist Robert Kleiner and his colleague, anthropologist Seymour Parker, have responded to what is a highly inconsistent, even contradictory, literature on the relationship between social mobility and mental illness by designing and carrying out a major research enterprise. Kleiner and Parker have added a Durkheimian dimension, that of anomie, to the earlier concentration upon simple movement, either up or down in the social order. They have asked their questions about the social and psychological correlates of social mobility before the fact, and they have sought their answers among the Negro population of Philadelphia, where they interviewed almost 3000 persons.

Their conclusions diverge from Durkheim's theory, which assumed an invariant relationship between social mobility, anomie, and a form of deviant behavior, specifically suicide. Kleiner and Parker demonstrate that mobility and mental illness are correlated when they occur at some strata in the social status hierarchy, but not at others. Their research, which is more fully reported in their book, *Mental Health in an Urban Negro Community* (1966), is a model for an attempt to integrate social structural and social-psychological variables in the investigation of mental illness.

3.9   Social Mobility, Anomie, and Mental Disorder

Robert J. Kleiner and Seymour Parker

The need for a comprehensive understanding of social mobility and related social-psychological phenomena becomes increasingly more salient with the progressive industrialization and urbanization of American society. A complex technology that requires role specializations and adaptations to these specializations is invariably associated with socially specified educational, occupational, and other prestige hierarchies. In this paper, "social mobility" refers to the individual's movement, relative to parental position, up or down the graded steps of any of these hierarchies.

Numerous efforts have been made to study the amount of social mobility in our society, but relatively little is known about the social and psychological concomitants of such movement. For example, considerable attention has been directed toward determining relationships between mobility and changes in political outlook or attitudes toward minority groups; other studies have shown that problems of mental health are intimately related to the amount of mobility experienced by the population under consideration. However, little conclusive evidence has been gathered relating the effects of upward or downward mobility to the individual's interpersonal relationships or to his mental health.

The present paper has two broad aims: (1) to examine the relationship between social mobility and mental disorder, and (2) to determine whether this relationship can be further attributed to various social-psychological phenomena that characterize the sample populations. Although data on the epidemiology of disease are valuable in themselves, attempts at causal explanations usually require a consideration of additional characteristics of population subgroups with different illness rates. Rather than merely to demonstrate the existence of such characteristics, it is important to link them temporally to the disease process by theoretical formulations. A method developed to investigate such temporal relationships (Parker & Kleiner, 1966) will be applied to data analyzed in this paper.

This attempt to examine some social-psychological concomitants of social mobility and mental disorder may also be relevant to an understanding of other social and political factors associated with mobility. With this larger perspective in mind, we have derived a series of hypotheses from sociological and psychological theory concerned with deviant behavior in general (Durkheim, 1951).

The importance of utilizing sociological and psychological concepts from a common frame of reference is self-evident. Most existing epidemiological research has concentrated on determining the distribution of mental disorder in various populations. Social-psychological factors have been employed usually as post hoc explanations of the results (see review in Kleiner & Parker, 1963). In a recent review, Dunham (1964) noted the inconclusive nature of the relevant epidemiological literature. He particularly emphasized that "many of the epidemiological studies by sociologists have supplied data on one level of organization [the sociological] and then have made an interpretation of these data on another level of organization [the psychological]." He regarded this "as a logical error and one that makes it quite difficult to assess the significance of the present state of knowledge in this area." McClosky and Schaar (1965) pointed out that a failure to incorporate psychological factors into the research design also characterized most studies relating anomie (or social normlessness) to various manifestations of deviant behavior.

This inconsistency in approaches to studying the epidemiology of mental disorder is reflected in research relating mental disorder and social mobility. Warner (1937) assumed that many mental ailments were atttributable to upward and downward mobility in American society. Implicit in his reasoning were further assumptions of a direct relationship between social mobility and interpersonal disturbances, and between the latter factor and mental illness. Blau (1956) reviewed the area of social mobility and interpersonal relations and cited empirical studies showing that socially mobile individuals (in either direction) manifested more racial prejudice (Greenbaum & Pearlin, 1953) and greater concern over their health (Litwak, 1956) than nonmobile persons. Blau concluded that these types of behavior resulted from interpersonal disturbances which interfered with social integration. A similar position was taken by Janowitz and Curtis (1957).

Lipset and Bendix (1963) suggested that extreme social mobility was often accompanied by discrepancies or inconsistencies among a person's various statuses (for example, high educational and low occupational status), which caused role conflict and interpersonal disturbances. All of these studies suggest that mobility results in a disturbance of one's social integration, but the validity of this hypothesis is still at issue (Tumin, 1959; Simpson, 1963).

Research relating social mobility more directly to mental disorder is also inconclusive and contradictory. Tietze, Lemkau, and Cooper (1942) reported that the inverse relationship they found between schizophrenia and social class could not be explained by high rates of downward mobility. Similar results were noted by Lapouse, Monk, and Terris (1956), Hollingshead and Redlich (1955), and Clausen and Kohn (1959): in none of these studies were mentally ill respondents characterized by particularly high rates of mobility in either direction.

Some studies, however, have confirmed a positive relationship between mental illness and mobility. Lystad (1957) noted that schizophrenic patients were more downwardly mobile relative to their fathers than a control group of neurotics matched for occupational achievement. In a study of a nonhospitalized population in New York City, Srole, Langner, Michael, Opler, and Rennie (1962) found that a relatively large proportion of individuals with severe psychiatric symptoms were downwardly mobile occupationally. Further analysis of the same data (Langner & Michael, 1963) corroborated Srole's findings.

Jaco (1959) reported that communities with high rates of mental disorder were characterized mainly by downward mobility. In a study conducted in England, Morris (1959) noted a heavy concentration of schizophrenic patients in his low-status group. Since the fathers of these patients were randomly distributed throughout all social classes, this concentration indicated that the patients had been downwardly mobile.

Some of the studies mentioned found no relationship between social mobility in general and mental disorder, and others noted a positive association between *downward* mobility and illness. This inconsistent picture is further complicated by studies showing a positive relationship between *upward* mobility and mental illness. Although Hollingshead and Redlich (1954) found no significant relationship between mobility and mental disorder, they noted that most of the patients who did change social position were upwardly mobile. Hollingshead, Ellis, and Kirby (1954) explored mobility and diagnosis at two different status levels. At the lower level they found no relationship between mobility and illness, but at the higher position neurotics were more upwardly mobile than nonpatients, and schizophrenics were the most upwardly mobile of all groups. The authors concluded that neurotic and schizophrenic individuals at relatively high status levels were strivers who had actually experienced more upward movement from parental level than had nonpatients.

Ellis (1952) determined the occupational mobility of sixty career women relative to their fathers' levels. The upwardly mobile women manifested significantly more severe psychosomatic symptoms than nonmobile subjects. A relationship between upward mobility and psychosomatic symptoms was confirmed by Ruesch (1946, 1956) and Ruesch, Jacobson, and Loeb (1948).

The studies mentioned in this review permit few conclusive generalizations about a relationship between social mobility and mental disorder. The widely varying criteria often used to define social mobility and mental illness render the results of many studies incomparable. For example, the data analyzed by Srole et al., and by Langner and Michael, were based on "diagnoses" made from questionnaire responses of a general community population—medically diagnosed patients were not considered. This approach was unlike that taken by Hollingshead and Redlich and other investigators cited above. Langner and Michael's utilization of a composite index to measure mobility also differed from the methods employed in other studies. In addition, these investigators determined a respondent's social status level with a different index than that used to determine parental level. Such methodological inconsistencies among studies indicate the unreliability involved in drawing general conclusions from their findings.

The variability in existing definitions of mobility is even more compounded by problems involved in measuring status itself (see review in

Kleiner & Parker, 1963). A single status measure such as education or income may be employed as the basis for determining mobility, or a composite status index may be utilized. The researcher must decide what criteria of mobility are most significant for his problem. A further difficulty suggested by the literature is that the nature of the relationship between social mobility and mental disorder differs, depending on the status level and the diagnostic group being analyzed. These problems emphasize the importance of studying samples large enough to permit careful controls in data analysis. In this respect, too, existing studies differ widely and are often seriously deficient.

A final problem (referred to earlier) is that very few epidemiological investigations of social mobility and mental illness have made systematic attempts to examine the social-psychological factors underlying the relationship between these variables. Perhaps these data would be more consistent if we understood the social-psychological concomitants of mobility and how these factors varied with changes in the direction of mobility and the social context in which it occurred. Mobility in one social context (for example, accompanied by migration or in interracial situations) may have very different implications and effects than mobility in another context.

The concept of social mobility in itself may be too complex a structural factor and too variable in its psychological implications to relate to mental disorder in a simple manner. A more sophisticated typology of mobility, encompassing additional aspects of the social situation and/or associated social-psychological factors, may yield greater consistency in research findings.

The inconsistent results reported in the literature and the lack of studies incorporating social-psychological variables into the research design led us to explore more fully the relationship between social mobility and mental disorder (Parker & Kleiner, 1966). In this effort, we utilized various ideas about goal striving and certain aspects of level-of-aspiration theory developed by Lewin and Escalona (Escalona, 1940; 1948; Lewin, Dembo, Festinger, & Sears, 1944). Our basic research design involved comparing a community and a mentally ill population (described more fully in the second section of this article). Individuals in our patient sample saw a more open societal opportunity structure, were characterized by higher goal-striving stress,[1] perceived larger discrepancies between

---

[1] Our measure of goal-striving stress was conceptualized in terms of the interaction of these different social-psychological components: the discrepancy between level of aspiration and achievement, estimate of chances of reaching the aspired goal, and the degree of involvement in the aspired goal.

their own general achievement level and that of an informal reference group,[2] and showed lower self-esteem than community respondents.

Although this pattern of responses differentiated ill and community respondents, we could not determine directly whether these characteristics were antecedents of mental disorder or merely consequences of the illness process. In an effort to resolve this problem, we developed a method to investigate more thoroughly the temporal sequence between these response characteristics and mental disorder. This method was intended to reduce the possible effect of illness on responses to our questionnaire instrument. It involved (1) determining the relative yields, or rates, of mental disorder for various subgroups in the community population (for example, sex or age subgroups, breakdowns by mobility type, and so on), and (2) ascertaining whether a high yield community subgroup showed a greater prevalence of the response characteristics observed for the mentally ill than did a low yield community subgroup. Implicit in this reasoning was the assumption that characteristics differentiating the community and ill samples would also discriminate (but not as strongly) between high and low yield community subpopulations.

If, for example, males were found to be over-represented and females under-represented in the ill sample, compared to their distribution in the community sample, community sample males would be considered to constitute a high yield subgroup and females a low yield subgroup. Further, we would predict that the high yield respondents (males) would be more prone than the low yield respondents (females) to manifest the illness-linked response characteristics noted above (that is, perception of an open opportunity structure, high goal-striving stress scores, large reference group discrepancies, and low self-esteem). Since the community respondents were not mentally ill and had no recent history of psychiatric contact, if a high yield community subgroup was more prone to manifest any one of these illness-associated characteristics, this factor could be considered a potential antecedent of illness.

Using this rationale, we divided the community sample into different occupational mobility subgroups (upwardly mobile from parental position, nonmobile, and downwardly mobile) and determined the relative rates, or yields, of mental disorder for these subgroups.

When occupational status position was held constant, or controlled, we found high illness rates for the downwardly mobile at the lowest occupational level [3] and for the upwardly mobile at the high end of the status

---

[2] A reference group represents an existing group of people (or set of values) by means of whose performance or opinions one evaluates himself.

[3] An individual's mobility status was based on the difference between his own

scale. We therefore predicted that individuals in these two high yield community mobility subgroups would manifest more of the illness-associated responses noted above than their nonmobile status peers. Subjects in both of these high yield subgroups perceived the opportunity structure as relatively more open, had higher goal-striving stress scores, and showed lower self-esteem than nonmobile subjects at the same two status levels. No differences between high and low yield mobility groups emerged when reference group discrepancy was considered, however.

The ability of these social-psychological variables to account for mobility-associated illness rates was a dramatic confirmation of their predictive power and affirmed the effectiveness of the yield procedure. The analyses using status controls showed that mental illness was not invariably related to mobility itself, but rather to particular response patterns of social-psychological variables associated with the three types of mobility at different status levels.

The relationship between illness and these social-psychological factors indicated that the results might be relevant to the body of theory on anomie and deviant behavior (Durkheim, 1951, pp. 241–276; Merton, 1957, pp. 131–194). It appeared that a series of predictions congruent with the findings reported above could be derived from this frame of reference.

Durkheim noted that suicide rates tended to increase during periods of economic depression and prosperity. The existence of high rates in both types of situations indicated that physical deprivation or poverty in itself was not the most important contributory factor. He concluded that each type of economic crisis situation was accompanied by disturbances in the "collective order" in which the individual was involved. Durkheim reasoned that the structure of human nature made the individual's needs and desires "insatiable" unless subject to an "external regulatory force." Normative regulation by the society (the controlling influence of psychologically significant social groupings to which the individual belonged) provided this restraining force on aspirations. Without this normative regulation, the society could be characterized as "anomic."

Using more modern sociological terms, Merton (1957, pp. 225–386)

-----

occupational level and that of either parent (which ever was higher). If his own level was higher, he was called upwardly mobile; if the levels were the same, he was called nonmobile; and if he was lower, he was called downwardly mobile. Utilizing this method and instituting occupational status controls meant that respondents already at the lowest occupational level could not themselves be upwardly mobile from a lower parental level, and those at the highest status level could not be downwardly mobile from some higher parental position.

called these social groupings the significant reference groups that supplied the individual with guidelines for judging his performance and setting realistic aspirational levels. Group norms about appropriate degrees of comfort and reward helped a person adjust to his place in the existing status hierarchy. Insofar as one was integrated with significant social groups, he internalized what he considered to be legitimate lower and upper limits to goals that were potentially attainable to someone in his position.

Durkheim reasoned that during an economic crisis society was disturbed (that is, abrupt status transitions disrupted the individual's integration with social groups that had previously provided consensus about the range of legitimate striving). When the regulatory force was shattered, the individual experienced "de-regulation" or anomie. The downwardly mobile individual in this situation would have to reduce his requirements, his desires, and so on. Durkheim felt that some individuals were able to exercise this restraint, but that others failed to adjust to the new situational requirements. He postulated a similar process operating in the upwardly mobile person: the disturbance in group relations occasioned by the transition in status would loosen restraint on the individual's aspirations. The failure to perceive realistic limitations in social situations would cause continual striving for unlimited goals. In both instances weariness and disappointment resulted from "the futility of an endless pursuit" and, according to Durkheim, constituted the preconditions of anomic suicide. Within this context we shall see whether characteristics attributed by Durkheim to socially mobile groups with high rates of anomic suicide are associated with socially mobile groups characterized by high illness rates.

Durkheim's approach allows us to formulate four hypotheses about characteristics of socially mobile groups with high rates of mental disorder:

1. Socially mobile individuals will show less integration with significant reference groups than those who have been nonmobile.
2. Socially mobile individuals will be less likely than socially nonmobile individuals to perceive realistic limitations on their ambitions.
3. Socially mobile individuals will have higher status aspirations and ambitions than those who have been socially nonmobile.
4. Socially mobile individuals will have lower self-esteem than those who have been socially nonmobile.

There is one difference between Durkheim's approach and that utilized in the present study. Durkheim based his theoretical elaborations and implicit predictions on assumptions about the nature of social mobility.

However, we made predictions about socially mobile groups only after determining some of the characteristics of the patients and establishing a relationship between illness and mobility.

PROCEDURE

The data for this paper[4] were collected in the context of a larger study investigating the relationship between mental illness and such social-psychological factors as goal-striving stress, reference group behavior, and self-esteem (Parker & Kleiner, 1966). Interviews were obtained from a mentally ill and a community sample. Respondents were selected according to the following criteria:

1. Mentally ill sample ($N = 1423$): a respondent had to be Negro, between 20 and 60 years of age, residing in Philadelphia, who was born (and whose parents were born) within the continental United States. These respondents had been diagnosed by psychiatrists as needing treatment. They were either new admissions or readmissions to selected inpatient and outpatient, public and private psychiatric facilities in Philadelphia during the period March 1, 1960, to May 15, 1961. The ill sample was drawn in order to represent the entire spectrum of diagnoses and treatment facilities.

2. Community sample ($N = 1489$): a respondent had to be Negro, between 20 and 60 years of age, residing in Philadelphia, who was born (and whose parents were born) within the continental United States. These respondents had no known recent history of psychiatric treatment (that is, within a year prior to the interview).[5]

In order to determine whether the psychiatric sample was representative of the larger, potentially eligible patient population, demographic data were gathered on eligible-but-noninterviewed admissions to all psychiatric facilities in Philadelphia during the specified 15-month period. Our interviewed ill sample was representative of the total potentially eligible ill population ($N = 2491$) with respect to sex, age, occupation, education, and migratory status.

The initial objective for the community sample was 1500 interviews, with a 1/200 probability of selection for a given individual. The sampling

[4] Supported by Research Grant MH-10690, National Institutes of Health, Public Health Service, Bethesda, Maryland. The community survey was conducted by National Analysts, Inc., Philadelphia, Pa. The authors wish to express their appreciation to Miss Judith Fine for her invaluable assistance in preparing this manuscript for publication.

[5] Only fifty-six community respondents had *any* history of previous psychiatric contact.

procedure was divided into a five-stage design, based on stratified proportionate sampling.

All interviewers for both samples were Negroes. The study instrument
was a 206-item questionnaire, designed for a person-to-person interview.
The study was introduced to the interviewee as part of an investigation of
the attitudes and health status of the Philadelphia Negro, conducted
jointly by the respective institutions with which the authors were then
affiliated.[6]

In analyzing questionnaire data in the original larger study, we noted
that rates of mental disorder decreased for the downwardly mobile and
increased for the upwardly mobile as one ascended the occupational status
hierarchy. At the lowest occupational level the illness rate for the downwardly mobile was higher than that for the nonmobile, and at the highest
status level the rate for the upwardly mobile exceeded that for the nonmobile subjects. Because of the changing relationship between direction
of mobility and illness rates as status varied, we decided to analyze only
those cases at the extreme ends of the status scale. The seven-step occupational scale utilized in the original study was collapsed into three categories: (1) a low-status occupational group (unskilled), (2) a middle-
status group (semi-skilled), and (3) a high-status group (skilled and white-
collar). In this paper, only males in the low- and high-status occupational categories will be considered. Community sample males in these
two occupational groups totaled 377 cases, and mentally ill males totaled
347 cases.

Mobility status was determined by taking the difference between a
subject's own occupational level and that of his father or mother (whichever was higher). If his achievement level was higher than his parents',
he was categorized as upwardly mobile. If it was lower, he was considered
downwardly mobile, and if his occupational level was the same as that
of his parents, he was considered nonmobile.

In developing the hypotheses of the present study, we considered the
question of one's integration with significant social groups. Racial identification (identification with other Negroes) was taken as an operational
measure of this concept. Racial identification was defined in terms of
three hypothetical situations designed to elicit respondents' positive or
negative attitudes toward other Negroes.

Each respondent designated both his reaction, and the reason for his
reaction, to the three hypothetical situations (six questionnaire items).
Responses to selected pairs of these items were categorized as "Positive

[6] The Pennsylvania Department of Public Welfare and the Jefferson Medical
College of Philadelphia.

Identification," "Weak Identification," or "Ambivalent Identification." If both responses to a pair of items indicated positive attitudes toward other Negroes, the respondent was said to have "Positive Identification." If both responses indicated negative attitudes, he was said to have "Weak Identification." If one response indicated a positive and the other a negative attitude, he was categorized as having "Ambivalent Identification."

The questionnaire items were paired for analysis according to the following scheme:

Set 1: Reaction to a friend's passing as white versus reaction to a favorable headline about Negroes.

Set 2: Reaction to an unfavorable headline about Negroes versus reaction to a favorable headline about Negroes.

Set 3: Reaction to a friend's passing as white versus reaction to an unfavorable headline about Negroes.

Set 4: Reasons for reactions to items specified in Set 1.

Set 5: Reasons for reactions to items specified in Set 2.

Set 6: Reasons for reactions to items specified in Set 3.

The only response categories selected in defining type of racial identification in the six sets of questions were those that showed a systematic relationship to status position. For any of the six questions, a respondent might have given a response to one item that varied with status and a response to the paired question that did not. Such a respondent was excluded from the analysis because his specific response configuration could not be classified. The reduction in sample size due to this problem limited our analyses to such nonparametric procedures as the sign test.

An illustration may clarify our categorization of responses. Each respondent was asked how he would feel if a friend wanted to pass as white, and also how he would react to the newspaper headline, "Negro Seized in Camden" (see Set 3, above). If he would be angry with the friend who wanted to pass as white but would feel little or no discomfort about the headline, he was classified as having "Ambivalent Identification." Anger about a friend's passing would reflect an affirmation of his own identity with other Negroes—a positive attitude. His lack of feeling about the unfavorable headline would indicate an implicit assumption that Negroes usually commit crimes and that the arrested Negro was probably guilty —a negative attitude.

A respondent who would be angry with a friend for passing as white but who would also experience a rather strong degree of discomfort at the unfavorable headline was considered to have "Positive Identification." A subject who would have mixed feelings about a friend's passing as

white and who would have little or no reaction to the unfavorable headline was said to have "Weak Identification."

In presenting the data, we shall first compare the mentally ill and
community samples on a given measure. The downwardly mobile and
nonmobile community respondents at the low occupational level and
the upwardly mobile and nonmobile community subjects at the high end
of the occupational scale will then be contrasted. Only the latter two
comparisons will specifically test the four hypotheses derived from
Durkheim's theory.

RESULTS

Before we can test our hypotheses, we must establish that a relationship
exists between social mobility and rates of mental disorder. The illness
rates for the mobility groups at the low- and high-status occupational
positions are presented in Table 1. The downwardly mobile have a
higher illness rate than the nonmobile subjects at the low-status occupational level. At the high-status position the illness rate for the upwardly
mobile is higher than for the nonmobile.

The percentage distributions of these mobility groups in the ill and
community samples are also shown in Table 1. The distributions of
mobility types in the ill and community samples differ significantly both
at the low- and high-status occupational levels ($P < .001$ and $< .01$,
respectively). Having established that the upwardly and downwardly

TABLE 1. Occupational Status, Social Mobility, and Mental Disorder

	Illness rates (number ill/ 100 community)	Community sample (percent)	Ill sample (percent)	Significance (by χ^2)
Low-status occupational level				
Nonmobile	70	70	48	$< .001$
Downwardly mobile	175	30	52	
Total n		271	275	
High-status occupational level				
Nonmobile	40	38	22	$< .01$
Upwardly mobile	85	62	78	
Total n		106	72	

mobile groups have higher illness rates than their nonmobile status peers, we may test our hypotheses.

Hypothesis I Our first hypothesis predicts that socially mobile individuals will show less integration with significant reference groups than will nonmobile individuals. Using type of racial identification (described earlier) as our operational measure of integration, we expect in this context that more mobile than nonmobile respondents will show "Weak or Ambivalent" racial identification, and that more nonmobile than mobile subjects will be characterized by "Positive" racial identification. Before testing Hypothesis I, we must establish that these patterns of racial identification are themselves related to mental illness. It has been established that the relationship between illness and mobility in itself and between illness and the direction of mobility varied with occupational

TABLE 2. RACIAL IDENTIFICATION BY OCCUPATIONAL STATUS AND SOCIAL MOBILITY[a] (IN PERCENTAGES)

	Community sample				Ill sample			
	Low-status occupational level		High-status occupational level		Low-status occupational level		High-status occupational level	
	Non-mobile	Mobile downward	Mobile upward	Non-mobile	Non-mobile	Mobile downward	Mobile upward	Non-mobile
Set 1								
Weak/ambivalent	52	64	65	57	45	44	67	67
Positive	48	36	35	43	55	55	33	33
Total *n*	81	36	34	21	65	67	21	9
Set 2								
Weak/ambivalent	43	52	69	65	57	54	80	68
Positive	57	48	31	35	43	46	20	32
Total *n*	148	63	56	34	119	134	46	16
Set 3								
Weak/ambivalent	66	78	84	66	72	67	93	80
Positive	34	22	16	34	28	33	7	20
Total *n*	97	40	37	24	72	73	26	10
Set 4								
Weak/ambivalent	49	71	69	73	69	80	79	83
Positive	51	29	31	27	31	20	21	17
Total *n*	111	52	46	15	95	93	38	12
Set 5								
Weak/ambivalent	56	79	81	73	68	80	85	65
Positive	44	21	19	27	32	20	15	35
Total *n*	135	53	52	22	101	101	40	11
Set 6								
Weak/ambivalent	71	92	82	68	76	70	92	72
Positive	29	8	18	32	24	30	8	28
Total *n*	121	60	45	16	88	85	45	16

[a] Summary of significance, by sign test: nonmobile, ill versus community: ten of twelve in expected direction, $P < .02$; upwardly mobile, ill versus community: all six in expected direction, $P < .02$; community respondents, high versus low yield mobility subgroups: eleven of twelve in expected direction, $P < .01$.

level (Parker & Kleiner, 1966). Therefore, in this article we shall limit the ill-community comparisons on racial identification patterns to the non-mobile respondents at each status level, in effect eliminating the influence of mobility factors.

Racial identification patterns shown by nonmobile subjects for each of the six sets of items at the low and at the high ends of the occupational scale provide twelve tests of differences between the community and ill samples. Ten of these twelve comparisons show a greater prevalence of "Weak or Ambivalent" racial identification among the patients (by sign test, $P < .02$; see Table 2). Conversely, the community sample is characterized by more "Positive" racial identification. We conclude that the patients, compared to the community respondents, are less integrated with the broader Negro community.

Hypothesis I predicts that downwardly mobile community subjects at the low end of the occupational scale will show less integration than non-mobile community subjects at that position, and similarly for upwardly mobile and stable subjects at the high end of the scale. Eleven of the twelve tests of these expectations are in the predicted direction (by sign test, $P < .01$). Hypothesis I is therefore confirmed.

We have established that when mobility is controlled (that is, when only nonmobile respondents are considered), the same differences observed between the ill and community samples also discriminate between high and low yield mobility subgroups in the community sample. An important and related issue may be raised at this point. Mental disorder has been shown to vary with different combinations of direction of mobility and occupational status position. To what extent do various combinations of these factors correlate with different patterns of racial identification? Do upwardly mobile ill and community subjects at the high-status occupational level differ in patterns of racial identification in the same manner as downwardly mobile ill and community individuals at the low-status level?

At the high-status occupational level the upwardly mobile patients express more "Weak or Ambivalent" racial identification than the upwardly mobile community subjects, for all six sets of items (by sign test, $P < .02$). However, at the low-status position the downwardly mobile patients, compared to the downwardly mobile community subjects, show more "Weak or Ambivalent" identification in three sets of items, and more "Positive" identification in the other three sets.

Thus, our operational measure of social integration discriminates systematically between the high-status upwardly mobile in the ill and community samples, but it does not discriminate between the low-status downwardly mobile in these two samples. Social integration clearly varies with changes in illness status, direction of mobility, and status achievement. The lack of systematic ill-community differences at the low-status occupational position also suggests that problems of integration with the Negro community are more salient among the upwardly mobile than among the downwardly mobile, a conclusion consistent with the research literature (Frazier, 1957; Parker & Kleiner, 1964, 1966). This does not necessarily mean that racial identification is not involved in the development of mental illness among the downwardly mobile. The answer to this question may lie in a consideration of a total constellation of relevant factors.

Hypothesis II Our second hypothesis predicts that socially mobile respondents will be less likely than nonmobile subjects to perceive realistic social restraints on their goal striving. We expect socially mobile individuals who manifest "Weak or Ambivalent" racial identification response patterns to minimize or underestimate the importance of race as a barrier to goal achievement. But the nonmobile subjects who show "Positive" identification with the Negro community should perceive race as a realistic barrier to goal achievement.

Again, a precondition for testing this hypothesis is to determine whether perception of race as a barrier is related to illness. Table 3 presents distributions of responses to the question, "Has race been a barrier to achievement?" for the ill and community samples and for mobility subgroups in the community, at two occupational status levels. More ill than community respondents say that race constitutes a slight barrier, or no barrier at all, to goal achievement. This difference emerges

TABLE 3. Perception of Race as a Barrier to Goal Achievement, by Occupational Status and Social Mobility (in Percentages)

	Illness status				Community sample			
	Low-status occupational level[a]		High-status occupational level		Low-status occupational level[a]		High-status occupational level[b]	
	Community	Ill	Community	Ill	Non-mobile	Mobile downward	Mobile upward	Non-mobile
Yes, very much of a barrier; yes, somewhat of a barrier	44	28	40	34	49	39	35	49
Yes, slightly; no barrier at all	56	72	60	66	51	61	65	51
Total *n*	256	275	100	74	188	79	61	39

[a] By χ^2, $P < .001$.
[b] Probability of obtained patterns occurring together $< .05$.

at both ends of the status scale but is significant only in the low-status occupational group (by χ^2, $P < .01$).

Since we have established an association between mental illness and perception of race as a barrier to achievement, we may test our second hypothesis. We predict that the downwardly and upwardly mobile groups at the low and high ends of the occupational status scale will be less inclined than their nonmobile status peers to perceive race as a barrier to achievement. More socially mobile than nonmobile respondents at both occupational status levels see race as a slight barrier or no barrier at all (probability of the two patterns occurring together $< .05$). These results tend to support Hypothesis II.

Hypothesis III Our third hypothesis predicts that socially mobile individuals will have higher status aspirations and ambitions than those who have been socially nonmobile. This expectation is based on the premise that an individual who is less socially integrated and who is minimally aware of limits of barriers to his striving will set higher goals and attach more importance to attaining these goals than an individual

TABLE 4. OCCUPATIONAL STATUS ASPIRATIONS, BY OCCUPATIONAL STATUS AND SOCIAL MOBILITY (IN PERCENTAGES)

	Illness status[a]				Community sample[b]			
	Low status occupational level		High-status occupational level		Low-status occupational level		High-status occupational level	
	Community	Ill	Community	Ill	Non-mobile	Mobile downward	Mobile upward	Non-mobile
Choice 1								
Bricklayer @ $120/wk	57[c]	38	29	29	61	48	27	33
Teacher @ $90/wk	43	62	71	71	39	52	73	67
Total n	268	278	100	83	188	80	60	40
Choice 2								
Machine operator @ $100/wk	65[c]	44	53	45	66	62	49	58
Government clerk @ $80/wk	38	56	47	55	34	38	51	42
Total n	268	275	101	80	188	80	61	40
Choice 3								
Factory worker @ $80/wk	75[d]	62	59	56	77	69	55	64
Sales (department store) @ $60/wk	25	38	41	44	23	31	45	36
Total n	265	275	97	77	187	78	58	39

[a] Probability of all five analyses showing expected pattern, by sign test, $< .03$.
[b] Probability of all six analyses showing expected pattern, by sign test, $< .02$.
[c] By χ^2, $P < .001$.
[d] By χ^2, $P < .01$.

who is more socially integrated and who does perceive realistic barriers to his achievement.

Two measures of goal striving were analyzed. The first measure was a series of three questionnaire items in which the respondent chose between a white-collar occupation associated with a relatively low income and a blue-collar occupation associated with a higher salary. We assumed that individuals at a given status level who selected the white-collar occupation despite the wage penalty attached to this choice were characterized by higher status aspirations than individuals choosing the blue-collar job. Our second measure of goal striving was derived from a question asking the respondent to state whether his current ambitions were "Higher," "The same," or "Lower" than in the past. This questionnaire item reveals nothing about a respondent's absolute aspirational level, but it does indicate his involvement in current goal striving. Those with higher present than past ambitions are presumably reflecting their concern with, or involvement in, their current ambitions.

A pattern analysis of the blue/white-collar occupational choices provides us with six tests of ill-community differences (that is, three comparisons at the low-, and three at the high-status occupational position). More ill than community respondents prefer the white-collar occupations in five of the six comparisons (by sign test, $P < .03$; see Table 4). One comparison does not discriminate between the ill and community samples.

Within each occupational preference situation, the patients show a significantly greater preference than the community subjects for white-collar occupations (by χ^2, $P < .01$). In terms of this operational measure of goal striving, the mentally ill manifest higher status aspirations than the community respondents.

Hypothesis III predicts that both downwardly and upwardly mobile community subjects will show higher status aspirations than their nonmobile counterparts. This expectation is confirmed for all six blue/white-collar choices (that is, three at each status level; by sign test, $P < .02$).

Data on perception of current, compared to past, ambitions were also analyzed. The ill and community samples were contrasted, as were the different mobility subgroups within the community sample. The distributions of ill and community responses on this item differ significantly at the low- and high-status positions (low-status occupational level, $P < .01$; high-status level, $P < .05$). In both analyses more patients than community subjects report lower current than past ambitions.

Within the community sample, contrary to expectations based on the yield of mental disorder, more socially mobile than nonmobile respondents report higher present than past ambitions. These differences are not significant, however.

In summary, as predicted by Hypothesis III, upwardly and down-wardly mobile community respondents at both occupational status levels have higher status aspirations, and possibly tend to attach more importance to reaching current goals than do nonmobile individuals at these status positions. The raising of present ambitions in the high yield community groups may be an antecedent condition of illness; the lowering of ambitions among the patients may represent a consequence of the illness process.

Hypothesis IV Our final hypothesis predicts lower self-esteem for socially mobile than for nonmobile subjects. Durkheim reasoned that anomic, mobile individuals became dissatisfied with their achievements. We assumed, in addition, that these individuals experienced lowered self-esteem.

The self-esteem measure utilized in this study was the individual's estimate of his current achievement on a self-anchored generalized striving scale. Each respondent specified what would constitute for him the "best" and "worst" way of life. These descriptions provided him with anchor points at either end of a ten-step scale on which he selected the step that best represented his present general achievement position. We assumed that the closer he placed himself to the "worst way of life," the lower his self-esteem, and conversely, the closer he placed himself to the "best way of life," the higher his self-esteem.

At both the low- and high-status occupational levels, significantly more ill than community subjects place themselves at low positions on this ten-step scale (by χ^2, $P < .001$ for both status levels; see Table 5). We con-

TABLE 5. Perceived Achievement on Self-Anchored Striving Scale, by Occupational Status and Social Mobility (in Percentages)

	Illness status				Community sample			
	Low-status occupational level[a]		High-status occupational level		Low-status occupational level		High-status occupational level	
	Community	Ill	Community	Ill	Non-mobile	Mobile downward	Mobile upward	Non-mobile
Low perceived achievement	7	26	4	32	9	9	3	3
Medium perceived achievement	38	45	26	41	31	48	27	20
High perceived achievement	55	29	70	27	68	43	70	77
Total n	267	275	101	79	197	81	60	40

[a] By χ^2, $P < .001$.

clude that the patients are characterized by lower self-esteem than community subjects.

In light of this relationship between self-esteem and mental illness, we may evaluate our final hypothesis. We predict that the downwardly mobile will show lower self-esteem than the nonmobile subjects at the low-status occupational level, and that the upwardly mobile will show lower self-esteem than the nonmobile subjects at the high end of the status scale. At the low-status occupational position, the downwardly mobile place themselves in middle-range positions on the ten-step scale, and the nonmobile place themselves in high positions. The differences between these groups are significant (by χ^2, $P < .01$). The same pattern of differences emerges for the upwardly mobile and the nonmobile at the high-status occupational position. Therefore, the socially mobile do have lower self-esteem than the nonmobile subjects, as predicted by Hypothesis IV.

The data presented in this section have demonstrated that the mentally ill, compared to the community respondents, manifest more "Weak or Ambivalent" racial identification, deny more strongly that race has been a barrier to achievement, maintain higher status aspirations, and have lower self-esteem. We have also shown that socially mobile individuals possess more of these illness-associated characteristics (which are implicitly attributed by Durkheim to anomie) than nonmobile subjects.

DISCUSSION AND CONCLUSIONS

In this paper the four factors derived from Durkheim's description of the anomic situation (lack of integration with significant reference groups, inability to perceive realistic barriers to achievement, high status aspirations, and low self-esteem), have been related to type of social mobility experience and to high rates of mental illness. Downwardly mobile individuals at the low-status occupational position and upwardly mobile individuals at the high-status position are characterized by higher illness rates than their nonmobile status peers. These socially mobile respondents also manifest relatively high levels of the four characteristics associated with the anomic syndrome, which indicates the relevance of these factors to an understanding of mental illness and Durkheim's "anomic suicide."

Our findings firmly support Durkheim's inference that the upwardly mobile, as well as the downwardly mobile, reflect the anomic situation. Other recently reported data (Parker & Kleiner, 1966) also support Durkheim's insights: although upwardly mobile patients had experienced more upward movement (that is, greater success) than their upwardly mobile community counterparts, they were still considered to be more anomic. The similarity between the conditions associated with mental illness and anomic suicide indicates that the theory of anomie may be relevant to a broad range of deviant behavior.

We have established a relationship between each of these four anomic-related factors and individuals who were already mentally ill, but data on high and low yield community subgroups suggest that these factors are also *antecedents* of mental disorder. The four factors characterize both mentally ill subjects and community respondents in subgroups associated with high yields of illness.

Throughout this paper we have entertained the assumption that the yield procedure we have developed would help identify antecedent conditions of mental disorder. We must emphasize, however, that any variables that discriminate between high and low yield community subgroups are only *possible* antecedents. This cautionary note must be injected since the data were collected at one point in time, and the logic of the yield procedure necessitates the *inference* of a time sequence. Longitudinal studies must ultimately be conducted to determine whether, and to what degree, such potential preconditions of illness are in fact antecedents. Community population subgroups with no history of psychiatric treatment, but differing with respect to illness-linked characteristics, must be studied over a period of time to see whether they eventually manifest an increase in psychiatric symptoms and develop mental illness. These studies could be carried out over five- to ten-year periods, since disorders like schizophrenia occur primarily among young people.

This paper has also illustrated the usefulness of racial identification as an operational measure of social integration in our study population. The conclusion that the larger Negro community generally constitutes an important reference group for a given Negro individual does not seem particularly surprising. In our larger study, however, we utilized an additional measure of social integration which failed to distinguish between high and low yield community subpopulations. This underscores the importance of selecting reference groups of particular significance to the population under consideration (Parker & Kleiner, 1964, 1966).

Some findings from our larger study (Parker & Kleiner, 1966) deviate from Durkheim's theory. Nonmobile subjects at the middle-status occupational level had a higher illness rate than upwardly mobile subjects at this status position and also manifested higher levels of most of the anomic-related factors analyzed. Since Durkheim assumed an *invariant* relationship between social mobility, anomie, and deviant behavior (suicide), his approach could not predict or explain our findings. He did not attempt to determine empirically the association between these anomic factors and suicide or mobility. The relationships that have emerged in the present study among mobility, anomic-related responses, and our criterion of deviant behavior (mental illness), indicate that Durkheim's assumption of such an *invariant* association is untenable. Mobility is apparently associated with anomic factors in some social contexts (for example, at low- and high-status occupational positions coupled with extreme mobility) but not in others (at the middle-status occupational level, for example).

These findings underline the importance of incorporating sociological and social-psychological variables into a research design intended to investigate deviant behavior. Sociologically conceptualized variables (independent variables) may be associated with mental disorder and other deviant behaviors (dependent variables) only when particular social-psychological conditions (intervening variables) are present. Changes in these social-psychological conditions imply concomitant changes in the relationship between the sociological and behavioral variables.

An overview of existing research on the relationship between mental disorder and such sociological phenomena as migration and social class reveals numerous inconclusive and even contradictory findings. The application of the type of research design utilized in the present study might help to order such findings and incorporate them within a broader conceptual framework. If different sociological variables are found to be related to mental disorder, and to one another via their association with social-psychological variables, our understanding of the total impact of sociological variables will be enlarged. A more intensive consideration of intervening social-psychological variables related to mental disorder may also deepen our understanding of such other forms of deviancy as suicide and criminal behavior.

Our results suggest a similarity in some concomitants of mental disorder and suicide. However, we do not know under what conditions pressures toward deviancy will eventuate in one or another of these behaviors. We should emphasize that our methodological procedure does not imply the reductionistic fallacy of explaining factors conceptualized at one level of analysis in terms of concepts formulated at another level. Although such levels must be kept conceptually separate, knowledge of their interrelationships is necessary for a more complete understanding of their influence on behavior.

REFERENCES

Blau, P. M. Social mobility and interpersonal relations. *American Sociological Review,* 1956, **21,** 290–295.

Clausen, J. A., & Kohn, M. L. Relation of schizophrenia to the social structure of a small city. In B. Pasamanick (Ed.), *Epidemiology of mental disorder.* Washington, D.C.: American Association for the Advancement of Science, Publication Number 60, 1959. Pp. 69–95.

Dunham, H. W. Anomie and Mental Disorder. In M. B. Clinard (Ed.), *Anomie and deviant behavior: A discussion and critique.* Glencoe, Ill.: The Free Press, 1964. Pp. 128–157.

Durkheim, E. *Suicide.* (Transl. by J. A. Spaulding & G. Simpson.) Glencoe, Ill.: The Free Press, 1951.

Ellis, E. Social-psychological correlates of upward social mobility among unmarried career women. *American Sociological Review,* 1952, **17,** 558–563.

Escalona, S. K. The effect of success and failure upon the level of aspiration and behavior in manic-depressive psychoses. In *University of Iowa studies in child welfare: Studies in topological and vector psychology I,* Volume 16, Number 3. Iowa City, Iowa: University of Iowa Press, 1940. Pp. 199–302.

Escalona, S. K. *An application of the level of aspiration experiment to the study of personality.* Teachers College, Columbia University Contributions to Education Number 937. New York: Bureau of Publication, Teachers College, Columbia University, 1948.

Frazier, E. F. *Black bourgeoisie.* Glencoe, Ill.: The Free Press, 1957.

Greenbaum, J., & Pearlin, L. I. Vertical mobility and prejudice: A socio-psychological analysis. In R. Bendix & S. M. Lipset (Eds.), *Class, status, and power: A reader in social stratification.* Glencoe, Ill.: The Free Press, 1953. Pp. 480–491.

Hollingshead, A. B., & Redlich, F. C. Schizophrenia and social structure. *American Journal of Psychiatry,* 1954, 110, 695–701.

Hollingshead, A. B., & Redlich, F. C. Social mobility and mental illness. *American Journal of Psychiatry,* 1955, **112,** 179–185.

Hollingshead, A. B., Ellis, R., & Kirby, E. Social mobility and mental illness. *American Sociological Review,* 1954, **19,** 577–584.

Jaco, E. G. Social stress and mental illness in the community. In M. B. Sussman (Ed.), *Community structure and analysis.* New York: Thomas Y. Crowell Co., 1959. Pp. 388–409.

Janowitz, M., & Curtis, R. *Sociological consequences of upward mobility in a U.S. metropolitan community.* Working Paper One, the Fourth Working Conference on Social Stratification and Social Mobility, International Sociological Association, December 1957.

Kleiner, R. J., & Parker, S. Goal-striving, social status, and mental disorder: A research review. *American Sociological Review,* 1963, **28,** 189–203.

Langner, T. S., & Michael, S. T. *Life stress and mental health: The midtown Manhattan study.* Vol. 2. Glencoe, Ill.: The Free Press, 1963.

Lapouse, R., Monk, M. A., & Terris, M. The drift hypothesis and socio-economic differentials in schizophrenia. *American Journal of Public Health*, 1956, **46**, 978–986.

Lewin, K., Dembo, T., Festinger, L., & Sears, P. S. Level of aspiration. In J. McV. Hunt (Ed.), *Personality and the behavior disorders: A handbook based on experimental and clinical research*, Vol. 1. New York: Ronald Press, 1944. Pp. 333–378.

Lipset, S. M., & Bendix, R. *Social mobility in industrial society*. Berkeley and Los Angeles: University of California Press, 1963.

Litwak, E. *Conflicting values and decision making*. Unpublished doctoral dissertation, Columbia University, 1956.

Lystad, M. H. Social mobility among selected groups of schizophrenic patients. *American Sociological Review*, 1957, **22**, 288–292.

McClosky, H., & Schaar, J. H. Psychological dimensions of anomy. *American Sociological Review*, 1965, **30**, 14–40.

Merton, R. K. *Social theory and social structure*. (Rev. ed.) Glencoe, Ill.: The Free Press, 1957.

Morris, J. N. Health and social class. *Lancet*, 1959, **1**, 303–305.

Parker, S., & Kleiner, R. J. Status position, mobility, and ethnic identification of the Negro. *Journal of Social Issues*, 1964, **20**, 85–102.

Parker, S., & Kleiner, R. J. *Mental health in an urban Negro community*. Glencoe, Ill.: The Free Press, 1966.

Ruesch, J. *Chronic disease and psychological invalidism: A psychosomatic study*. New York: American Society for Research in Psychosomatic Problems, 1946.

Ruesch, J. Social technique, social status, and social change in illness. In C. Kluckhohn, H. A. Murray, & D. M. Schneider (Eds.), *Personality in nature, society, and culture*. New York: Alfred A. Knopf, 1956. Pp. 123–136.

Ruesch, J., Jacobson, A., & Loeb, M. B. *Acculturation and illness*. Psychological Monographs, General and Applied, Volume 62, Whole Number 292. Washington, D.C.: The American Psychological Association, 1948.

Simpson, R. L., & Miller, H. M. Social status and anomia. *Social Problems*, 1963, **10**, 256–264.

Srole, L. Anomie, authoritarianism, and prejudice. *American Journal of Sociology*, 1956, **62**, 63–67.

Srole, L. Social integration and certain corollaries: An exploratory study. *American Sociological Review*, 1956, **21**, 709–716.

Srole, L., Langner, T. S., Michael, S. T., Opler, M. K., & Rennie, T. A. C. *Mental health in the metropolis: The midtown Manhattan study*. Vol. 1. New York: McGraw-Hill, 1962.

Tietze, C., Lemkau, P., & Cooper, M. Personality disorder and spatial mobility. *American Journal of Sociology*, 1942, **48**, 29–39.

Tumin, M. M., & Collins, R. C., Jr. Status, mobility, and anomie: A study in readiness for desegregation. *British Journal of Sociology*, 1959, **10**, 253–267.

Warner, W. L. The society, the individual, and his mental disorders. *American Journal of Psychiatry*, 1937, **94**, 275–284.

chapter four

Social Deviance and Mental Illness

4.1 Introduction

The record of history is saturated by man's expression of concern over the deviations of his fellow men—with rebels, heretics, perverts, eccentrics, criminals, and so on. Because every society has established a normal, natural and, thus, entirely proper, way of doing things, every society has had to deal with the improper conduct of persons who deviate from the "proper" religion, politics, law, or morality. History, too, records a continuing concern with the reasons why men deviate. Thus, history tells us not only of grim or triumphant episodes in which a society has taken vigorous and concerted action against deviants, but also of the untiring inquiry of many men into the motivation underlying man's conformity, or his dissent and search for freedom. The history of any country offers many examples, as in Spain where the Inquisition is an illustration of the former and Unamuno's *Against This and That* exemplifies the latter.

"Social deviance" is the currently fashionable term by which the social and psychological sciences refer to such diverse categories of deviators as alcoholics, social nudists, criminals, delinquent juveniles, homosexuals, narcotics addicts, "beatniks," Black Muslims, and prostitutes. Although the utility of any term that relates to such a variety of persons and behaviors is questionable, it appears that the term is most generally applied to persons whose conduct violates the shared and sanctioned expectations of society, as they are expressed either in law or in custom. Therefore, it is often stated, there is a core of similarity among all "social deviants."

Faced with such a mixed bag of "deviants," many questions readily emerge. For example, to what extent is deviance "consciously elected" as by, say, call-girls, and to what extent is it "imposed"? Can the severe deviance of criminals be considered under the same heading with the lesser nonconformance of persons in nudist colonies? Is there not a vast difference between the secretive or apologetic deviance of alcoholics or narcotics addicts, and the defiant, unrepentant superiority of deviants in the "gay" world or in some religious cults? In short, there is much to question in the current broadside employment of the term social deviance.

Nonetheless, the term is in use, and widely so. We want to turn our attention here to a contrast in views about the nature of persons who are commonly known as "social deviants," a contrast that has basic relevance to an understanding of mental illness. Out of a welter of conflicting, ambiguous, and overlapping views about the mental health status of "social deviants," it is possible to discern two contrasting perspectives, which we might call the "social system" perspective and the "psychiatric" perspective.

The social system perspective is most regularly seen in the work of sociologists. Here, "social deviance" is examined in terms of its consequences for the social structure. Although some sociological writers assume that social deviance is impelled by, or correlated with, psychopathology, this approach is typically overtly unconcerned with the "mental health" of the deviant. In some instances, however, it is implicit in this perspective that the deviant is every bit as normal psychologically as is the nondeviant. In the psychiatric perspective, the emphasis is upon the psychological structure of the deviant individual. Here, it is often assumed that social deviance is, virtually by definition, evidence of psychopathology, and treatment is often directed toward ridding the deviant person of his "need" to be deviant. It should be added that not all sociologists ignore the mental health of social deviants or assume that such persons are "normal," and not all psychiatrists subscribe to any simple position that deviant behavior is, ipso facto, "sick" behavior. But neither have we merely set up straw men; these extreme polar positions not only exist, they are common.

These contrasting perspectives tend to be perpetuated by the absence of crucial operational tests of the mental health of socially deviant populations. If we can assume that there are valid and reliable means by which the mental health or illness of a person can be measured (and it is by no means certain that such means exists), then some critical questions should be asked. For example, are specific "social deviants" more or less mentally ill than some "normal," (that is, nondeviant) comparison population? Is there any such comparison population? Would nondeviant siblings of the social deviants suffice? The only certain answer is that difficult methodological problems exist. A second set of questions would ask whether social deviants are more or less mentally ill than they would have been had they never become deviant. This, too, is a critical question, asking whether a deviant role is more or less stressful than a nondeviant one. But, here, the methodological problems are still more formidable. And, were we to continue in this vein, we could produce many more relevant questions and encounter a like number of problems.

The chapters that follow will not provide definitive answers, nor will they lay to rest many of the methodological problems. They will, however, provide an introduction to some of the conceptual differences between the social system and the psychiatric perspectives. In different ways and with differing explicitness, the authors of these chapters ask, What sense does it make to regard social deviants as persons who are mentally ill? Are there more rewarding ways to examine social deviance?

4.2 Orientation

Alcoholism is one of the world's most vexing social problems, one that has resisted moral and medical prescriptions. This article gives us an insight into the problem of alcoholism, and, while it will not provide "solutions" to the problem, we nonetheless recommend it to anyone who wishes to think more clearly about the subject.

Craig MacAndrew's treatment of the question of whether, or in what sense, alcoholism is a disease, is a deft combination of serious purpose and a light touch. His essay not only casts suspicion upon the cherished notion that alcoholism is a disease, it also challenges— and does so very persuasively—the common belief that we know an alcoholic when we see one. MacAndrew argues for a return to basics, or more specifically, to an operational definition of alcoholism.

4.2 On the Notion that Certain Persons Who Are Given to Frequent Drunkenness Suffer from a Disease Called Alcoholism

Craig MacAndrew

While alcohol is a demonstrably toxic substance (a "poison"), it has also been termed the world's original miracle drug—both a brew of the devil and a gift of the gods, mankind's scourge and its liberator. Its ingestion by some persons has been variously termed a failure of will, a symptom (of sundry different things), a "runaway symptom" that has taken on disease significance, and a disease proper. It has been argued at one time or another that its ingestion prevents, constitutes, and causes psychosis. Its sale within the confines of this republic has been transformed within most reader's lifetimes from the status of a federal offense—indeed, it is the only substance the manufacture, sale, and transport of which has been specifically prohibited by constitutional amendment—to a source of astronomical state and federal revenue. Even skid rows, while seen by most as a blight on the landscape of an opulent society, have been construed by some latter-day discussants as blessings in disguise (for, the argument goes, were their inhabitants unable to channel their primitive aggression and dependency drives into the impotent alienation of Skid Row, they would provide fertile recruitment material for authoritarian political movements; see Rosenman, 1955). It would appear, then, that for all our efforts we have failed to achieve even the semblance of consensus concerning either the words we use to depict, or the ways we think about, the relation between man and alcohol.

In the following pages I shall limit my remarks to the notion of "alcoholism"—a relatively recently introduced, variously defined, and even now only sometimes accepted, designation of one course this relationship may assume. Rather than engage in the dubiously profitable and unavoidably tedious analysis of the numerous definitions of alcoholism that have been variously recommended,[1] my concern will be to explicate what such a notion is doing in the world and why it is that only now, at this time, the notion of alcoholism has come to be accorded its present

---

[1] Compilations of such definitions abound. While incomplete, two of the better compendia are those of Bowman and Jellinek (1941) and Jellinek (1960). A useful historical survey of eighteenth- and nineteenth-century European medical thought on the subject is contained in Marconi (1959).

limited but growing respectability. In focusing the discussion in this manner I do not propose to ignore the substantive question concerning "what alcoholism really *is*." Rather, I shall argue that insofar as this question assumes the existence of, and thus requires as the condition of an adequate answer the enumeration of the essential features of, a "substance" which is coordinate with the substantive expression "alcoholism," the question itself is based upon a misunderstanding. I take it to be a peculiar form of provincialism to assume that every quirk of our idiom is mirrored in the real world. While I shall not, then, be in quest of the nature of some coordinate substance, I do hope that the present explication will yield some understanding of why the efforts of those who have so quested have resulted in such a welter of conflicting thoughts about and definitions of the substantive expression that is my topic.

  Let me begin with a brief statement of the general orientation that informs the present discussion—an orientation that derives from the work of Alfred Schutz (1962, 1964), the later Wittgenstein (1953, 1956), and from many hours spent in analysing the status of the social sciences with my colleague, Harold Garfinkel. If over the course of their history, the several disciplines that are engaged in the attempt to construct a science of social life have advanced one truly radical insight into the nature of man, it is that the comprehension of the temporally emitted sounds and movements of men as events of human conduct is possible *only within the context of the relations-between-men-in-a-society*. Call this our fundamental insight. And if we, the flesh and blood members of these several disciplines, are properly to be faulted, as I believe we are, for the manner in which we have typically handled our basic insight, our error can scarcely be said to lie in having accorded it premature acceptance. The "evidence" (if one wishes to speak in this manner) is clearly overwhelming. Nor, since the force of our insight lies precisely in its ubiquitousness, can we properly be charged with having overextended its legitimate domain of applicability. The grounds for criticism are to be found not in the direction of reckless abandon, but of undue caution. Specifically, I would argue that our fault resides in having failed to take seriously the more radical consequences that are inexorably entailed in its wholehearted acceptance. For if we take our fundamental insight in full seriousness, we must recognize—and not just programmatically or as it serves our ad hoc purposes—that pristine and thus unsullied facts do not exist either in our world or in anyone else's world. Stated positively, we must appreciate that all facts are necessarily and from the outset *preinterpreted* facts, rooted in what Whitehead once termed "the whole apparatus of common-sense thought." And since all facts come to us "pre-coded," if we are to be true to our fundamental insight we must come to appreciate and to take fully into account the fact that the social sciences, *qua* positive sciences, require a prescientific determination of their "objects."

I am not recommending, then, that we are to be faulted because in dealing with prescientifically determined "objects" we begin our enterprise "somewhere in the middle"—one has, after all, to begin someplace, and if our fundamental insight is correct, this is where we must necessarily begin. Rather, I am suggesting that our difficulty lies in the fact that in the course of so doing we have unblinkingly presupposed precisely that which our fundamental insight recommends as most urgently in need of analysis in its own right. I say "most urgently" because in implicitly assuming the nonproblematic character of our point of departure "and-all-that-has-gone-before," we thereby gloss the absolutely crucial problem of explicating the very grounds that alone can provide a science of social life with its rational foundations. And in directing ourselves to the task of supplying correctives to this otherwise unspecified stock of common understandings that we possess prior to the initiation of our inquiries, and which in composite constitutes our everyday version of social reality, we place ourselves in the peculiar and, with rare exceptions, only superficially examined position of claiming that *qua* social scientists we are somehow capable of being "in the world, but not of the world."

While the difficulties with such a claim are both numerous and monumental, one such difficulty may be posed as follows: What guarantee have we that the products of our inquiries will be immune to whatsoever consequences might derive from the fact that, in simple truth, we are no less "of the world," and are thus no less subject to the force of our fundamental insight, than are those whom we study? Where this puzzle is addressed at all, it is customary for it first to undergo a "procedural" translation and come out something as follows: How do we come to count (what are our *grounds* for counting) the actual findings of social scientific inquiry as warranted findings? The guarantee demanded by *this* question, our methodologists are wont litanously to proclaim, resides in our subscription to "the correct rules of scientific procedure." That is, we deem our findings to be warranted findings by virtue of the fact that our actual inquiries are both informed by, and are conducted in accordance with, what we together with our colleagues presently count as correct scientific procedure. The difficulty here lies not in the answer—which is unexceptionable—but in the fact that the radical character of our original question has been lost in its "procedural" translation. Indeed, since "the subscription to the correct rules of scientific procedure" itself begins "somewhere in the middle," *viz* in the middle of a discipline of accredited practitioners busily engaged in conducting research aimed at supplying correctives to what we together with our nonprofessional fellows already know as competent members of the society in which we live our lives, and within and upon which we do our science, it begs the very problem it purports to settle.

In social inquiry it is simply not the case that in doing our research and in formulating our theories of a given phenomenon, state of affairs, person, or culture we have put our priorly existing common understandings out the door and had done with them. Fidelity to our fundamental insight entails the recognition that "what everybody knows" is ubiquitously present in inquiry from the first vague glimmering of the problematic nature of a given phenomenon or state of affairs—which, with greater or lesser modification, is taken as "the problem that initiates inquiry"—to our presentation of the finished product of that inquiry. In a word, *our prior knowledge is not first cast out and only later, if ever, readmitted; it is present at every point along the line.*

Paraphrasing the post-Tractatus Wittgenstein, it is not enough simply to recognize ("in passing," as it were) that this prior knowledge functions as a scheme of interpretation, that it is codified in our language, and that thus both in asking questions (raising "puzzles") and in giving answers (providing "solutions") we must use this language "full blown." Rather, having accepted that this "knowledge at hand" is the primordial stuff of our enterprise, we must recognize that any fundamental clarification of the actual activities in which we are engaged amounts, in large measure, to getting clear about its *use.* As Whitehead (1949, p. 110), with his characteristically pithy elegance, has put the matter, " . . . common sense thought . . . is the datum from which [inquiry] starts, and to which it must recur . . . you may polish up common sense, you may contradict in detail, you may surprise it. But ultimately your whole task is to satisfy it." [2]

Turning now to our subject, what do we know—what does Anyman know—of the relationship between man and alcohol that causes him to be puzzled? More to the point, what is the nature of the puzzle confronting common sense for which the notion of alcoholism has been introduced as a solution? Certainly "alcoholism" is the solution to some puzzle, but *what* puzzle? It is my contention that a realistic comprehension of our actual doings—both conceptual and empirical—with the notion of alcoholism is contingent upon the clarification of this matter.

Let me begin my exegesis of what I take to be the nature of this puzzle

[2] This insight is not, however, of contemporary vintage. Hume, for instance, in his introduction to *A Treatise of Human Nature* wrote: " 'Tis evident that all the sciences have a relation, greater or less, to human nature; and that however wide any of them may seem to run from it, they will return back by one passage or another."

with an essential ingredient of the folk wisdom concerning the relationship between man and alcohol, *viz*, that, "There are some people who just can't handle their liquor." In speaking thusly, I take it that we are giving voice to our observation that for some of us the ingestion of alcohol gives rise to troubles, not the least of which concern the trials and tribulations thus created for sundry innocent second parties. This, I submit, is a fact of social life which is objectively verifiable in the sense that it is "there for anyone to see who would but look." I take it to be a fact of similar status that among those for whom the ingestion of alcohol has this visible trouble-evoking propensity, there exists a subclass of persons who, despite an awareness of the deleterious consequences that they, no less than their fellows, recognize as a common (if not an inevitable) accompaniment of their ingestion of alcoholic beverages, do not direct their conduct in accordance with this recognition. Indeed, and again "as everybody knows," for many members of this subclass, the frequency of drunkenness and/or the amount of alcohol ingested per drinking episode actually increases in the face of this awareness.

I suggest that it is the recognized existence of this subclass of drinkers—drinkers who continue to drink even in the knowledge (1) that while their biographies may not inevitably terminate in ruination thereby, they will with unsettling frequency assume (or continue their present) downhill course, and (2) that the longer they continue to drink, the greater the likelihood that such will be the case[3]—which constitutes for common sense a puzzle of some appreciable moment. How are we to make sense of the fact that there are people in the world who, while seemingly like us in other respects, engage in a project that is so patently pernicious?

Behind a veil of obviousness lurks the absolutely fundamental fact that *every* society is predicated upon the unquestioned assumption that its members, in their overwhelming majority, are not only competent to conduct their everyday affairs in accordance with whatsoever their society counts as correct forms of conduct, but where a choice is possible (as in the present case it seems so self-evidently to be) will freely *elect* to do so. Put differently, every society assumes that its members, in their overwhelm-

---

[3] Although this point scarcely needs documenting, consider that ultimate ruination—"premature" death. In the tightest study to date, Tashiro and Lipscomb (1963) found that, for a sample of Caucasian males admitted to one or another treatment facility in the state of California in the early to mid-1950s, the average annual death rate over a two- to five-year period was at least 2½ times greater than the expected California age-specific death rate for Caucasian males. Especially striking is the authors' breakdown of the causes of alcoholics' deaths: that category with the largest number of entries (24 percent of the total) was "death due to violent causes" (motor vehicle accidents, falls, and the like).

ing majority, are responsible for their doings, which is to say that they are *moral* agents. I say, "in their overwhelming majority," because it is also everywhere recognized that in no society is the socialization process so wholly efficacious as to produce members who, without exception, do all the things they are supposed to do and refrain from doing all the things they are supposed not to do. Every society, that is, recognizes that it has its deviants; and it has been a perennial task of every society in one way or another to mitigate the disruptive consequences that are contingent upon the existence of these deviants in their midsts. It has always been thus, and doubtless it always will be. But, barring recourse to the morally unsanctionable (and thus over the long haul, self-defeating) doctrines of strict liability or capricious despotism, every society, in order to act in a manner which its members will regard as proper, must have available an acceptable rationale that relates whatsoever action it takes to the publicly appreciated comprehension of the wellsprings of the deviant conduct to the management of which its action is directed.

Until very recent times, our attempts to bring the chronic drunkard's seemingly irrational project back under the purview of common sense rationality have been fashioned preeminently on the basis of a single conceptual resource derived from the view of the person as a moral agent —the notion that being-in-the-world-*drunk* is an enjoyable, or at least in some sense a gratifying, state of affairs. Unheedful of the longer range, we have held, such drinkers drink in order to obtain some form of transitory gratification. While the specific nature of the gratification thus obtained has been variously rendered, our attempts to come to terms with the chronic drunkard, *qua* deviant, have consisted precisely in the invocation of one or another version of short-term gain as the counterweight to the publicly appreciated likelihood of long-term loss. Until most recent times, this general formulation has provided the rationale for our efforts at social control as well. Specifically, this conception has informed us that such drinkers are to be comprehended neither on the grounds of an inability to refrain from, nor an inability to appreciate the nature and consequences of, their continued drinking, but as persons who, acting in full knowledge, *choose to so indulge themselves.* Put differently, the notion of short-term gain has informed us that such drinking—indeed, that *all* drinking—is neither a "happening to" nor the manifestation of an error of judgment, but an intended doing from which the doer could refrain *if he so desired.*

Now, because the kind of drinking pattern with which we are here concerned is deemed both avoidable, and in sundry respects troublesome to self and/or to others, it is properly an accountable matter as well. Note, however, that when an accounting is called for in situations such as this, what is at issue is not an explanation, but a justification. The context of discourse is not that of dispassionate inquiry, but of the assessment of one's blameworthiness; and in this latter context to "know" is not necessarily to forgive. Thus, Peters observes (1958, p. 31), "A motive is not necessarily a discreditable reason for acting, but it is a reason asked for in a context where there is a suggestion that it might be discreditable." In effect, then, in calling the chronic drunkard to account, that is, in asking him "why," a charge is being made against him and a defense is being called for. And because the drinker himself is typically incapable of providing "good reasons" in defense of his continued trouble-making (about which, more later), he is deemed properly deserving of censure and/or punishment.

How then to handle the troublesome drunkard who will not refrain from such wanton self-indulgence? By adding externally imposed penalties to the already existing inherent long-term penalties that accompany the continuing exercise of his propensity to drink; and this on the entirely reasonable assumption that by so increasing the tax upon such conduct the existing balance between short-term gain and long-term loss will be tilted once and forever in favor of the life of moderation and good sense.

The logic underlying such a policy is as impeccable as it is simple. It contains but a single difficulty. However, this difficulty is overriding: when put into operation, the policy has proven to be considerably less than totally efficacious. And, no doubt in exasperation over the failure of punishment to dissuade, such ventures into social engineering have cyclically given way to periods of relative "do-nothingism." But for society to turn its collective back and allow the chronic drunkard to "stew in his own juices" is not simply to admit the failure of a specific policy; it is to raise the gravest questions concerning the very legitimacy of the whole conception of moral agency from which its punitive policy derives. And, since there is a profound sense in which the common sense theory of action, with its core doctrine of personal agency, has a monopoly on morality, any admission of final failure would not mean simply that its monopoly had been successfully challenged by a rival ethic that differed only in certain particulars from itself; the legitimacy of the whole moral stance would lose its self-evident character. Small wonder, then, that periods of laissez-faire have ever given way to the refurbished efforts of social activists—only to be defeated as had been their predecessors by the Chaplinesque recalcitrance of those whom they would seek to correct. The common sense wisdom was clearly on the hook, and with each failure, the hook dug in a bit deeper.

Let us, at this point, step back for a moment and see where we stand. It has been argued that the in sundry ways troublesome, yet self-evidently avoidable conduct of certain drinkers can be comprehended by common sense only by imputing an overriding gratificatory quality to their drunken state; that social policy that is predicated upon such a version of the actually existing state of affairs has historically consisted in the imposition of additional penalties on such continued drunkenness in the belief that the drinker, *qua* reasonable man, will thereby come finally to conduct himself in comport with a thus heightened appreciation of the fact that it is in his own best interest to refrain from such a further self-indulgence; and that the various applications of such a policy have, by and large, failed to dissuade the chronic drunkard from his chosen course. It has also been recommended that in construing the habitual drunkard as "one of us," and thus as morally accountable for the troubles his continued drunkenness evokes, we are, in effect, making a charge against him, and that in inquiring of such a one why it is that he continues to drink we are not searching for an explanation in anything like the scientific sense of that term, but are allowing him the opportunity to present us with "good reasons" by recourse to which he might justify himself.

I want now to examine the possibility of such a defense more closely. In the most general terms, a charge may be challenged (opposed, defended against) in one of two ways. One may either deny the facts upon which the charge is based or, as Hart (1951, pp. 147–48) has so neatly put it, one may plead "that although all the circumstances on which a claim could succeed are present, yet in the particular case, the claim or accusation should not succeed because other circumstances are present which bring the case under some recognized head of exception, the effect of which is either to defeat the claim or accusation altogether, or to 'reduce' it so that only a weaker claim can be sustained." Since, in the present case, neither the chronic drunkard's continued drinking per se nor the troubles contingent upon such drinking are typically in dispute, it is upon the compellingness of the plea of exceptionality that his defense must turn.

I would now argue that in allowing the chronic drunkard this opportunity to justify himself, we are actually engaging in an empty formality. What, after all, could a convincing justification possibly look like? At base, it would require a demonstration of the existence of a compelling discrepancy between his (subjective) and our (external) evaluation of the conduct in question. Such a demonstration could, at least in principle, take either of two forms: While accepting responsibility for his doings (which is the sine qua non of any justification), the accused could either (1) deny the moral and/or rational propriety of the proscription which he admits having violated, or he could (2) accept the legitimacy of the proscription and plead some manner of "special circumstances of the occasion" in his defense. Neither form of justification however, will do. The first alternative would inevitably meet defeat at the hands of an indignant public's prior consensus to the effect that only a fool (or worse!) would deny that such habitual drunkenness *is* wrongful. And the second alternative is flatly irrelevant to the matter at issue since the charge concerns not the exceptional, but the *chronic* character of the transgression. Clearly, then, no defense that is based upon a denial of the blameworthy nature of such continued drunkenness will suffice either as an adequate defense for the chronic drunkard or as a viable rescue operation for common sense.

There is another and final possibility, however. Since the policy of penalization is, after all, an elementary derivative of the conventional theory-in-use, one might argue that this policy could not have failed so consistently and so notoriously were this theory itself not somehow gravely at fault. Surely, it would seem, the dilemma presented by the repeated failures of rationally derived social policy *is* of sufficiently scandalous proportions to warrant a radical reexamination of the root assumptions of our common sense theory. Could it be that the chronic drunkard is other than the conventional understanding assumes him to be and that the bind in which common sense finds itself derives from an erroneous assumption that he is to be explained on its terms? Could it be, that is, that the difficulty derives from the unstated and thus un-examined belief that such drinkers are in fact "like us" in being able on the exercise of our individual discretions either "to take it or leave it alone?" In a word, could it be that we are dealing here not with an avoidable, but with an unavoidable course of conduct?

If such a defense could be sustained, it would have an initial strategic advantage that is denied, by definition, to the defense of justification. In accepting the wrongful character of his conduct, the drunkard openly acknowledges his allegiance to the operative morality. The implications of such a strategy are metamorphic, for in proposing that such drinking is indeed wrongful, but unavoidable, one is at the same time proposing that the chronic drunkard is not a rebel, but a victim; that one is here dealing not with acts of willful self-indulgence but with an affliction of the innocent.

Such a challenge to the received opinion had its late eighteenth- and early nineteenth-century precursors in the persons of such luminaries as Drs. Benjamin Rush (1811) in the United States, Thomas Trotter (1810) in England, and C. von Brühl-Cramer (1819) in Germany. But while their writings received some attention, their message attracted scant support, and it was not until the late nineteenth century that articles with such titles as "The Treatment of Inebriety As a Disease" (Edwards,

1896), "Drunkenness a Curable Disease" (Keeley, 1892), and "Alcoholism: The Treatment and Cure of the Disease" (Taylor, 1894), began to appear with any frequency in the professional literature.

It was during this period, too, that *The Journal of Inebriety* (the organ of a very small minority within the American medical profession who held that "inebriety is a disease") began publication. Its limited effect, however, was for the most part in a direction quite opposite from that intended. By the time it finally gave up its always financially precarious existence at about the beginning of World War I, it had become the target of occasional, severe, and broadly acclaimed criticism from other members of the medical profession, the clergy, and the public at large. Thus, recalls one of the journal's co-founders (quoted in Jellinek, 1960, p. 3), "A Brooklyn clergyman on one occasion offered prayers in his church that these infidel efforts to dignify vice might be neutralized and pointed out with great emphasis the evidence of Satan in the promotion of these efforts." The readership of the journal remained small from beginning to end, and its final demise, if noticed at all, was greeted less with sorrow or jubilation than with a yawn. And thus the first organized attempt in this country to see the chronic drunkard as a victim rather than a culprit passed from the scene leaving scarcely a trace.

Then came the War, America's entrance into which provided the prohibitionists—who had long been both active and consequential in America's politics—with their first national opportunity. "There is nothing to understand except one thing," declared Senator Myers of Montana, "and that is that bread will help us win the war more than whisky. That is the only thing that is necessary to understand." Against such an argument, the brewers' contention that beer was "liquid bread" proved unavailing, and wartime prohibition was passed by Congress in the name of Victory. Although the war ended before this legislation could be put into effect, in the wake of victory came the Eighteenth Amendment and shortly thereafter, the passage of that much-amended, multisectioned and altogether wondrous morass of compromise and ambiguity upon which its enforcement was to rest—the Volstead Act.[4] Once this act was passed, its circumvention became, if not the new national pastime, certainly an engaging project for countless thousands. As a wag of the time had it, "The history of the United States can be summed up in eleven words: 'Columbus, Washington, Lincoln, Volstead, Two flights up and ask for Gus.' " However this may be, the ineptitude,

[4] While replete with the typically encountered array of prejudices that contemporary British intellectuals seem wont to bring to their writings on American social history, A. Sinclair's monograph (1962) contains a wealth of source material on this and related matters.

laxity, and corruption with which the enforcement of the Eighteenth Amendment proceeded did result, within a decade, in a situation in which the number of going speak-easies approximated the number of saloons in operation on the eve of its passage. Prohibition's doom was finally sealed in the presidential election of 1932. Roosevelt (the wet candidate) called for its outright repeal, and Hoover (the moist candidate) stood for its resubmission to the states. Thus forsaken, it was the prohibitionist (as Will Rogers noted) who had truly become Roosevelt's "forgotten man." Roosevelt was, of course, elected, and with his election came the passage and speedy ratification of the Twenty-first Amendment, the force of which was to repeal the Eighteenth.[5] And thus the "experiment, noble in motive" was at an end. A policy predicated upon and sustained by moral indignation had again come a cropper, but this time in a manner far more visible than any previous attempt. Indeed, public involvement in the pros and cons of prohibition was such that the scandal could be glossed no longer. Something had to give.

The traumatic impact of the depression on such of the received verities as thrift and diligence, the Darrowian character of New Deal (and most post-New Deal) political-social rhetoric, the growing reverence for Science and its Works, the popularization and Americanization of selected conceptions and misconceptions of the cultural relativists and of such figures as Freud and Marx are only a few among the forces that contributed to the continued weakening of the moral stance which, with the failure of the Eighteenth Amendment, was already in acute disarray. And with the erosion of organized moral indignation, the way was open for what, in a country dedicated to change and thus only dimly aware of its past, came to be termed the "new approach" to the chronic drunkard—the notion that he is afflicted with the disease of alcoholism.

Having departed the arena of the politics of indignation, the study of the effects of alcohol on man was transformed almost overnight into an area of practical inquiry. With the increased public recognition and consequent concern regarding the role of drunkenness in traffic accidents, the courts cried out for objective procedures that would yield "scientific" de-

[5] In the light of present protestations, it is perhaps instructive to note that in the debates over prohibition it was the typically liberal wets who argued that, "You can't legislate morality," while, *pari passu*, the typically conservative drys argued that you could. Nor was either side much concerned with its (polemically inspired) rape of economic realities. While the drys had promised that the enactment of prohibition would in some unspecified manner eliminate the ups and downs of the business cycle, once the depression came, the wets argued that reopening the breweries would, by providing additional employment opportunities, contribute substantially to its alleviation.

terminations of such legal categories as "under the influence." Although the courts had finally to settle for determinations of blood-alcohol level —a related, but essentially different thing—the development of even these procedures required a greatly expanded understanding of such things as alcohol metabolism. And attempts to establish relationships between such blood-alcohol levels and various sensorimotor capacities (not to mention judgment and conduct proper) entailed the investigation of aspects of man's relation to alcohol that had scarcely been addressed before. Thus, it should not surprise that the "new approach" came to be peculiarly and properly associated with a university research center—Dr. H. W. Haggard's laboratory of applied physiology at Yale University. The "Yale group" constituted a center for and the clearinghouse of research, the content of which soon spread far beyond an original focus on alcohol metabolism. Nor was their concern limited to empirical inquiry: they conducted a highly influential annual educational program for community leaders—the "Yale Summer School of Alcohol Studies"—and were the original sponsors of the National Council for Education on Alcoholism, both of which did much to popularize and give credence to the "new approach." And as this was going on, the now-famous self-help fellowship known as Alcoholics Anonymous was created. Based polemically (but not procedurally) on the slogan that alcoholism is "an allergy of the body and an obsession of the mind," it achieved undeniable (but indeterminate) success in making "dry alcoholics" out of wet ones. As word of AA's success spread, it gradually came to be much publicized and celebrated, for its members constituted living proof that the chronic drunkard was not necessarily lost beyond all hope of redemption. And certainly, anything the untutored layman could do, the practitioner of scientific medicine could do better. Or so, at least, it was assumed.

The climate was ripening fast, and when, in 1946, the Presbyterian Church of the United States at its one hundred and fifty-eighth General Assembly voted to accept the proposition that "once drinking has passed a certain point, alcoholism is a disease; that is, the drinking cannot be stopped by mere [sic] resolution on the part of the drinker [quoted in Roueché, 1960, p. 108]," the larger acceptance of the "new approach" became but a matter of time. How far things had come from the period but a few years previous when "a constitutional explanation of vice" had been held to border on the heretical! After this church action, itself a sign of the changing climate and not its cause, things fell ever more rapidly into place. The bandwagon was rolling, and in short order all that remained was for the American Medical Association and the American Hospital Association to proclaim the official standing of the "new approach." And this they proceeded to do in 1956 and in 1957 respectively. Thus, less than half a century after the *Journal of Inebriety* had passed from the scene, its message having fallen on either indifferent or militantly antagonistic ears, the conception of the habitual drunkard as the innocent victim of a bona fide medical illness had carried the citadels and was in process of carrying the nation. And, if present indications offer any clue to what the future holds, it seems destined to carry the world as well. Not long ago, for instance, a research clinic with which the writer was affiliated recently received a letter from the Organizing Secretary of the Zambian National Council on Alcoholism announcing that his organization was about to conduct a survey on the prevalence of alcoholism amongst the Zambian citizenry. Indeed, the last to join the chorus could well be the slavish ideologues of "History's Vanguard Party." As recently as the Twenty-first Russian Party Congress, M. Suslov (the party's leading theoretician) remained adamant concerning the culturally vestigial character of "the problem."

While the local medical consensus concerning the propriety of the notion that "alcoholism is a disease" continues to grow, there is precious little agreement among the parties to this consensus as to the nature of this disease. It is to this lack of univocality that I now turn. While specifications of the etiology of the disease, alcoholism, may, in principle, posit the universal character of alcohol's "fatal attraction," since everybody knows that "only some of those who drink become alcoholics," all conceivable versions of universalism must be eliminated from consideration. The disease notion must, then, posit one or another theory of differential vulnerability. Such theories may be conveniently subdivided on the basis of whether the victim is held to be the unfortunate possessor of some manner of differentially vulnerable body or of some manner of differentially vulnerable psyche. There are numerous versions of both alternatives available to choose from. And herein lies the difficulty, for not one of them may properly be said to rest upon a hard core of supporting evidence. Furthermore, what evidence has been advanced in support of one or another of them is in *every* case moot. Indeed, if empirical corroboration were truly our guide and not simply our shibboleth, we would be forced to conclude that, in respect to empirical warrant, the present day proponents of the disease formulation are scarcely better off than were the editors of the *Journal of Inebriety* some fifty years ago! This being the case, the conclusion seems to me inescapable that in officially proclaiming that "Alcoholism is a disease," whatever else the proclaimers may be doing, they are *not* announcing a discovery of fact. And if this is so, it follows that the acceptance presently accorded this proclamation can only be explained in terms of the greater receptivity of the audience to which it is addressed. In a word, *the success of this latest venture in medical designation is a social-historical attainment and not a scientific achievement.*

If we are unable to set forth a series of criteria, the differential presence or absence of which constitute the necessary and sufficient conditions for the existence of the disease, alcoholism, it is apparent that the designation lacks what might be called a "fixed meaning." Ought we conclude, then, that we are using a word whose meaning we do not know and that we are thus talking nonsense? Only the most radical denotationist would so recommend. There is greater wisdom, I believe, in Wittgenstein's answer (1953, p. 37) to the general form of this question: "Say what you choose, so long as it does not prevent you from seeing the facts. (And once you see them there is a good deal you will not say.)" In answering thusly, I understand Wittgenstein to be recommending that we depart from the denotationist framework altogether and look instead to the role that the notion of alcoholism is employed to perform, for it is here that the relevant facts are to be found.

What role, then, does the notion of alcoholism play in the world? Its role is, of course, to solve the puzzle that originally attracted attention, *viz,* that the self-evidently avoidable and variously injurious conduct of the chronic drunkard is not "shaped up" by the application of negative sanctions as one would reasonably expect were such conduct in fact the avoidable conduct of a normally prudent man, which it had historically been understood to be. Since an adequate solution to this puzzle must refute the hitherto accepted assumption that such continued drunkenness is avoidable, alcoholism's role must be to rationalize its unavoidable character. And when we say that "Smith is an alcoholic," or in other words, that "Smith suffers from the disease of alcoholism," I submit that we are doing just that.[6]

But whence comes the compellingness of such an "explanation"? On this point, I would quote from a closely reasoned essay on the "definition of alcoholism" by Mark Keller (1960), the editor of the *Quarterly Journal*

---

[6] Actually, we are of course doing a great deal more than this. Not only are we recommending that such drunkenness is unavoidable and that moral judgments are, in consequence, both factually irrelevant and essentially improper, we are at the same time recommending a rival procedure—medical treatment—for the management of the chronic drunkard. In general, however, the results of such treatment are not sanguine, and I would agree with J. A. Smith (1957, p. 736) that "It is unlikely that any other diagnostic group has been so variously, frequently, and briefly 'cured' as alcoholics." As of this writing, the therapeutic effectiveness of medical treatment constitutes a most fragile defense for the disease notion.

of *Studies on Alcohol* and one of the leading exponents of the notion that "Alcoholism is a disease." While candidly admitting that neither physical nor biochemical instruments or tests exist by which a diagnosis of alcoholism can be verified, Keller argues (p. 128) that such a diagnosis can be established "by adequate anamnesis." Recognizing that neither the absolute quantity of alcohol consumed per unit time nor the quantity of alcohol consumed relative to the social and/or dietary standards of the community[7] are adequate yardsticks for establishing the existence of the disease, Keller recommends the following definition: "Alcoholism is a chronic disease manifested by repeated implicative drinking so as to cause injury to the drinker's health or to his social or economic functioning." For Keller, then, the matter of "ill effects" is clearly of the essence, and about these ill effects he says the following:

The key criterion, for all ill effects, is this: Would the individual be expected to reduce his drinking (or give it up) in order to avoid the injury or its continuance? If the answer is yes, and he does not do so, it is assumed—admitting it is only an assumption—that he cannot, hence that he has "lost control over his drinking," that he is addicted to or dependent on alcohol. *This inference is the heart of the matter. Without evident or at least reasonably inferred loss of control, there is no foundation for the claim that "alcoholism is a disease"* [p. 132; emphasis supplied].[8]

If "loss of control" does constitute the essential foundation for the claim that "alcoholism is a disease," and if, as is clearly the case, the existence of this "loss of control" cannot be independently determined but must be inferred on the basis of the failure of the chronic drunkard to comport himself in the manner of a prudent man, it seems to me that we cannot escape the conclusion that the disease formulation is a circular one. For, as I have already argued, it is precisely the unreasonable character of the chronic drunkard's project that makes him problematic to common sense in the first place. The argument reduces to this: because no one who is "sound of mind and body" would conduct himself in the irrational manner of the chronic drunkard, anyone who does so conduct himself must be other than sound of mind and/or body, that is, must

[7] The notion of "deviance from community social and/or dietary standards" constitutes the core of the World Health Organization's attempt to resolve the matter. Seeley (1959) has written a devastating critique of this essentially misguided attempt at quantification.

[8] "Except," Keller adds, "in the medical dictionary sense of diseases (of the nervous or digestive system, for example) caused by alcohol poisoning—a sense which leaves out of account a vast part, quite likely the most part, of the alcohol population."

be diseased; and the presumptive evidence for the existence of said disease consists in the discovery ("by adequate anamnesis") of just such irrational conduct.

But is the chronic drunkard in fact the complete and total "judgmental dope" which the sundry versions of unavoidability must, by definition, consider him to be? While I shall not attempt to answer this question here, the matter is far too important to be settled by theoretical election, and before one forecloses the issue he might well ponder, for instance, the conclusion of Gerard, Saenger, and Wile (1962, p. 95) based upon their detailed follow-up study of fifty-five abstinent alcoholics:

They believed that the pain and suffering which they experienced in their alcoholism became so bad that they had to stop drinking. Though certain individuals, such as priests, general physicians, or friends may have been acknowledged by them as helpful through giving them support, financial or moral, at a crucial point in their lives, when the need to give up drinking was impressed upon them by circumstances to which their drinking problem had led them, they did not credit these persons with, nor is there any reason for us to believe that these persons had a deep personal impact on their lives, which either led them to the decision to become abstinent or sustained them in their abstinence. . . . Similarly, the activities of the Connecticut Commission on Alcoholism—either inpatient or outpatient—if they were regarded as helpful, were regarded as helpful not in the sense of professional assistance helping them to initiate abstinence, but (with some exceptions) rather as a setting in which they could get kind treatment and medical support when they were in a state of ill health or on the verge of DTs or sick with a hangover, etc.

The question of the chronic drunkard's capacity to exercise discretion aside, I turn finally to the matter of the substantive import of the general position I have here advanced. In a very real and an entirely legitimate sense, it is a fact that there exist in the world a large number of people about whom it is correct to say, "They are alcoholics." It has been my contention, however, that the *grounds* that in any individual case make this designation a *correct* designation do *not* reside in some empirically well-documented professional-theoretical version of the "alcoholic personality," the "alcoholic body," or some combination of the two.

Still, one must not conclude from this that the social world in which these recognition and designation procedures are employed and from which they derive is Pirandelloesque. Organized social life would be literally impossible if everyone subscribed to the maxim, "Right you are if you think you are." Rather, there *is* a social order, and, returning to our fundamental insight, every social event must be construed as an event within that order. This entails (among other things) that the recognition and designation procedures actually in use are not only socially employed, but are socially sanctioned as well. With this in mind, I recommend the following formulation: *One is an alcoholic by virtue of the fact that a bona fide member of the medical profession, acting in his capacity as a member of that profession, has so designated him.*[9]

While there is a rich but ill-organized literature—both folk and theoretical—on the general topic of sanctioned entitlement, I know of no empirical study addressed specifically to the actual procedures used by medical practitioners in determining the warranted applicability of the designation "alcoholic" to a series of individual cases. And neither, apparently, does the Surgeon General of the United States Public Health Service, who, after consulting with the staff in the National Office of Vital Statistics on this matter, was informed that "while the Standard Nomenclature of Diseases does list the various types of alcoholic conditions, definitions are not given and it is not possible to know the criteria used by physicians in completing death certificates. (Nevertheless) the condition entered on the death certificate is accepted as final by the National Office of Vital Statistics . . . the lack of precision . . . arises from the fact that there is no generally accepted clear-cut definition of what constitutes chronic alcoholism [Surgeon General, 1956, pp. 4–5]."

I submit, in conclusion, that a truly operational definition of the alcoholic must await the procedural account of how this discrimination is in fact accomplished within a social order of everyday activities, and under the auspices of the members' common sense knowledge of, and motivated compliance with, that order in the various situations in which practical circumstances dictate that such a determination is relevant. Such an investigation would clearly seem to be the next step. Indeed, logically, it would seem to be the first step.

REFERENCES

Bowman, K. M., & Jellinek, E. M. Alcohol addiction and its treatment. *Quarterly Journal of Studies on Alcohol,* 1941, 2, 98–176.
von Brühl-Cramer, C. *Uber die Trunksucht und eine Rationelle Heilmetode. Derselben.* Berlin: 1819.

[9] The late E. M. Jellinek (1960, p. 12), like Keller an eminent spokesman for the notion that, "Alcoholism is a disease," arrived at much the same conclusion in his final work. "It comes to this, that a disease is what the medical profession recognizes as such. . . . the medical profession has officially accepted alcoholism as an illness, and *through this fact alone* [emphasis mine] alcoholism becomes an illness, whether a part of the lay public likes it or not, and even if a minority of the medical profession is disinclined to accept the idea."

Edwards, O. C. The treatment of inebriety as a disease. *Montreal Medical Journal,* 1896, **27,** 736–737.

Gerard, D. L., Saenger, G., & Wile, R. The abstinent alcoholic. *Archives of General Psychiatry,* 1962, **6,** 83–95.

Hart, H. L. A. The ascription of responsibility and rights. In A. G. N. Flew (Ed.), *Logic and language.* Oxford: Basil Blackwell and Mott, 1951. Pp. 145–166.

Jellinek, E. M. *The disease concept of alcoholism.* New Haven: Hillhouse Press, 1960.

Keeley, L. E. Drunkenness, a curable disease. *American Journal of Politics,* 1892, **1,** 27–43.

Keller, M. Definition of alcoholism. *Quarterly Journal of Studies on Alcohol,* 1960, **21,** 125–134.

Marconi, J. T. The concept of alcoholism. *Quarterly Journal of Studies on Alcohol,* 1959, **20,** 216–235.

Peters, R. S. *The concept of motivation.* London: Routledge & Kegan Paul, 1958.

Rosenman, S. The skid row alcoholic and the negative ego image. *Quarterly Journal of Studies on Alcohol,* 1955, **16,** 447–473.

Roueché, B. *The neutral spirit: A portrait of alcohol.* Boston: Little, Brown & Company, 1960.

Rush, B. *An inquiry into the effects of ardent spirits upon the human body and mind, with an account of the means of preventing, and of the remedies for curing them.* New York: Cornelius Davis, 1811.

Schutz, A. *Collected papers. I. The problem of social reality.* The Hague: Martinus Nijhoff, 1962.

Schutz, A. *Collected papers. II. Studies in social theory.* The Hague: Martinus Nijhoff, 1964.

Seeley, J. R. The W. H. O. definition of alcoholism. *Quarterly Journal of Studies on Alcohol,* 1959, **20,** 352–356.

Sinclair, A. *Prohibition: The era of excess.* Boston: Little, Brown & Company, 1962.

Smith, J. A. Psychiatric treatment of the alcoholic. *Journal of the American Medical Association,* 1957, **163,** 734–738.

Surgeon General, United States Public Health Service, Personal communication to J. Hirsh. Quoted in J. Hirsch, Public Health and social aspects of alcoholism. In G. N. Thompson (Ed.), *Alcoholism.* Springfield, Illinois: Charles C Thomas, 1956. Pp. 3–102.

Tashiro, M., & Lipscomb, W. R. Mortality experience of alcoholics. *Quarterly Journal of Studies on Alcohol,* 1963, **24,** 203–212.

Taylor, C. Alcoholism; the treatment and cure of the disease. *Therapy Gazette,* 1894, **10,** 238–240.

Trotter, T. *An essay, medical, philosophical, and chemical on drunkenness, and its effects on the human body.* London: Longman, Hurst, Rees and Orme, 1810.

Whitehead, A. N. *The aims of education.* New York: New American Library of World Literature, 1949.

Wittgenstein, L. *Philosophical investigations.* New York: Macmillan, 1953.

Wittgenstein, L. *Remarks on the foundations of mathematics.* New York: Macmillan, 1956.

4.3 *Orientation*

The rising problem of drug addiction in contemporary life has been the subject of numerous professional articles and books, as well as having received considerable attention in the popular press. The problem has come into sharper focus in recent years because of the discussions about whether or not society should allow relatively uncontrolled distribution of LSD. In this case, the drug's most ardent supporters are asking that each individual be allowed to have his own psychotic-like experience, free from the more pressing dangers of immediate addiction from the use of habit-forming narcotics.

In this article Edwin M. Schur writes about addiction and the question of whether or not continued use of narcotics and barbiturates is indicative of mental health problems. His information is current, and he writes with clarity and purpose. As Schur points out, any view of the relationship of mental illness to addiction must also take into account the social setting in which addiction occurs. A psychiatric explanation by itself is insufficient, even in those cases where the addict exhibits obvious personality disturbance.

4.3 The Addict and Social Problems

Edwin M. Schur

There is considerable dispute as to whether or not drug addiction[1] constitutes a mental illness or symptom of such illness. In part this disagreement simply reflects problems involved in the analysis of social and psy-

---

[1] The present discussion is limited to addiction to opiates—which involves tolerance and physical dependence as well as psychological habituation. (On the nature of these drugs and of the addiction process, see Chein, Gerard, Lee, & Rosenfeld, 1964; *Drug Addiction,* 1961; Lindesmith, 1947; New York, 1963; Nyswander, 1956; Schur, 1962.)

chological pathology generally—such as the difficulty of transcending culture-bound definitions and establishing objective diagnostic criteria. Awareness that the "deviant" nature of offending behavior often is relative to particular sociocultural conditions, and that the drug user's deviance in our society is therefore partly "caused" by processes of socio-legal definition, has challenged conventional psychiatric theories of addiction. At the same time, explanations of addiction demonstrate not merely differences among the theoretical orientations of divergent disciplines, but also covert or even overt rivalries and clashes of interest among the adherents of particular approaches and therapeutic techniques. Furthermore, ambivalence in public attitudes about addiction significantly shapes our thinking about the drug problem, as may the current state of information, dominant values, and social power of the relevant practicing professionals, such as lawyers, doctors, and law enforcement personnel. The very ramifications of the narcotics problem itself, as it has been developing in modern American society, have forced some rethinking of earlier overly simplified "causal" theories. Likewise, the extremely poor success record of conventional therapy has sparked a search for new approaches. Increasingly there is acceptance of the general viewpoint to be stressed in this article—that with respect to opiate addiction *medical, social,* and *legal* aspects are crucially interrelated; that all three perspectives must be considered in an assessment of the "causes" of our current addiction problem, and likewise that all three must be taken into account in any comprehensive effort to treat that problem.

Much of the recent policy-oriented discussion of addiction (and as we shall see, the "policy" aspects are extremely germane to etiological analysis) has centered around the question: Is addiction a *crime or disease?* But in this debate, "disease" has really meant "symptom," for psychiatry (which tends to view addiction as merely symptomatic of underlying psychopathology) has provided the primary support for the disease argument. The dichotomy of "bad" or "sick" has not been entirely satisfactory to sociological students of the problem. On the one hand, they recognize the socially harmful consequences of policies defining addiction as a crime (see below), while, on the other hand, believing that significant aspects of the narcotics situation are inadequately considered if the problem is conceived of as "essentially" being one of psychologically diseased individuals. Some alternative perspectives are possible. As will be made clear below, addiction can be seen primarily as *social* rather than individual pathology. Or, theoretically, one could view it *simply as deviating behavior,* avoiding all implications of necessary pathology. Alternatively, one may construe the very fact of full addiction—involving actual physical dependence on the drug with a characteristic abstinence syndrome following withdrawal—as constituting *physiological* pathology, a phenomenon of roughly the same order as diabetes. This analogy was sharply drawn several years ago in a satiric comment in a psychiatric journal, entitled "The Land of Insulin Addiction," in which the author pictured a country where insulin-taking is a crime, where all insulin "addicts" therefore become criminals in order to support their habit, and where special police units are formed to track down addicts and combat the traffic in insulin (Davidson, 1959). We know, however, that a pharmacophysiological process alone is not sufficient to account for persisting opiate addiction (involving relapse following withdrawal from drugs); an independent or accompanying psychological craving for the drug must also be present. In connection with the interpretation of inherent (rather than symptomatic) pathology, it is noteworthy that addiction sometimes is created through medical administration of opiates for relief of pain; yet again, we know that not all individuals so treated become long-term addicts—something more is needed. Furthermore, this particular path to addiction probably has occurred in only a small proportion of present addiction cases in this country.

PSYCHOLOGICAL AND SOCIAL VIEWS
OF ADDICTIVE PATHOLOGY

Psychiatric Theories

If the notion that physiological addiction is an illness in its own right has not been widely accepted, there is a vast body of literature asserting that such addiction is symptomatic of underlying psychological disturbance and, also, that particular personality types are psychologically predisposed to drug-taking. While specific psychiatric and psychological interpretations may differ in certain respects, there appears to be considerable consensus as to the dominant "clinical picture" in addiction cases. The addict is found to be immature and overburdened by feelings of inadequacy. He is bent on self-destruction, yet at the same time narcissistically preoccupied with his own gratification. The addict's life becomes a self-enclosed system centered around the search for and use of drugs, and with no room for the normal sexual and social contacts of the interpersonal world. His great dependence on drug sources together with his insistence upon immediate gratification of his demands suggest a reversion to infancy (Nyswander, 1956).

Psychoanalytic interpretations sometimes relate drug addiction to such matters as unconscious homosexuality, phallic symbolism (for example, of the syringe), and the Oedipus Complex. An especially dominant theme is oral fixation: ". . . addicts are persons who have a disposition to react to the effects of alcohol, morphine, or other drugs in a specific way, namely, in such a way that they try to use these effects to satisfy the archaic oral longing which is sexual longing, a need for security, and a need for the maintenance of self-esteem simultaneously . . . [Fenichel, 1945, p. 376]." According to such formulations, it is the person for whom the drug has a special significance, for whom it holds out the best means of satisfying needs normally met by sexual and other object-relationships, who becomes an addict. As Fenichel (1945) goes on to state:

Patients who are ready to give up all object libido necessarily are persons who never estimated object-relationships very highly. They are fixated in a passive-narcissistic aim and are interested solely in getting their gratification. . . . Interests in reality gradually disappear, except those having to do with procuring the drug. In the end, all of reality may come to reside in the hypodermic needle. The tendency toward such a development, rooted in an oral dependence on outer supplies is the essence of drug addiction. All other features are incidental [p. 377].

For present purposes, there is no need to explore at length such psychodynamic explanations. This material is included merely to illustrate some of the basis for interpreting personality traits seen in already-addicted individuals as being of etiological significance, and hence for considering psychotherapeutic intervention to be indicated. Other "incidental features"—such as the effects on the individual's personality of protracted drug-taking, and particularly of playing the role of "addict" with all that this implies (sociologically and psychologically, in our society)—tend to receive little attention. This kind of reasoning can be pushed quite far indeed, as in one recent analysis where the statement is made that the female addict's frequent resort to prostitution to obtain money for drugs "further suggests a tendency to devalue the female role [Laskowitz, 1961]."

Attempts to classify the diagnosed personality characteristics found in samples of known addicts have provided support for the clinicians' claims of basic psychopathology in addiction. One influential early report found 86 percent of the addicts studied to have been affected "with some forms of nervous instability before they became addicted," the largest category comprising "care-free individuals, devoted to pleasure, seeking new excitements and sensations, and usually having some ill-defined instability of personality that often expresses itself in mild infractions of social customs [Kolb, 1925]." Other studies have used the term "psychopathic personality" or "psychopathic diathesis or predisposition" in diagnosing addicts (Felix, 1939). In one relatively recent psychiatric study employing a control group of nonaddicts (control groups were conspicuously absent in some of the early researches), *none of the addict subjects was considered to be normal* (Gerard & Kornetsky, 1955). But the meaning of these findings was thrown into question by the fact that more than 50 percent of the controls (drawn from the same ethnic and racial groups and from the same areas of residence in New York City as those from which the addicts had come) were held to show signs of serious psychological disturbance—over one-fifth being diagnosed as overtly or incipiently schizophrenic. As one commentator has pointed out, this latter finding may well "suggest that deviation from middle-class personality patterns is widespread in the neighborhoods and groups from which the addicts were drawn [Clausen, 1957, p. 252]."

Criticisms of the Psychiatric Approach

In a now classic critique, sociologist Alfred Lindesmith (1940) insisted that the psychiatric approach to addiction was inadequate because it failed to develop a specific, self-consistent, and universally applicable theory of addiction. It evaded the problem of explaining how some otherwise "normal" persons (found even in most of the psychiatric surveys) become addicted. Nor did it explain cross-cultural and group variations in addiction rates. Noting the absence of control groups in early studies, Lindesmith pointed out that even if control groups were used the problem would remain that psychiatrists study the addict only after addiction, and therefore are unable unequivocally to separate those traits resulting from addiction from those that caused addiction. Furthermore, there was reason to feel that attitudes disapproving of addiction often colored the diagnosis. Lindesmith referred to

. . . the unspoken assumption . . . that any trait which distinguishes addicts from nonaddicts is *ipso facto* a criterion of abnormality. . . . Addicts are said to become addicted because they have feelings of frustration, lack of self-confidence and need the drug to bolster themselves up. Lack of self-confidence is taken as a criterion of psychopathy or of weakness. But another person becomes addicted, it is said, because of "curiosity" and a "willingness to try anything once" and this too is called abnormal. Thus self-confidence and the lack of self-confidence are both signs of abnormality. The addict is evidently judged in advance. He is damned if he is self-confident and he is damned if he is not [p. 290].

It is of course true that some degree of circularity and "judging in advance" are necessarily involved in much psychiatric diagnosis. In many instances it is the "symptomatic" deviating behavior itself that largely determines (at least initially) a clinical finding of "disturbance" or "abnormality." And in cases of voluntary submission to observation, analysis or therapy, perhaps the very fact of such submission can be held to indi-

cate the individual's own recognition of such "disturbance"—although
such self-evaluations are heavily determined by public attitudes and prevailing theories. Nonetheless, such circularity becomes perhaps more
questionable (especially with involuntary "patients") as the analyst resorts
to increasingly vague diagnostic labels. In the case of addiction, diagnoses
are typically quite vague—the blatantly circular term "addict personality" has even been used at times—and often the evaluated individuals
are not voluntary "patients." One certainly senses, from some psychiatric
reports, the therapist's assumption that anyone taking up drugs must, by
definition, have been a disturbed individual. (In this connection, we
might wish to consider the recent statement by one New York addict
that drugs were so widely prevalent in his neighborhood that the only
boy who did not try them was mentally retarded! See Larner & Tefferteller, 1964, p. 252.) It has also been suggested that psychiatric assessments
sometimes exaggerate the positive gratifications addicts receive from opiates. The authors of a major New York study have recently pointed out
that even if physiological dependence alone is insufficient to explain continuing addiction, a theory of "kicks" grossly misrepresents the motivation of long-term (and perhaps even beginning) addicts (Chein et al.,
1964). Even theories emphasizing "escape"—and most psychodynamic explanations seem to focus on this in one way or another—seem questionable when one considers the serious social hardships and severe psychic
strains facing the addict in present-day American society (to be discussed
further below).

Area Studies

Another approach to the "causes" of addiction is represented by the
considerable research on the nature, extent, and spatial and social distribution of drug use in major American cities. These various area studies
have produced strikingly consistent evidence of the relationship between
the city's socioeconomic structure and the distribution of known cases of
addiction. As an example of such findings, Chein et al. (1964), reporting
on their extensive interdisciplinary research into juvenile drug use in
New York stated that

. . . juvenile drug use is not randomly distributed over New York City. It is
heavily concentrated in certain neighborhoods. These are not a cross-section of
the city's neighborhoods, but rather they are the ones which are economically
and socially most deprived. Even within the relatively few [census] tracts in
which we found the vast majority of cases, the tracts of highest drug use can
be distinguished from those with lower rates of juvenile drug use by a variety
of social and economic indexes. The tracts with the greatest amount of drug use
are those with the highest proportions of certain minority groups, the highest

poverty rates, the most crowded dwelling units, the highest incidence of disrupted family living arrangements, and so on . . . [p. 78].

As well as this socioeconomic and geographic concentration, these researchers found high drug-use neighborhoods to be characterized by a special "cultural climate" (pp. 78–106) believed conducive to experimentation with drugs. This climate consisted of a generalized outlook on life that might be summarized as pessimistic antisocial hedonism. And it is quite clear, from ecological surveys and other studies of drug use, that there exists in large metropolitan centers today not only such an outlook (which may lead to experimentation and addiction) but also a distinct addict subculture—an entire way of life that has developed around actual drug distribution and use—the significance of which will be considered further below.

There is a familiar problem posed by such research findings: not all individuals in the high drug-use neighborhoods become users or even adopt the prevailing antisocial and pessimistic attitudes. Seeking to explain the existence of non-drug-using "squares" in the very areas of high drug use and a well-developed addict subculture, Chein and his associates refer (on the basis of a comparison of a group of addicts with one of matched nonaddicts) to certain family background factors:

> In contrast to our control cases, the addicts were reared in a family milieu which, in terms of our psychological theorizing, we would regard as contributing to the development of weak ego functioning, defective superego, inadequate masculine identification, lack of realistic levels of aspiration with respect to long-range goals, and a distrust of major social institutions. Moreover, each of the hypotheses was supported within each ethnic group separately—native Whites, Negroes, and Puerto Ricans [p. 268].

Although the implication here is that some individuals are psychologically predisposed to drug use and others are not, the same authors are also aware of the importance of the sheer availability of drugs, which is fully documented in their work. And presumably, even within particular neighborhoods, variations in "opportunity structures," patterns of associations, and reference-group orientations may be of significance in determining variations in individual "susceptibility." At any rate the interrelation of social and psychic factors in this matter seems evident. As Clausen (1961) has properly stressed, "personality is not independent of environmental influences and, by and large, the influences that permit heroin to be available to a teen-ager and that permit a high proportion of adolescents to become members of street-corner society also create psychological needs and vulnerabilities which enhance the value of narcotics to the person [p. 205]." The ecological studies, then, provide a basis for concluding that addiction is as much a symptom of social pathology as of individual pathology, and that amelioration of the problem rests significantly upon large-scale socioeconomic reforms as well as upon direct treatment of individual and family pathology.

A PROCESSUAL APPROACH: LINDESMITH'S THEORY

Still another approach to the causation of addiction may be termed processual. In his early critique of psychiatric theories, Lindesmith (1947) objected to the fact that they cannot be applied to all cases of addiction. He therefore sought to develop a theoretical formulation that would include all cases, on the assumption that the only true causal statement is one that is universally applicable to all instances of the phenomenon being explained (clearly a rather different premise than that employed in much etiological research, where association between variables is stated in terms of probability). Lindesmith began his research with a working hypothesis, which he revised to take account of negative cases whenever he encountered them. His final thesis, to which no exceptions could be found, was that "the knowledge or ignorance of the meaning of withdrawal distress and the use of opiates thereafter determines whether or not the individual becomes addicted [p. 69]." (This refers to the persistence of a craving for the drug after withdrawal; continued use may result in physical dependence on the drug, regardless of the presence of this knowledge.) A major shortcoming of this "theory" is apparent in that it provides no basis for predicting which particular individuals are likely to become addicted. But it does highlight the fact that becoming addicted always involves going through a type of learning process, and it suggests that a special psychological predisposition may not be necessary. It is evident that in our present narcotics situation the process of "learning to be an addict" will usually involve a great deal more than simply acquiring knowledge about the drug and the withdrawal symptoms—which knowledge, in any case, may be rather widespread.

Deviance as a Labeling Process

To adopt a processual perspective on the addiction problem, one does not need to accept Lindesmith's specific explanation of addiction. More important, is the general stress on a learning process, which suggests important lines of analysis usually ignored in approaches focusing on either personality or socioeconomic characteristics of individual addicts. Sociologists concerned with the analysis of deviant behavior have recently displayed a strong interest in the societal reaction to deviance, a matter that has often been overshadowed by concentration on the motivation and behavior of the deviating individual himself. As Howard S. Becker

(1963) suggests, "deviance is *not* a quality of the act the person commits, but rather a consequence of the application by others of rules and sanctions to an 'offender.' The deviant is one to whom that label has successfully been applied; deviant behavior is behavior that people so label [p. 9]." Any analysis that avoids the implications of this point cannot really expect to come to grips with the social psychology of the addict. The addict's deviance can be represented as a "career" (Goffman, 1961) which is continuously developing through his interaction with significant others—their reactions to (and treatment of) him "cause" his behavior and outlooks every bit as much as do his basic "characteristics." This point is stated well by Lemert (1964):

> . . . with repetitive, persistent deviation or invidious differentiation, something happens "inside the skin" of the deviating person. Something gets built into the psyche or nervous system as a result of social penalties, or "degradation ceremonies," or as a consequence of having been made the subject of "treatment" of "rehabilitation." The individual's perception of values, means, and estimates of their costs undergoes revision in such ways that symbols which serve to limit the choices of most people produce little or no response in him, or else engender responses contrary to those sought by others [pp. 81–82].

The societal definition of addiction as deviant (and criminal, under present American policy) must then be seen as shaping the very nature of that condition and the meaning it holds for the individuals involved.

It has recently been argued that since deviance is essentially a matter of societal definition, relative to time and place, and since some cases of addiction in our own society seem patently "nondeviant," it is questionable whether it is appropriate to apply to addiction the blanket label of "deviance"—let alone either "crime" or "illness" (Lindesmith & Gagnon, 1964). One must be alert to the possibility that different etiological explanations may be required to cover different types of addiction—even within a single society. And one can always raise the question whether a particular form of behavior *should* be labeled and treated as deviant (though there are definite limits on the contribution of the scientist, *qua* scientist, in answering such questions). But one of the central facts about drug addiction in the United States today is that, by and large, it *has* been labeled deviant *and criminal*. (The major exception is the "addict" created through long-term administration of opiates in the treatment of cancer and other physical illnesses. Well-to-do individuals and doctors, who may manage to keep their addiction hidden and to obtain supplies without difficulty, do evade at least some of the implications of society's negative definition of the addict. Nonetheless, their addiction, if disclosed, will still be considered "deviant" and possibly even criminal.) On the societal level, as well as on the individual level, this labeling process is of great sociological significance. It may well be that many of the individuals succumbing to addiction in our society are in some ways more disturbed or disadvantaged than otherwise similar individuals who do not succumb, although one cannot entirely ignore the alternative explanation that in the areas of high-drug use addicted individuals are simply more fully socialized into a prevailing (although deviant, by dominant standards) pattern. Yet the broader dimensions of the addiction problem cannot be understood without an effort to bring the elements of social reaction and public policy directly into the analysis.

As Clausen (1957a) has stated, "The prevalence and consequences of addiction in any society depend as much upon the social and legal definitions placed upon the nonmedical use of narcotics as upon the nature and effects of narcotics or the nature of the persons who became addicted [p 34]." Sociologists, and certainly psychologists and psychiatrists, have not shown much inclination for considering legal policies as "causal" factors in deviance. Informal, rather than formal, mechanisms of social control have been of central concern in sociological analysis. The sociologist often seems to have inferred from evidence of law's questionable deterrent effect (for example, studies of capital punishment, the unenforceability of prohibition, and so on) that law by itself has little social effect of any sort. Yet even laws that fail to deter the proscribed behavior may have considerable impact in shaping that behavior. The "criminalization of deviance"—through the enactment of a law "against" a particular form of deviating behavior—may have far-reaching consequences, many of which may be dysfunctional from the standpoint even of dominant values and institutions (Schur, 1965). All of these considerations point, in the case of addiction, to the importance of examining current narcotics laws and enforcement policies.

SOCIETAL REACTION AND ADDICT BEHAVIOR

Laws and Enforcement Policies

Technically speaking, it is not a crime in this country to be a drug addict, but it is the practical effect of current narcotics policy (stemming largely from the restrictive interpretation given the federal Harrison Act) to make it so (see Lindesmith, 1965; New York, 1963; Schur, 1962). Psychiatrist Karl Bowman (1958) has described the process as follows: "A law which was designed as a revenue law has been pushed forward and extended so that we have nonmedical persons telling doctors how to practice medicine and interfering with the legitimate and humanitarian care of sick persons [p. 171]." Under existing state and federal legislation, the addict cannot legally possess the drug to which he is addicted. Likewise, while it may be legal for a doctor to prescribe small amounts of a narcotic for an addict under certain circumstances, the legal position of the medical practitioner regarding any such prescription at any other time than when incidental to institutional withdrawal treatment of the addict is not at all clear:

> The physician has no way of knowing *before* he attempts to treat, and/or prescribe drugs to an addict, whether his activities will be condemned or condoned. He does not have any criteria or standards to guide him in dealing with drug addicts, since what constitutes bona fide medical practice and good faith depends upon the facts and circumstances of each case . . . [p. 78].

Although current laws provide severe penalties for unauthorized possession, sale, or transfer of addicting drugs, most nongovernmental observers agree that this repressive approach has not significantly curbed addiction. Yet these laws have greatly influenced the overall development of the drug problem. In the absence of a legal way of satisfying his demand, it is natural for the addict to seek out illicit drug sources. The strong demand for narcotics provides the incentives for a thriving underworld traffic in the drugs. This supply-and-demand cycle is believed by many disinterested students of the problem to be virtually invulnerable. Because of the strength and continuous nature of the demand, no amount of enforcement effort can realistically be expected to cut off all ways of making the drugs available illegally.

We can see in this situation one instance of a more general type of sociolegal problem involving the exchange of socially disapproved goods or services between consenting adults. Other examples are abortion, prostitution, homosexuality, and gambling. The attempt to control such behaviors through the criminal law gives rise to what the present writer has termed "crimes without victims" (Schur, 1965). Because of the lack of a complaining "victim" in the illicit drug transaction, evidence against drug traffickers is extremely difficult to obtain. Even with special investigative techniques—such as the use of addict stool pigeons and narcotics agent-decoys—no significant incursion is made into the well-organized network of underworld drug distribution. Despite the occasional exposés of "dope rings," the brunt of enforcement efforts is felt by addicts themselves and small-time pushers or peddlers. The higher-ups in the illicit traffic, themselves rarely addicted, seem relatively free from interference. In short, we find in the drug addiction situation an example of virtually unenforceable law. And, as one legal expert (King, 1956) has asserted, "It is precisely our law enforcement efforts, and nothing else, that keep the price of drugs, nearly worthless in themselves, so high as to attract an endless procession of criminal entrepreneurs to keep the traffic flowing."

Secondary Deviation

In addition to failing to curb addiction, present policy drives most narcotic addicts into a life of crime (the reference here is to other offenses besides the mere possession and use of drugs). It should be emphasized that there is no evidence whatsoever that the effects of narcotics on the individual (now widely recognized to be depressant) lead to criminal behavior; nor is there any indication that the personality characteristics of addicts conduce to such behavior. On the contrary, most addict-crime is evidently attributable to the economics of the drug situation. Prices charged for illicit drugs are such that few long-time addicts can support their habits through ordinary sources of funds. Once such funds prove inadequate, criminality is almost bound to follow. This explanation is supported by the fact that addicts invariably commit cash-producing offenses (typically theft among the males, prostitution among the females). Evidence from the New York studies (and from research in other cities as well) points to a close association between drug use and "crime for profit" (with low rates of offenses against persons and other noncash-producing violations occurring in high drug-use areas), and to the conclusion that, "the user, juvenile or adult, engages in the illegal activities in which he does become involved, not for 'pleasure' or because of any basic depravity, but mainly because he needs the cash to meet the high cost of black market drugs" (Chein et al., 1964, pp. 167–168). Indeed, the need to engage in income-producing criminality "becomes an important determinant of the drug-user's life style and of his associations. Arguing against this position, Federal Bureau of Narcotics spokesmen insist that currently (in contrast with findings in early research) most addicts have records of criminal or delinquent activity antedating the onset of addiction. Since drug use is concentrated in those urban areas in which crime and delinquency are also prevalent, very likely there is some truth to this claim. Nonetheless, there is no disputing the point that once one becomes addicted in the United States today there is almost no alternative to engaging in petty theft or prostitution to support one's habit. It seems evident, then, that the addict's criminality must largely be characterized as "secondary deviation"—as a mode of deviant behavior adopted because of the problems created by societal reaction to the initial deviance (Lemert, 1951, 1964).

Elements of secondary deviation can also be seen in the development of specialized addict subculture. Very likely it is true that there are psychological gains the addict may derive from association with similarly addicted individuals. And there is considerable psychiatric literature suggesting ways in which the drug-centered way of life provides functional equivalents of more "normal" ways of satisfying basic human needs. Quite apart from such psychological mechanisms, it may also be true that certain features or types of addict subculture that are grounded in general sociocultural conditions may be only incidentally associated with drug use. This is suggested, for example, by Harold Finestone's analysis of a "cool cat" pattern found among young male Negro addicts in Chicago. Noting that the basic features of this pattern (speech, dress, general "cool" approach to life, and so on) apparently existed prior to the members' introduction to heroin, Finestone (1957) attributes the pattern's development to the various frustrations experienced by these youths through segregation and discrimination in the larger society. The "cat" as a social type, he asserts, "is the personal counterpart of an expressive social movement." There is also, in various sociological analyses of delinquency, the more general assertion that drug addiction is a "retreatist" form of adaptation by socially disadvantaged youth to disparities between dominant cultural goals and available avenues for the achievement of such goals. Other analysts, however, have criticized the applicability of the "retreatism" label to addiction—partly on the ground that this theory places undue emphasis on the drug's euphoric effects and "escape" potential, which in fact sharply recede in the course of long-term addiction (Lindesmith, 1964).

Notwithstanding the possible role of the above-mentioned general factors in addict subculture, some of its features clearly involve defense and reaction against society's specific hostility toward and persecution of the addict. For the addict who must rely on illicit drug supplies, involvement in such a subculture becomes almost inevitable. Through his recourse to the illicit traffic, the addict necessarily engages in frequent interaction with peddlers and pushers and may very likely become a pusher himself in order to support his habit. Whatever the psychic gains derived from association with other drug users and total immersion in the drug-distributing and drug-consuming world, such immersion is also clearly to the practical advantage of the addict who wishes to ensure a constant source of supply (Faris & Dunham, 1939). Furthermore, there is a directly defensive (that is, anti-enforcement) aspect of this subculture, reflected in addict argot, in the development of neighborhood "grapevine" communications systems, in mechanisms for protecting against informers, and in various other devices and behavior patterns (Fiddle, 1963).

The need to involve oneself in the transactions of an underworld market, to engage in criminal activities, and constantly to avoid law-enforcement interference as well as exploitation and harm from underworld sources (for example, receiving watered-down drugs, being named by an informer, being dealt a fatal overdose) inevitably affects the addict's self-image. The addicted individual, spending so much of his time and energy in these activities can scarcely help beginning to feel that society is his enemy—and perhaps even that he is an enemy of society. Almost unavoidably, a self-fulfilling prophecy mechanism is set in motion: not only do "respectables" view him as a criminal, but also he finds that increasingly he is in fact beginning to act like one. In part, the world of addiction becomes his entire way of life because respectable society has closed off other social worlds.

The British Experience

Evidence concerning the behavior of addicts in Great Britain and of physician addicts in the United States provides a broadened perspective on addiction and related problems. Although the United Kingdom has enacted statutory controls over possession and handling of dangerous drugs, the treatment of addiction has remained a medical matter (Lindesmith, 1965; New York Academy, 1963; Nyswander, 1956; Schur, 1962). Doctors are warned to exercise caution in the prescribing of narcotics, but they are in fact permitted (within broad limits) to prescribe drugs for addicts. The practitioner decides what treatment a particular addict shall receive and "treatment" is interpreted broadly— to permit ambulatory as well as institutional management, and to allow even extended administration of drugs where that is believed to be medically advisable. Under this policy, the addiction situation in Britain has remained benign; there are probably fewer than a thousand opiate addicts in the United Kingdom. Furthermore, there is practically no illicit traffic in opiates, since provision of low-cost drugs (and the addict qualifies as a patient under the National Health Service) largely eliminates the incentives for such trafficking.[2]

[2] A recent news account cites the report just issued by a British interdepartmental committee on addiction, which notes increases in addiction since 1959, and which calls for tighter controls over prescribing of narcotics. *The New York Times,* Nov. 25, 1965, p. 22. In this connection, the following points should be noted: (1) While there may have been an actual increase, it is also possible that the apparent increase may be partly attributable to improved reporting procedures. Responsible students of the problem have always allowed for a certain amount of "hidden addiction" in Britain. (2) Increased publicity about the "British approach" has attracted to Britain some Canadian addicts, and possibly some American ones, thus contributing to a real increase. (3) There apparently has been no substantial development of either illicit traffic or addict-crime. There

In this kind of situation, the behavioral correlates of addiction are pronouncedly different from those typically seen under repressive addiction policy. It is not a crime to be an addict; the addict commits an offense only if drugs he possesses were obtained illegally. The addict need not become a thief or prostitute to support his or her addiction, and hence addict-crime is practically nonexistent. Nor is there any incentive for the addict to himself "push" drugs. Under such policy, development of specialized addict subculture is slight; there is no practical need to associate with other addicts, and there is less need (than exists under anti-addict pressures) for interpersonal support from fellow addicts. This is not to suggest that the addict in such a situation is "the same as everyone else." Occupational adjustment may often be impaired (although there have been many instances cited of capable and productive work by long-term addicts, provided their supply was insured); and usually heterosexual activity is greatly restricted (because of the drug's severe inhibition of sexual drive, which operates to produce impotence in many male addicts).

However, the primary correlates of addiction (mainly the effect on sexual functioning, and some minor physiological disturbances) must be distinguished sharply from the secondary aspects of addict behavior. It seems clear that addict-crime, the development of a criminal self-image, involvement in illicit trafficking, probably involvement in addict subculture are to a considerable extent functions of society's response to the condition of addiction. Although there is much dispute about its relevance to the American situation, the British experience is at least useful for analytic purposes in highlighting this distinction. Furthermore, British policy has seemed to many students of the American drug problem to reflect an approach grounded in humanity and common sense. It is noteworthy that what have here been termed secondary correlates of addiction are found to be largely absent among physician-addicts in this country. One study of such addicts revealed that they "almost never associated with other physician-addicts, or did not do so knowingly. They did not have any occasion for doing so, either for the purpose of getting drugs or for passing time, for emotional supports." Likewise, it may be noted that the physicians interviewed did not make use of the special addict argot so prevalent in American underworld-linked addict circles (Winick, 1961). The nature of the addict's drug sources and his overall sociolegal status appear to be the crucial determinants of subcultural involvement. Similarly, there is every reason to

---

appears to be little basis in this report for any generalizations about "failure" of the British approach.

believe that the self-image of the physician-addict is quite different from
that of the subcultural-addict. Although the mere knowledge that one
is addicted to narcotics will undoubtedly affect the self-conceptions of
any individual, the physician-addict will in most instances not view
himself as a criminal, whereas other addicts in the United States can
hardly avoid doing so.

TREATMENT AND RELAPSE

Although there has been considerable medical and psychiatric treatment of individual addicts in this country, until recently, as least, such
efforts have met with only slight success. Withdrawing the addict from
drugs is not difficult, but a real "cure" in which the confirmed addict
overcomes his craving for the drug and remains abstinent over a long
period of time is not frequently attained. The relapse rates for patients
at specialized treatment facilities (usually offering a comprehensive
program of medical care including at least some form of psychotherapy)
have been extremely high, and it is now widely recognized that extensive
after-care (including practical guidance as well as psychological counsel-
ling) is a necessary supplement to institutional treatment. Crucially
implicated in the process of relapse are many social pathological features
of the community to which the addict typically returns on release from
the hospital. In the light of such difficulty, and given the long-term
addict's likely commitment to a deviant way of life, conventional
therapeutic procedures often prove inadequate. Community-based treatment programs (Freedman, Brotman, & Meyer, 1962; Freedman, Sager,
Rabiner, & Brotman, 1963) pooling the knowledge, skills, and facilities
of the hospital and the neighborhood social agency, and perhaps employing what has been termed "storefront psychiatry" (Hentoff, 1965),
seem to hold out special promise. Such relating of individual treatment
to a broader environmental context seems an important first step in
attempting to deal with the complex of individual and social problems
surrounding addiction.

An interesting challenge to conventional therapy may be seen in
the work of Synanon House, a completely voluntary program in which
the addict lives and works with former addicts in a milieu expressly and
fully dedicated to the eradication of "criminal addict" behavior and
value patterns (Yablonsky, 1965). Following withdrawal (which is
accomplished with little or no medication, but with strong group support), the member works in the organization (advancing through a
system of graded work statuses) and participates in "synanons"—brutally
candid group discussion sessions in which members are encouraged to
vent their hostilities and are forced to recognize the "rationalizations"

involved in drug-centered behavior and outlooks. Although the program has been charged with being a "protective community" rather than a true therapeutic community—because the extent to which it prepares members for a full life in the outside world is not clear (Sternberg, 1963)—there seems little doubt that Synanon has managed to keep substantial numbers of addicts off drugs for long periods of time. And whereas the severe forms of "attack therapy" (synanons with a small *s*) employed in this program have been criticized as having dysfunctional and self-destructive effects, it is interesting that Synanon's explicit demand that the individual, in effect, "shape up" or get out seems to have had some effectiveness in maintaining abstinence where more orthodox therapeutic approaches have frequently failed. Whatever its limitations, a program such as Synanon's has the great merit of providing a comprehensive basis for a total reassessment and reorganization of the individual addict's behavior and outlook on life. As one perceptive discussion of relapse (Ray, 1961) notes, "The ex-addict who is successful in remaining abstinent relates to new groups of people, participates in their experience, and to some extent begins to evaluate the conduct of his former associates (and perhaps his own when he was an addict) in terms of the values of the new group [p. 136]."

As already suggested above, some specialists involved in therapy with addicts assert that advances in treatment technique have been hampered by the restrictive policies embodied in recent American drug laws and regulations. It is neither possible nor appropriate in this brief article to discuss the various arguments advanced in favor of and in opposition to the numerous proposals for revision of these laws and regulations (see Chein et al., 1964; Lindesmith, 1965; New York Academy, 1963; Nyswander, 1956; Schur, 1962). However, it should be emphasized that the desire to reduce pathology currently associated with addiction and to enhance overall treament effectiveness are the chief motivations underlying these reform proposals. Most of the proposals urge greater latitude for the medical practitioner in treating the addict, especially with respect to prescribing of drugs for addicts and undertaking effort at ambulatory treatment. The pressure for such experimentation has grown rapidly in very recent years, and various pilot projects designed to test the feasibility of such procedures are now under way. One study in which heroin addicts are being maintained on the less dangerous drug methadone has, in the early stages of research, shown quite promising results (Hentoff, 1965).

In connection with efforts to expand the medical profession's role in managing addiction, it is important to recognize that just as individual pathology does not exist in a social vacuum, therapy itself also reflects and is dependent upon prevailing social conditions and definitions. The problem posed by the probability of addicts' returning to a drug-oriented sociocultural milieu following hospital treatment has already been cited. There has also been a developing awareness by therapists that their efforts with individual addiction cases might be greatly enhanced if the involvement of addicts in illicit traffic and other secondary deviation could be eliminated or reduced. An undercutting of the economic incentives for this traffic through legal prescription of low-cost drugs would be a major step in this direction. Notwithstanding the objection of some practitioners that these sociolegal aspects do not lie at the "core" of the problem (that is, the underlying pathology of which addiction is but a symptom), many now question whether individual therapy can have much meaning within the overall context of a "war against the addict" atmosphere. Because of the strong negative effects on the addict's self-image of current social definitions and repressive policies, a revision of these definitions and policies may be necessary if efforts at long-term "cure" are to become meaningful.

Relating to this point is the question of "compulsory therapy." Given present American policies, most institutional treatment of addicts occurs under some degree of compulsion. While some specialists assert that an authoritarian regime is useful in treating addicts, and perhaps this argument has particular validity in connection with after-care (Diskind & Klonsky, 1964), others would insist that in the long run the addict simply cannot be "cured' against his will. This is the basic objection (although there are others as well) raised against the "civil commitment" laws recently enacted in some jurisdictions and proposed in others. Under this scheme—which is described by its proponents as a "medical approach" to the curing of addiction—certain selected addict-offenders will have the option following arrest of undergoing institutional treatment rather than imprisonment, with the criminal charges held in abeyance pending evaluation of treatment success (Lindesmith, 1965; Schur, 1965). Although it appears that this approach does accept the importance of "treating" addicts rather than simply punishing them, and while some ,individual addicts will undoubtedly be handled more humanely than under previous policies, critics insist that the context of compulsion will vitiate even well-meaning treatment efforts. The specific settings within which such treatment is attempted, and the training and attitudes of personnel involved in such programs, may be crucial in determining effectiveness (although in any case, the civil commitment laws do nothing to undercut illicit traffic, reduce repressive law-enforcement measures, and so on). Experience has shown that "treatment" in a prison-like milieu may not only be ineffective; it may actually reinforce a deviant or criminal self-image. As one girl drug addict noted (Hughes, 1961), it was on release from the Lexington, Kentucky (United States Public Health Service), hospital that she first became convinced she was an incurable addict: "I felt beaten, when I got out of there; really beaten [p. 232]."

SUMMARY AND CONCLUSION

This review of addiction and related social problems should make clear the limitations of a monistic "individual pathology" approach. Individual susceptibility appears to be inextricably linked with particular sociocultural conditions. From a certain standpoint, "treatment" of these conditions is indicated as the ultimate means of ameliorating the problem. Social psychiatric perspectives are extremely useful in highlighting the interrelationships between pathological elements exhibited by the individual addict and those centered in the community and the society. But an approach through social psychiatry will be inadequate if it does not also take account of the role that societal definition itself has played in exacerbating these particular problems. Even if we accept the appropriateness of considering drug addiction to be deviant behavior within the context of modern American society, it is important to recognize that many of the behavior patterns found associated with it in that society represent secondary rather than primary deviation.

From this perspective, how we answer the question of whether addiction constitutes or reflects mental illness may depend largely on exactly which conditions we are attempting to explain. If we seek only to locate determinants of the individual's reliance on drugs, then perhaps a combination of such factors as family background, socioeconomic and ethnic status, and patterns of interpersonal association will largely suffice. On the other hand, if we seek a more comprehensive understanding of the "addiction problem" (or of a behavioral complex we might describe as "the addict and his problems"), then an additional and rather different type of determinant demands our attention. At the beginning of their important research report, Chein et al. (1964) state that they had begun their study with no preconceptions and further that "we did not start with any suspicion that the law might be in any way contributing to the existence of the problem [p. 6]." Through close observation of the actual drug situation, they found that dysfunctions of existing drug policies could not be ignored. In their concluding remarks they state

We are not suggesting that the typical addict would lead a sane, respectable, productive, and responsible life if the drug were legitimately accessible or, for that matter, if he had never had access to the drug in the first place. Our point is that whatever chance he may have had to make something of his life, whatever modicum of human dignity it may have been possible for him to extract from it, virtually disappear once he has become an addict. This is not because of any intrinsic effect of enslavement to the drug, but because he is enslaved to a drug the possession of which and traffic in which is subject to vigorous persecution. By far the worst consequences of addiction are associated with its illegality [pp. 350–351].

This is a perspective which enforcement officials in the United States still by and large resist, and which the medical profession (including some psychiatrists) is only now beginning to appreciate. The attitudes and practices of such interested professionals (which are highly influential in shaping "public opinion") must also be considered significant "determinants" of the narcotic problem (Schur, 1964). As medical ambivalence toward the addict (Freedman et al., 1963) is overcome, and as the medical profession in this country moves toward an acceptance of greater responsibility for the management of the addict and his problems, we can expect to see increased pressure for policies that will serve to reduce the secondary aspects of the addiction situation. Such policies could also generate an atmosphere in which an increasingly wide variety of treatment approaches might hold out some realistic hope of more effectively controlling the primary deviation—the individual's addiction itself.

REFERENCES

Becker, H. S. *Outsiders: Studies in the sociology of deviance.* New York: Free Press, 1963.

Bowman, K. Some problems of addiction. In P. Hoch & J. Zubin (Eds.), *Problems of addiction and habituation.* New York: Grune and Stratton, 1958.

Chein, I., Gerard, D. L., Lee, R. S., & Rosenfeld, E., with the collaboration of D. M. Wilner. *The road to H: Narcotics, delinquency, and social policy.* New York: Basic Books, 1964.

Clausen, J. A. Drug addiction. In R. Merton & R. Nisbet (Eds.), *Contemporary social problems.* New York: Harcourt, Brace and World, 1961.

Clausen, J. A. Social and psychological factors in narcotics addiction. *Law and Contemporary Problems,* 1957, **22,** 34–51. (a)

Clausen, J. A. Social patterns, personality, and adolescent drug use. In A. Leighton, J. A. Clausen, & R. N. Wilson, *Explorations in social psychiatry.* New York: Basic Books, 1957. (b)

Davidson, H. A. The land of insulin addiction. *American Journal of Psychiatry,* 1958, **116,** 559–560.

Diskind, M. H., & Klonsky, G. A second look at the New York State Parole drug experiment. *Federal Probation,* December 1964.

Drug addiction: Crime or disease? Interim and Final Reports of the Joint Committee of the American Bar Association and the American Medical Association on Narcotic Drugs. Bloomington, Ind.: Indiana University Press, 1961.

Faris, R. E. L., & Dunham, H. W. *Mental disorders in urban areas*. Chicago: University of Chicago Press, 1939.

Felix, R. H. Some comments on the psychopathology of drug addiction. *Mental Hygiene*, 1939, **23**, 567–582.

Fenichel, O. *The psychoanalytic theory of neurosis*. New York: Norton, 1945.

Fiddle, S. The addict culture and movement in and out of hospitals. United States Senate, Committee on the Judiciary, Subcommittee to Investigate Juvenile Delinquency. *Hearings*. Part 13, New York, September 20–21, 1962. Washington, D.C.: Government Printing Office, 1963. Pp. 3154–3166.

Finestone, H. Cats, kicks, and color. *Social Problems*, 1957, **5**, 3–13.

Freedman, A. K., Brotman, R., & Meyer, A. A model continuum for a community based program for the prevention and treatment of narcotic addiction. Paper presented at annual meeting of American Public Health Association, Miami Beach, Florida, October 1962.

Freedman, A. M., Sager, C., Rabiner, E., & Brotman, R. Response of adult heroin addicts to a total therapeutic program. *American Journal of Orthopsychiatry*, 1963, **33**, 890–899.

Gerard, D. L., & Kornetsky, C. Adolescent opiate addiction: A study of control and addict subjects. *Psychiatric Quarterly*, 1955, **29**, 457–486.

Goffman, E. The moral career of the mental patient. In Goffman, *Asylums: Essays on the social situation of mental patients and other inmates*. New York: Doubleday Anchor Books, 1961.

Hentoff, N. The treatment of patients (Profile of Marie Nyswander, M.D.). *The New Yorker*, June 26 & July 3, 1965.

Hughes, H. M. (Ed.) *The fantastic lodge: The autobiography of a girl drug addict*. Boston: Houghton Mifflin, 1961.

King, R. Testimony before United States Senate, Committee on the Judiciary, Subcommittee on Improvements of the Federal Criminal Code. Hearings on the causes, treatment, and rehabilitation of drug addicts. Part 5, Sept. 19–21, 1955. Washington, D.C.: Government Printing Office, 1956. P. 1379.

Kolb, L. Types and characteristics of drug addicts. *Mental Hygiene*, 1925, **9**, 300–313.

Larner, J., & Tefferteller, R. *The addict in the street*. New York: Grove Press, 1964.

Laskowitz, D. The adolescent drug addict: An Adlerian view. *Journal of Individual Psychology*, 1961, **17**, 68–79.

Lemert, E. M. *Social pathology*. New York: McGraw-Hill, 1951.

Lemert, E. M. Social structure, social control, and deviation. In Clinard (Ed.) *Anomie and deviant behavior*. New York: Free Press, 1964.

Lindesmith, A. R. The drug addict as psychopath. *American Sociological Review*, 1940, **5**, 914–920.

Lindesmith, A. R. *Opiate addiction*. Bloomington, Ind.: Principia Press, 1947.

Lindesmith, A. R. *The addict and the law*. Bloomington, Ind.: Indiana University Press, 1965.

Lindesmith, A. R., & Gagnon, J. H. Anomie and drug addiction. In M. Clinard, *Anomie and deviant behavior*. New York: Free Press, 1964.

New York Academy of Medicine, Committee on Public Health, Report on Drug Addiction. II, *Bulletin of the New York Academy of Medicine,* 2nd series, **39,** July 1963. Pp. 417–473.

Nyswander, M. *The drug addict as a patient.* New York: Grune and Stratton, 1956.

Ray, M. The cycle of abstinence and relapse among heroin addicts. *Social Problems,* 1961, **9,** 132–140.

Schur, E. M. *Narcotic addiction in Britain and America: The impact of public policy.* Bloomington, Ind.: Indiana University Press, 1962.

Schur, E. M. Attitudes toward addicts: Some general observations and comparative findings. *American Journal of Orthopsychiatry,* 1964, **34,** 80–80.

Schur, E. M. *Crimes without victims: Deviant behavior and public policy—Abortion, homosexuality, drug addiction.* Englewood Cliffs, N.J.: Prentice-Hall, 1965.

Sternberg, D. "Synanon House—A consideration of its implications for American correction. *Journal of Criminal Law, Criminology, and Police Science,* 1963, **54,** 447–455.

Winick, C. Physician narcotic addicts. *Social Problems,* 1961, **9,** 174–186.

Yablonsky, L. *The tunnel back: Synanon.* New York: Macmillan, 1965.

4.4   Orientation

The social order of contemporary society is uniquely reflected in our system of law and order and our views of criminals. In a democracy, the legal system is responsive to changes in social norms and, because of many recent court decisions, many old and unanswered questions about the causes of criminal behavior have reappeared to demand more adequate explanations.

In the following article, Troy Duster addresses himself to the perplexing question of whether or not it is possible for a mentally healthy member of society to commit a crime. If not, then are all criminals psychologically disturbed and in need of treatment? Duster points out the often contradictory views about criminals and the causative explanations for their behavior held by psychiatrists, psychologists, sociologists, the courts, and the larger social order. The criminal's mental health may be viewed in several different ways during the course of his relationship with the legal-judicial system and, accordingly, may be offered differing modes of treatment as corrective therapy for his deviant behavior.

4.4 Mental Illness and Criminal Intent

Troy Duster

Mental illness and criminal intent are incompatible in Western civilization. If a life has been taken, or if someone has been sexually assaulted, a criminal act has not been committed unless the perpetrator of the act is mentally responsible.[1] This incompatibility has been the source of a critical problem of explanation and treatment. It must both be explained and acted upon how a mentally healthy member of society could *healthily* decide to commit a criminal act. Once pathology of the mind is excluded as a possible explanation of crime, men are left searching for reasons that contain the fewest possible residues of the idea of sickness.

The difficulty, of course, is that the violation of rules in any culture can hardly be regarded internally as "healthy," reasonable behavior decided upon as the normal and rational course. It is one thing for an observer of cultures like Durkheim to speak of the functional and cohesive role of crime (especially the punishment of crime). It is quite another matter for men acting in that culture to interpret and treat unlawful behavior in these terms. Few societies have difficulty imputing sickness or some kind of aberration to the law violator. Western man, however, faces an important dilemma in dealing with the problem, and that is simply to explain crime without imputing illness.

The attempt to discern the intent of action has become the most important theoretical element in the courtroom practice of law (Hall, 1960). Although this has been popularized by the mass media's saturation with courtroom procedure in criminal law, there are ramifications of the idea of criminal intent that escape ordinary attention and which reach far beyond the official administration of justice. Some of the important consequences of this absorption with establishing *mens rea* versus mental illness are felt not only in the way social workers, probation officers, judges, and police see and treat people, but it is also a critical base to an understanding of how the typical normal member of the society, and therefore, behavioral scientists, make sense of crime. To say that an objectionable act is provoked by mental disturbance is to give not only an explanation, but to chart as well the possible avenues to treatment,

[1] The M'Naghten Rule of 1843 established the basis for the plea of insanity as a legitimate defense for the accused. See Daniel M'Naghten's case in Johnston, Savitz, and Wolfgang (1962), pp. 42–46.

correction, and change. To say that certain criminal acts are provoked by mental illness is therefore to channel the way in which men can conceive of the correction and rehabilitation of criminals. This is only one example of subtle consequence of how men deal with the dilemma in the interpretation of criminal behavior.

It is important to state at the outset that the whole class of persons who may be called criminals (violators of the criminal law) is such a conglomeration of heterogeneous elements as to make simple, inclusive statements about the whole class impossible. There are professional criminals who treat crime as an occupation and a way of life. There are one-time violators who otherwise regard criminal activity as abhorrent. There are serious violators who commit felonies, petty thieves and shoplifters who commit misdemeanors, and there is the distinction between those who get caught and those who do not. This is only a partial list of important variations among "criminals." It would be impossible to deal with all of the significant variations as separate categories, and equally impossible to try to discuss them all under one banner, in one article. Instead, this article will address itself in a general way to serious crimes that are usually called felonies, and to those who get caught.

As has been indicated, if a man is a criminal, he is mentally healthy in the eyes of the law. However much the layman may agree with this when he is impaneled for jury duty, he is hard-pressed to go along with it in his explanations of everyday life. Nonetheless, legal interpretation has its own impact, and Western men do try to live with the idea of a mentally healthy criminal. The attempts to explain how this could come about are varied, and each is of significance for how the criminal is perceived and treated.

THE CRIMINAL AS IMMORAL

The first significant resolution of the problem is to regard the criminal as mentally capable and responsible, but antagonistic to the contemporary moral order. Thus, the murderer "knows" what he is doing. He "knows" that his actions violate the moral code of others, but he feels that he can and should commit the act anyway. He may reach this conclusion by asserting a contrary morality, but the essential point is that he refuses to subscribe to moral dictates that hold others in check. For the murderer, the classic statement of this would be Raskolnikov's transcendent morality in *Crime and Punishment*. He *decided* that he could commit murder. The rational thought processes that produced this conclusion document the mentally healthy and responsible character of his act, and for that he was held accountable.

Raskolnikov's reasoning, or some facsimile of it, is imputed to the criminal who is thought to be mentally healthy, but immoral. It is not so much that criminals are said to explicitly engage in abstract philosophical meditation about the ethical issues, but that they do come to a position of a contrary morality that is rationally acted upon. The moral interpretation of criminality carries with it the stigma of any activity cast in moral terms. Between the state of physical fitness and the state of physical illness, men believe that passage can occur both ways. One who has been ill can become well, and vice-versa. However, as Harold Garfinkel (1956) has noted, between the state of being moral and the state of being immoral, a barrier to passage has been erected that precludes the movement of the individual back and forth (as is possible with physical illness). Once the murderer has committed the act, he is permanently stigmatized as a kind of person who must be held suspect. The ex-convict faces the insurmountable problem of a continual confrontation with a hostile society that firmly believes that he is "morally capable" of that act again, and again. The ex-convict is therefore treated in such a way as to prevent his movement back into moral normalcy by the very devices that have been used to explain his behavior. For example, at that point in time when the drug addict was transformed into a moral deviant in the eyes of the public around 1920, he was for the first time excluded from the possibility of movement back into nonaddicted society (Terry & Pellens, 1928). The intensity of moral conviction and the force of moral reaction guarantee this.

The moral interpretation of criminality has long historical roots, and successfully infuses all other views of crime to some degree. To the extent that it is explicit, it undermines the concept of rehabilitation. In prisons, it can make little sense to try to rehabilitate a man who is regarded in the larger society as immoral, because even if the individual is successfully changed, his return to normal society cannot be accepted. The rejection of the ex-convict is documented by every ex-convict who goes into the world unannounced and tries to secure employment, irrespective of his "moral conversion." This problem emerges again and again in every other view of the criminal.

THE CRIMINAL AS PSYCHICALLY INADEQUATE

To regard the criminal primarily as one with a personality disorder is to risk getting too close to the area of mental illness. It takes a great deal of skill and agility to impute psychic disturbance, and yet not taint the individual with the imputation of mental illness. Yet, this is exactly the present situation in American courts and prisons. Treatment programs in prisons focus around the attempt to reorganize the psychic makeup of the inmate. Therapy sessions center upon the inadequacies of the in-

mate's personality, inadequacies which in the eyes of the therapist produced the criminal behavior in the first place.

In order to be able to live with the idea that the criminal is mentally
responsible, although psychologically inadequate, it is usually necessary to
impute to him the rational cognitive process. Thus, he must also be
thought of as a bit immoral, if not evil, as will be illustrated below. He
may have this "morbid and unhealthy need for antisocial behavior," but
it is not a compulsive thing. He "can" control these impulses. The fact
that he can but does not control them means that the inadequate personality suddenly becomes adequate in making a judgment about right and
wrong, or good and evil. It is inevitable that this particular route of interpretation carries with it an imputation of immorality. Inmates are
poignantly aware of this, and report that while they may be told repeatedly of their personality problems, what they "really hear" is a statement
about their moral inferiority. Irrespective of whether the criminal is regarded as immoral or inadequate, the rehabilitation problems are identical when the society at large refuses to allow the normal return of the
ex-convict. However, which one is more important at a given time is dependent upon that point in the sequence of the administration of justice
that is uppermost. Whereas the morality issue is more important in the
judicial process leading up to imprisonment, the psychological issue assumes primacy in the rhetoric of rehabilitation. For the police, the prosecuting attorney, the judge, and the jury, the guilty defendant is first of all
guilty of a moral breach. Each in his turn may acknowledge that the
accused has "personality problems," but the *focus* of the accusation is in
moral territory. (Otherwise, he may be too close to mental irresponsibility.) However, once convicted and imprisoned, the focus shifts to the
personality dimension. Treatment and rehabilitation programs begin with
the assumption that the inmate can be helped to restructure and rebuild
his inadequate psyche. As has been suggested, when access routes to normal life are cut off for the ex-convict, no amount of sophisticated and
successful therapeutic treatment can rehabilitate him.

In sum, the interpretation of the criminal as personally inadequate
(deficient personality, psychic disturbance) tends almost always to carry
with it a large measure of the imputation of immorality. As such, each
of those consequences discussed in the preceding section about what happens to the criminal when he is regarded as immoral apply to some extent
here. The difference is primarily one of the way in which selected persons
can treat the criminal if they choose to do so. They may respond to him
as "curable," and subject him to therapeutic measures designed to effect
a change. The residue of moral judgment makes failure in this area the
documentation of the moralists' charges, and the therapists must contin-

ually confront this issue in themselves as well as in others. If the law-breaker is simply and completely immoral, then there is a tendency to regard his rehabilitation as hopeless. If, however, he is suffering from a disturbance of personality, there may be access to change, health, and thus, correction.

THE CRIMINAL AS A VICTIM OF EXTERNAL FORCES

There is an almost opposite interpretation which focuses upon the *conditions* in which the criminal exists. This is the more sociological view, still a minority position, but held by an increasing number of lay-men. The particular orientation or bias leads these observers to see forces outside the control of the individual as more determinant factors in ex-plaining criminal behavior. Laymen of this persuasion explore and em-phasize the broken home, poverty and the attendant lack of recreational facilities, pernicious influences in the community, and so on. Sociologists have emphasized the social systems that surround the individual. Thus, the condition of poverty provides the context for the development of the culture of poverty. The peer group emerges as a dominant theme in the explanation of criminal behavior (Cohen, 1955; see also Cloward & Ohlin, 1960). The individual is seen as a malleable substance, formed and di-rected by these external forces. It is important to recognize that individual will and responsibility make few appearances in this conceptualization. The adequacy of the personality or the moral character of behavior come into question only with regard to the relevant social system. In the cul-ture of poverty, theft from the owner of a small, struggling store may be regarded as very immoral behavior, while theft from a large chain depart-ment store is treated as a matter of course. It is common enough knowl-edge that there is honor among thieves, but men often neglect to make the next logical conclusion. As for adequacy of personality, that too is determined within the limits of the relevant system in which the individ-ual acts. One performs adequately in the role of a bureaucrat in organ-ized crime or as a professional thief, and the issue of a basically anti-social, rebellious personality, hostile to authority, need never be raised from this orientation.

Accordingly, the analysis of organized crime in sociology begins with very traditional assumptions about how any normal bureaucracy works. Rather than positing a pathology or an abnormality, the concepts that are used to characterize and explain a syndicated crime operation are pre-cisely those that fit when describing the Pentagon, a legitimate business corporation, or the line of command in an army regiment. Indeed, what is remarkable to those who have studied organized crime from this per-spective is the degree to which these concepts fit (Tyler, 1962, pp. 227–

366). The individual occupying an organizational role in the Mafia discharges his obligations with the same dedication to procedural rules as any other bureaucrat. His mobility in the organization reads like a chapter from Whyte's *Organization Man,* his view of why he ought to discharge his duties could come from Blau's *Dynamics of Bureaucracy;* and Barnard's *Functions of the Executive* just as easily apply to Capone as to Charlie Wilson. At this level of analysis, say sociologists, it adds little to an understanding of the behavior in question to impute mental abnormality.

In the heyday of organized crime in Chicago in the 1920s, judges, senators, newspapermen, and city clerks were all on the payroll of the Capone organization (Tyler, 1962, pp. 138–139). Bootlegging was a serious and dangerous business, as evidenced by more than 200 gangland killings in Chicago over a four-month period (Tyler, 1962, pp. 138–139). (The only thing sensational about the St. Valentine's Day massacre was that seven men were killed at one standing, and the world press play to it.) Torrio and Capone carried out the production and distribution of alcohol with efficiency that is not characteristic of the mentally deficient or disturbed. In values, motives, and ideology, one can speculate just how far Capone was from the typical successful American businessman. Gang murders were only a small part of the total operation, and it is too easy to make the mistake of concluding from these other activities that there is a difference that shades into all areas. More will be said about this subject later, but there is an interesting parallel here with the layman's tendency to regard the serious attempt at suicide as an indicator of mental illness. He also tends to regard the attempt at (or completion of) murder in the same light, despite the fact that the attempt itself may be the only behavior that can be characterized as distinctive. The obvious cautionary note is that mental disturbance is probably a more generic or diffuse thing which is reflected in more than a single act or even a single set of acts.

Organized crime is only one area of criminal activity that lends itself to traditional sociological techniques of explaining and interpreting behavior. For example, the social systems approach is equally usable in interpreting behavior within an occupational or career setting. The professional criminal who makes crime "a way of life," or perhaps makes crime his occupation, is engaged in the occupational role in a remarkably normal, patterned way. As Sutherland (1937) pointed out in his discussion of the professional thief, such occupations come complete with a code of ethics, specialized language, pecking order, and ideology. Once again, there is a literature in sociology on the occupation as a career, and the parallels are more striking than are the differences between criminal occupational careers and noncriminal ones.

The major point of this orientation to crime, it seems, is that the participants are very very normal in their ways of coping with the world. They can hardly be called "hostile to authority" in a generic sense, in that they respond to the bureaucratic superior in the same way as any noncriminal bureaucrat. As long as the observer is capable of seeing the criminal in terms of a social system parameter, he sees normality, and not pathology. Clearly if the *behavior* is compared to the *activity* of the middle class, the differences are striking. But if we address the *forms* of interaction, the man in organized crime or the independent professional criminal is identical with the "normal" citizen of everyday life. There is nothing in the manner or style of the criminal that sets him off from his fellowman. It is debatable as to whether the substance of behavior is sufficient to set off qualitative distinctions. In the Eichmann trial, the defense argued strongly that Eichmann's instrumentality in the slaughter of hundreds of thousands of Jews was purely bureaucratic. As such, the manner and style of his activity was to be viewed in these terms, and the substantive issue of *what* he did was to be treated as secondary, if not tangential or totally irrelevant. His ultimate guilt was established for the court by the argument that he was responsible for the substantive moral decisions.

The sociologist's suggestions for the way in which the society achieves "rehabilitation" of this kind of criminality is accordingly quite different. Instead of focusing upon the individual and the problem of reconstructing him, the emphasis is upon either (1) modifying or changing the social conditions that have ordinarily enveloped him, or (2) changing the way in which the society regards that setting.

In the first instance, the change of the ex-convict's environment can be partially effected by making sure that he does not return to his old neighborhood, his old community, and the culture of his criminal past. Prisons in this country now emphasize this strategy for parolees. However, for reasons that were discussed earlier, the ex-convict is often channeled by the society in such a way that he normally and naturally gravitates back to his old environment. That is, the societal reaction is so strong and so moral, and the stigma of being an ex-convict so great, that the individual has little choice in selecting alternative environments for his acceptance. He can expect rejection in all environs but one, that from which he developed as a person.

Another tactic would be the attempt to change the old environment itself. This is clearly the more difficult task. Law enforcement authorities say that they pursue this policy to some extent when they make raids on bookie joints, Sin Areas, marijuana parties, and the like. A wave of public indignation may follow a newspaper's exposé of a Calumet City, in which case the Sheriff's police are designated to go and "clean up" the area. These Sin Areas are usually in big cities, and those familiar with metropolitics know that the "cleanup" is more rhetorical than real in its consequences. The residents are not really committed to these "reforms," and this tactic is conceived in and rooted to failure.

If this first alternative is a difficult, if not impossible chore, then the other major alternative which the sociologist envisions seems unthinkable. How does one go about the task of effecting attitudinal change or institutional receptivity? Yet, the rehabilitation of the criminal is inextricably intertwined with his reception in the society. It is imperative that the prospective employer, prospective mate, prospective insurance man, prospective anyman receive the ex-criminal as though rehabilitation were possible, if not a fact, and as though no stigma were attached to past associations, *if* the ex-criminal is to have any chance for rehabilitation.

The theoretical issues involved for sociology and social anthropology are certainly significant. There exists a category of strong moral judgment, with full moral rejection of a segment of the stigmatized population. During the last century, the history of the conception and treatment of mental illness underwent remarkable changes. In 1860, mental illness was burdened by the imputation of immorality through the idea of the individual's free will to choose among alternatives. Even today, many families are ashamed of a case of mental illness in the family, whereas they will announce physical illnesses publicly as a matter of course. (These same physical illnesses, by the way, were conceived in moralistic terms in the eighteenth century and before; and men were then ashamed of such sickness or of any association with it.) With the passage of time, and with the coming of the "enlightenment," the West began to disassociate morality from mental illness, just as it had done previously with physical illness.

It seems legitimate to consider the possibility, then, that conceptions of crime and criminality will follow the same path. To be sure, crime is regarded as activity hostile to the society; but so too is the behavior of the mentally ill. If the behavior of the latter were thought of as constructive and beneficial, men would find a new label for it, reward it, and abandon an orientation of sickness. It is suggested therefore, that the objective antisocial character of behavior is no guarantee of its moral rejection. It is conceivable that crime could go the way of physical and mental illness in an enlightened society, where the solution is cast in remedial terms, but where the society's members themselves recognize the need to change their moral conception of the problem *so that remedy is possible.*

SOCIETAL AMBIVALENCE, INCONSISTENCY,
AND THE PROBLEM OF TREATMENT

At the beginning of this article, I indicated that Western minds are pulled back and forth between two incompatible poles with regard to the criminal population: "One must be mentally healthy in order to commit a crime, but the commission of a crime reflects an unhealthy mental state." On the one hand, the criminal is said to be mentally balanced, and therefore capable of and responsible for his actions. On the other hand, his criminal behavior is popularly and professionally conceived as a reflection of a disorder of personality. This is a dilemma that is partially resolved by compartmentalizing one horn of the dilemma for a period of time. For example, it is typical to regard the criminal as mentally healthy and responsible during the period of apprehension, prosecution, and conviction. The police, the prosecuting attorney, the judge, and the jury all have a tendency to view the criminal as mentally normal, sane, and responsible. However, after conviction, and beginning with incarceration, the imputation shifts, and the criminal is suddenly regarded as psychologically disturbed. The warden, the prison psychiatrist, and to some extent the custodial staff tend to view the inmate as one possessed with some kind of mental problem. Upon release from the prison, the ex-convict meets a combination of these imputations. The parole officer, the halfway house administrator and staff, and the receiving community and family are likely to exhibit a large measure of ambivalence and ambiguity toward the ex-convict.

During the entire first stage of his contact with the agents of law enforcement, the accused rarely finds his psychological normality questioned. The police handle him in such a way as to reinforce the idea of his reasonability and rationality. The whole notion of a modus operandi in police work illustrates very clearly how the police investigators impute sanity and reason to the culprit. Once apprehended, the accused person is treated by his captors as responsive to reason. The prosecuting attorney, for example, offers a "reasonable" deal to the accused. He is presented with the alternative of pleading guilty to a lesser charge, or he risks facing prosecution and conviction for the full charge if he upsets the judicial normality and pleads "not guilty." It is not only the prosecuting attorney who treats the accused as a reasonable man, but the public defender as well who offers a deal based on the most rational and calculated factors (Sudnow, 1965). In Sudnow's study of one public defender's office, this procedure is well illustrated (Sudnow, 1965). The typical pattern is for the public defender to explain why the accused ought to be rational and agreeable, accept the deal offered, and plead guilty to the agreed-upon charge. If there is any question about the imputation of psychic disturbance, it occurs only when the accused refuses to accept the defender's advice and pleads "not guilty." Otherwise, that possibility is never seriously entertained by the administrators of justice, at least insofar as it is reflected in behavior directed toward the accused.

Once he is placed behind prison bars, however, the convict finds that his psychic makeup is problematic. It is the focus of continual interpretation and reinterpretation. It is, as well, the primary basis upon which explanations of his behavior revolves. This is the case for both past behavior and present activity in the institution. When the treatment staff of the prison frames a question as to why the criminal act was committed, the tendency is to reconstruct the inmate's motivation in such a way that it reflects psychic disturbance. For example, what the police and judge were willing to regard as a normal, legitimate, rational thought process in the decision to steal, the prison treatment staff may reinterpret as the rebelliousness of a basically antisocial person. The same behavior that the police choose to slap down as the rational, understandable, but objectionable machinations of a wise ass, the treatment staff choose to regard as pathological in its hostility to authority, a quality of an aberrant personality. Therapy sessions, both group and individual, are thereby directed toward an attempt to better understand the inmate's psychic problem. This is a relatively recent development. It is an unmistakable trend, however, with the more self-consciously progressive prisons in the more self-consciously progressive states placing greater and great emphasis upon a therapeutic community. The new "rehabilitation centers" for drug addicts are in the vanguard. In the older traditional prisons, the inmates had a saying which symbolized the best way to get out: "Do your own time!" The phrase captured the attitude that each inmate should mind his own business and choose either to work off his own good time or not, but that he not interfere in the parole chances of others. The inmates in the newer rehabilitation prisons also have a favorite saying which they feel symbolizes the best way to get out: "If you wanna walk, you gotta talk!" Simply put, this means that the inmates recognize that the treatment staff wants them to be obviously engaged in the therapeutic community. While engagement is indicated by the degree and quality of expressiveness about one's own psychic condition, it is also important that the individual be expressive about *other* inmates' problems and conditions in the group therapy sessions.

It must be remarkable to the inmate, then, when at the point when he is to be considered for parole, the sociological interpretation of criminal activity emerges as the dominant theme. The parole board suddenly wants to know what kind of social system setting awaits the parolee.

Concern is expressed that the prospective parolee sever all associations with the criminal community, and proceed to a new environment. The assurance that he can obtain gainful employment is the single most important thing among factors in the receiving community. This reflects more than the fear that idle hands are the devil's plaything, but also great concern for the meaning and consequences of practical problems of financial stability. This is to begin to treat the individual criminal as once again a normal, rational member of society, motivated by the same goals as typical others. As Merton (1957) suggested many years ago, the normal and rational response to frustration in the achievement of goals by legitimate means may well be the pursuit of illegal means. That parole boards place such a premium upon the availability of an occupation is strong evidence that they have suspended the explanatory mode of psychic disturbance as the central problem. If this were not the case, the parole board would need only address itself to the mended or unmended character of the inmate's personality. (If it is mended, then he should be able to go out into the world and *cope* with reality . . . and so on.) There would be no need to treat the nature of the situation in the receiving community as critical to the decision to parole.

Once back into the community, the ex-convict finds many supervisory authorities imbued with a sociological determinism: What kinds of friends does he see? What kinds of places does he frequent? In selected communities, parolees do meet for a counseling or therapy session, but the focus may be upon the exchanges that occur in the community. The parole officer's training is more likely to be in sociology than in psychology, and the review board that considers parole violations is likely to look at the *conditions* in which the violator lives, rather than the way in which he manages the world. That is not only easier to observe, it can also be used as an indicator of personal stability. However, the ex-convict is continually confronted by an extremely hostile society. As far as the typical member of society is concerned, the quality of being once-imprisoned for a crime is never irrelevant. The prospective employer, prospective mate, prospective lender or creditor all treat the history of criminality as a quality possessed by the person, not simply as a product of varying social conditions. Therefore, even when the ex-convict changes all of his social conditions, he remains suspect *as a person*. There is a large residue of sentiment about this even among those marginally committed to an environmental or sociological determinism.

THE SOCIAL CONTEXT OF THE PROBLEM
OF CRIMINAL INTENT

In the courtroom practice of criminal law, the ability to establish or undermine the existence of criminal intent in the action is critical. The basis upon which the plausibility of intent rests is the common social reality of "reasonable," "normal," and "typical" men (Schutz, 1962). As an example, we can look at how the social milieu of the act determines whether it will be regarded as crime or illness.

In police precinct X, a woman is booked for her third offense within a year's time. The prosecuting attorney decides to take the case to court and secure a conviction. The woman is accused of stealing a piece of jewelry worth approximately $650. She has three children, no husband, and obtains sporadic employment from week to week as a menial household service worker, with extended periods of layoff. The judge listens to the prosecuting attorney present his case, especially the evidence that bears directly upon the commission of the act. All are satisfied that the act was committed. The next problem is to establish whether the act was committed with criminal intent. The important point here is that the judge will listen with great interest and attentiveness to the prosecution's case about the family and occupational condition of the accused. The woman was in need. The motive is set for a reasonable man (or woman) to act in such a way as to gratify that need. The judge can, in a sense, enter the world of the accused, empathize with her decision as a rational one, and pronounce her guilty of the intention to commit the crime. It is important to recognize the judge's ability to impute reason. The woman is fined either $500 or sentenced to 30 days.

In police precinct Y, a woman is booked for her third offense within a year's time. The prosecuting attorney decides to take the case to court and secure a conviction. The woman is accused of stealing a piece of jewelry worth approximately $1400. She has two children, and a husband who is a corporation executive with an income of $175,000 per year. The judge listens to the prosecuting attorney present his case, especially the evidence that bears directly upon the commission of the act. All are satisfied that the act was committed. The defense attorney acknowledges that the act was committed. The next problem is to establish whether the act was committed with criminal intent. In this instance too, the judge listens with great interest to the familial and occupational condition of the accused. She was not in need. Any reasonable man can see that she was not stealing for the money, which is the only "reasonable need" residing in the minds of normal people. The need to possess a stolen artifact for its own sake is something entirely different. The social reality is that this desire is thought to be a reflection of an aberrant state of the mind. Whereas the judge could empathize with the reasonable need of the reasonable woman with no husband and no money, he finds it impossible to understand any *criminal intent* in the desire to possess an object that could easily be purchased across the counter by the husband. Upon further inquiry, he discovers that the husband has indeed purchased many such items of jewelry for the woman. This is "clearly" a case of illness, kleptomania, and not criminal intent, theft. The woman is committed to outpatient status with a psychiatrist whom she is to see once a week for a year.

The interpretation does not always go in favor of the upper-middle class and against the lower classes. A 12-year-old lower class urban-dwelling Negro boy is caught by the police smoking a marijuana cigarette in a raid upon a party. The juvenile authorities investigate, and after determining the age of the boy and the nature of his family and home life, decide to drop the case. They do not even bother to file a petition. The boy's father is employed by the railroad, and is seldom home. His mother is contacted, informed, and warned verbally. Nothing more is done, and the authorities resignedly contemplate the inevitable pathway to trouble that they feel the boy will follow.

A 12-year-old middle class suburban-dwelling white boy is caught by the police smoking a marijuana cigarette in a raid on a party. The police are shocked. The juvenile authorities investigate, and after determining the age of the boy and the nature of his family and home life, decide to pursue the case.

They find a typical middle-American suburban home life, family intact, stable income. The juvenile authorities "cannot understand" how a boy from such a home could find himself in such a situation. The parents are drawn into the case and informed of its gravity. (It is explainable if not normal and reasonable that the other boy should be in that situation, but *not this boy.*) Very few interpretations are open to the authorities, and the one which they choose is psychic disturbance. Because they can not comprehend another social reality where it would be "normal" for this kind of youth to do what he did, sickness is the only explanation possible. The boy is remanded to a psychiatrist's care for a period of weeks. A petition is filed, and remains with him until he becomes an adult.

Despite every attempt in democratic societies to minimize extraneous considerations, the law does not, nor can it exist in a vacuum. It may be a nation of laws and not of men, but the law is always interpreted in terms of the meanings that "reasonable" men can bring to it. Judges and juries bring to the court a certain view of what is reasonable behavior. Action that is unreasonable and incomprehensible (kleptomania, for example) is treated in law as an indicator of psychic imbalance. As has been suggested, the problem of the social context of law is crucial, since the same behavior may be regarded as theft when social conditions encompassing the behavior can be given a more "reasonable" meaning. For the social scientist, the problem is to uncover and explain the distribution of social meanings as they vary from one social system to another. From this perspective, the administration of justice is simply one more system, and has no greater legitimacy in defining the ultimate quality of "reasonable" behavior than any other system.

So far, the problem of the criminal's mental health has been treated from the point of view of contrasting social systems. Those in the larger society who surround the criminal population may have a view of what constitutes mental illness that has little to do with the conception of mental illness among criminals. It is instructive to return to the analogy of the layman's interpretation of the serious attempt at suicide. Since most men must pursue the daily task of living, they find it difficult to empathize with the decision to end one's own life. "Anyone who tries to commit suicide must be crazy!" However, among those who recover from or are rescued from a suicide attempt, most that we know about return to routine mundane everyday life as though nothing occurred. Except for the specific behavior connected with the would-be suicide, the individual's actions do not permit an interpretation of mental abnormality. Occasionally, individuals who attempt suicide are placed in the mental patient's ward of a hospital for several days' surveillance, but they usually do not stay for more than a week. This is true despite the fact that the general population is quick to impute mental illness to anyone who seriously attempts suicide.

For the criminal, the situation is very similar except that he is incarcerated for long periods. His specific criminal activity may be interpreted as an indicator of mental disturbance by others, but that is untrue not only within the criminal "community"; a member of the general population is also incapable of making any such assessment by looking merely at the criminal's other behavior. It is acknowledged and documented by the continual questions that ex-convicts must answer on applications for employment, drivers' licenses, passports, and the like. If their mental disturbance could be detected simply from observing their behavior, there would be no need for continually calling attention to the stigma.

MENTAL ILLNESS AND SOCIAL THEORY IN CRIME

We have come a long way since the days of Lombroso's criminology. Few of us regard the shape of the head as the most important determinant of whether a man will pursue a life of crime. Phrenology is in disrepute, if not completely dead. There are theories, however, that begin with the assumption that criminal behavior is to be explained by addressing a property of the individual. There are other theories that trace the explanation to the assumption that forces external to the individual account for crime. Indeed, it is possible to arrange theories of crime along a continuum of this sort: at one end, the individual as the complete agent of his action, possessed of either free will or compulsion, but at the very least, the motivated center of action; at the other end there are theories that see the individual as nothing more than a grossly malleable substance wafting back and forth in the social currents of the time and the space most immediately pressing.

I think it is reasonable to present the proposition that the closer a theory comes to the individual-autonomy end of the continuum, the more likely is that theory to contain the imputation of mental abnormality. The obverse is also true. Theories on the other end of the continuum that deal, for example, with a qualified economic or social determinism, will rarely entertain the possibility of mental illness as an important ingredient in criminal behavior. Forces and conditions like poverty or the peer culture impel the adaptive and "mentally normal" responses of crime.

The question to be raised about these theories is twofold. First, of what significance is each to the discipline of which it is a part? Second, what are some of the consequences for a society that adopts one over another in preference for the explanation of crime?

In sociology, recent theories of crime that have emphasized the response of social systems developed primarily from an increasing concern for theory in the sociology of deviance. At the turn of the century, research in deviance centered primarily around individuals who constituted "social problems." Sociology during this period sponsored longitudinal and case studies of prostitutes, alcoholics, tramps, and the like. Because such studies focused upon the individual deviant, they tended to emphasize the unique and idiosyncratic qualities of the deviant, an analytic technique that acted as a roadblock to a broader understanding of deviance in its other forms. Mental illness is a kind of deviance that should prove to be the most fruitful subject matter for social theories of order and disorder. The reason is that it is a form least tied a priori to substantive problems. Drug addiction, for example, is always associated with the empirical issue of drug use, irrespective of the social group that is using or interpreting. The same is true for prostitution and alcoholism. While it is true that the various *meanings* of these activities vary from group to group, one can still determine whether or not drug addiction is a deviance problem in a particular group. Mental illness, however, will always be an issue to be dealt with by a community. The same thing can be said for crime, or perhaps a more universal concept, deviance. The community must handle deviance as a generic problem of social control. It seems both natural and inevitable then, that the trend in social science theories will be a broader incorporation of theories of mental illness (lay and professional) into the newly emphasized concern for social reaction to deviation.

REFERENCES

Cloward, R., & Ohlin, L. *Delinquency and opportunity: A theory of delinquent gangs.* Glencoe, Ill.: The Free Press, 1960.

Cohen, A. K. *Delinquent boys, the culture of the gang.* Glencoe, Ill.: The Free Press, 1955.

Garfinkel, H. Conditions of successful degradation ceremonies. *American Journal of Sociology,* 1956, **61,** 420–424.

Hall, J. *General principles of criminal law.* (2nd ed.) Indianapolis, Ind.: Bobbs-Merrill, 1960.

Johnston, N., Savitz, L., & Wolfgang, M. (Eds.) *The sociology of punishment and correction.* New York: John Wiley & Sons, 1962.

Merton, R. K. *Social theory and social structure.* (Rev. ed.) Glencoe, Ill.: The Free Press, 1957.

Schutz, A. *Collected papers.* Vol. 1. *The problem of social reality.* The Hague: Martinus Nijhoff, 1962.

Sudnow, D. Normal crimes: Sociological features of the penal code in a public defender office. *Social Problems,* 1965, **12,** (3), 255–276.

Sutherland, E. H. (Ed.) *The professional thief.* Chicago: University of Chicago Press, 1937.

Terry, C. E., & Pellens, M. *The opium problem.* New York: Bureau of Social Hygiene, 1928.

Tyler, G. (Ed.) *Organized crime in America.* Ann Arbor, Mich.: University of Michigan Press, 1962.

4.5 Orientation

Although the actor is not commonly thought of as a deviant in the same sense that a criminal or homosexual is so regarded, actors are often stereotyped as improper, immoral, or, at the very least, unconventional people. In addition, we often hear that actors are emotionally unstable people who—if they can afford it—regularly take their problems to psychiatrists.

Peter McHugh, in his study of fifty professional stage actors, finds
that there is some substance to these beliefs, for actors do sometimes
appear to behave in bizarre and irresponsible ways. McHugh does
not look for the sources of this behavior in actors' emotional disturbances, however; rather, he seeks an explanation in the nature of
the social conditions within which actors must live. He argues that
the critical problem facing actors is uncertainty, and he believes
that actors come to terms with the uncertainty in their lives by
forming a group that can be characterized as "collegial." McHugh's
analysis cannot answer many of the questions that might be asked
about the mental health problems of actors—as, for example, how
they resolve their identity problems—but his perspective upon the
link between the life conditions of actors and their group practices
is both intriguing and illuminating.

4.5   Structured Uncertainty and Its Resolution: The Case of the Professional Actor

Peter McHugh

An actor being interviewed at home by a newspaperman:

Yes, we have orgies here all the time. Pot, LSD, everything. Then the next
day the maids clean up, and we have to throw out all the people who couldn't
make it to the street the night before.

The same actor after the newspaperman has left:

Have you ever given an interview and seen how it turns out? They put in
what they want, or the better ones leave out what they want. Look, reporters
have an idea what actors are like, so why argue? Just feed the machine. Say
whatever will get you through it, and don't worry about paying the check,
because you will have to pick it up.

His statement to the journalist was a misrepresentation, in the sense
that it was "objectively" false, but it was not a lie because actors think
that kind of behavior appropriate when dealing with the public.

At a black tie dinner:

HUSBAND: Shit on you.
WIFE: Fuck you.
HUSBAND: "Too"?
WIFE: My husband's finally admitted he doesn't know the difference be-
tween shitting and fucking.

A vulgar exchange, but it is more informative to disclose that no one, including husband and wife, thought anything was wrong—not in choice of language or the relations it depicts.

Finally, in gathering of actors killing time before a rehearsal:

> He won't be very helpful to us, playing those tiny parts. Not only that, he's sick. I don't know why he doesn't do something about it, pull himself up, make the most of what he has.

This proposition, acceptable perhaps to those in bureaucratic and professional settings, caused the group of actors to disband. Something was wrong.

If we can learn about the conditions in which professional stage actors must live, we may unravel why these conversations occurred as they did —why a man would say he sponsors orgies when he doesn't, why no one at the dinner expressed surprise or disgust, why actors would be startled to hear someone suggest self-improvement.

These conditions will be described in some detail in order to show how very uncertain they are, so uncertain that there is no a priori reason to expect actors to form a group at all. But we shall discover that actors nevertheless do form a group, a rather rare one for an industrial society. It is this special group that shapes the behavior of actors, behavior that from any other perspective would seem bizarre, irresponsible, anomic. Following this, it will be argued that the uncertainty of conditions and special group form are compatible with one another, and so actors' behavior is signally appropriate to their situation.

PROCEDURE

Data were gathered by depth interviews with fifty male actors, observation of their rehearsals, and participation with them out of hours (rehearsals and out of hours activities included females). Actors were selected to participate in the interviews only if they had earned at least half their income from the stage in the previous two years, thus insuring their dependency on the stage for a livelihood. Females were not interviewed because they are not expected to be the primary source of income and familial status in our society. Consequently, those interviewed do not represent the total membership of Actors Equity Association, the stage union, but they are not meant to, because many on the union roll work elsewhere and so do not meet the basic criterion of uncertainty.

Access was gained through the investigator's friends in the theater, an important detail in light of the findings. These friendships had developed over many years, and were of immeasurable help in providing entry to rehearsals and out of hours interaction. It is a mark of their cooperation that several actors themselves suggested that the study be done, and a mark of their veracity that the straight interview materials were not contradicted by the direct observations.

Interviews were partially structured. The same questions were asked of each subject, but for most questions there were no fixed alternatives to limit responses. Leads that developed in particular interviews were followed up. Participation out of hours took place over the course of several years, and included interactions such as parties, meals, and conversations.

Raw responses have been coded and tabulated on the assumption that so-called qualitative data can be counted. Verbatim materials are presented when necessary for illustration.

I should stress again here that the aim of this paper is to describe uncertainty and its consequences for social organization and behavior, rather than to capture acting as a whole. A great deal about the history of the craft, and peripheral aspects of the general life of actors, has therefore been omitted.

I shall begin with a description of the uncertain socio-economic and technical conditions of professional stage acting, and then go on to describe the social organization of the craft. A third section will suggest that the kind of social organization existing in those conditions is not entirely fortuitous.

UNCERTAIN OCCUPATIONAL CONDITIONS OF ACTORS

To begin with, the socioeconomic position of actors fluctuates very greatly, in both the long and short run, and so it is difficult for them to anticipate their place in society. Second, the technical procedures available to actors at work are vague in principle and ambiguous in application, and make it equally difficult for them to predict their effectiveness on the job. We shall take up socioeconomic and technical uncertainty in turn.

Socioeconomic Uncertainty

Here we shall portray the amount and kind of social mobility actors undergo, the proportion of time they spend without work, and the social precariousness of celebrity. Actors average about four jobs per year, and they lose five for each job they obtain. Thus, their competence is reviewed about twenty-five times a year. These are very meaningful encounters, for they require face-to-face participation by the applicant: He must "read" for parts in the presence of writers, directors, and producers. In many cases he is asked to return several times. The milieu in which these readings occur directly confronts an actor with his

TABLE 1. Socioeconomic Conditions of Actors

	Actors ($N = 50$)
Average number of jobs, past year	4.3
Average number of jobs lost, past year	20.3
Number working less than fifty weeks	44
Number working less than thirty weeks	33
Mobility	
Perceived upward mobility	
Possible upward mobility, as median income	$92,000
Probable upward mobility, as income	Don't know
Perceived downward mobility	
Likelihood of remaining at possible peak	
"Very likely"	0
"Somewhat likely"	1
"Somewhat unlikely"	7
"Very unlikely"	42
Total	50
Likelihood of remaining at probable peak	
"Very likely"	0
"Somewhat likely"	4
"Somewhat unlikely"	28
"Very unlikely"	18
Total	50
Actual mobility	
Percent increase in income:	
After 5–10 years	220%
After 10–20 years	24
After 20+ years	−21
Occupational income	
$ 0–999	8
1,000–4,999	31
5,000–9,999	2
10,000–19,999	3
20,000–49,999	3
50,000–	2
Total	50
Number recognized as member of occupation out of hours	24

own small chance of success. They take place in a theater or an office suite at an appointed time, but when the actor arrives he discovers that there are ten or twenty or thirty others there too, all with similar appearance, style, age, and so forth. It does not take a lightning calculator to compute the probabilities in these cases. When one adds the fact that an actor's agent, supposedly on his side, may have sent a couple of others in an attempt to get his 10 percent (actors call these types "flesh peddlers"), readings indeed become a whimsical affair. The actor is forever presenting himself for a job, exposing himself to evaluation by others, and this usually occurs when he is out of work. The result is failure four times out of five.

Although an actor has several jobs in the course of a year, he is not always working. Only 12 percent work fifty weeks of the year; fully two-thirds are employed less than thirty weeks. These periods can hardly be called leisure or vacation, however, since the unpredictable longevity of a show makes it impossible to plan them in advance, and naturally the actor is not paid when he is not working. As a result, actors are always in the market for work. When they have a job, the tendency for shows to be short-lived pressures them to be on the lookout for the next time; when they are without work, the start and term of their next employment are similarly tenuous. Insofar as society makes regular work an important value, this condition poses the actor with important problems of self-regard, not to mention the matter of sheer economic survival.

These uncertain structural factors, created by the economics of the theater, are reflected in the actor's own view of his career prospects. When asked how much money they might *possibly* make at their career peak, actors speculate a median of $92,000 per year. Yet when asked how much they will *probably* make, in order to bring the pie back down from the sky, actors find it so difficult to give an answer that two out of three say that they do not know. The import here is that a "career" has no practical meaning, for it is without a prospective contour. Actors cannot specify what a career looks like, cannot describe a typical future for a member of their occupation, and so cannot anticipate one for themselves. They can guess an upper range of achievement, exemplified by their ability to speculate about possible income. They cannot, however, go on from there to formulate their own *particular* chances by first consulting what they understand to be the typical career ladder, by assessing their own capacities, and then putting the two together by relating the typical pattern to their self assessment. They cannot respond to what is probable, as opposed to what is merely possible, because the channels of upward mobility are one dimension of an unpredictable future. According to one actor: "Hell, I could make a million dollars. I could make a thousand dollars. I could make ten thousand dollars. Take any number you want and put it down. But this I know . . ." He went to his desk and exhibited his tax return. His total income for the previous year was $736.45, which leads us to consider actors' feelings about downward mobility.

They expect to be downwardly mobile. Actors think it "very unlikely" that they will remain at their *possible* peak, and "somewhat unlikely" that they will remain at the *probable* peak (whatever it may be, since they cannot predict it). Their responses to potential upward and downward mobility suggest that actors do not know what to expect in the way of a career peak, except to say that they will not stay up there. "We'll have to do a benefit for him" is heard over and over again with reference to the man who puts nothing away in the face of likely downward mobility.

Now what of actual mobility? Regardless of what they say, what happens to actors in fact? According to Table 1, income rises for twenty years, then decreases, with much the greatest increase coming between the fifth and tenth years in the business. Theodore Caplow (1964, p. 75) points out that earnings always drop at the end of a career, but these data indicate that the decrease for actors begins after only twenty years, not ordinarily the end of a career. We can combine Caplow's statement with these findings by suggesting that actors peak out much earlier than those in other occupations. One clear reason for this is the smaller number of parts available to those in middle age.

Note, too, that these actors, who were selected for their dependency on the stage, are concentrated in the $1000–$4999 category. Unfortunately, Table 1 cannot show whether those in the lower ranges have always been there, but actors will say that there is a good deal of fluctuation in the inhabitants of a category from one season to the next. And actors who have been relatively successful at some earlier point say that they maintained their peak for a very short time, and then experienced a swift slip downward (the term "roller coaster" turned up regularly in these interviews). Income is cyclic rather than linear, requiring continuous adjustment and readjustment in living style. A chart of a single actor's career, for example, would be as likely to show its high point immediately before or after its low point as anywhere else, reinforcing his conception of the future as unpredictable.

As a final aspect of socioeconomic uncertainty, it is important to know about actors' celebrity. Celebrity expresses how the public thinks of actors and what the actor must contend with when he is thrown together with persons not in his business. Almost half the actors state that they have been recognized as actors outside of working hours. Most of the actors so identified were known as a generic occupational type, that is, actor, but three were identified as specific persons, which is sui generis an aspect of fame or notoriety (this distinction being contingent on whether the occupation has high or low prestige). Whatever the identification, a stare will follow, and in stores this is often accompanied by the removal of valuable objects from reach. But actors do not think of themselves as so childlike that they will break things, or so poor that they will steal them, with the result that handling the discrepancy between self and social treatment becomes a regular facet of such encounters. Most of them do this by adopting an air of perfect executive propriety, detached sensuousness, or sagacity, depending on their age and appearance vis-à-vis the other party. Needless to say, they have had the training to be good at this, but they still must *do* it.

The personally identified actor has even greater problems in this regard, because the public thinks of him as being just like the parts he plays— in Goffman's terms, they confuse doing with being (Goffman, 1961, p. 100). In one instance, a comedian found it impossible to give directions to household help, because they thought him a funny dope. Another actor, accosted at a restaurant, was punched several times on the shoulder, knocking his spoon out of the soup, all the while being smiled at and called by his first name. Of course, the public thinks he will be gratified by this sort of thing, but every actor denies it. In fact, most of the celebrated ones refuse to go out in public if they can help it, since they expect that their private space will be violated if they do. Even the least obnoxious sort of confrontation, like being asked for an autograph, is usually accompanied by some undercutting statement to the effect that it is for a daughter or a niece, someone who is young and impressionable enough to be fooled by counterfeit. From the point of view of the actor, people around him lose their poise without knowing it; since they do not know it, they expect him to cooperate in an affront to himself.

Technical Conditions

Other uncertain aspects of the actor's environment are the technical exigencies within which he must perform. There are two of these, the first having to do with his own rules for working up a performance, the second with his relation to the audience as he presents that performance. Below is an illustration of these vagaries:

Q. Suppose you follow all the rules you have learned, in acting classes or from reading, in some scene. What happens usually?

A. (Laugh). What rules? Classes help to loosen you up, and the reading helps to loosen you up in theory so you can loosen up in classes, but they don't tell you how to actually do a scene. What happens usually is the scene flops. Go and get another suggestion, it is impossible to rely on "The" or "a" method.

(A reference to the Actor's Studio in the first instance, and to the bromide that every actor has a method in the second.)

Q. How do you know someone has offered a good suggestion?

A. Well, you can't always know. Sometimes a suggestion is made that just clicks, and everyone knows it's a good one.

Q. What do you mean, "just clicks"?

A. It sounds right. Everyone can agree that it's right, and then you try it out and it turns out to be right. The audience likes it.

Q. Can you tell beforehand that it will be right, in any sure way?

A. No, you have to try it out to be sure, but there is a feeling beforehand. Of course, sometimes there's no feeling beforehand, yet it turns out right. I don't know, it's just a matter of experience and trying things out.

This interview, and the tabulation of responses in Table 2, suggest that the actor is faced with vague and indeterminate technical standards before he steps on a stage, and that this burden is amplified by absence of audience feedback once the actual performance begins. We shall discuss these in turn.

Indeterminate standards of technical competence   When asked about what they do at work in order to create a performance, actors (1) find it difficult to specify what they should do *beforehand* to bring off a successful result ("No, you have to try it out . . ."); (2) say they are likely to fail even when they act in terms of (some unspecified) success rules ("What happens usually is the scene flops . . . It is impossible to rely on 'the' or 'a' method"); (3) discover success and failure through general approval-disapproval rather than by calculated observation ("Everyone can agree that it's right . . . The audience likes it").

Actors' technical rules are clearly not rationalized in the bureaucratic sense, with the result that they may vary in application even when the tactical demands of the situation remain the same. There is not a set of means that permits an actor to plan a performance so as to produce a certain effect. Similarly, the difference between success and failure is hard to determine even after the fact—after the task has been performed and must be regarded as a finished product. He can only gain the closure permitted by ad hoc and generalized approval which does not help to locate specific and thus remediable sources of error.

One-way communication between actor and audience   One reason for the finding above involves the one-sided relation between actor and audience: the audience "sees" the actor, but cannot be seen in return. With the exception of a comic line, there is no reciprocal interaction between the two, yet the audience engages in a *concomitant and continuous review* of the actor's effectiveness. The activities of many other oc-

TABLE 2. TECHNICAL CONDITIONS OF ACTORS

Indeterminate standards	Actors (N = 50)
"Can you say beforehand what you should do on the job, in order to bring about the results you want?"	
Always	4
Some of the time	20
Seldom	22
Never	5
Total	50
"When you do follow some plan to bring about the results you want, how often does it work?"	
Every time	1
Most of the time	22
Less than half the time	25
Never	2
Total	50
"Is there any way of checking up on work already done that tells you if you've been successful?"	
Yes, cites abstract rules	22%[a] (11)
Yes, cites change in performance of play	10% (5)
Yes, cites approval-disapproval	84% (42)
No	10% (5)

[a] Total percentages greater than 100 because respondent can mention more than one alternative.

cupations are reviewed while they occur (diagnostician, beautician, salesman, for example), but in these cases the audience is also visible, so the worker may discover at any point how efficiently he is communicating his work to his audience. Actors and other performers are disadvantaged in being judged simultaneously with the assembly of their performance, while at the same time they are not permitted much feedback. Responsive adjustments while the "interaction" is taking place are therefore difficult because the client is invisible and his reactions are silently imposed. In this respect, professional stage actors have less access to the hidden backstage, where they may privately adjust their act to situational and audience demands, than does Goffman's metaphorical actor of everyday life (Goffman, 1959, pp. 106–141).

In summary, the socioeconomic and technical conditions of acting increase the uncertainty of a member's position in society and decrease the calculability of his effectiveness at work. The actor moves unpredictably from job to job. Vertical mobility may be great, it may not, there being no way to tell—the only sure thing is a rapid descent. The time he spends out of work poses problems of worth in terms of the value of regular employment, because joblessness cannot be planned in advance and is not considered a routine reward for services rendered. And his treatment by the public is out of harmony with his own sense of self. On the technical side, indeterminate standards make it difficult to predict the consequences of alternative ways of doing things. Work turns into a series of trials where even error is not clear, and certainly not the obvious effect of a specific act, while the asymmetry of communication and judgment leaves actors without cues at the critical moment of performance.

These conditions raise a serious question: Are actors anomic, a mere conglomerate that survives only because the public demands entertainment, or do actors form a group, with shared norms and interaction? Structured uncertainty could be resolved by the sentiments and forms of interaction between actors, or it could so permeate their activities that the label "actor" designates a mere aggregate of persons. We must ask whether socially organized behavior accompanies these conditions, or if instead we observe a formless collection of bodies.

We can begin to answer this question by using actors' occupational identification as a measure of groupness. Should we discover some identification, we may reasonably describe acting as a subculture, one that maintains some viable level of cohesion, and go on to investigate what kind of group it is.

Table 3 suggests that actors identify with their occupation.

First, they say that the job of another person is the most important determinant of their treatment of him, that is, their social preceptions incorporate occupational differences. Second, they say they would become an actor if given another chance to choose—a rather positive view of their occupation. Finally, these feelings are reinforced by their interaction patterns, which are restricted primarily to others in their occupation. Thus, to the degree that occupational identification implicates a subculture, actors are more like a group than an aggregate. Our next step will be to delineate the kind of group it is, what it establishes as appropriate behavior, and how that behavior helps to resolve uncertainty.

GROUP PRACTICES AND SENTIMENTS

I shall turn now from the socioeconomic and technical conditions of acting, over which the membership can have little control of a direct sort, to the internal norms for technical and interpersonal activity that actors

TABLE 3. Actors' Identification with Their Occupation

Recognized differences between occupations
  "Which of these are important to you in deciding how to act
  with other people?"

The money they make	22%[a]
Their education	12%
The job they have	70%
Their personality	36%
The kind of family they have	10%
None	6%

Occupational choice
  "If you had it to do over again, would you become an actor?"

Yes	27
Probably	11
Probably not	9
No	3

Interaction

Proportion of friends who are actors	72%
Proportion of casual interaction with actors	54%
(cup of coffee, chat for a minute, and so on)	

---

[a] Total percentages greater than 100 because respondents can mention more than one alternative.

as a group construct and enforce. Table 4 summarizes these data, and illustrative responses are included in the discussion.

Technical Practices

Actors are all equals on the job, too. I have gotten good advice from bad actors, and bad advice from good actors, so I always listen and take it seriously no matter who makes the suggestion. Sooner or later one will work. Something happens, and the performance goes better.

Actors solicit suggestions from every quarter on the job. They do not assess the worth of a suggestion by distinguishing the size of part or public reputation of the player who initiates it ("No matter who makes the suggestion"). Moreover, since an actor has no explicit set of rules that tell him beforehand that a suggestion will work, he looks to others in the cast for agreement that it is a good one ("Everyone can agree its right"). If an actor gains this consensus, he tries that out ("You have to try it out to be sure"). If he thinks the audience is not properly affected, he returns to his colleagues for another suggestion and tries that out ("Go and get another suggestion"). This is an ad hoc trial and error procedure that utilizes cast consensus as the yardstick for choosing between alterna-

TABLE 4. GROUP PRACTICES AND SENTIMENTS

Technical practices		
Source of suggestions ("Where do you go to get a suggestion?")	Status-linked (depends on size of part, past success of initiator) 12	All actors 38
Validity of suggestions ("Where do you go to decide if a suggestion is a good one?")	Status linked 9	All actors 41
("When can you be sure that a suggestion was a good one?")	Before the fact 5	After the fact 45
Interpersonal sentiments		
Looking for work	Competitive 8	Cooperative 42
Dislike	Individually controllable 6	Situationally determined 44
Public acclaim	Relevant to actors' relations with one another 13	Irrelevant to actors' relations with one another 37

tives. But the point here is that validation by group consensus tends to *diffuse* the error of a particular actor by absorbing it into the group as a whole—he cannot in this circumstance be held responsible or blamed when a mistake is made, and cannot be regarded as a hero when a success occurs. Diffusion differs greatly from the explicit, hierarchically organized rules and roles that predominate in bureaucracies and professions, where members can locate the specific source of error in any instance, and then hold that source accountable. The efficacy of an actor's suggestion can be discovered only retrospectively, owing to the joint effects of indeterminate standards and asymmetrical review, and so, in retrospect, the identity of its initiator tends to get lost in time. But more than that, a consensus technique magnifies the effect by losing him in space as well, since validation by consensus intervenes between the suggestion and the trial. The whole group takes responsibility for the consequences.

Sentiments of Interaction

Actors also exhibit a normative structure for other problematic activities that are job-related but not directly concerned with actual performance: job seeking, dealing with like and dislike, and responding to public acclaim.

1. They cooperate rather than compete with one another when looking for work:

> I always tell someone a job is coming up, even if I'm up for it myself. Why not? It never makes any difference, you either get the job or not. It doesn't depend on who the rival is so much as what the director wants, and when I lose out one time I get the part the next time. I think most of us feel this way. No, I wouldn't call the competition "cutthroat."

2. Actors treat dislike as unchangeable and situationally determined, not to be controlled by the individuals involved:

> Sure, there are people I don't like. But nothing can be done, it's just "personality conflict." In the service we used to get transferred when that happened, but in the theater you just go ahead and pay no attention since nothing can be done about it. It's the fault of the person doing the disliking as much as the person disliked . . . I like most everyone, and when I don't it's personality conflict and nothing can be done.

3. Actors refuse to accept public acclaim or prestige as a determinant of their relations with one another on and off the job:

> Some actors get high-falutin' when they make it big, or even when they land in a hit, but there aren't many. Face it, work and friendship are two entirely different things, and we all know there are good actors who don't make it, so public recognition is unimportant so far as actors themselves are concerned. Oh, we're all happy when somebody does well, but it doesn't have any effect on the kidding, say, that actors do to one another. Besides, today's flash is tomorrow's poop, and everyone is aware of that.

Actors are confronted with differentiation, as in public acclaim and personal animus, but to them it is an epiphenomenon, the immutable product of situational happenstance. They need not evaluate an act as if the individual is to be blamed or praised, with the result that a particular behavior does not become invidiously attached to the person who originates it. These sentiments, based on normative dissociation of act from actor, make it possible to enforce horizontal rather than vertical relationships. Interaction can be egalitarian, a style which deflects the emergence of stratification as an important dimension of behavior.

Thus, technical rules stress the development of consensus, while interpersonal sentiments are egalitarian. These are characteristics of *collegial* social organization, as opposed to the bureaucratic and professional kinds.

It is a type that has received little attention since Max Weber (1947), who discussed it as a form of organization that limits monocratic or bureaucratic authority: "Legitimate acts require the participation of all members [p. 395]," "Acts of authority must be carried out only after previous consultation and vote [p. 393]," and "there is concern with uniformity of opinions and attitudes [p. 396]." We might add that among actors, insofar as they furnish a collegial contrast to bureaucracy, there is little emphasis on step-by-step formulae that delimit a recognizable series of points for the assembly of the end product. This absence of formula and assembly points means that there is a comparable diminution of hierarchically organized statuses, for there are too few rules to induce an internal division of labor—there are not enough distinctions to tell the members what the statuses are, or could be. Nor is there the individual autonomy and responsibility in actors' collegiality which is so characteristic of the professions: suggestion and trial is a procedure requiring validation by colleague agreement before a particular proposal can be considered legitimate. Among actors, authority resides in the whole group, whereas in other endeavors it is vested in roles within the group. As a result, interaction on and off the job does not exhibit the finite stratified perspective typical of other occupations. If there is little emphasis on making distinctions, there is correspondingly little grist for stratification.

COLLEGIALITY AND UNCERTAINTY

Having described the occupational conditions and group organization of acting as, respectively, uncertain and collegial, it remains now to put them together. Is there a relation between the two, a compatibility between the form of the group and the conditions in which it exists?

First, the parametric uncertainty of potential and actual mobility is mitigated by refusing to act in terms of public acclaim. The individual actor, facing an unpredictable socioeconomic future, is provided with continuing support by the group, however his public status may fluctuate. If instead there were a parallel stratification system among actors that required comparable changes in treatment and self every time a change in public status occurred, uncertainty would impair continuous interpersonal behavior. In the latter scheme of things, the occupation actor would probably designate no more than random collisions of disparate men. The need to act on the unpredictable would obviate the development and persistence of norms that could be regularly applied and mutually expected, circumstances that are necessary to sustained concert among persons. Among other things, the dissonance of celebrity engenders this disdain for the public ranking system, with the result that actors are not likely to act on, or even care about, outside criteria of success anyway. Since the public and private definitions of acting and actors are exactly opposite, a man can easily misrepresent himself to the public without any apparent purpose except to do it. In fact, our actor's remarks to the newspaperman were fully *responsible* ones, if by that we mean responsibility to one's own. As the public and its journalist surrogate are the violators of one's private self, not to mention fickle arbiters of employment and performance, it becomes a duty, not a choice, to portray one's life for the public as at odds with one's life for the group. Being forced to participate in two worlds, our actor accomplished this by contradicting them, and kept them separated in so doing.

The actor's view of animosity is equally compatible with uncertainty. As an ascriptive quality, one beyond the capacity to change, an actor need not conclude that some act by those involved could rectify the conflict, and so he need not define and deal with exceptions to egalitarianism. An actor does not have to think anyone is at fault. To the extent this characteristic is shared, it inhibits the growth of an esteem system, a system which would demand a routine search for invidious comparisons and lead him back to stratification and the contingencies of uncertainty. Thus, when one actor talks about bootstrap betterment the rest become uncomfortable, because it implies that the individual does not merely have a place in the world, but is morally required to do something on his own to improve it.

After a first glance, it is not so surprising that actors adopt a cooperative rather than adversary system in looking for work. Some actors, for example, will go for a reading, discover what the production staff wants, and then telephone an acquaintance who seems to fit the bill more precisely. Such collaboration may decrease the chance of a single actor for a single job, yet the over-all effect, besides an increase in collegiality, is to enlarge the amount of information that any one actor can possess. This may, on balance, outweigh the increased competition, since all will know where the opportunities are, and where they are not, with the result that the actor is probably rejected less often and accepted more often. Thus, besides supporting the collegial system, cooperation tends to overcome the secrecy that would make things even vaguer than they are.

It has already been suggested that consensus at work diffuses failure and success into the group as a whole. Given the uncertainty of conditions between audience and performer and the large amounts of error that ensue, consensus is a way of concealing fallibility, but it also supports the general egalitarianism exhibited in actors' sentiments of interaction. No one may claim sole responsibility for what he has done, nor must he accept sole responsibility for what he has not done, with the result that

a particular triumph belongs to all. Actors probably could not survive as
a group if they had to recriminate, there being so much error and so little
technique for locating it that they would not have time for anything
else. Consensus is a fitting motif for going right ahead when goals are
coming no closer to realization.

Thus, collegial social organization is an ensemble format for egalitarianism and consensus, with little emphasis on hierarchies of rules and
distinctions of authority. In this type of organization there is just one
kind of member, not many kinds—once admitted, one member is the
same as everyone else, and will continue to be, since there is no important
way of evaluating him. One is a member and that ends it. Collegiality
is a gyroscopic device that washes out the effects of environing uncertainty,
because actors can respond to nominal criteria of membership that are
met simply by being a professional stage actor, rather than to complicated
and unpredictable shifts in socioeconomic status or technical fortune.
The point of reference for membership—whether or not one possesses
the specific quality "actor"—is totally encompassing, open-armed, so one
need not find his place by addressing multiple foci that change in unknown ways and can be discovered only after the fact. A success here, a
failure there; acclaim now, ignominy then—none of these call for adjustment by actors, because one is a colleague regardless, entitled to all the
claims and perquisites of any other member. When one actor is asked for
his autograph, he is careful to pass the request around to the others,
especially if they have suffered reverses.

The idea of a collegial subculture suggests the appropriateness of certain other actions we have not directly considered: de-individuation, ex-
pansive behavior, and passion, all antithetical to the bureaucratic version
of social life. Whatever he may do, a collegial member continues to be
supported by his group. Error is, as we have said, diffused rather than
specified; egalitarianism emphasizes what is held in common rather than
what is special about the individual; single focus membership excludes
any behavior other than occupational identification as irrelevant criteria
of unity. Consequently, acts that would be deviant in some other kind of
group—the dinner conversation that we began with—can be perfectly
acceptable among actors. The individual participant is permitted a wider
band of normatively acceptable behavior because a particular act does not
call its initiator or recipient into question as a bona fide member. Thus,
no one at the party thought anything was wrong because (1) sexual
behavior between man and wife is irrelevant to their group identity, and
so (2) a public statement of such behavior, whether true or untrue, is
possible without changing their standing in the group. Nothing was im-
minent in that conversation because it was not grave. It was not grave

because the language employed, and the action it depicted, occurred in a context of collegiality.

IMPLICATION

The stress in social science on explicit rules of calculation, performance, and evaluation may have led us to assert that these are necessary conditions of social order, that their absence will lead to anomie. Similarly, we may have concluded that the individual behaviors that are associated with those conditions are the only appropriate ones, and that their absence is evidence of psychological debility, obtuseness, and lack of control.

But the existence of such rules, and the individual behaviors they prescribe, may be no more than numerically predominant empirical phenomena in the professional and bureaucratic organizations we usually study. If the actor's case is a valid one (and here I am not referring to any but professional stage actors), there are circumstances where uncertainty does not lead to anomie, where a detailed set of rules and positions are not necessary to order, where broad-gauged behavior and unconcern with reputation are not signs of demoralization. Calculation, differential authority, and stratification are minor subcultural imperatives and not reflected in the behavior of actors; if they were, sooner or later there would be no group left to enforce them. A structure of invidious distinctions, the creation of a paradigm of individual accountability, would in the uncertain world of the actor require pervasive, instantaneous, but unpredictable shifts in action, role, and self-image. Acting is a vague and amorphous business, but the kind of solidarity it exhibits enables the craft to persist as a group endeavor. Collegiality resolves uncertainty by ignoring its effects.

REFERENCES

Caplow, T. *The sociology of work.* New York, McGraw-Hill, 1964.

Goffman, E. *Presentation of self in everyday life.* Garden City, N.Y.: Doubleday Anchor Books, 1959.

Goffman, E. *Encounters.* Indianapolis, Ind.: Bobbs-Merrill, 1961.

Weber, M. *The theory of social and economic organization.* (Transl. by T. Parsons & A. M. Henderson.) Glencoe, Ill.: The Free Press, 1947.

4.6 *Orientation*

It is said that prostitution is one of the oldest professions and, therefore, must provide useful social functions to have survived various attempts at its banishment throughout the ages. The writings of novelists and historians have often concentrated on the role of prostitutes in affecting the lives or political careers of important persons, but there is no evidence of previous attempts at scientific inquiry into the personal lives of prostitutes or the social purpose they fulfill in a complex society.

The article by James Bryan focuses on the problem that prostitutes must simultaneously live in two worlds—the square world of "everyday" life and the "working" world filled with "Johns," pimps, other prostitutes, and a variety of persons existing in the shadows of city life. The conflicting nature of these dual roles presents problems for prostitutes and has a bearing on factors affecting their mental health. Bryan's subjects in his pioneering studies are high-class "call girls" in Hollywood and Chicago—girls who build up a select list of expensive clientele and who maintain a standard of living that is beyond the reach of most women. He provides us with fresh insights into the lives of socially deviant women, and a way of understanding how they are indoctrinated into a profession that is confronted with nearly universal public disapproval.

4.6 Occupational Socialization and Interpersonal Attitudes: A Partial Failure in the Acculturation of High-Class Prostitutes[1]

James H. Bryan

Although the study of sustained illegal and immoral behavior is of theoretical concern to those interested in deception, passing, and stigma

[1] Part of this study was supported by the Graduate School, Northwestern University. Thanks are due to Professors Howard S. Becker, Perry London, and Lee Sechrest for their critical comments of earlier manuscripts of this chapter. I am indebted to Vivian London for her editorial help, and to Alice Vicks for her considerable aid in the analysis of the data.

effects, virtually no systematically gathered data exist concerning those individuals who commit such acts successfully, that is, without eliciting public attention. That such information is lacking is surprising insofar as the concept of duplicity and stigma is theoretically important to both psychology and sociology, as it pertains to deviation, psychopathology, and the unconscious. Witness, for example, the Freudians' concern with repression and insight, self-duplicity if you will (Reiff, 1959), or Mowrer's (1961, 1964) conceptions regarding guilt, redemption and confession. Substantially all humanistically oriented psychologies have, to varying degrees, preached a doctrine prescribing honesty as the psychically preferred mode of life. While psychologies appear to differ as to what one might be honest about, there appears to be virtual unanimity regarding the merits of intrapersonal and interpersonal intimacy. Furthermore, Goffman (1959) has proposed to analyze the interaction of self and situation on the basis of the ecology of role performance and self-revelation.

While both psychological and sociological orientations place emphasis upon the importance of public awareness of deviant behavior, their hypotheses concerning the ultimate consequences of interpersonal honesty are antithetical. Psychology has tended to give little theoretical weight or valence to the impact of the consequent social processes following public knowledge concerning misbehavior.[2] Mowrer (1961, 1964) apparently is concerned with the impact of public knowledge upon the deviant actor, giving both considerable theoretical weight and positive valence to the process of public confession. The everyday behavior of practitioners suggests, however, that most support honesty and discourage "passing" behaviors, at least on the part of such norm breakers as ex-mental patients. It is assumed that the psychic taxation of passing exceeds the social humiliation of stigma. Patients are instructed to be discrete but honest.[3] Sociologists, however, argue that it is exactly the stigma effects, as opposed to personality factors, that "locks" one into a particular deviant role, the enactment of which is increasingly required within and across situations (Cohen, 1963; Glaser, 1965; Kituse, 1962). Indeed, it has been asserted (Scheff, 1963) that "mental illness" obtains stability only as a result of public disclosure.

Unfortunately, most of those studies concerned with socially deviant

[2] In this context the public refers to two or more actors not bound by the ethics of confidentiality. Experimental psychology has, of course, concerned itself with the parameters affecting the reinforcement of behavior.

[3] An interpretation of the official sanctioned behavior of the stigmatized vis-à-vis the public at large can be read in Goffman (1963).

behavior of the criminal variety have contaminated dishonesty with stigma, passing with unhappiness, personality characteristics with situationally controlled role behavior. The arrested and the psychiatrically supervised have provided the bulk of the systematically gathered information pertaining to deviant acts and actors. In spite of the methodological, legal, and professional difficulties apparently confronting the investigator of tabooed behavior, the unconfounding of these theoretically important variables can only be accomplished through field studies of deviant individuals, groups or acts, heretofore not publicly discredited or revealed (see Becker, 1963).

The few such studies that have been completed using such respondents have yielded a rich harvest. The information that has been gathered on samples other than those under the direct control of social regulating agencies (police and psychiatrists) has proved theoretically important. Hooker's (1961, 1965) work on the "normal homosexual," Lindesmith's (1955) on the heroin addict and Becker's (1964) on the marijuana smoker are exemplary.

The writer has been conducting, for the past several years, studies on the individual and cultural variables that may support and sustain the activities of the high-class prostitute by using respondents, by and large, free of both police and psychiatric supervision.[4] This sample appears to be an ideal target group for such field studies; first, because the high-class prostitute is available for study, and second, because she is often involved in both immoral and criminal behavior—the latter including such felonies as counterfeiting, burglary, and smuggling (in the current sample, over 25 percent had, at one time or another, engaged in felonious activities). This population, therefore, is an accessible criminal population available for psychological and sociological scrutiny.

Traditionally, psychological orientations to the study of the prostitute have shown considerable homogeneity. Twentieth-century theorizing concerning this occupational group has employed, most often, a naive version of Freudian or neo-Freudian theory. The description of the prostitute reads much like a catalogue of psychological horror stories. She has been described as masochistic (Benjamin & Ellis, 1955; Glover, 1953), of infantile mentality (Benjamin, 1951), unable to form mature interpersonal relationships (Hollander, 1961), a latent homosexual (Caprio & Brenner, 1961), regressed (Glover, 1953), emotionally dangerous to males (Karpf, 1953), hateful of men (Glover, 1953), hostile (Glover, 1953; Oliver, 1955),

---

[4] The study of high-class prostitutes is part of a series of larger studies on socially deviant behaviors and is being undertaken in conjunction with Professor Perry London of the University of Southern California, and Dr. David Rosehan of the Educational Testing Service.

and as normal as the average woman (Robinson, 1929).[5] The "call girl," the specific focus of this chapter, has been described by Greenwald (1960) as possessing a confused self-image, excessively dependent, demonstrating gender-role confusion, aggressive, lacking internal controls, and masochistic.

The exclusive use of motivational models in attempting to predict behavior, and the consequent neglect of situational and cognitive processes, has been steadily lessening in the field of psychology (for recent trends in personality theory, see Sanford, 1963; Miller, 1963; Milgram, 1965). Their inadequacy as models for understanding deviance has been specifically explicated by Becker (1963, 1964).

The present investigation has employed an alternative model for the conceptualization and study of deviant behavior by focusing upon the interpersonal processes that help define the deviant role, the surroundings in which the role is learned, and limits upon the enactment of the role. As Hooker (1961) has indicated regarding the study of homosexuals, not only must the personality structure of the participants be considered, but one must also view both the theoretical structure of their community and the pathways and routes (that is, training periods) by which one learns and enacts the behavior. The importance of such "training periods" has also been indicated by Maurer (1940) in his study of the con man, and by Sutherland (1937) in his report on professional thieves. More recently, Becker (1963) has outlined those learning sequences necessary for development of the steady use of marijuana.

In general, sociological notions, such as those presented by Goffman (1963), Reiss (1961), Sutherland and Cressy (1955), and Sykes and Matza (1957), indicate that these learning experiences pertain not only to the acquisition of necessary skills, but also to the ideological commitments and values of the "deviant" group in question. It is said that when behavior is stigmatized, the deviant group will propagate attitudes and moralities counter to dominant cultural values. While individual deviants are thought to vary in their degree of socialization, professionals are developed (Goffman, 1963). The ideologies of deviant groups, according to Becker (1964), "tend to contain a general repudiation of conventional moral rules, conventional institutions, and the entire conventional world." Further, students agree that deviant groups stress in-group loyalties and minimize the moral nature of their transgressions (Sykes & Matza, 1957). The learning of this ideology is said to be the turning point

[5] For a review of the speculation concerning the motivational properties of prostitutes see V. L. Bullough, "Problems and methods for research in prostitution and the behavioral sciences. *Journal of the History of Behavioral Sciences,* 1965, 1, 244–251.

of the deviant's career (Goffman, 1963). While it is commonly thought that prostitutes' ideologies play an important role in the continuation of their behavior, these beliefs have rested as much on faith as on fact. The perspectives of prostitutes have generally been ignored in favor of motivational states and, when not ignored, are often inferred from very limited samples or anecdotal material.

The specific purpose of this article, then, is to provide information concerning entrance into and training for high-class prostitution, with special emphasis upon the professionally prescribed versus individually held ideologies. This particular emphasis appears appropriate insofar as "official" ideology and accompanying changes in self-concepts provide a major focal point in contemporary sociological theories of deviation.

The respondents, from which the data were collected, were fifty-two prostitutes, who volunteered to be interviewed, who were not paid for the interviews, and who, with one exception, defined themselves as "call girls." No member of the sample was under the supervision of the police, and only eight were found within the context of the psychiatric hospital. The subjects ranged in age from 18 to 40, the median age at the time of interview being 22.[6] Their clients were typically obtained through individual referrals, primarily by telephone. They enacted the sexual contract in their own or their clients' place of residence or employment. The respondents did not initiate contact with their customers in settings such as bars, streets, or houses of prostitution, although they might meet them by prearrangement at any number of locations. With five exceptions, the minimum fee charged per sexual encounter was $20.[7] As an adjunct to the call girl interviews, three pimps and two "call boys" were interviewed.

Thirty-nine of the respondents worked primarily in Los Angeles, six in Chicago, three in Las Vegas, and one each in San Francisco and Miami. Many of the respondents, however, had worked in more than one city.

All but two interviews were recorded on tape, and all respondents had prior knowledge of this procedure. The interviewing was, most often, at

[6] The mean age of the respondents at the time of initial interviewing was 24.5, the standard deviation = 5.69.

[7] One respondent, at the time of interviewing, was charging a minimum fee of $10 per contact. The remaining four had, earlier in their careers, worked $10 "tricks." It might also be noted that this definition departs somewhat from that offered by Clinard (1957). He defines the call girl as one dependent upon an organization for recruiting patrons and one who typically works in lower class hotels. The present sample is best described by Clinard's category, high-class independent professional prostitute. Respondents were obtained primarily from referrals from previous informants.

the girls' place of work and/or residence. Occasional interviews were conducted in the investigator's office, and one in a public park. Interviews were semi-structured and employed open-ended questions.[8]

THE SOCIAL SYSTEM OF CALL GIRLS

The Entrance

The decision to become a call girl and the subsequent entrance into the occupation appear to be casual events, often occurring at a time of financial need. The decision to begin is by no means necessarily followed by action; some of the girls in this study had aspirations to become call girls long before the opportunity to do so arose (see theoretical discussion in Cloward, 1962).

The median age of entrance into the occupation was 20 years. The two- or three-year lag that typically occurs between leaving high school and being "turned out" (becoming a prostitute) implies that entrance into the occupation follows abortive attempts to manage "square" jobs. Indeed, while the evidence is spotty, the data support the not surprising notion that the prospective call girl has had difficulty within the usual vocational contexts.

Immediately prior to the "turning out" period, all but four girls were acquainted with individuals directly engaged in the business of prostitution. As one might expect, without such personal contacts, transcending the secrecy surrounding the occupation is, at best, difficult, and, at worst, impossible.

I had been thinking about it [becoming a "call girl"] before a lot . . . thinking about wanting to do it, but I had no connections. Had I not had a connection, I probably wouldn't have started working. . . . I thought about starting out. . . . Once I tried it (without a contact). . . . I met this guy at a bar and I tried to make him pay me, but the thing is, you can't do it that way because they are romantically interested in you, and they don't think that it is on that kind of basis. You can't all of a sudden come up and want money for it, you have to be known beforehand. . . . I think that is what holds a lot of girls

[8] The quantitative analyses to be reported throughout the article are not always based upon responses of the entire fifty-two girls. The reduced size of the sample is primarily due to the fact that all the tapes have not as yet been transcribed. In some instances, the respondents were not asked the question, as it had a low priority within the interview schedule, or if asked the question, refused to answer it. The shortage of sample size is most apparent for the computation of the median number of sexual partners the respondents had prior to entering "the life."

back who might work. I think I might have started a year sooner had I had a connection.

The girls' initial liaison is almost invariably another "working girl" (call girl) or a pimp. The four exceptions to this had connections with customers. Never has it been reported that the initial contact was an individual in such peripherally involved occupations as cab driving, modeling, or photography. While unquestionably such institutions may serve as pathways for entrance, the degree to which they do so for girls entering prostitution at this level appears limited. The aspiring call girl's initial contact furthermore will be one that is involved in prostitution at the call girl level; it will not be a streetwalker, a streetwalker's pimp, or a "house" girl. It is extremely rare, in fact, that social mobility is "upward"; house girls or streetwalkers do not become call girls.[9]

Approximately 50 percent of the sample reported that their first liaison was with another "working girl." The nature of their interpersonal relationships was quite variable. In some cases, for example, the girls had been long-standing friends. Most, however, had known each other less than a year and did not appear to have had a very close relationship in the sense of biographical information exchanged.

Whatever the nature of the relationship between novice and professional, whenever the latter agrees to aid the beginner, she also implicitly assumes responsibility for the training of the girl. This is evidenced by the fact that only one such female contact referred the aspirant to another for any type of training.

If the original contact was not another "call girl" but a pimp, a much different relationship is developed, and career progression follows a somewhat different, albeit stereotyped course. The male, like his female counterpart, may undertake the training of the girl; or, unlike his female opposite, refer the girl to another "call girl" for such training. Either course is equally probable. Referrals, when employed, are typically to friends, and in some cases, wives or ex-wives.

The Training: Social Structure and Content

Once the almost necessary contact is acquired and the decision made, the next step in career sequence is very predictable.[10] The apprenticeship

___

[9] The use of "upward" implies that call girls have higher status than other types of prostitutes. This is certainly true from the call girl's perspective. The nature of status hierarchies and their underlying dimensions will be presented in a forthcoming paper.

[10] The predictability of the career sequence as well as the formality of the

is typically served under the direction of another call girl, although the novice may be occasionally supervised by a pimp. Of those subjects serving such training periods, which includes over 80 percent of the current sample, approximately three-fourths worked under the supervision of another "working girl."

The place of training is, like the future place of work, an apartment. While most often it is the trainer's place of residence, it occasionally will be an apartment rented for the sole purpose of turning "tricks" (that is, fulfilling the sexual contract).

Although the data are not extensive, the number of girls being trained simultaneously by a particular trainer has not been reported to be greater than three. The time spent in such training has been indicated to extend up to eight months, but the average duration seems to be only two or three months. The trainer controls all referrals and appointments, and novices seemingly do not have much command over the type of sexual contract negotiated or those circumstances surrounding the enactment of the agreement.

The structure of the training operations, when the respondent is under the direction of a pimp, seems quite parallel to those described above. The girls are trained in an apartment in the city where they intend to live. If the pimp and girl anticipate living together, typically a "trick pad" will be rented. This appears to be not only because of the inconvenience of having an extra male present during working hours, but also because of the widely held and apparently mistaken belief that clues that suggest the presence of other men displease the great majority of customers (Winick, 1961–1962).

When specifically questioned as to the contents of the teaching, most respondents indicated that the *acquisition of skills, rather than ideology,* comprised the bulk of the learning process. While the details of such skill training have been presented elsewhere (Bryan, 1965), in general, techniques concerning solicitation, pitches, sexual hygiene, proprieties concerning collecting the fee, and other skills pertaining to the problematic situation are taught. Occupationally sanctioned morality seems to be directly taught with less regularity. The prostitute is occasionally taught, however, that customers are exploitative, exploitable, and foolish. Further, girls are informed of the virtues of their colleagues, although there appears to be less emphasis upon the development of the latter than the former set of interpersonal attitudes. Justifications, often moral in nature, are offered for exploiting those who "should" be exploited, while

training may vary considerably across geographies. The remarks of the following section apply primarily to the Los Angeles call girl.

rationales are proposed for aggrandizing those with whom cooperative behavior is required.[11]

What is omitted from training should be noted. Most often there seems to be little instruction concerning sexual techniques as such, most likely due to the extensiveness of the girl's previous sexual history. The novice prostitute is typically no novice to sex. Indeed, the median number of heterosexual partners experienced by the girls prior to becoming a professional prostitute was twelve.[12] Thus, there is little need or "technical training" in this phase of the occupation, and the opportunities for acculturation may thereby be reduced. If there is instruction in sexual acts, it typically concerns the practice of fellatio. Further, and surprisingly, there appears to be little concern regarding techniques of passing, either with the context of the sexual contract or more generally with the community at large.[13] There is virtually no attention to the generation of socially acceptable explanations for the girl's apparent high income, unique hours, and peripatetic habits. Apparently, there is no necessity to concern herself with legitimizing her behavior. The reasons for such cavalier indifference will be discussed later. Further, there appears little effort, except as described above, to directly teach a counter-morality. This does not mean that there is none of a well-defined sort, but rather that it does not appear to be taught with the same emphasis or at the same time as the functionally important skills.

There is evidence (Bryan, 1965) that the primary function of the apprenticeship for the novice is gaining access to customers; for the trainer, the advantage of convenience and income. The latter obtains 40 percent of the novice's income and simultaneously maintains liaison with her reputedly fickle customers. Training, either ideological or technical in nature, appears to be of little import. Indeed, no respondent has reported that the termination of the apprenticeship was the result of adequate training. While disruptions of this relationship may be due

[11] The position that customers are foolish or fools is similar to the position attributed to the con man with regard to the "mark" (See Goffman, E., 1962).

[12] These calculations are based upon a limited sample of the respondents ($N = 21$). The selection of these particular respondents was based upon considerations other than pre-occupational sexual activities. The remaining interviews have either not been analyzed for this specific information or the respondents were unwilling to indicate such numbers, more often due to a hesitation to give unreliable guesses than embarrassment concerning such activity.

[13] Obviously, the initial screening of customers is concerned with maintaining secrecy. With this exception, however, techniques of passing are not taught.

to personal or impersonal events, its expiration is not directly due to the development of sufficient skills.

The Ideology and Counter-Morality

While the data pertaining to ideologies are necessarily impressionistic, certain roughly specifiable criteria were used to select that material relevant to occupational perspectives. First material was chosen that was used by the girls in such a manner as to explain and justify the occupation of prostitution. Responses had to be known to the majority of respondents; consensus was apparent. Certain views were also repeatedly attributed to or given by members considered "pro," part of the "in-group," of those who had been in the profession for a lengthy period. For example, not infrequently, a respondent would indicate how one should perceive, feel, or act, if one were to be a real professional. Hence, attributed professional views, if there was agreement as to their nature, were used as the basis for inferring occupationally sanctioned ideologies.

A major element in the occupational perspective, indicated by virtually all respondents, was that prostitution served important social functions because of the male's extensive and varied sexual needs, protecting both individuals and social institutions alike from destructive ruptures.

. . . we girls see, like I guess you call them perverts of some sort, you know, little freaky people and if they didn't have girls to come to like us that are able to handle them and make it a nice thing, there would be so many rapes and . . . nutty people really.

. . . I think that a lot less rapes and murders would occur if it were [legalized].

I believe that there should be more prostitution houses and what have you, and then we wouldn't have so many of these perverted idiots, sex maniacs, all sorts of weird people running around.

Marriages are thought to be more enduring because of prostitution:

I could say that a prostitute has held more marriages together as part of their profession than any divorce counselor.

Respondents also commonly indicate that prostitutes serve as important psychotherapeutic agents, giving comfort, insight, and satisfaction to those men too embarrassed, lonely or isolated to obtain inter-personal gratification in other ways.

I don't regret doing it because I feel I help people. A lot of men that come over to see me don't come for sex. They come over for companionship, someone to talk to . . . They talk about sex . . . A lot of them have problems.

While the foregoing positions are commonly stated, the professional, as opposed to the novice, holds additional views. Both trainers and professionals appear to encourage a view that makes exploitation of the "John" less morally reprehensible. The customer is exploitative, hence should be exploited. "Johns" are to be cultivated through extensive contacts, such that repeated "scores" can be made, often to the customer's disadvantage. In general, the professional devalues men as a whole. This position is often felt by the girls to be the natural outcome of sustained acts of prostitution whereby extensive experience with customers is thought to produce the "hard and cold" girl who has developed a "very crude attitude toward the profession" with the end result of being "bitter and hating men clients." Of the conceptions held by the girls of the consequences of being a prostitute, perhaps this is the one that produces the most personal anxiety.

The prostitute should see her customers as exploitative, cutting each corner of the financial contract, and herself as a potential victim: "so the trainer taught me to get my money out in front a lot of time . . . if you accept clothes from them, they'll buy you a $10 dress and the whole deal is worth fifty."

In addition, girls recognize occupationally sanctioned attitudes toward women and colleagues alike. They sometimes say that the "in-group" is unique, special, more honest: "I feel that people in the life are more honest with themselves and with others."

Occasionally the trainer will exhort the novice to join the "in-group." As one prostitute of two weeks explains her reaction to her trainer's exhortations to "Get with it; do what we do": "It has to do with being a swinger or hip. Going out and more or less cheating on your boyfriend or carousing around with a fast crowd and looking hot . . . I won't do it."

Another view, popular at both the novice and professional levels, is that interpersonal relationships between the sexes are, in essence, acts of prostitution. This position stems from the assumption that within such relationships, gains are often derived from intentional manipulations, deceptions and sex. The housewife, then, is no less guilty than the prostitute. ". . . Actually all women are whores in my opinion whether they get married for it or whatever it is. There are just different ways of being a whore." The square's hypocrisy may be further compounded by envy. "They [the public] resent them because the working girl [call girl] can do things that other women can't do."

In sum, the professional perspective argues that customers can and should be exploited and that the role of the prostitute is no more honest and helpful than that of women outside of the profession. Furthermore, since it is a necessary, indeed therepeutic, practice, prostitution should not be stigmatized, and one should not look down upon oneself for being a prostitute. These simple rules may, perhaps, serve as justification for exploitation, sustain what cooperative behavior is necessary for occupational functioning, and reduce both the public and personal stigma, real or potential, that is attached to the actor.

Individual Attitudes

Given the validity of the inferences concerning these perspectives, the question remains as to how much impact they have upon the individual respondent.[14] The interview material suggests that individual respondents do not, in fact, personally endorse the above-mentioned perspectives. While the respondents know them, they do not believe them. For example, many of the individual respondents, not surprisingly, refuse to stereotype the customer: "I've never found two alike." Or stereotyping may be more benign than that suggested by the occupation's ideology. "Most of them are very, very nice people, like overly nice." Reality soon appears to break down the ideology, occasionally to the discomfort of the actor: "Even though they're tricks, and I hate tricks, they are still people and they have as many hangups a lot of times as I do. Therefore, I have been able to empathize with them in most cases, which is bad when you try to take somebody for all they're worth. It gives you guilt feelings." Not infrequently, personal friendships with customers are reported: "Some of them are nice clients who become very good friends of mine." However while friendships are formed with "squares," personal disputations with colleagues are frequent. Speaking of her colleagues, one call girl says that most "could cut your throat." Respondents frequently mentioned that they had been robbed, conned, or otherwise exploited by their call girl friends. Interpersonal distrust among call girls appears to be considerable. While respondents tend to deny that they or their fellow workers fulfill the usual conceptions of the tight-skirted, hip-swinging, customer-rolling street walkers, they do characteristically indicate that their relationships with other call girls are marked by interpersonal conflict, disloyalties, and mutual exploitation.

To more formally assess individually endorsed attitudes, we administered a rating scale to the last twenty-eight respondents, all currently active in prostitution. Each was asked to rate, on the semantic differential, herself, other call girls, women-in-general, Johns, and men-in-general

[14] It may be that the inferences are unreliable, reliable but invalid, or valid but method specific. To the degree that inference concerning such ideologies lead to valid predictions, evidence is garnered that such inferences are correct and that such occupational socialization has occurred. Conversely, the failure of such predictions suggests the conclusion that either the original inferences were incorrect or that such perspectives have little impact upon the individual actor.

(Osgood, 1957).[15] If occupational socialization occurred, then individually held attitudes toward such groups should be predictable from the occupational ideology. The three audiences of primary concern were: self, Johns, and other working girls. These groups were chosen because they appeared relevant to the girls' occupational success and because occupationally supported perspectives pertaining to them existed. If occupational socialization does occur, on the basis of the described ideology, we can predict that the distribution of attitudes toward these groups would not only not be random, but that particular groups would be more favorably evaluated than others. If the ideological justifications have the effect of reducing the girls' personal distress, the self should be rated, relative to other groups, as more worthwhile. Conversely, due to the Johns' "perverted" sexual nature and economic avarice, they should be held in relatively low esteem. Other call girls, some contact with whom is necessary in the daily round of affairs for most call girls, should be held in greater esteem than the customer. In addition to these groups, girls were also asked to rate women-in-general, and men-in-general. These ratings allow us to avoid confounding attitudes toward specific groups with those toward a specific gender. Additionally, in light of the perspective that all women are, in spirit if not in practice, prostitutes, the latter ratings also served as an additional test of the effects of socialization.

In the present study, three dimensions of attitude were measured: activity, potency, and evaluation. Insofar as the counter-morality has rather clear cut implications for evaluative perspectives, this dimension is of primary concern. In the analysis of the data, however, all dimensions were included, thus providing evidence that discriminations were being made not only across groups but across dimensions.[16]

While mean differences were found in the ratings of the groups, the rank ordering of the groups on the basis of evaluative ratings were not predictable from the occupational ideology. While the call girl rated

[15] The respondent rated each group on the following bipolar items: Good-bad, cruel-kind, valuable-worthless, fast-slow, passive-active, dull-sharp, hard-soft, large-small, weak-strong. These nine items have been shown previously to load on one of three factors subsequently labeled evaluation, activity, potency. The first three items load heavily on evaluation, the next three on activity, and the remaining on the potency dimension (Osgood, Suci, & Tannenbaum, 1957). For a more detailed description of the scoring procedures, see Bryan (1966).

[16] The method of analysis employed analysis of variance for correlated measures. See Winer (1962). Statistically reliable differences were found in the ratings of Groups ($F = 3.30$, $df = 4$), Dimensions ($F = 8.66$, $df = 2$), and Groups by Dimensions Interactions ($F = 3.78$, $df = 8$). Differences between mean ratings of the two groups was assessed by the Newman-Keuls method.

herself significantly more worthwhile than her colleagues, her ratings of self did not differ, on the evaluative dimension, from her ratings of men-in-general, women-in-general, or Johns. Only call girls were rated as being significantly less worthwhile than the self. Further, the only other group that was rated reliably as being more worthwhile than call girls were Johns. Indeed, customers were evaluated by the call girl as being as worthwhile as herself, and as significantly better than her colleagues. This particular ranking could not have been predicted from knowledge of occupational beliefs. The ratings of men-in-general and women-in-general fell just short of being reliably different than ratings of call girls.

It might be noted that call girls rate themselves as being significantly more active than either Johns or women-in-general. These findings suggest that Johns are seen as more passive than most males, and the self as busier and more active than most women.

The impact of the socialization aside, if the prostitute is exposed to some sort of uniform ideological training, then attitudes toward these groups, whatever their various nature, should be correlated with opportunities for learning. One, admittedly crude, measure of such opportunity is the time the respondent has been working as a prostitute. During the course of the interview, each respondent was asked how many months she had been working as a prostitute, and this estimate was then correlated with ratings of the groups for each dimension.

The only statistically significant correlation is the positive correlation found between time in the profession and esteem of men-in-general.[17] This correlation may be the result of attrition based upon negative attitudes toward men, subsequent changes in attitudes toward male noncustomers resulting from occupational experiences, or from chance artifacts within the data. The position held by at least some call girls however, that the longer a girl is in the occupation the harder, colder, and more hateful of men she becomes, is clearly refuted. At least for girls who stay in the "life," the current ratings do not indicate such changes in attitudes.[18]

[17] For a more complete description of the correlations found, see Bryan (1966). These findings may reflect nothing more than the respondents' adoption of the oft-discussed double standard. Whether it is generally true that women tend to rate men more worthwhile than women is still a moot point. For positive evidence, see McKee and Sherriffs (1957). For negative evidence, see Nunnally (1961). The latter investigator used the same type of questionnaire as did this author.

[18] The product-moment correlation between months in the profession and ratings of self, other call girls, and customers were .01, .03, and .00 respectively.

DISCUSSION

The available data suggest that prostitutes do not undergo occupational socialization and that sustained prostitution is not dependent upon adoption of particular interpersonal attitudes. While evidences of a "counter-morality" are ubiquitous within the interview, most respondents personally reject, both verbally and through rating scales, those evaluative dimensions of the interpersonal attitudes apparently supported by the occupation. (That this finding is not likely due to sets for socially desirable responses when talking with a "wise square" is suggested by the frequency of other "confessions" given pertaining to other criminal and immoral behavior.)

While the data indicate that there are differential attitudes toward the relevant audiences, correct predictions as to their nature were not deduced from knowledge of the occupational ideology. The respondents know the ideology but they do not endorse it. It is, of course, possible that the description of the occupational perspective may be incorrect, but the consensus in both the scientific and lay literature as to its nature hints otherwise. If the occupationally sanctioned ideology is as described, why do so many know the perspectives and yet not adopt them privately?

It seems reasonable to assume that such ideologies serve a variety of purposes for both the individual prostitute and her related audiences, and do so with varying importance over time. For example, the belief that in-group affiliations are more real, warm, honest, and right than other relationships provides for more cooperative and consequently more lucrative business, isolates the novice from influences hostile to prostitution, and provides a group in which passing and duplicity are not required of the actor. Additionally, the myth of the male's exploitative nature suits not only the economic aspirations of the novice, but also those of her trainer (Bryan, 1965). The belief that women are hypocrites and that prostitution provides a valuable social service may not only reduce moral conflicts, but serve additionally as a defense against public stigma. It has heretofore been assumed, however, that the functions of these perspectives are served with equal efficiency across the individual prostitute's career span. It appears more likely, in light of the current data, that such orientations are learned during the initial few months of her career and during her apprenticeship period, and may be taught directly by the trainer. While the professional ideology is learned and perhaps serves a function during this apprenticeship period, it is doubtful that it remains of equal importance throughout the call girl's career.

Once entrance into prostitution has been accomplished, there are many reasons to reject such beliefs. First, prostitution at the call girl level, particularly for pimpless and madamless girls as in this study, is loosely organized. While training periods do exist, the training appears more oriented toward the acquisitions of skills than ideology. Cooperative interaction with colleagues is required for only short periods of time and usually within restricted circumstances. For example, the most frequent activity of this nature is that of "putting on a show." This refers to two girls simulating homosexual activities while the customer observes. These activities, however, most often last but a short time. Additionally, many girls are usually available to a particular prostitute for this purpose, each being an actor of equal utility. No critical dependencies upon particular individuals are developed.

The everyday interaction of the call girl with her colleagues dramatically belies notions concerning her good character. Respondents are suspicious of one another, being less concerned with competition than with simple exploitation.[19] Interview data, as well as personal observation, demonstrate that extensive disloyalty and exploitation characterize the interpersonal relationships among call girls, as one girl suggests: ". . . But yet there's never a real close friendship. . . . I mean they will do anything for each other. But still at times when they're taking pills and things, they'll go against you . . . they'll slit your throat at times."

There is evidence, furthermore, that suggests that the personal acceptance of an ideology is, under certain circumstances, considerably dependent upon the affect attached to its sponsor (Elms & Janis, 1965). In light of the conflict between girls, such negative affect may mitigate against personal incorporation of the counter-moralities.

If the adoption of counter-moralities is a function of public visibility and consequent stigma, then socialization is necessarily intertwined with success in passing and the consequences of public revelation. Two questions arise. Is prostitution heavily burdened with reproach, and does the individual prostitute personally encounter such reproach in her everyday affairs? The findings of J. Nunnally (1961) that the general public holds the mental hospital attendant in higher esteem than the psychoanalyst makes any a priori assumptions of stigma or status somewhat suspect. (It is interesting to note the absence of systematically gathered data pertaining to public attitudes toward prostitutes.) Furthermore, despite general cultural sanctions, the everyday life of the call girl is, to a great extent, designed to avoid public revelation, and she is generally successful in this effort. If stigma is present, it is easily avoided. Passing is simple

---

[19] W. C. Reckless (1950) has suggested that competition disrupts group cohesiveness among streetwalkers. Competition appears to play a minor role in determining relationships among call girls in the present sample.

because so few care. Those who should care, do not. Of those who do care, most approve. Of those who do not approve, most do not care. With remarkable uniformity, respondents have indicated that there is little need to be concerned with biography control and stigma management. There are few pressures to generate a fictitious existence for purposes of family, friends, or interested parties. This need is not engendered simply because of the indifference, the resignation, or the moral support of the significant others. If perchance someone does care and might not approve, customers are readily available to provide testimonials as to the girls' moral and legal legitimacy.

Additionally, unlike the physically disabled, the heroin addict, or the effeminate homosexual, the call girl's public visibility is easily controlled. First, there are no physically obvious signs revealing that which should not be, and those sterotypes regarding dress, manner, and character of the prostitute are easily manageable. There are, then, no telltale signs readily apparent, either through stereotype or fact, of this deviant group. Further, the girl earns a living in a "back region" setting (Goffman, 1959), not being forced to deal with the day-to-day money earning activities where biographies are demanded and accounts checked. Her public appearances then can be, and often are, restricted in geography and infrequent in number.

Moreover, much of the interaction of John with girl is specifically oriented toward the reduction of the stigma attached to both roles, each pretending that the other is fulfilling a role more obscure than that which is apparent. While explicit role definitions (whore and John) are rare, when they do occur, they are delicately put, for motives more benevolent than otherwise. The call girl rarely experiences moral condemnation through interpersonal relations, thus reducing the need for justification. This may further lessen the impact of attempts at occupational socialization.

SOURCES OF STRAIN

While it has been argued that stigma, passing and duplicity are of no great moment in the life of the call girl, there are springs of personal distress that are related to occupational functioning. A major source of anxiety revolves around an act, one of the few of its kind, which is often required of the girl and which is clearly inappropriate in terms of culturally prescribed gender role behaviors. The act of consequence is that of telephoning the prospective client. To so aggressively sell yourself, to be asked to count immodestly your feminine and sexual attributes, and to reduce so markedly the fiction of masculine pursuit, turning it rather into its opposite, imposes a most frequent source of strain. While moral transgressions appear to be of little concern, such grossly inappropriate gender role behaviors are often a considerable source of embarrassment to the girl.

Also, sexual activities may in and of themselves produce anxiety. While "perversions" may give rise to amazement at best, revulsion and fear at worst, they are not by and large a significant source of personal distress. Individual encounters with customers requiring such acts live long in the memory, but these, most often well-known, clients can be avoided. Rather, it is the more common, less avoidable and less "perverted" sexual activity that is of concern; that of fondling and kissing. Objections to such activities may have economic basis (it takes longer to fulfill the contract), but another hypothesis appears more probable in accounting for these results. Such activities are frequently reported by the girls to imply a love rather than a business relationship. This, then, is giving too much, reflecting an excess in terms of the sexual contract, an asymmetry in the reciprocity relationship. Generally, the managing of this type of sexual activity, simply because of its frequency, gives rise to more anxiety than demands of anal intercourse, fellatio, and the more obvious "perversions."

The major sources of personal distress appear to be, on the one hand, the transgressions of gender role dictates, and on the other, differential expectations with regard to sexual behavior and its trappings of romance. Distress appears to be infrequently generated from moral transgressions.

While the individual call girl does not suffer from anxiety produced by passing or other duplicities, nor does she necessarily adopt an ideology alienating her from the "square" world, this does not mean that the respondents meet, by and large, those clinical stereotypes of the mentally healthy.

Perhaps the most telling source of evidence relevant to their personal adaptation is that pertaining to suicide attempts. Fifty-five percent of the respondents indicated that they had, with serious intent, attempted suicide.[20] While young women of this age are more likely to attempt

[20] This percentage is based upon a total N equal to 47. The problem of sampling bias is particularly acute with regard to this point. The respondents generally knew, prior to volunteering for the interview, that the interviewer was by profession a "mental helper" of some variety. This introduction may well have introduced a sampling bias such that those individuals who either desired some professional help or who had previously had such help would more frequently volunteer than respondents with no such desires or experiences. Certainly such a sample would yield data grossly overestimating the prevalence of "mental illness" within the population of call girls. Of the forty-eight respondents from which the data are available, 27 percent indicated a desire for some psychotherapeutic intervention; of the forty respondents for whom

suicide than either males of the same age, or females of a different age, the frequency of such attempts among the current sample is obviously extremely high (Stengel, 1964).[21] It should be noted however, that most girls and most attempts by the same girl were made prior to entrance into prostitution. It should be noted that these differences were not statistically reliable. Obviously more of the girl's life had been spent outside prostitution than within the occupation. Assuming that suicide attempts are equally likely during the adolescent and early adult years, then findings regarding pre- versus during-prostitution suicide attempts are hardly surprising. One can speculate further that the home life and the corresponding social life of the respondents produced more personal stress than that encountered after having left such controlling circumstances. Answers are not available at this time.

These findings then replicate those of Greenwald (1960), which suggested high suicide attempt rates among girls working in New York City, and further suggests that such attempts reflect personal difficulties existing prior to entrance into the occupation. It is not yet possible from the available data to determine those occupational variables associated with either reducing, stabilizing, or increasing the personal distress of the individual call girl. They are however, drawn from a population that appears to suffer considerable unhappiness.

While the practice of prostitution may be illegitimate, the aspiration to and the psychological rewards of competence are not. The interpersonal relations between John and girl may, in fact, sustain her enactment of the deviant behavior. [If college students believe their own self-flattering *deceptions* of others, that is, if the "conner" learns to believe the con (37), there is little reason to doubt that the play-love of John and girl may have positive feedback upon the latter's own self esteem.] Whether such mechanisms as these or many others support and sustain the psychic tranquility of the call girl is as yet unknown. Outside of hunches, primarily psychoanalytic in nature, regarding the motivations underlying sustained prostitution, little else is known. Studies of the interpersonal, cognitive, and situational determinants of such behavior remain to be completed.

---

information is accessible, 37 percent previously had sought some psychological aid but were not seeking such help at the time of interview. Whether this reflects the characteristic adjustment of this population remains to be seen.

[21] It should be noted that there were no statistically reliable differences in reported suicide attempts from respondents seeking and not seeking psychological help. χ^2 corrected for continuity, < 1, $df = 1$, $N = 44$. Exaggerations in such reports for purpose of therapeutic gains, therefore, seem somewhat unlikely.

As yet, there are insufficient data to indicate why the call girl does not experience more personal strain while fulfilling the occupational role. Apparently, an ideology is not needed to counteract the stigma or guilt. There does not appear to be much condemnation from either the self or the society, and the counter-moralities are not required. What sustains the girl within the occupation remains to be determined, but speculations might be offered. First, reported income is quite high and greatly exceeds her worth on the legitimate market, a point that Davis (1937) made long ago. The frequently stated source of worry among the general population is infrequently faced by the individual call girl (Gurin, Veroff, & Feld, 1960). Perhaps more important, however, is the fact that it appears very difficult to function inadequately within the occupation. Negative feedback from the customer to the girl is quite rare, while tangible signs of her adequacy, both sexual and otherwise, are frequent. While she may occasionally feel guilty, the call girl rarely reports being unable to cope with her vocation. On the contrary, she often feels that she is among the most skilled and the most adequate of the occupation.

REFERENCES

Becker, H. S. *Outsiders: Studies in the sociology of deviance.* New York: Free Press, 1963.

Becker, H. S. (Ed.) *The other side.* New York: Free Press, 1964.

Benjamin, H. Prostitution reassessed. *International Journal of Sexology,* 1951, **26,** 154–160.

Benjamin, H., & Ellis, A. An objective examination of prostitution. *International Journal of Sexology,* 1955, **29,** 100–105.

Bryan, J. H. Apprenticeship in prostitution. *Social Problems,* 1965, **12,** 287–297.

Bryan, J. H. Occupational ideologies and individual attitudes of call girls. *Social Problems,* 1966, **13,** 441–450.

Bullough, V. L. Problems and methods for research in prostitution and the behavioral sciences. *Journal of History Behavioral Sciences,* 1965, **1,** 244–251.

Caprio, F., & Brenner, D. *Sexual behavior: Psycho-legal aspects.* New York: Citadel Press, 1961.

Clinard, M. D. *Sociology of deviant behavior.* New York: Rinehart & Co., 1957.

Cloward, R. H. Illegitimate means, anomie, and deviant behavior. In B. H. Stoodley (Ed.), *Society and self.* New York: Free Press, 1962. Pp. 360–379.

Cohen, A. K. The study of social disorganization and deviant behavior. In R. K. Merton, L. Broom, & L. S. Cottrell (Eds.), *Sociology today.* New York: Basic Books, 1963.

Cressy, D. R. Social psychological theory for using deviants to control deviation. In *Proceedings of the Conference on the use of products of a social problem in coping with the problem.* Norco, Calif., July, 1963.

Davis, K. The sociology of prostitution. *American Sociological Review,* 1937, 2, 744–755.

Elms, A. C., & Janis, I. L. Counter-norm attitudes induced by consonant versus dissonant conditions of role playing. *Journal of Experimental Research in Personality,* 1965, 1, 50–60.

Gergen, K. J. The effects of interaction goals and personalistic feedback on the presentation of self. *Journal of Personality and Social Psychology,* 1965, 1, 413–424.

Glaser, D. Criminality theories and behavior image. *American Journal of Sociol.,* 1965, 61, 433–441.

Glover, E. The abnormality of prostitution. In A. M. Krich (Ed.), *Women.* New York: Dell Publishing Co., 1953.

Goffman, E. *The presentation of the self in everyday life.* New York: Doubleday Anchor Books, 1959.

Goffman, E. On cooling the mark out: Some aspects of adaptation to failure. In A. M. Rose (Ed.), *Human behavior and social processes.* Boston: Houghton Mifflin Co., 1962. Pp. 482–505.

Goffman, E. *Stigma.* Englewood Cliffs, N.J.: Prentice-Hall, 1963.

Greenwald, H. *The call girl.* New York: Ballentine Books, 1960.

Gouldner, A. The norm of reciprocity: A preliminary statement. *American Sociological Review,* 1960, 25, 61–178.

Gurin, G., Veroff, J., & Feld, S. *Americans view their mental health.* New York: Basic Books, 1960.

Hollander, M. H. Prostitution, the body, and human relations. *International Journal of Psychoanalysis,* 1961, 42, 404–413.

Hooker, E. The homosexual community. *Procedings XIV International Congress of Applied Psychology,* 1961, 40–59.

Hooker, E. An empirical study of some relations between sexual patterns and gender identity in male homosexuals. In J. Money (Ed.), *Sex research: New development.* New York: Holt, Rinehart and Winston, 1965.

Karpf, M. Effects of prostitution on marital sex adjustment. *International Journal of Sexology,* 1953, 29, 149–154.

Kitsuse, J. I. Societal reaction to deviant behavior: Problems in theory and method. *Social Problems,* 1962, 9, 247–257.

Lindesmith, A. R. *Opiate addiction.* Evanston, Ill.: Principia Press, 1955.

McKee, J. P., & Sheriffs, A. C. The differential evaluation of males and females. *Journal of Personality,* 1957, 25, 356–371.

Maurer, D. W. *The big con,* New York: Signet Books, 1940.

Milgram, D. Some conditions of obedience and disobedience to authority. *Human Relations,* 1965, 18, 57–76.

Miller, D. R. The study of social relationships: Situation, identity, and social interaction. In S. Koch (Ed.), *Psychology: A study of a science*. Vol. 5. New York: McGraw-Hill, 1963.

Mowrer, O. H. *The crisis in psychiatry and religion*. Princeton, N.J.: D. Van Nostrand Co., 1961.

Mowrer, O. H. *The new group therapy*, Princeton, N.J.: D. Van Nostrand Co., 1964.

Nunnally, J. C. *Popular conceptions of mental health*. New York: Holt, Rinehart and Winston, 1961.

Oliver, J. F. *Sexual hygiene and pathology*. Philadelphia: J. B. Lippincott Co., 1955.

Osgood, C. E., Suci, G. J., & Tannenbaum, P. H. *The measure of meaning*. Urbana, Ill.: University of Illinois Press, 1957.

Reckless, W. C. *The crime problem*. New York: Appleton-Century-Crofts, 1950.

Reiff, P. *Freud: The mind of the moralist*. New York: Viking Press, 1959.

Reiss, A. The integration of queers and peers. *Social Problems*, 1961, **9**, 102–120.

Robinson, W. J. *The oldest profession in the world*. New York: Eugenics Publishing Co., 1929.

Sanford, N. Personality: Its place in psychology. In S. Koch (Ed.), *Psychology: A study of a science*. Vol. 5. New York: McGraw-Hill, 1963.

Scheff, T. J. The role of the mentally ill and the dynamics of mental disorder: A research framework. *Sociometry*, 1963, **26**, 436–453.

Southerland, E. H. *The professional thief*, Chicago: University of Chicago Press, 1937.

Southerland, E. H., & Cressey, D. R. *Principles of criminology*. (5th ed.) Philadelphia: J. B. Lippincott Co., 1955.

Stengel, E. *Suicide and attempted suicide*. Baltimore: Pelican Press, 1964.

Sykes, G., & Matza, D. Techniques of neutralization: A theory of delinquency. *American Sociological Review*, 1957, **22**, 664–670.

Winer, B. J. *Statistical principles in experimental design*. New York: McGraw-Hill, 1962.

Winick, D. Prostitutes' clients' perception of the prostitute and themselves. *International Journal of Social Psychiatry*, 1961–1962, **8**, 289–297.

4.7 Orientation

Bohemians and their way of life are not a new phenomenon. Each generation in America seems to find a new way of rebelling, Bohemian fashion, against what are considered to be unjust social mores or the restrictive middle class values of the larger society.

In this article, L. Douglas Smith presents the results of an intensive study of the "Beats" from the North Beach area of San Francisco, a colony which was subjected to considerable public exposure and comment in 1958 and 1959. It is a psychological study in which the central question is whether the movement represents positive social deviance or a problem in collective pathology. In presenting his information, Smith represents a group of social scientists who find that the mirror image of contemporary social problems is often reflected in the social causes supported by deviant groups, and that there are often larger benefits to be gained from their rebellion.

4.7   The "Beats" and Bohemia: Positive Social Deviance or a Problem in Collective Disturbance? [1]

L. Douglas Smith

Bohemia, at different points in history, may lie in Greenwich Village, North Beach, The Left Bank, or Venice West. The people who are identified as Bohemians—Baudelaire, Poe, Utrillo, Kerouac, O'Neill— change. The ideas expressed and championed by Bohemians—Democracy, Communism, Pacificism, Freudianism, Existentialism, Positivism, Theism, Atheism—also change to some extent. However, the general *Geist,* and the behavior that reflects this spirit, remains the same through the history of Bohemia. It is a spirit of cynical, iconoclastic, rebellious, nonconformity to the currently accepted values, mores, and behavior of the rest of society. As far as the rest of society is concerned, Bohemians drink too much, talk too much, make love too frequently and too indiscriminately, are addicted to narcotics, and do not bathe often enough.

The center and meeting place of the Bohemian community is, typically, a coffeehouse. It is located in a district where the buildings are old and run down and the rents are cheap. The non-Bohemian inhabitants of the district are usually only marginally related to the rest of society in terms of their cultural, racial, or national backgrounds. The Bohemians stand in sharp contrast to their neighbors. They are, usually, products of the mainstream of society, coming from upper and middle class families, well educated, expressing a lively interest in the arts, philosophy, and other intellectual pursuits. While his neighbor is trying to attain and

[1] I wish to acknowledge a debt of gratitude to the authors and publishers for permission to use copyrighted material from The Real Bohemia, by Francis J. Rigney and L. Douglas Smith, copyright 1961 by Basic Books, Inc., Publishers, New York.

adopt the values and other trappings of the major culture, the Bohemian is trying to divest himself of these values and trappings.

Why does the Bohemian denounce and disown the values and behaviors of his cultural origin? Is it because he has special insight and critical faculties which allow him to see the sham and hypocrisy of society? Or is it because he has a character disorder and is unable to internalize cultural values and function within the social system? In an attempt to understand the nature and character of Bohemians, the present author took part in a study of the Bohemian community of San Francisco's North Beach in 1958 and 1959 (Rigney & Smith, 1961).

The study consisted of the observation and analysis of the social behavior, interview material, literary productions, and test responses of fifty-one (thirty-three men and eighteen women) of the approximately 180 Bohemians living in North Beach during this period. Each of the fifty-one subjects participated in from four to eight hours of individual testing, including the Rorschach, selected cards from the Thematic Apperception Test (TAT), the Minnesota Multiphasic Personality Inventory (MMPI), and the California Psychological Inventory (CPI); in addition, each subject was given a lengthy life history interview. One member of the research team (Dr. Rigney) acted as a "participant observer" at many of the social functions held in the community. The tests were scored and interpreted by the present author and many were submitted to other clinical psychologists for their views and interpretations. (A more detailed account of the research methodology and findings may be found in Rigney & Smith, 1961.)

Although Bohemians have been living peacefully in the North Beach area for many years, it was in 1958 that they began to receive a great deal of attention from the press, and the notoriety from this resulted in increased attention from the public and the police. As the newspapers chronicled the exploits of these members of the "beat generation," or "beatniks" as they were termed, a stereotype was formed. The newspapers began to picture the North Beach Bohemian as a shaggy, unkempt, unwashed, drug-using, poetry spouting, free-living, free-loving delinquent. The philosophy of the beat generation was depicted as one of nihilism, apathetic withdrawal from society, emotional noninvolvement, but including a frantic search for sensory stimulation and excitement. This philosophy, it was suggested, was the result of a generation of people disillusioned by the values of a materialistic and conforming society and living in the menacing shadow of "The Bomb." But many saw this philosophy as merely an excuse to avoid social responsibility and lead an uninhibited, wanton life. The patois of the Bohemian ("cool," "dig," "like," "man") was regarded as a verbal attempt to avoid meaningful communication. Overall, the idiosyncratic dress, behavior, attitudes, and mores of these Bohemians were viewed not as nonconformity, but as slavish devotion to the standards of a cult, the rebellion of adolescents in a frenzied search for identity.

The present article addresses itself to the problem of distinguishing the Beat phenomenon as either a problem in collective disturbance or as a sign of positive social deviance. These categories, of course, are not mutually exclusive, and the assignment of the Beats to one or the other depends on one's perspective, values, and orientation.

Most writers agree that the Beat Bohemians are an alienated sub-culture in American society. McGee (1962) indicates that the Beats are a disorganized group manifesting alienation and anomie, or a lack of structure and norms with which the individual in the group can guide his behavior. The alienation of the Beats is demonstrated by their feelings of powerlessness, meaninglessness, cynicism, and isolation. A person so alienated from society feels himself to be a pawn being manipulated by forces beyond his control; he may be aware of the rules by which the game is being played, but he does not understand these rules, he does not believe that the game is really being played by these rules, and he does not think very highly of the rules anyway. An individual or group so afflicted should behave in a highly random, irrational, and disorganized manner. However, a group that had no guidelines or norms for their behavior would have little positive effect upon society. Society's only reaction to such a group would be to isolate and control it. For some, the sole contribution of the Beats to American culture was that of reading poetry to jazz, and for many, this is of dubious value. In the past, Bohemians have been leaders or, at least, in the vanguard of those bringing about cultural changes. If we assign the Beats to Bohemia we must, if only on the basis of historical precedent, take a closer look for more important and lasting contributions of the Beats to American culture.

It would appear that the Beats were one of the first groups of modern times who could criticize the "American Way of Life" without being denigrated with the label of "Communist." They showed that it was possible to disapprove of the "system" without being organized and directed by a foreign power. By espousing and practicing racial brother-hood, pacifism, and what may be more sensible approaches to drug addiction and sexual morality, they have taken stands on issues that are now more openly supported by more responsible groups and individuals. Goodman (1960) adds that "they are a kind of major pilot study of the use of leisure in an economy of abundance." In my view, the major contribution of the Beat Bohemian, at this time, is that he has questioned, publically, passionately, and persuasively, a system of values that all too many of us have accepted without a murmur of protest.

While the question of the positive influence of the Beat Bohemian on our culture is one that is still open to discussion and debate, the question of the Beat phenomenon as one of collective disturbance is more easily answered. Goodman suggests that the Beat is a product of the middle class system, dominated by his mother and with a weak identification with his father. He further indicates that the Beat has withdrawn from the values of the middle class home but has not grown into other worthwhile values. In a study of the case histories of fifty-one North Beach Bohemians it was discovered that the majority of this group were products of middle or upper class homes and had been exposed to the value system of middle class American society. The degree and area of rejection of these values varied from individual to individual. There were serious artists and writers, who, while dressing casually in the Beat fashion and occasionally seeking new experiences from drugs, followed rigorous schedules and devoted most of their time to their work. These also seemed to lead fairly conventional sex lives, being either married or mostly celibate. There were unwed mothers who spent most of their time and energy in supporting and caring for their children. There were also married mothers who spent much of their time and energy in supporting and caring for both their husband and their children, but who also had occasional and controlled experiments with narcotics. At the other extreme, there were men and women whose behavior and appearance evidenced little or no guidance by middle class standards, but whose extreme unhappiness and misery could have derived from the fact that they still evaluated themselves by these standards.

While there was little evidence of strict adherence to parental moral codes, the Beat Bohemians seemed to be involved in a search for a better model of identification than that provided by their parents and a moral code that would guide their relations with other people as people, but not with other people as society. Some of the poetry they wrote suggests an identification with Christ, whom they saw, with his gentle ways, sandaled feet, beard, tolerance for others, his simple life, and his disregard for some of the social conventions of the times, as the prototype of the Beat Bohemian.

The high degree of communality among those interviewed and tested was quite impressive. They all seemed intelligent, sensitive, displayed an active interest in one or more art forms, and were nonconformists in terms of one or more of the standard American values. Equally impressive, however, was the amount of variety and individualism they displayed; they very definitely had not been stamped from the same mold. An analysis of the test results of the fifty-one subjects revealed the presence of subgroups of people having similar patterns in their MMPI profiles. This discovery led to a "Bohemian typology" consisting of six types, four male and two female. These types were named the "Passive Prophets," "Earnest Artists," "The Lonely Ones," "Tormented Rebels," "Beat Madonnas," and the "Angry Young Women." [2]

These six categories can be grouped under two major headings according to the degree of psychopathology present in their MMPI profiles. Three groups, the Angry Young Women, the Tormented Rebels, and the Lonely Ones, have MMPI profiles indicative of psychopathology or character disturbance to a marked degree and suggestive of an inability to function under conditions of social stress. The other three groups, the Beat Madonnas, the Passive Prophets, and the Earnest Artists, have MMPI profiles suggestive of only mild character disturbance at the most and indicating that these people had the capacity to adjust to most social demands and the ability to function under most conditions of normal stress.

TORMENTED REBELS

The Tormented Rebels exemplify the popular conception of the Beatnik. In their personal lives and behavior they are rebellious, nonconforming, iconoclastic, sexually promiscuous, heavy drinkers, frequent users of drugs (usually marijuana), and usually unemployed. Each has artistic pretensions (poets, writers, musicians, actors), but ratings of their abilities range from "tops" to very poor. They are intellectually ambitious, wishing to do something creative, but their enthusiasms burn out quickly and their artistic output is irregular. Their relationships with others, particularly with women, were judged to be shallow, erratic, and exploitive.

Clinical analysis of the test results of the Tormented Rebels was in

[2] The MMPI profile criteria, established for each group, were as follows: Tormented Rebels: F over 65, D below 60, Pd, Mf, and Sc over 70, Ma over 65. The other scales could vary, but only one other clinical scale could exceed 70. The Lonely Ones: F, D, Pd, Mf, Pt, and Sc all over 70. The other scales could vary. The Angry Young Women: Pd, Pa, Sc, and F all over 70; Mf below 50. The other clinical scales had to be above 60. The Earnest Artists: Mf above 65; Ma was allowed to exceed 70, but all the other scales had to be below 70, with Pd, Sc, D, and Pt below 65. The Passive Prophets: Pd and Mf above 65; Ma was allowed to exceed 70, but all other clinical scales (and F) had to be below 65. The Beat Madonnas: Pd and Ma were the only clinical scales allowed to exceed 70, and Pd had to be above 65, Mf had to be below 50; Sc, Pa, Pt and D had to fall below 65.

complete agreement with observations of their behavior and the interview material. Many of their test responses were unusual and suggested a lack of concern for convention and social reality. Their major interest seems to be in the immediate satisfaction of their own needs, with little thought or consideration for the needs of others or the consequences of their behavior. One man, in responding to the TAT, wrote the following story:

This man has killed the woman he loves in a fit of jealousy and rejection. After strangling her he has fondled her lustily. He now regrets his action, fearing the consequences of discovery and prosecution. Although he has no regrets (he would do it again) he wishes she were alive and responsive. He is a victim of emotions and circumstances.

While the tests supported the view that they were rebellious, nonconforming, irritable, unable to bind tension or delay gratification, and shallow in their interpersonal relationships, they also gave some clues as to the sources of their attitudes and behavior. These were disturbances in parent-child relationships and a consequent failure to establish a strong masculine sexual identification. In the Thematic Apperception Test, mother-son relationships were pictured as scenes of unhappiness and grief, with the mother viewed as a shallow, self-centered person who lacked understanding. The fathers appeared as distant and authoritative. Problems in sexual identification appeared in their responses to the Rorschach where one man saw the inkblots as a series of portrayals of the undeveloped sexual organs of young girls and boys. Another gave this response:

It's a dilly. I'll give it to you straight. It's a mother and father pulling apart in two opposite directions. The figure in the center is split and he has his hands upraised in protest . . . a person wearing a dress . . . or maybe not . . . wearing either woman's or man's attire . . . the mother is pulling it into the feminine world. The child is uncertain which role to assume. . . . The parents don't realize the suffering of the child or its desires . . . a perfectly normal attitude for parents to have.

In the Tormented Rebels it is quite possible that social protest and nonconformity to social norms and standards are manifestations of severe psychological disturbance.

LONELY ONES

Another group of men who appeared to be suffering from severe personality problems were the "Lonely Ones." These men are "Beat" in the sense of beaten down; they are lonely, unattached, aloof, preoccupied wanderers, and filled with dispair. In an attempt to cope with crippling anxiety, all of the men in this group used both alcohol and drugs; five were alcoholics, three were addicts (heroin), and seven of them had been patients in mental hospitals. The test results indicated that they have a great deal of difficulty in establishing relationships with other people, and those that are established are strongly motivated by dependency. They seem to distrust women, only three of the eleven had married, and only one was married at the time of the study; six of them had had homosexual relationships. Their artistic productions (six were writers, three were painters, and two were jazz musicians) varied in both quantity and quality, and their output seemed related to the degree of severity of their symptoms. When their tensions were under control they could be fairly productive, but when they were not, all work ceased and they sought relief in alcohol, drugs, or hospitalization.

The most striking feature about these men, and the one that most differentiated them from the Rebels, was the high degree of passivity and ambivalence with which they met the world. These qualities are vividly portrayed in their TAT stories. One man wrote the following:

Two lovers facing some insurmountable inadequacy between them. It is not sexual, but rather exposed in the light of sex. She is taut, unsatisfied, sees no solution except the blankness of the wall. He is distraught, ashamed, undecided. They are sensitive.

Another characteristic of these men is their distrust of close relationships with others and their failure to find satisfaction in their relations with people. In response to another TAT picture showing a man and a woman together, one man wrote:

He is accustomed to being self-contained and has just admitted to a guilt feeling. She is a girl whom he just met and she is trying to console him without any real conviction, and he has just realized her basic lack of concern and is angry with both himself and her for having revealed himself to her. He will leave and she will be relieved that he has.

As this story suggests, these men find little comfort in intimate relationships; instead they feel misunderstood, rejected, and betrayed.

ANGRY YOUNG WOMEN

The "Angry Young Women" are also characterized by severe personality problems. Like the Lonely Ones, they are crippled by tension and anxiety. But their behavior alternates between explosive, hostile outbursts and depression, hopelessness, and self-pity. Unlike the men, they drink sparingly and are not drug users. Most of their rebelliousness and acting-out behavior is expressed in their sex lives. They appear to seek tenderness and love in their sexual relations, but they equate sexuality with violence, and their affairs end unhappily. They try to play the martyr role, frequently giving the impression that they have been put upon, taken advantage of, and hurt. Their love affairs are disappointing to them and usually end by the boyfriend's walking out, leaving them despondent, demoralized, and sometimes, pregnant. The Angry Young Women are attracted to the Rebels and the Lonely Ones, and they all seem to be looking for closeness and tenderness, yet they are unable to accept it when they find it and they are unable to give it in return. By selecting their lovers and companions from among people like themselves, they run no risk of finding tenderness and love, but they do find a substitute in the form of sexual relations and physical contact.

The attitudes of the Angry Young Women toward interpersonal relationships in general, and sexual relationships in particular, were revealed by their responses to the projective tests. One girl responded to the Rorschach with the following:

Looks like different kinds of animals . . . fighting or fornicating. Having great . . . some great thing is happening to them. Elephants or rhinoceroses . . . two large creatures . . . joined together physically and spiritually.

Another girl wrote the following TAT story:

Louise came home to find her lover had fled from her possessiveness . . . she flipped, calmly put the gun neatly in her purse and left to seek him . . . finding him in the place . . . she shot 3 times, fell to the ground, wept, recovered, put the gun to her temple and ended it . . . finally.

Parental relationships were also difficult and strained. One girl responded with the following to the Rorschach:

Mother and daughter on two different circuits or universe . . . searching for one another . . . No real communication . . . They're not really connected. They're searching for contact and communication. The dark represents a barrier. Growing away from one another . . . If it continues they will be worlds apart.

To the "sex" card of the TAT another girl wrote, "The father has killed his daughter."

Another girl wrote the following story to the same picture:

This virile old father of course thinks incest abhorrent; however, his wife is old and weary, his daughter fresh and beautiful. He's having trouble in this scene, but he'll make it . . . a good cat. Obviously that intelligent if he'll hang a painting and read those books.

The six women in this group were better known for their displays of emotion than they were for their artistic abilities. Although they described themselves as painters, actresses, poetesses, or writers, none were particularly productive and they were given low ratings in both the quantity and quality of their artistic work.

For the Lonely Ones, the Tormented Rebels, and the Angry Young Women, Bohemianism is a mode of social adjustment. For them, Bohemia is a marginal society, a permissive "open air mental hospital," where demands on personal behavior and conformity to social norms are markedly less than those made in standard middle class society. Many of the individuals in these three groups had gravitated to North Beach and the Bohemian existence because they were unable to function anywhere else in our society. In North Beach they found companionship, tolerance, freedom, and an opportunity to play social roles that were not available to them elsewhere. In addition to this, they had the opportunity to work and display whatever talent they possessed, and some of the individuals in these groups were quite talented and creative, although somewhat erratic in their artistic output.

The seeds of their maladjustment were planted early, and, for many, blossomed during adolescence, under the stress of puberty. Many of them felt cheated and embittered by life; they had been caught and twisted by forces beyond their control. The Tormented Rebels and Angry Young Women seem to have problems of impulse control. They act out sexual, aggressive, and dependency impulses in ways that are not acceptable to the rest of society. Their anger and rebellion toward society seem to be a neurotic outgrowth and displacement of their anger toward their parents.

The Lonely Ones, however, crippled by anxiety and fear, have withdrawn from society; even their adjustment to Bohemia is tentative and transitory. They fade in and out of Bohemia like gray shadows against the wall. When they are feeling fairly well they "make the scene"; when they are not feeling well they hole up in their rooms or go to the mental hospital. But even when they feel well, their behavior is bizarre and unusual enough not to be acceptable in anything other than a very tolerant community. One man, blatantly schizophrenic, delusional and hallucinating, functioned and was accepted in this community for seven years following his escape from a mental hospital.

The individuals within these three groups have severe disturbances in interpersonal relations; they are alienated from other people, and their alienation from society is secondary to this. They came to North Beach, not in the spirit of social protest, but out of the necessity for personal survival. The choice of the Bohemian existence is forced upon these people; it is the only way they can function as members of society.

EARNEST ARTISTS

The other three groups display less pathology in their test responses and greater control in their overt behavior. The seven men in the Earnest Artist group are, by far, the most productive on the Beach, they are serious about their artistic endeavors and quite industrious. They are gain-fully employed (musicians, janitors, and so on), and in addition receive money for their artistic productions. They tend to enjoy high status in the Bohemian community. They are well known within the group, pop-ular, and are spokesmen and leaders in matters of significance to the com-munity. They demonstrate discretion and control in their use of alcohol and drugs (almost all had tried marijuana or peyote; three had tried heroin, one jazz musician had been addicted to heroin many years earlier, but all were "clean" at the time of the project). Four of the men were married, three were not; all had had sexual relations with women and some had had homosexual relations also. Their life histories, while not without periods of stress or emotional disturbance, are generally more stable and contain less acting-out behavior than the histories found in the previous groups. Their arrival in North Beach was not as the result of a frantic escape from society or a search for "kicks," but, rather, the culmination of a search for an artistic community where they could work and study.

Their test results reflected this greater integration and control. The tests revealed a tendency for them to approach problems rationally and intellectually rather than with blind emotionality. Although their rela-tions with others are somewhat cold and distant, they are not self-centered and exploitive. The men in this group display more social re-sponsibility, although they are quite critical of many social institutions. One man in responding to the TAT wrote

I feel that I am supposed to feel that the younger man is feeling shame for some schmutzing deed, shame brought on by the noble words of his noble and long-suffering mother; but I have seen this scene enacted too frequently in movies, plays, bad novels, and high-pressure sermons, and too seldom in life, to feel anything about it other than mild amusement.

Another wrote

The older man is one who has lived a full and wise life, perhaps in the field of science or the humanities; he is passing his wisdom on to a young man who will not accept the burden that his elder has taken upon himself. . . .

Their muted tones of social criticism and control over their deviance from social norms are due, perhaps, to the greater degree of inner peace and tranquility they experience. Unlike the Rebels and the Lonely Ones, they are not compulsively driven to prove their masculinity and their intellectual capability. One of the TAT responses of this group was

This is a healthy situation . . . a young man . . . perhaps an artist, has just thrown open the windows of his studio and is taking the fresh air and looking into the sky . . . with anticipation. Though he is at peace . . . he feels that there is something there he cannot yet see.

PASSIVE PROPHETS

The Passive Prophets are similar to the Earnest Artists in that they exercise greater control over deviant behavior. The five men in this group drink sparingly, and only occasionally "experiment" with the milder drugs (marijuana and peyote). In terms of their artistic-occupational endeavors, they are largely nonproductive, they are writers who seldom write, actors who rarely act, artists who do not paint. Their major preoccupation is commenting, in a dogmatic and pedantic fashion, upon the social scene. Their main product is words. They are witty, cynical, intellectually pretentious, and verbose. Their responses to the TAT were on the order of the following:

Here are two philosophers having a profound conversation regarding the nature of freewill versus determinism. The older man has convinced the other that his theory about determinism is more valid.

Watson Lautrec, world's foremost authority on Mongolian Pornography, came home from a busy evening of research at the local branch library, and discovered, much to his delight, a beautiful nude woman asleep in his bed. He was so astonished that he rubbed his eyes to see if it were not just some trick of fancy.

In their relations with others they are, like the Earnest Artists, controlled in their emotions and distant, but they are also self-centered and somewhat exploitive. Since their words have little retail value, they live off others, wives, girlfriends, or just plain "scrounge" from friends. The quality of overcontrol, intellectualizing, and distant interpersonal relations comes out in this TAT story:

This couple have just about come to the end of their relationship. She has no desire to have sexual relations, although the man still possesses a strong desire to make love to her. They have had to stay together in this room because they are on a trip intending to get a divorce and have stopped off at some friends' home. And do not wish their situation to be known to them. She is unconsciously attempting to hurt him by sleeping nude, knowing he will have the desire to manifest a sexual advance, and then be rejected by her.

Although at the time of the study the men in this group demonstrated control over their emotions and behavior, for some this had not been the case in the past, and neurotic acting out had been a feature of their behavior. This group did not seem to have the comfort and inner peace of the Earnest Artist group. The Passive Prophet longs for intellectual recognition, but seems to be blocked in producing anything by which he can achieve this recognition.

BEAT MADONNAS

The Beat Madonnas, like the previous two groups of men, exercise some control over their behavior and they are the housewives of North Beach. However, they add "Kulture" and "Kicks" to the typical *Hausfrau* interests of *"Kinder, Kirch, und Küchen."* Of the eight women in this group, five were married and worked to help support their husbands and/or children. Their husbands were of the Earnest Artist variety of Bohemian. All of the women in this group have some artistic or creative outlet (they are dancers, writers, painters, or actresses). However, none seem particularly interested in achieving fame or fortune in her field and each tends to see her efforts as a hobby or pleasant spare time activity, subordinate to the maintaining of a home or helping her husband in his field.

All of the Beat Madonnas drink, but with control; two had tried peyote, five tried marijuana, and three had tried heroin (one of these was addicted for a year while still a teenager). In their sexual behavior they seem to be less promiscuous and certainly more discreet than the Angry Young Women. All indicated that they had premarital sexual experiences, but only two indicated that they had had an illegitimate pregnancy. None of them reported having extramarital affairs.

Their responses to the projective tests indicated that these girls were much less intellectualizing and overcontrolled than the men in the Earnest Artist and Passive Prophets groups. While they are in close touch with their feelings, they exercise some control and do not act out on the basis of emotions alone. Some of their responses to the TAT reflect these qualities.

The mood is one of depression, dejection and hopelessness. . . . This is my brief story . . . A woman feeling alone . . . unwanted and unloved feels like hiding at this moment . . . perhaps she will stay like this or perhaps she will take a deep sigh and start to do something to change the things that are oppressing her.

It is evening and autumn in a large city. The sun has just gone down and the lights are beginning to show. The man is sitting in the window, watching . . . with much pleasure. Perhaps he will later take a walk through the evening crowds, people going to the theatre, etc., etc. . . .

Like the Earnest Artists, the Beat Madonnas are not driven compulsively to act out neurotically or impulsively, they are more at peace within themselves.

The young girl is sitting on the floor in her friend's apartment listening to a moving piece of music on the phonograph. She is carried off into another world by the music.

The Beat Madonnas are much more conventional in their attitudes toward sex than any other group studied and there were indications that they had some inhibitions and feelings of guilt concerning this area of life. Some of these feelings are revealed in the following TAT stories:

The man has feelings of guilt after having been to bed with the woman who is asleep. He feels unclean and just wants to get away, his mind is filled with many thoughts and he is unable to move to the door at this second. In a moment he will walk out into the cold night and continue to walk to a quiet lonely place and think until daybreak.

This could be entitled "Sir! How dare you think that of me!" . . . A girl has come to a producer's apartment to render a reading of "East Lynn" and is shocked when the producer has more basic desires than of judging her acting ability.

The life histories of at least some of these women suggested, however, that sometime prior to their coming to North Beach their behavior was less conventional and under less control, but even then their behavior lacked the self-destructive quality found in the histories of the Angry Young Women.

These last three groups did not come to North Beach seeking asylum and escape from a cruel or indifferent society. Their coming to Bohemia may have been an act of rebellion, but it was a rational and deliberate rebellion. These people appeared to have internalized some set of standards which served to guide and control their behavior even in this permissive and, reportedly, licentious society. Some of the men in this group seemed to have formed some degree of identification with a parent, probably their mother. This identification expressed itself as artistic interest, rather than compulsive heterosexual and/or homosexual behavior.

CONCLUSIONS

The results of this research suggest that most of the questions that can be raised about the Beats and Bohemia can best be answered only with a qualified yes or no. Many of the people we encountered in this segment of Bohemia displayed signs of severe psychological disturbance, and much of their deviant behavior derived from this disturbance. However, we cannot dismiss the whole group as a bunch of nuts and crackpots, since there were many who behaved in a rational, organized, and purposeful manner. Whether or not their behavior, or any part of their behavior, represents positive social deviance is even more difficult to answer. We must first look at the areas in which they deviate. Deviations in dress, manner, and speech can be dismissed as superficial and of little consequence. The important areas of their deviance seem to lie in the fact that they were largely nonproductive in a production-and-success oriented society, that they practiced racial tolerance, or racial indifference, in a society where racial discrimination is still the norm in either overt or covert behavior, they were pacifists in a nation that maintains one of the strongest military forces in the world, they used narcotics which are illegal and vigorously suppressed, and they practiced sexual freedom in a society where monogamy and stringent sexual morality are the ideal, if not the norm. Let us discuss each of these in turn.

In American society, for a person to be accepted as an artist, poet, writer, or composer, he must either be making a great deal of money at it or it must be only a hobby or sideline to some other major occupational role. In Bohemia he is regarded as a writer even if he has never published a book, an artist even if his pictures are unsold, a composer even though his tunes are not whistled or hummed, or a poet even if his verses do not rhyme. It is true that many idlers and wastrels hide under these titles, but it is also true that many hard working, serious, and talented men and women are practicing their arts even though their efforts go unrecognized and unrewarded by society. For this latter group this class of behavior represents a positive social deviance.

For most Bohemians, racial tolerance is merely a matter of evaluating other human beings on the basis of qualities other than skin color or ancestry, but for some it is a matter of compulsive "crow-jimism." For the first group, the practice of racial tolerance is a sign of positive social deviance. For those in the second group, it is a sign of psychological disturbance, but I feel that it is certainly no more pathological than the violent displays of racism accepted as the norm in many parts of America today.

Their beliefs in pacifism may be motivated by personal cowardice, by denial and repression of their own feelings of hostility, or by true altruistic concern for other human beings. It would seem to me, however, that, whatever their motivation, pacifism is more a sign of sanity and responsible social behavior than the advocation of destruction and war.

Narcotics seem to be employed by many Bohemians to find peace and to supply tranquility to a troubled mind. For others it is a source of exciting new experience and release from inhibitions for a jaded personality. Still others experiment with drugs in an attempt to widen and deepen their experience of art, symbolism, and reality. For this latter group, the use of drugs could conceivably represent a manifestation of positive deviant behavior.

Freedom and license in sexual behavior undoubtedly represent different things to different Bohemians. For some it is blind rebellion against parental and societal norms for conduct. For others it is a shallow substitute for warmth, love, physical closeness, and acceptance. For still others it is necessary proof to quiet nagging doubts regarding their worth and masculinity. Finally, for some it is one expression of the love they felt for another human being.

Most Bohemians manifest some evidence of direction and guidance in their conduct in most areas. For some the direction comes from rebellion and negativism toward social standards. For others it is the result of rational consideration and reflection upon alternatives of moral behavior, the individuals sometimes deciding for and sometimes against societal norms. But for only a few is their behavior so chaotic that it could be determined only by the impulsive whims of the moment.

Bohemia is a venerable and necessary institution in Western civilization. It serves as a self-supporting asylum for the emotionally disturbed, a training school, workshop, and experimental laboratory for the artistic, a spawning and testing ground for new and radical social ideas and practices, and a voice of criticism and dissent in a conforming society.

Although the North Beach Bohemian group has done much protesting, this was rarely done in any organized or directed fashion. In no sense could they be thought of as a "protest movement" that had banded together for the purpose of making their complaints and criticisms heard. Their motivations for coming to this community varied from individual to individual, but there are communalities in attitudes and behaviors; and they protested in unison, but not in coordination, and they were without organization and leadership in their protests.

The voice of the Beat Bohemian has apparently passed from the American scene. Although many of the original group still live in North Beach or in nearby Sausalito and they lead much the same life as they did nine years ago, they no longer receive the notoriety they once did. The attention of the police, press, and public in San Francisco is now focused on another North Beach phenomenon, the topless swim club and other bare-bosomed entertainment. However, the influence of the Beat is still being felt in society, particularly on the college campus, where students seem to have adopted, openly, the values, mores, and behavior of the Beats. Many of the issues, questions, and criticisms raised by the students today are the same as those that concerned the North Beach Bohemian a decade ago.

REFERENCES

Goodman, P. *Growing up absurd.* New York: Vintage Books, 1960.
McGee, R. *Social disorganization in America.* San Francisco: Chandler Publishing Co., 1962.
Rigney, F., & Smith, L. *The real Bohemia.* New York: Basic Books, 1961.

chapter five

Nature-Nurture and Perspectives on Pathology

5.1 Introduction

Repeated pronouncements to the contrary notwithstanding, the so-called nature-nurture controversy remains very much alive. As those who delight in quoting the Greeks seldom fail to point out, the fundamental opposition of man's nature and his environment intrigued the ancients as much as it does modern geneticists. And, the puzzles of classical times have continued to be puzzles. John Locke's seventeenth-century phrasing of environmentalism spoke of the infant as being *tabula rasa*. Ashley-Montagu represents a common modern view that babies are not simply born blank, they are born innately good. Man, many would have it, is never born bad —his environment makes him so. Gobineau and Galton are among the most notorious of those who took an opposing view, seeing man's nature as set, not infinitely malleable. Contemporary versions of this view continue to appear, as for example, in the recent conclusion of the eminent ethologist, Konrad Lorenz, who has found that man shares with animals "an instinct of aggression." What is more, the controversy is not without its political overtones, for, as Pastore ("The Genetics of Schizophrenia") has shown, political liberals almost unanimously have environmentalist views, whereas conservatives are often hereditarians.

Present scientific consensus has it that the conflict between nature and nurture is no more than the collision of two illusions—that all genotypes

594

are influenced by the environment, and that the only proper understanding resides in the interaction of the two. That is, man—whatever his primate nature may be—can only be understood in the context of his relations with other men in a social and cultural environment. This perspective, the social system perspective, has become dominant, and as it has done so, the biological nature of man has been neglected. It has been said that if one gives a small boy a hammer, he will find that everything needs hammering. The social system perspective, too, can be employed with uncritical enthusiasm. Nietzsche warned us of the "dogma immaculate of perception," and we would do well to remind ourselves that the social system perspective is not the only perspective that can be taken upon man's mental disorders.

We do not want to throw out the force of the social world. Far from it. This whole book is devoted to explicating the force of this perspective. We continue to believe, for example, that social systems do indeed have the power to program man to suffer all manner of disorders, including what we call the neuroses. But, for more serious disorders, such as the psychoses, particularly that chimera called schizophrenia, we urge a second look. We would caution the sciences of man as a social and psychological being not to forget that man is also an animal, and that man's immense plasticity and sensitivity to his social and cultural surroundings should not becloud the fact that he is also a host for microorganisms, the victim of sundry toxins, and that his primate heritage includes heritable disorders of many sorts. Furthermore, men *differ* in all these regards.

In the articles that follow, we will begin with a discussion of genetics and psychopathology (Murray and Hirsch). Those who lack familiarity with genetics will find a basic introduction in this article. We move next to a discussion of sexuality, first in animals (Whalen) and next in humans (Rosen). In both instances, we are concerned with dimensions of the nature-nurture puzzle. For our final concern, we examine schizophrenia. First we hear from John Weakland, a prominent adherent of the Bateson family system approach to schizophrenia. As with the approaches of Lidz and Wyman, the Weakland-Bateson view is a social system—or family system—perspective. Our last article is radically different. Bernard Rimland argues, both humorously and persuasively, that schizophrenia should be seen, not as having its origins in the social world of man, but in man's biology. We believe that Rimland's challenge to psychogenesis—and the social system perspective—is not to be shrugged off. The biogenesis of schizophrenia must be taken seriously, and not only by biochemists and geneticists, but by social scientists as well. Only then will our perspective on mental illness be complete.

5.2 *Orientation*

Most professionals in mental health fields, imbued as they are with psychosocial explanations of mental illness, possess little knowledge of the genetic basis of disordered behavior, let alone an understanding of the basic principles of human genetics that have been discovered in recent years. "The purpose of this article," to quote the authors, "is to examine some of the evidence relating to hereditary factors in psychopathology, and to suggest some new directions, based on modern concepts in behavior genetics, that might be followed in future research."

Harry G. Murray and Jerry Hirsch provide us with a clear and concise description of the important research on hereditary and psychopathology. They preface their presentation with a highly readable summary of basic behavior genetics to place their concluding material in proper perspective. This chapter is primary reading for anyone who has not kept himself current in the field of the genetic basis of psychopathology.

5.2 Heredity, Individual Differences, and Psychopathology

Harry G. Murray and Jerry Hirsch

The layman has known for centuries that "insanity runs in families." In the last fifty years, this observation has been confirmed by evidence of a more objective sort; we now know that several types of mental disorder are transmitted along family lines. However, the question of whether mental disorders are transmitted by genetic or by cultural channels has been a source of heated controversy, and this controversy has in turn been a source of unnecessary restrictions in genetically oriented research on psychopathology. The purpose of this chapter is to examine some of the evidence relating to hereditary factors in psychopathology, and to suggest some new directions, based on modern concepts in behavior genetics, that might be followed in future research. As a background to this discussion, it will first be necessary to review some basic principles of genetics.

HEREDITY AND INDIVIDUAL DIFFERENCES

Heredity is both a conservative agent, which ensures the continuity of species and the resemblance of parent and offspring, and an agent of innovation which generates widespread diversity both within and between species. Our primary emphasis in this chapter will be upon the differentiating role of heredity and its relevance to individual differences in human behavior.

Genetics may be broadly defined as the study of relations between genotypic and phenotypic levels of biological organization. An organism's *phenotype* includes all of its morphological, physiological, and behavioral traits. Underlying this phenotype is a *genotype,* the organism's complete endowment of genes and chromosomes, which is received at conception and subsequently replicated in every cell of the body. The primary data of genetics are phenotypic variations, or individual differences, among organisms (for example, variations in coat color in mice, variations in IQ in man); and the methods of genetics are designed to evaluate the manner and extent to which these variations are related to genotypic diversity. Modern genetics assumes that an organism's phenotype is a joint product of its genotype and its environment, and that individual differences are a function of both genotypic and environmental differences among organisms.

Behavior-genetic analysis is the approach to the study of organisms and their behavior that combines the concepts and methods of genetic analysis, based on knowledge or control of ancestry, with the concepts and methods of behavioral analysis from psychology and ethology, based on knowledge or control of experience. It makes an important contribution to psychology and related disciplines in its treatment of individual differences in human and animal behavior. The usual approach in psychology and psychiatry is either to disregard individual differences completely, by treating them as random deviations in the behavior of a hypothetical average organism (represented by such convenient abstractions as the group learning curve, and "the schizophrenic . . ."), or to attribute individual differences exclusively to differential environmental influences. This approach is inappropriate whenever all organisms of all species do not obey the same general laws, or when organisms raised in the same environment do not exhibit the same behaviors. Behavior genetics treats individual differences as biologically inevitable facts of life, and attempts to understand the relations between genotypic and phenotypic diversity.

Genes and Gene Action

The functional unit of heredity is the *gene*. There are probably between 10,000 and 50,000 genes in every human cell (Spuhler, 1948), each of which occupies a specific locus or region on one of forty-six chromosomes. The *chromosomes* are threadlike structures which occur in homologous pairs in the nucleus of the cell. Genes exist in alternative forms, called *alleles,* which represent differences in the chemical effects of a gene. Some genes have several alleles, while for others only two have been identified. At a chromosomal locus each gene exists in duplicate, in that separate alleles of the gene, which may be the same or different, occupy corresponding regions on the two homologues of a chromosome pair.

Chromosomes consist of three chemical substances: proteins, deoxyribonucleic acid (DNA), and ribonucleic acid (RNA). DNA is believed to be the fundamental material of the genes. According to Watson and Crick (1953), the DNA molecule consists of two long strands twined about each other in the form of a double helix. Although it is not yet possible to translate individual genes into structural units of DNA, it has been suggested that the hereditary instructions carried by a gene are coded in the linear arrangement of chemical bases along the strands of the DNA molecule.

Genes exert their effects by regulating the synthesis of proteins in the cell cytoplasm. The major class of proteins in which gene action has been analyzed is the enzymes, which control the rates of chemical reactions carried out by the cells. These reactions combine in a series of steps to carry out the complex metabolic and physiological processes of the body. The manner in which genes and their primary products influence the development of human intelligence, personality, and psychopathology is not understood in detail, but it must be assumed that the pathways between genetic and behavioral levels are complex and indirect, involving a large number of genes and a complicated network of physiological processes.

The Transmission of Genes

The mechanisms by which genes are transmitted from parent to offspring ensure substantial genotypic variability among members of sexually reproducing species. The principles of gene transmission, therefore, provide our most fundamental basis for understanding and dealing adequately with individual differences in human behavior.

We have described chromosomes as threadlike structures which occur in homologous pairs in cell nuclei, genes as specific chromosomal loci concerned with specific chemical activities, and alleles as the alternative ways in which the chemical activity may be carried out. Genes are transmitted from parent to offspring by way of *gametes,* or sex-cells. Gametes are formed by the division of somatic cells, a process known as *meiosis.* The essential result of meiosis is that the two members of a chromosome pair separate, each going to a different gamete. Thus, human gametes contain twenty-three unpaired and nonhomologous chromosomes. Reproduction occurs when a female gamete (called an ovum) is fertilized by a male gamete (sperm) to form a *zygote.* This union combines two sets of unpaired chromosomes to form one set of paired chromosomes, one member of each pair being of maternal origin and one being of paternal origin. In this way each parent contributes 50 percent of his own genotype to each offspring.

Since the zygote receives a paired set of chromosomes—each parent contributing one member of every pair—it also receives a pair of alleles at every chromosomal locus. If both homologues of a chromosome pair carry the same allele at a particular genic locus, the individual is said to be *homozygous* for that gene. If different alleles are received at a particular locus, the individual is said to be *heterozygous* for that gene. As an illustration we can consider a gene with two alleles, T and t, which in humans controls the ability to taste phenylthiocarbamide (PTC). To homozygotes with the alleles TT, the compound has a bitter taste in solution, whereas to homozygotes of genotype tt, it is tasteless. The fact that heterozygotes are phenotypically indistinguishable from TT homozygotes indicates that the activity of the T allele masks that of t, preventing the latter from expressing itself in heterozygous combination. Masking alleles are said to be *dominant* over the alleles whose effects they cover, while masked alleles are said to be *recessive.* For some genes neither of two alleles is dominant, so that the heterozygote shows a form of the trait that is approximately intermediate between the homozygous forms.

We have noted that the two homologues of a chromosome pair segregate to different gametes during meiosis. Thus, an individual who is heterozygous for the taster gene (Tt) can produce two types of gametes with respect to that gene, that is, gametes carrying the T allele and gametes carrying the t allele. A mating between two such heterozygotes (Tt x Tt) can produce offspring of three different genotypes, namely TT, Tt, and tt, in the expected ratio 1:2:1, as each parent will produce both types of gametes in equal numbers and these will combine randomly in the formation of zygotes. The expected ratio of tasters to nontasters among the offspring is 3:1. The expected ratios of genotypes and phenotypes among the offspring of other types of matings can be calculated by entering the types of gametes produced by male and female parents along separate axes of a 2 x 2 table, and representing genotypes of the offspring

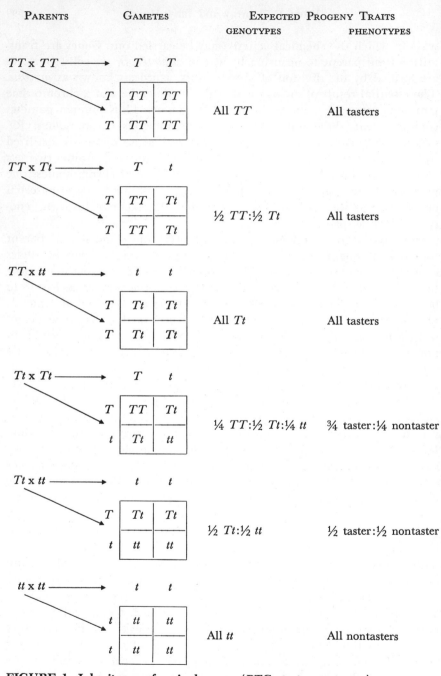

PARENTS	GAMETES	EXPECTED PROGENY TRAITS	
		GENOTYPES	PHENOTYPES

TT x TT ⟶ T T

	T	T
T	TT	TT
T	TT	TT

All TT — All tasters

TT x Tt ⟶ T t

	T	t
T	TT	Tt
T	TT	Tt

½ TT:½ Tt — All tasters

TT x tt ⟶ t t

	t	t
T	Tt	Tt
T	Tt	Tt

All Tt — All tasters

Tt x Tt ⟶ T t

	T	t
T	TT	Tt
t	Tt	tt

¼ TT:½ Tt:¼ tt — ¾ taster:¼ nontaster

Tt x tt ⟶ t t

	t	t
T	Tt	Tt
t	tt	tt

½ Tt:½ tt — ½ taster:½ nontaster

tt x tt ⟶ t t

	t	t
t	tt	tt
t	tt	tt

All tt — All nontasters

FIGURE 1. Inheritance of a single gene (PTC: taster-nontaster).

by cells. The expected outcomes of several types of matings are shown in Figure 1. Observations of this sort on pea plants were the basis of Mendel's first law of inheritance, the *law of segregation.* Mendel postulated that each phenotypic trait of his plants was governed by a separate pair of "elements," which somehow divided and then recombined when a plant produced offspring. We now know that these elements are the allelic forms of genes, and that meiotic cell division is the basis of their segregation.

Mendel's second law of inheritance, the *law of independent assortment,* describes the simultaneous inheritance of two or more traits. During meiosis the segregation of homologous chromosomes to gametes occurs independently for each pair of chromosomes, so that all combinations consisting of one homologue from each chromosome pair are equally likely in the gametes. Thus, alleles located on separate chromosome pairs also segregate independently to gametes, and traits related to them combine independently in the offspring. For example, an individual heterozygous for each of two genes located on different pairs of chromosomes (for example, *TtAa*) will produce four types of gametes with respect to the two genes, namely *TA, Ta, tA,* and *ta.* A mating between two double heterozygotes (represented by a 4 x 4 table in Figure 2) will produce offspring of

TtAa x *TtAa* ⟶	*TA*	*Ta*	*tA*	*ta*
TA	*TTAA*	*TTAa*	*TtAA*	*TtAa*
Ta	*TTAa*	*TTaa*	*TtAa*	*Ttaa*
tA	*TtAA*	*TtAa*	*ttAA*	*ttAa*
ta	*TtAa*	*Ttaa*	*ttAa*	*ttaa*

Expected distribution of genotypes and phenotypes, assuming dominance at both loci:

PIGMENTED TASTERS	ALBINO TASTERS	PIGMENTED NONTASTERS	ALBINO NONTASTERS

$$9\begin{cases}1\ TTAA \\ 2\ TTAa \\ 2\ TtAA \\ 4\ TtAa\end{cases} : 3\begin{cases}1\ TTaa \\ 2\ Ttaa\end{cases} : 3\begin{cases}1\ ttAA \\ 2\ ttAa\end{cases} : 1\ \{ttaa$$

FIGURE 2. Mating of double heterozygotes for two independent genes.

nine different genotypes. If T and t are the alleles of the taster gene, and A and a are the alleles of the gene that produces albinism in man (AA and Aa individuals have normal pigmentation, aa's are albinos), the expected distribution of phenotypes is a 9:3:3:1 ratio of pigmented tasters, albino tasters, pigmented nontasters, and albino nontasters.

The principle of independent assortment of chromosomes guarantees genotypic variability among members of a species, because it maximizes the likelihood that gametes will receive unique sets of chromosomes. A species with two pairs of chromosomes, Aa and Bb, will produce gametes containing four alternative sets of homologues, namely AB, Ab, aB, and ab; while three pairs of chromosomes (Aa, Bb, and Cc) will produce eight alternative gametes: ABC, ABc, AbC, Abc, aBC, aBc, abC, abc; and four pairs of chromosomes will produce sixteen types of gametes. In general, n pairs of chromosomes produce 2^n alternative gametes. Man, with twenty-three chromosome pairs, produces gametes with any of $2^{23} = 8,388,608$ alternative sets of homologues. Thus, when a pair of parents have two offspring (other than monozygotic siblings) the probability that the second will have the same genotype as the first is $(\frac{1}{2}^{23})^2$, or less than one chance in 70 trillion. The probability that unrelated individuals will have the same genotype is effectively zero.

Thus it becomes clear why individual differences are found in human populations. Humans are intrinsically variable before they undergo differentiating experiences, and individual differences in behavior are inevitable when unique genotypes encounter different environments. Thus, our answer to the question, "What do genes determine?," is that genes provide an a priori basis for phenotypic diversity in animal and human populations. We must remember, of course, that genes, not behaviors, are inherited. The task of behavior genetics is to discover what role inherited gene differences play in observed behavioral differences.[1]

Polygenic Inheritance

So far, we have assumed that phenotypic traits are determined in either-or fashion by single genes. Although the variation of some traits has been found to be governed by single genes (for example, in humans, ability to taste PTC, albinism, blood types), others have been found to

[1] This discussion has assumed the integrity of the individual chromosome from one generation to the next. Actually, in the course of meiosis, chromosomes sometimes break, exchange parts, and then recombine—a process known as *crossing-over*. This process increases the potentialities for genotypic variation, because it permits the alleles of genes located on a particular homologue to segregate independently.

depend on the combined effects of a number of genes acting together. These are called *polygenic* traits, and the complex of genes involved is known as a polygenic system. Generally, single-gene traits are those that can be classified into a few sharply defined qualitative categories (for example, taster versus nontaster), whereas polygenic traits show continuous variation on quantitative dimensions. The genes in a polygenic system may be located on the same or on different chromosomes. Each gene in the system is assumed to behave as a discrete unit and to obey the usual rules of transmission (for example, segregation, independent assortment, crossing-over). However, the contribution of each gene to variation of the trait is small and cumulative rather than all-or-none. The action of a polygenic system is analogous to the simultaneous tossing of a large number of coins, where the alleles of each gene (assuming only two per gene) represent heads or tails, and the value of the phenotype represents the number of heads. The result is continuous variation among members of a population.

Nature and Nurture in Modern Genetics

Forty years ago it was fashionable to classify all behavioral traits as either "due to heredity" or "due to environment." This dichotomy was the basis of the infamous nature-nurture controversy, which generated such absolute all-or-none statements as, "Our conclusion, then, is that we have no real evidence for the inheritance of traits" (Watson, 1930, p. 103); and, "There is no escape from the conclusion that nature prevails enormously over nurture . . ." (Galton, 1883, p. 241). Despite its persistence in some quarters the nature-nurture controversy is seen to be both fallacious and obsolete when considered in the light of modern genetic principles.

When applied to the individual organism, the question of whether a trait is "due to heredity" or "due to environment" is completely meaningless, because without heredity there is no organism, and without an "appropriate" environment the organism does not survive to display the trait. With respect to a population of individuals, however, it is meaningful to ask how much of the observed variation of a trait is related to genotypic differences among individuals, and how much to environmental differences. In the language of genetics this is equivalent to estimating the *heritability* of a trait—the percentage of trait variance that is attributable to genotypic differences among individuals. Even at this level we must not expect absolute answers, because heritability is a measure of the relationship between a trait and the population in which it is studied, not a constant property of the trait per se. Thus, the same trait that *must* have zero heritability in a clone (for example, a set of genetically identical plants or animals) *might* have substantial heritability in a heterogenic group of organisms. Similarly, human intelligence, as measured by a given test, may have quite different heritabilities in different populations (as a function of the range of genetic and environmental diversity that exists in those populations); and it may have different heritabilities in the same population under different conditions (for example, the equalization of educational opportunities should serve to *increase* the heritability of intelligence by minimizing environmental sources of variation). Although this principle is fairly obvious, it is frequently ignored, as in statements asserting that a particular trait is "60 percent genetic and 40 percent environmental." One important implication of the heritability concept is that we can understand the genetic basis of individual differences only by understanding the genetics of populations.

Genes in Populations

The term *Mendelian population* refers to a community of interbreeding individuals that is reproductively isolated from other individuals of the same species. Thus, rabbits inhabiting a forest in Norway, rabbits in Pennsylvania, Negroes in Rhodesia, and Caucasians in Rhodesia are four separate Mendelian populations, or isolated breeding units. Dobzhansky (1951, p. 15) has emphasized that a Mendelian population possesses "a corporate genotype," namely its genetic structure, which, although clearly a function of the genetic composition of its individual members, nevertheless obeys its own laws of functioning "distinct from those which govern the genetics of individuals." These laws of genetic structure are the subject matter of *population genetics,* which studies relations between the distribution of genes and the distribution of individual differences in trait expression in Mendelian populations. Of particular importance are mechanisms responsible for change in gene distributions, as these underlie the process of Darwinian evolution in natural populations, and provide a theoretical framework for analysis of the genetic correlates of individual differences in experimental populations.

The central concept of population genetics is that of the *gene pool,* which may be defined as the totality of alleles carried by members of a breeding population, or briefly, the population genotype. If we assume that matings among members of a population occur on a purely random basis, then the formation of a zygote represents the random combination of two samples of alleles from the gene pool. Thus, if alleles A and a of a gene have relative frequencies p and q in the gene pool ($p + q = 1$), the proportions of AA, Aa, and aa genotypes in the population will be p^2, $2pq$, and q^2 respectively—the binomial expansion of $(p + q)^2$. As long as matings occur at random among these genotypes, the relative frequencies of both alleles and genotypes will remain constant in succeeding generations of the population. This principle, known as the *Hardy-Weinberg law*, is a fundamental concept of population genetics, because it specifies a base-line against which the effects of change-producing mechanisms may be evaluated.

The mechanisms responsible for change in the genetic structure of a population include selection, mutation, inbreeding, and assortative mating. *Selection* refers to the existence of a correlation between genotype and reproductive capacity. If individuals of genotype *aa* tend to produce relatively few offspring, then the frequency of *a* alleles in the gene pool will decrease over successive generations in the population, and the distribution of *AA, Aa,* and *aa* genotypes and their correlated phenotypes will be correspondingly altered. *Mutation,* the inaccurate reproduction of a gene in cell division, may create new alleles in the gene pool or modify the relative frequencies of existing alleles (for example, if *A* mutates to *a* at a faster rate, than *a* to *A*). *Inbreeding,* or consanguineous marriage, the mating of blood relatives, and *assortative mating,* the tendency of either similar or dissimilar phenotypes to mate together, represent deviations from random mating in a population. The primary effect of inbreeding is to increase the probability that offspring will inherit the same genes from both parents. Thus, with respect to a particular locus, inbreeding will increase the frequency of homozygotes (*AA* and *aa*) and decrease the frequency of heterozygotes (*Aa*) in a population, without changing the relative frequencies of *A* and *a* alleles in the gene pool. However, if *AA* or *aa* genotypes are sexually infertile, inbreeding will facilitate natural selection and thereby produce indirect effects upon the gene pool. Assortative mating may facilitate selection in similar fashion by increasing or decreasing the frequency of the phenotype upon which mating is based. This result can occur, of course, only when the phenotypic trait is (1) to some extent heritable, and (2) correlated with reproductive capacity.

Much of our present knowledge of the role of genetic mechanisms in behavioral trait variation is based on laboratory studies of synthesized animal populations. Under constant environmental conditions it is possible to manipulate experimentally the genetic structure of laboratory populations, by procedures such as artificial selection, inbreeding, and hybridization, and to measure resulting changes in behavioral trait distributions. Tolman (1924), Tryon (1940), and Heron (1935), for example, each produced strains of "maze-bright" and "maze-dull" rats by selective breeding in successive generations of a foundation population in which maze learning ability showed continuous variation. The brightest and dullest animals of each generation were selected and intermated (that is, bright × bright and dull × dull) to produce the next generation. In succeeding generations of the population, the distribution of maze-learning scores became increasingly bimodal, indicating genetic control of individual differences. Similar experiments have demonstrated response to selection of both emotionality and activity level in rat populations (Hall, 1938; Rundquist, 1933, respectively); susceptibility to audiogenic seizures in mice (Frings & Frings, 1953); and locomotion with respect to both gravity and illumination in *Drosophila melanogaster* (Hirsch & Erlenmeyer-Kimling, 1961; Hirsch & Boudreau, 1958, respectively). In all of these studies, response to selection was gradual rather than discontinuous, indicating that a large number of genes were contributing to trait variation. Many investigators have demonstrated heritabilities by measuring behavioral differences among inbred strains of various species; these results are reviewed in Hirsch (1967). A few studies have employed more sophisticated breeding procedures, such as crossbreeding of selected and inbred strains, in order to analyze behavioral variation into more refined components. Hirsch and Erlenmeyer-Kimling (1962), for example, were able to measure the contributions of individual chromosomes to geotactic behavior (that is, locomotion with respect to gravity) in *Drosophila*.

Man, of course, is not a laboratory animal and cannot be subjected to breeding experiments. Nevertheless, valuable information may be obtained by studying relations between inferred properties of the genetic structure of human populations and the distribution of behavioral traits in those populations. Human races, for example, have been to a great extent reproductively isolated populations and differ in the relative frequencies of various alleles in their gene pools. Other partially isolated populations exist as a result of economic, religious, and geographic barriers. If human populations differ in the composition of their gene pools, then we might expect to find behavioral differences among them, including differences in the expression of psychopathology. Racial differences are already well documented for at least two psychological traits—color blindness and taste blindness for phenylthiocarbamide (Stern, 1960). Other resources for population genetic analysis are provided by small, geographically isolated populations, which usually show a higher incidence of inbreeding, and by study of fertility differentials and assortative mating in larger populations. Research in human behavior genetics, including that on psychopathology, has tended to de-emphasize population genetic concepts. Most studies have examined individual differences only within the restricted framework of the traditional family and twin methods, and have been preoccupied with the goal of demonstrating heritabilities of traits. A complete understanding of the genetic basis of human behavioral variation will require the extension of traditional methods and concepts to the broader framework of the Mendelian population.

HEREDITY AND PSYCHOPATHOLOGY

The literature on the role of heredity in mental disorder is very broad, and we shall make no attempt here to exhaustively review it. Evidence of hereditary involvement has been reported in several forms of mental retardation, in all major psychoses, in several neurotic reactions and personality traits, and in criminality and homosexuality. (For general reviews, see Kallman, 1953, 1959; Fuller & Thompson, 1960; Shields & Slater, 1961.) The most direct evidence of gene effects is found in the area of mental retardation, where, for example, phenylketonuria (PKU) is understood as the homozygous recessive expression of the gene that regulates phenylalanine metabolism; Down's syndrome (mongolism) is attributed to trisomy (triplicate homologues) of chromosome #21; and Huntington's chorea is recognized as a classical single-gene dominant character.

The present discussion will deal mainly with genetically oriented research on schizophrenia. Other disorders will be cited only to illustrate particular principles or to indicate generality of findings. Schizophrenia is the most common of the psychoses, and the problems and controversies involved in elucidating its relationship to gene differences may be characteristic of other disorders as well. Behavior genetic studies of schizophrenia may be classified with respect to methodology as (1) family studies, (2) twin studies, and (3) population studies.

Family Studies

Several studies have investigated the incidence of schizophrenia in the relatives of hospitalized schizophrenics. The most extensive family data are those of Kallman (1938), who examined nearly 13,000 relatives of 1087 schizophrenic patients. Kallman's findings are summarized in Table 1. The data shown are age-corrected estimates of the incidence of schizophrenia in various categories of relatives.[2] It may be noted that the expectancy of schizophrenia is higher in all categories of relatives than in the general population, and, more significantly, the probability of schizophrenia is positively correlated with degree of kinship (that is, degree of

---

[2] Actual incidence rates are often statistically corrected (for example, by Weinberg's abridged method) to account for the fact that some relatives, although not presently afflicted, have not yet lived through the manifestation period of schizophrenia (15 to 44 years of age) and might subsequently be diagnosed as schizophrenic.

TABLE 1. INCIDENCE OF SCHIZOPHRENIA IN RELATIVES
OF HOSPITALIZED SCHIZOPHRENICS (KALLMAN, 1938)

Relationship to index cases	Age-corrected incidence of schizophrenia (in percentages)
Unrelated (general population)	0.9
Nephews and nieces	3.9
Grandchildren	4.3
Half-siblings	7.6
Parents	10.4
Full-siblings	11.5
Children (one parent affected)	16.4
Children (both parents affected)	68.1

genotypic similarity) between relative and index case. These results, as well as the high incidence of schizophrenia in the children of two schizophrenic parents, are consistent with the view that gene differences play a role in the development of schizophrenia. The family data do not unequivocally establish this conclusion, nor do they provide much support for Kallman's hypothesis that schizophrenia is inherited according to a single-gene recessive paradigm. A monogenic recessive mode of inheritance predicts incidence rates of 25 percent in siblings of schizophrenics and 100 percent in the children of two schizophrenic parents, neither of which is approximated in Table 1. Kallman dealt with these discrepancies by postulating that the recessive allele related to schizophrenia shows reduced penetrance (that is, fails to express itself in all homozygous carriers). The trouble with post hoc manipulation of penetrance values is that, given enough degrees of freedom, one can account for any set of data in terms of a particular hypothesis. In the present context, Kallman's use of the penetrance concept can probably be interpreted as an indirect way of saying that environmental factors are also playing an important role. Böök (1953) has argued for a single-gene dominant model of inheritance for schizophrenia, but, again, has found it necessary to adjust penetrance values. While there could be a certain genotype that is predisposed toward schizophrenia, its phenotypic expression might be highly dependent upon the nature of the environment to which it is exposed during development.

Other investigators (for example, Elsässer, 1952; Rudin, 1916; Schulz, 1939) have generally confirmed Kallman's data, although Pollock and Malzberg (1940) found no tendency of schizophrenia to concentrate in families. Other family studies have demonstrated that although the incidence of manic-depressive psychosis is increased in relatives of affected persons (Slater, 1963; Kallman, 1953), manic-depressives tend not to have schizophrenic relatives and vice versa (Elsässer, 1952; Kallman, 1953). These findings suggest that schizophrenia and manic-depressive psychosis are genetically distinct rather than alternative expressions of a common genotype.

Kallman's findings have been widely criticized on methodological grounds, particularly with respect to diagnosis and sampling (Jackson, 1960; Pastore, 1949). The relative unreliability of psychiatric diagnosis is well known and need not be elaborated at this point. Diagnosis becomes even more precarious when the relatives of schizophrenic patients must be classified, either by a single interview, or, in the case of persons who have died or migrated, on the basis of testimony of friends, public officials, and other laymen. Further, as Rosenthal (1963) has pointed out, the diagnosis of nonhospitalized relatives introduces a "double standard" of classification, in that the criterion of hospitalization is imposed on the diagnosis of index cases but not of relatives. This situation could be rectified in two ways: (1) by imposing the hospitalization criterion on the diagnosis of relatives, a procedure which, if applied in Kallman's study, would have yielded markedly *lower* incidence rates in the relatives of schizophrenics; or (2) by removing the hospitalization criterion from the diagnosis of index cases, a more reasonable procedure, which is proposed in somewhat modified form in the final section of this chapter.

In addition to problems of methodology, a more general difficulty is involved in the interpretation of family incidence data. This is the obvious fact that members of a family tend to experience similar environments as well as to carry similar genotypes, so that family resemblance can just as plausibly be attributed to similarity of environment as to genetic similarity. Anyone wishing to argue along these lines could cite nutritional factors, reinforcement contingencies, or cultural patterns as possible shared environmental influences. Two important points should be stated in relation to this issue. First, and most important, Mendel's law of segregation of alleles provides a substantive and a priori basis for explaining the fact that *differences* as well as similarities are found among family members. Given only the unrefined notion of environmental similarity, it is difficult to explain how a pair of brown-eyed parents can produce a blue-eyed offspring, or why some family members develop schizophrenia and others do not. Second, family resemblance data represent only one source of genetic evidence, and must be supplemented by other observations. No geneticist would argue that family correlation alone is unequivocal evidence of heritability.

Twin Studies

One of the standard methods of human genetics involves comparison of the degree of intrapair phenotypic similarity of monozygotic (MZ) and dizygotic (DZ) twins. Monozygotic twins derive from the splitting of a single fertilized ovum, and therefore are genetically identical. Dizygotic twins result from the fertilization of two ova by two sperm and are no more alike genetically than ordinary siblings; that is, they share, on the average, 50 percent of a common set of alleles. The rationale of the twin-study method is that phenotypic differences between MZ co-twins should reflect environmental influences alone, whereas phenotypic differences between DZ co-twins should reflect the combined effects of hereditary and environmental factors. Thus, with respect to a particular trait, the degree to which DZ twins show greater intrapair dissimilarity than MZ twins should indicate the degree to which variation of the trait is genetically controlled. This inference is based on the assumption that MZ and DZ twins do not differ significantly in the degree to which members of a pair experience similar environments. The validity of this assumption is subject to debate, as described below.

Kallman (1946), Luxenburger (1928), Rosanoff, Handy, Plesset, and Brush (1934), and Slater (1953) have undertaken relatively large-scale twin studies of schizophrenia. The usual procedure in these studies has involved first obtaining a sample of mental hospital patients, each of which is (1) diagnosed as schizophrenic, and (2) known to be a twin; then locating the co-twins of these patients and classifying each pair of twins as monozygotic or dizygotic, and as concordant (both affected) or discordant with respect to schizophrenia. The intrapair similarity of MZ and DZ twins may then be compared in terms of concordance rate, or percentage of pairs classified as concordant. The results of the major twin studies of schizophrenia, summarized in Table 2, have consistently

TABLE 2. CONCORDANCE FOR SCHIZOPHRENIA IN MZ AND DZ TWINS (UNCORRECTED FOR AGE)

Investigator	Number of pairs		Percent concordant	
	MZ	DZ	MZ	DZ
Luxenburger (1928)	21	60	66.6	3.3
Rosanoff et al. (1934)	41	101	68.3	14.9
Kallman (1946)	174	517	69.0	10.3
Slater (1953)	41	115	68.0	11.0

revealed markedly higher concordance rates in MZ than in DZ twins, a finding that lends further support to the view that genetic factors are significant in the etiology of schizophrenia. It should be emphasized that the concordance rates shown in Table 2 are uncorrected for age, and therefore represent overly conservative estimates of the actual difference in MZ and DZ concordances. Kallman, for example, obtained age-corrected concordance estimates of 86.2 and 14.7 percent for MZ and DZ pairs respectively, and Slater reported comparable estimates of 76 and 14 percent.

For purposes of comparison, the results of twin studies dealing with other psychiatric disorders are summarized in Table 3. These results indicate that gene differences play a major role in the occurrence of manic-depressive psychosis and male homosexuality, but a somewhat more minor role in the occurrence of suicide and psychopathic personality.

The twin studies of schizophrenia seem to provide clear evidence that variation with respect to the categories "schizophrenic" and "normal" is partly under genetic control. However, these studies have not been immune to criticism. Jackson (1960) and Rosenthal (1963) have discussed problems of sampling and diagnosis in the major twin studies of schizophrenia. These include: (1) measurement error in both psychiatric diagnosis and zygosity determination; (2) existence of a double standard in the diagnosis of index and co-twins (discussed above in relation to family studies); (3) use of indirect information (for example, testimony of relatives, photographs) in both psychiatric and zygosity diagnoses of missing or dead co-twins; (4) possible "halo" effects resulting from lack of inde-

TABLE 3. CONCORDANCE RATES IN MZ AND DZ TWINS FOR SEVERAL PSYCHIATRIC DISORDERS

Diagnosis	Investigator	Percent concordant	
		MZ	DZ
Involutional psychosis	Kallman (1953)	60[a]	6
Manic-depressive psychosis	Rosanoff et al. (1935)	70	16
	Kallman (1950)	93	24
Psychopathic personality	Slater (1953)	25	14
Male homosexuality	Kallman (1953)	98	12
Suicide	Kallman (1953)	6	0
Alcoholism	Kaij (1957)	65	30
Hysteria	Stumpfl (1937)	33	0

[a] Age-corrected; all other values are uncorrected.

pendence of psychiatric and zygosity diagnoses (the same person has typically made both diagnoses); (5) biases in favor of locating concordant pairs; and (6) sampling biases with respect to (a) proportion of MZ and DZ pairs (fewer MZ pairs than the expected MZ:DZ ratio of 1:2; see Table 2), and (b) severity of illness (index cases were sampled only from hospital populations, so that less severely disturbed cases seen in private practice and outpatient clinics were overlooked). Rosenthal points out that some of these factors have probably produced overestimation of concordance rates while others have led to underestimation. For example, inclusion of only severely disturbed index patients should inflate the MZ concordance rate, as Rosenthal has elsewhere (1961) demonstrated that the incidence of schizophrenia is much higher in the co-twins of severely disturbed than of mildly disturbed index cases. However, the shortage of MZ pairs in the twin study samples may reflect a systematic error in the direction of classifying MZ pairs as DZ, which of course would serve to increase DZ concordance rates (and decrease the MZ-DZ discrepancy). It may be that these overestimation and underestimation factors balanced each other to some extent, whereas other factors probably introduced essentially random error (for example, 1 and 3 above), or did not differentially influence MZ and DZ concordance estimates (for example, 2 and 5). For these reasons it would probably be difficult to account for the highly consistent twin study findings solely in terms of methodological artifacts.

Several writers (for example, Jackson, 1960; Jones, 1955; Smith, 1965) have questioned the validity of the fundamental assumption underlying the comparison of MZ and DZ concordance rates, namely that MZ and DZ pairs share environmental influences to an equal degree. It is suggested that MZ co-twins (1) experience more similar environments than DZ twins (are treated more alike by parents, for example), and show characteristic intrapair relations that would tend to increase their phenotypic similarity (for example, form stronger bonds of attachment than DZ pairs). Other writers have cited environmental factors that might serve to produce *dis*similarities in MZ pairs; for example, MZ co-twins apparently experience more dissimilar prenatal environments than DZ twins, as evidenced by greater intrapair differences in birth weight (Price, 1950), and in later years tend to adopt complementary social roles such as dominance-submission (von Bracken, 1936).

Jackson (1960) has argued that the twin concordance findings can be explained solely in terms of shared environmental factors and unique intrapair personal relations in MZ twins. He assumes that persons who develop "confusion of ego identity" (inability to delineate clearly the boundaries of the self) are especially vulnerable to schizophrenia and suggests that MZ co-twins, as a result of such factors as similar parental treatment and strong mutual attachment, are particularly prone to identity-confusion problems. DZ co-twins are assumed to be treated less similarly and to be less prone to identity confusion.

Fortunately Jackson's psychodynamic interpretation of the twin data is subject to empirical test. If confusion of ego identity is common in twins, and particularly in MZ twins, then one would expect the *frequency* of schizophrenia (that is, its overall incidence as opposed to its intrapair concordance) to be higher in persons who are twins than in the general population, and higher in MZ than in DZ twins. Rosenthal (1960) tested these predictions but failed to confirm them; the frequency of schizophrenia was actually lower in MZ than in DZ twins, and lower in twins than nontwins. This result strongly contradicts Jackson's identity-confusion hypothesis, and at the same time tends to preclude other interpretations of the concordance data that depend on etiological agents assumed to be associated with monozygosity (for example, premature birth, retarded language development).

One very decisive way to further verify the genetic interpretation of the twin studies of schizophrenia would be to compare concordance rates for schizophrenia in MZ twins reared apart from birth and in MZ twins reared together. If concordance remains high for identical genotypes living in different family environments, then we have strong evidence of hereditary factors. Although no large-scale study exactly fitting these requirements has been undertaken, Kallman (1946) has reported data on 59 of his 174 MZ index twins who had been separated from their co-twin for at least five years (and on the average for 11.8 years) prior to hospitalization. The age-corrected concordance rates were 77.6 percent in the separated group and 91.5 percent in the nonseparated group (versus 14.7 percent in DZ twins reared together), indicating that concordance for schizophrenia continues to be associated with genotypic similarity even when environmental similarity is attenuated.

Population Studies

Very few studies of schizophrenia have been undertaken within the framework of population genetics. There is evidence that the frequency of schizophrenia differs among Mendelian breeding populations; for example, schizophrenia is reported to be less frequent than manic-depressive psychosis in the mental hospitals of India (Dhunjibhoy, cited in Klineberg, 1954), but more frequent in the United States (Coleman, 1964), and is found to be more frequent in the upper strata of American society than in the lower strata (Hollingshead & Redlich, 1958). Studies of small isolated populations have revealed similar results. Böök (1953) surveyed an isolated North Swedish community and estimated the incidence of schizophrenia to be 3 percent (versus the usual estimate of about 1 percent in larger populations), whereas Eaton and Weil (1955) found almost no schizophrenia but a high incidence of affective psychoses among the Hutterites, an isolated religious sect living in Canada and the northern United States. All of these findings are amenable to both genetic and environmental interpretations. It is interesting that Jackson (1960), a psychiatrist, and Shields and Slater (1961), both psychiatric geneticists, give completely opposite interpretations of the Eaton and Weil study, each consistent with the author's bias. Jackson cites the study as evidence against a genetic theory of schizophrenia, claiming without further explanation, that it ". . . does not lend itself to simple genetic explanations" (p. 49); while Shields and Slater assert that ". . . the only simple explanation seems to be the genetical one" (p. 321). This contrast exemplifies the dichotomous thinking so often applied to problems in this area. Jackson's interpretation reveals a lack of familiarity with the concepts of population genetics, which lead us to expect differences in the frequencies of various alleles in the gene pools of different Mendelian populations. Shields and Slater's conclusion reveals an unwillingness to recognize such alternative interpretations as regional, cultural, or environmental conditions.

Several investigators in different countries (for example, Böök, 1953; Essen-Möller, 1935; Kallman, 1946) have found that schizophrenics show reduced reproductive fertility. Kallman, for example, reported that catatonics and hebephrenics had a marriage rate of 39.1 percent (versus 71 percent in the general population) and a birth rate per marriage of 1.4 (versus 3.3 in the general population). These findings suggest that the gene or genes assumed to underly schizophrenia should be undergoing elimination from the gene pool; yet we have no evidence of a decline in the incidence of schizophrenia. There are several possible reasons for this apparent paradox. For example, it may be that natural selection against schizophrenia is being counterbalanced by such cultural changes as increased urbanization, which probably operates to increase the incidence of schizophrenia by imposing more stressful conditions. Also, urban society is probably less tolerant of deviant behavior than is rural society, so that maladjusted individuals are more likely to be hospitalized and labeled "schizophrenic." Gottesman (1965) explains the resistance of schizophrenia to natural selection in terms of a balanced polygenic system. That is, schizophrenia is assumed to depend on many genes in such a way that persons carrying more than a critical number of adverse alleles are afflicted and selected against, whereas persons carrying less than the critical dosage are said to be inventive, imaginative, and versatile (traits often identified with the schizoid personality syndrome) and therefore to enjoy a selective advantage which serves to balance the negative selection operating above the critical level. Finally, a survey by Goldfarb and Erlenmeyer-Kimling (1962) indicates that the fertility of schizophrenics (in New York State) has been increasing since the time of Kallman's survey of the same region, so that the difference between schizophrenics and the general population is decreasing.

RECENT TRENDS AND FUTURE PROSPECTS

The family, twin, and population studies, taken together, provide cogent evidence for the role of heredity in the etiology of schizophrenia. The fact that more than fifty years of research and polemics have been devoted to this preliminary goal of "proving heredity" attests both to the methodological difficulties encountered in this area and to the persistence of the unfortunate nature-nurture controversy. However, having now succeeded in demonstrating heritability, it should be possible in future research to ask more interesting questions and employ more fruitful modes of analysis. In what follows we shall examine several recent trends and suggest several reformulations (the latter based on concepts developed in the first section of this chapter), that may prove useful in future work.

A Dimensional-Polygenic Model of Psychopathology

An important problem in behavior-genetic analysis is that of selecting phenotypic dimensions that can be measured reliably and which are likely to have some biological significance. In dealing with complex behavioral observations such as personality and psychopathology, for which there are no physical scales or obvious natural units of analysis, the investigator usually has wide latitude in his choice of descriptive dimensions. For example, there are at least three general ways in which schizophrenia can be defined phenotypically for purposes of genetic research: (1) as an all-or-none category, (2) as a continuum from mild to severe, and (3) as a combination of several more basic phenotypic dimensions.[3]

Previous investigators have usually adopted the first of these alternatives; and it can be argued that this convention has been a source of methodological and conceptual difficulties. First, the categorical approach has been associated with the use of psychiatric diagnosis as a convenient

[3] Eysenck (1961), for example, has argued that psychiatric disorders should be treated as continuously distributed traits rather than as qualitative entities, and has shown that conventional diagnostic categories can often be differentiated in terms of a combination of factor-analytically derived dimensions.

all-or-none measure of schizophrenia. The unreliability of psychiatric diagnosis has been frequently demonstrated in empirical studies.[4] The use of subjective diagnosis in genetic research has precluded both accurate estimation of parameters and unequivocal evaluation of differences between geographical areas or between time periods in the expression of schizophrenia. Furthermore, the typological nature of the diagnostic system has restricted the examination of individual differences. It may be reasonable to treat disorders such as phenylketonuria as all-or-none phenotypes, but individuals diagnosed as schizophrenic show such a diversity of symptom patterns that a finer-grained descriptive system might be of value in genetic research. There is evidence, for example, that schizophrenics, as a group, show greater variability in some traits than do "normals." Shakow (cited in Yates, 1961, p. 55) found that the standard deviation of reaction times was approximately six times greater in a schizophrenic group than in a normal group, and Payne (1961) has reported similar but less extreme results for several intellectual abilities.

The all-or-none approach has also been a source of sampling problems in genetic studies of schizophrenia, because it has encouraged the practice of sampling index cases exclusively from mental hospital populations. This procedure, as previously noted, introduces both a sampling bias with respect to severity of illness and a double standard in the classification of index cases and their nonhospitalized relatives.

Finally, the convention of defining schizophrenia in all-or-none fashion has resulted in a preference for single-gene theories of inheritance, which are both empirically and intuitively inappropriate in the case of schizophrenia. Single-gene models are appropriate for sharply discontinuous traits whose alternative expressions are closely correlated with allelic variations at a single locus. We have already noted that available data on the intrafamilial distribution of schizophrenia (for example, Kallman, 1938) do not conform neatly to single-gene models. The persistent attempt to justify these models is misleading, because it carries the implication that schizophrenia, like phenylketonuria, Huntington's chorea, and other single-gene related traits, is in some sense unambiguously "hereditary." It is more reasonable to assume that the development of schizophrenia depends on a large number of genes. This assumption is supported by the

---

[4] Ash (1949) found that three psychiatrists asked to diagnose independently fifty-two patients showed unanimous agreement in only 20 percent of cases and majority agreement in 48 percent of cases. Other investigators have reported marked disagreement among hospitals (Hunt, Wittson, & Hunt, 1953) and among geographical areas (Hoch, 1957).

results of selection studies in animal populations, which indicate that polygenic inheritance is characteristic of behavioral traits, and has the advantage of not requiring exact correspondence between genotypic and phenotypic levels.

One possible solution to the problems described above is to deal with schizophrenia in a dimensional rather than all-or-none framework, by investigating various quantitative dimensions of the disorder as possible hereditary factors, and by employing psychological tests, physical measures and other objective devices as indexes of these dimensions. On logical grounds we might expect that simple or unitary traits would be more unambiguously related to genetic mechanisms than complex or compound traits. Also, a dimensional approach would (1) avoid the equivocalities and constraints of psychiatric diagnosis, (2) provide a finer-grained descriptive system, (3) permit sampling from the population at large, and (4) justify the use of parametric statistical procedures.

The feasibility of a dimensional approach in genetic research on schizophrenia is illustrated by the work of McGonaghy (1959). He investigated the possible hereditary basis of schizophrenic thought disturbance (that is, intrusion of irrelevant and illogical associations in thought processes), which is often said to be the core symptom of schizophrenia. An objectively and quantitatively scored test of irrelevant thinking was administered to the parents of ten hospitalized schizophrenics whose test scores had indicated a marked degree of thought disturbance. Although none of the parents were either hospitalized or clinically schizophrenic, at least one parent of each patient showed schizophrenic-like thought disorder, and twelve of the twenty parents (60 percent), as opposed to six of sixty-five controls (9 percent), scored in the schizophrenic range. Lidz, Wild, Schafer, Rosman, and Fleck (1963) and Rosenthal (1963) have replicated McGonaghy's procedure and obtained similar results. These findings imply that thought disturbance, as a symptom or dimension of schizophrenia, may itself be genetically transmitted, even when parent and offspring are discordant in terms of an all-or-none definition of schizophrenia.

The McGonaghy data suggest the possibility that other dimensions of schizophrenia, and of other psychopathologies, may also behave as separate hereditary factors. The problem then becomes one of identifying basic phenotypic dimensions that both contribute to psychopathology and show evidence of heritability, and of investigating the interaction of these dimensions with environmental and cultural factors. There is evidence that individuals in various diagnostic categories frequently obtain extreme scores on basic behavioral and physiological dimensions. For example, in terms of group averages, schizophrenics are reported to show slower reaction time (King, 1954), shorter memory span (as measured by the Wechsler digit span subtest, Payne, 1961), greater conditionability of the eyeblink response (acute cases only, Taylor & Spence, 1954), less perceptual size constancy (Raush, 1952), and more pronounced EEG abnormality (Freeman, 1958) than normals. Unfortunately, little interest has been shown up to now in investigating family and twin correlations with respect to these traits.

We may generalize this discussion by representing each phenotypic dimension of relevance to psychopathology by a dimension in a coordinate space. It is likely that variation along many of these dimensions is influenced by polygenic systems, so that thousands of genes contribute to variation in the space. The conventional diagnostic categories are represented as regions or partially overlapping subspaces of the n-dimensional space. This model is similar to Eysenck's (1961) model of psychopathology, except that the dimensions of the space are selected on the basis of their biological significance, that is, the segregation of similarities and differences along family lines, rather than their statistical purity per se.

In concluding this section, we should emphasize that the identification of biologically meaningful dimensions of psychopathology will not necessarily be facilitated by the exclusive use of conventional psychological tests. The trouble with general tests of personality and intelligence is that they measure too much. That is, because of their omnibus nature and their focus on social categories, we should not expect them to be very precise measures of biological differences, which, because of the mosaic nature of the human genotype, should prove to be relatively fine grained.

Individual Differences, Populations, and Psychopathology

Ernst Mayr (1958) has described two fundamentally different approaches or modes of thought in biosocial science, namely, "typological thinking" and "population thinking" (see Hirsch, 1962). The goal of the typologist is to discover laws that describe a "typical" or "representative" organism. It is often assumed that these laws will apply to all species. The typologist ignores individual differences by treating them as imperfect replicas of the type, or, in terms of Plato's allegory, as "shadows on a cave wall." Typological thinking is prevalent in psychology and psychiatry, where it is exemplified by performance curves based on group means, by psychiatric diagnostic categories, and by Harlow's dictum that, "The obligation of the theoretical psychologist is to discover general laws of behavior applicable to mice, monkeys, and man" (1949, p. 51). The basis of population thinking is the fact that in a Mendelian population no two individuals are genetically alike. The populationist takes individual differences as biological inevitabilities rather than as "error," and recognizes that different laws of behavior may be found in different populations and in different individuals. The population concept implies, for example, that, "It is not only wrong to speak of *the* monkey but even of *the* rhesus monkey" (Mayr, 1958, p. 352). Population thinking is illustrated by the approach of behavior-genetic analysis in which the individual differences present at the moment of fertilization (that is, prior to any differentiating experiences) are understood in terms of the mechanisms that produce genetic variation (for example, meiotic segregation and independent assortment) and the mechanisms that regulate variation in Mendelian populations (for example, selection, inbreeding). In this section we shall examine more closely the implications of population thinking for psychiatry and related fields, and shall describe recent methodological developments that may permit the implementation of a population-oriented approach in this area.

Williams (1956) has discussed the practical implications of hereditary variation and hereditary uniqueness in the treatment of physical and mental disorders. His basic argument is that because every human is genetically unique, and because genes regulate biochemical reactions, we should expect each individual to show a unique pattern or sum total of biochemical characteristics. If the individual is biochemically unique, then he must also have a unique set of nutritional needs; and to the extent that pathology, including mental illness, is biochemically mediated, it is necessary to consider these unique nutritional demands in order to arrive at an optimal method of treatment. Williams has successfully applied this approach in the treatment of genetically controlled alcoholism in rats. An important implication of the "genetotrophic" approach is that it may be possible, through an understanding of genetic uniqueness and through early detection of the individual's biochemical makeup, to successfully treat disorders related to the genetic endowment by controlling the individual's environment (the nutritional intake, for example).

The principles of genetics predict behavioral differences among populations as well as among individuals, as the gene pools of reproductively isolated populations (for example, animal species, human races) have evolved in different environments and therefore may have different compositions. Thus, it may be necessary for psychiatrists to deal with patients differentially as a function of their membership in Mendelian populations based on racial, economic, religious, and geographical boundaries. This principle may have relevance for one of the most perplexing problems in psychiatric research, that of identifying the physiological correlates of schizophrenia. The literature in this area (Brackbill, 1956; Freeman, 1958) is characterized by contradiction and failure to replicate. One obvious reason for this confusion is that the physiological basis of schizophrenia may be different in different Mendelian populations, in the same way that activity level is controlled by the gonads in laboratory rats, but by the adrenals in (reproductively isolated) wild rats (Richter, 1954). Studies of physiological processes in schizophrenia may have defeated their purpose by failing to differentiate individuals on the basis of population membership. Our knowledge of animal populations forces us to recognize the possibility of population differences, not only in the distribution and expression of psychopathology, but in its "causes" as well.

Research in human behavior genetics, including that on psychopathology, has usually examined individual differences only within family units or pairs of twins, and has deemphasized population-oriented approaches. One reason for this restriction has been the practical difficulties involved in obtaining data on large numbers of individuals, or entire populations, over several generations. Recently, however, progress has been made in developing methods that permit genetic analysis of individual differences on a population-wide basis, and which facilitate comparisons among populations and among generations of the same population. These methods, which are best represented in the work of Newcombe (1959, 1962), are based on the use of preexisting data contained in routinely collected records, and on the use of modern high-speed computers in storage and treatment of data. A great deal of genetically relevant information is contained in birth and death certificates, and in school, hospital, military, workmen's compensation, health survey, and other routinely collected and centrally stored records. However, in order to maximize the value of these data for genetics research, there must be methods whereby large numbers of individual records can be grouped efficiently into family units. Newcombe has developed a computer technique that permits the linkage of each and every birth record in a given geographical area and time period to the marriage record of the parents, thus yielding family groupings on a population-wide basis. The linkage operation is based on certain items of information that appear on both birth and marriage certificates (for example, family surname, dates and places of birth of parents). For each birth record, coded on magnetic tape, the computer rapidly searches its file of marriage records until a match is achieved. Once the initial linkage of birth to marriage records is completed, data from other sources on physical and mental traits of family members (for example, school records of intellectual abilities, hospital records of illnesses) can be linked, by the same linkage procedure, to the family units. The resulting pedigrees can also be extended to more distant relatives and to previous and future generations.

In addition to providing basic information on family correlations (for example, parent-offspring or sib-sib correlations with respect to various traits), segregation patterns, and assortative mating (that is, mother-father trait correlations) in human populations, the Newcombe technique is sufficiently flexible to be applicable to several other problems in human genetics. For example, it should be possible to extend the record linkage technique to twin study designs, as both the occurrence and type (MZ or DZ) of multiple birth is commonly recorded on the birth certificate (Powell, 1962). Similarly, by utilizing information pertaining to race, socioeconomic status, and religion contained in vital and health records, it should be possible to compare efficiently trait distributions in various subpopulations within a geographical area. Moroni (1962) has used techniques similar to those of Newcombe in a large-scale study of the effects of consanguineous marriage (inbreeding) in a human population. He made use both of records of consanguineous marriages maintained by the Roman Catholic Church in Italy since the year 1535, and of military conscription records of health and anthropometric traits. Cavalli-Sforza (1962) has reported a method for estimating mutation rates in human populations that utilizes routinely collected data. Finally, techniques like that described by Newcombe should be of particular value in assessing both the presence and possible selective effects of fertility differentials with respect to behavioral traits. Natural selection is a process that can be understood only in terms of the population as a whole, and its effects are probably so small in human populations that they can be detected only by studies that sample thousands of individuals and extend over several generations. Newcombe (1963) has proposed a study, potentially of these proportions, that is designed to assess the effects of the reported tendency of high-intelligence parents to produce relatively few children (Scottish Council for Research in Education, 1949). Newcombe's study utilizes computer record linkage, school records of students' intelligence-test scores, and, in an attempt to assess and correct for trends due to environmental factors, data from the vital statistics system on social conditions within family units.

The applicability of techniques such as those described above in genetic research on psychopathology will depend on the availability of relevant and reliable data from routinely collected records. Some possible sources of data include school, military, and mental hospital records of personality and intelligence testing, and, of course, hospital records of psychiatric diagnoses. Other data of great value might be made available if objective measures of various dimensions of psychopathology were included both in the regular initial assessment of incoming mental hospital patients, and in the national health surveys regularly undertaken in several countries.

Nature-Nurture Revisited

The history of the nature-nurture controversy is almost coextensive with the literature on genetic factors in psychopathology. We may now examine some possible "solutions" to the related problems of assessing the relative contributions of nature and nurture to mental disorder, and of disentangling the effects of genetic and environmental sources of variation. The most simple solution, as Thompson (1957) has noted, is to ignore the problem. This approach assumes, perhaps rightly, that the most useful role of the behavior geneticist, given present limitations, is to accumulate information on the transmission of traits along family lines without attempting to separate genetic and cultural bases of transmission. A second solution involves the attempt to isolate the genetic component of trait variance by the study of parent-offspring correlations for foster children versus biological children, or twins reared apart, or by the use of Cattell's (1960) multiple-variance method, which estimates nature-nurture ratios from trait correlations for pairs of relatives who differ to varying degrees in both genetic and environmental similarity. Another, and perhaps more efficient, technique of this sort is to employ parent-offspring correlations with relevant environmental variables "controlled" or "held constant" by the partial correlation procedure. For example, one might measure the correlation between fathers' IQ scores and sons' IQ scores with family socioeconomic status and other environmental variables partialed out. The square of this partial correlation coefficient could then be considered a somewhat "purified" estimate of the heritability of the IQ variable in the population and generation studied.[5]

A final approach to the nature-nurture problem is one that has been advocated by several writers (for example, Anastasi, 1958), and which seeks to answer the question of *how* genetic and environmental factors interact rather than *how much* they contribute to trait variance. Very little progress has been made in dealing with the problem of "interaction," either in genetics proper or in behavior genetics. One possible approach, in the context of psychopathology, might be to examine environmental and experiential differences within pairs of MZ twins who are *discordant* for schizophrenia or some other disorder. The environ-

---

[5] The possibility of using partial correlation in this way was suggested to us by Dr. John C. DeFries, Institute for Behavioral Genetics, University of Colorado—Boulder.

mental variables for which discordant pairs show differences (and concordant pairs do not) could be the ones that are crucial in determining whether or not a genetically predisposed individual manifests the trait of interest. In a study somewhat along these lines Rosenthal (1959) found that the affected member of MZ pairs discordant for schizophrenia tended to have a poorer premorbid social and sexual history than did the nonaffected member.

REFERENCES

Anastasi, A. Heredity, environment, and the question "how?". *Psychological Review,* 1958, **65,** 197–208.

Ash, P. The reliability of psychiatric diagnosis. *Journal of Abnormal and Social Psychology,* 1949, 44, 272–276.

Böök, J. A. A genetic and neuropsychiatric investigation of a North Swedish population. I. Psychoses. *Acta Genetica et Statistica Medica,* 1953, 4, 1–100.

Brackbill, G. A. Studies of brain dysfunction in schizophrenia. *Psychological Bulletin,* 1956, **53,** 210–226.

von Bracken, H. Vererbungheit und Ordnung in Binnenleben von Zwillingspaaren. *Zeitschrift für Pädag. Psychol.,* 1936, **37,** 65–81.

Cattell, R. B. The multiple abstract variance analysis equations and solutions: For nature-nurture research on continuous variables. *Psychological Review,* 1960, **67,** 353–372.

Cavalli-Sforza, L. L. Demographic attacks on genetic problems: Some possibilities and results. In *The use of vital and health statistics for genetic and radiation studies.* New York: United Nations, 1962.

Coleman, J. C. *Abnormal psychology and modern life.* (3rd ed.) Chicago: Scott, Foresman and Company, 1964.

Dobzhansky, T. H. *Genetics and the origin of species.* (3rd ed.) New York: Columbia University Press, 1951.

Eaton, J. W., & Weil, R. J. *Culture and mental disorders.* Glencoe, Ill.: The Free Press, 1955.

Elsässer, G. *Die Nachkommen Geisteskranken Elternpaare.* New York: Stechert-Haffner, 1952.

Essen-Möller, E. Untersuchungen über die Fruchtbarkeit gewisser Gruppen von Geisteskranken. *Acta Psychiatrica et Neurologica Scandinavica,* suppl. 8, 1935.

Eysenck, H. J. Classification and the problem of diagnosis. In H. J. Eysenck (Ed.), *Handbook of abnormal psychology.* New York: Basic Books, 1961.

Freeman, H. Physiological studies. In L. Bellak (Ed.), *Schizophrenia: A review of the syndrome.* New York: Logos, 1958.

Frings, H., & Frings, M. The production of stocks of albino mice with predictable susceptibilities to audiogenic seizures. *Behaviour,* 1963, **5,** 305–319.

Fuller, J. L., & Thompson, W. R. *Behavior genetics.* New York: John Wiley & Sons, 1960.

Galton, F. Inquiries into human faculty and its development. London: Macmillan, 1883.

Goldfarb, C., & Erlenmeyer-Kimling, L. Mating and fertility trends in schizophrenia. In F. J. Kallman (Ed.), *Expanding goals of genetics in psychiatry.* New York: Grune and Stratton, 1962, 42–51.

Gottesman, I. I. Personality and natural selection. In S. G. Vandenberg (Ed.), *Methods and goals in human behavior genetics.* New York: Academic Press, Inc., 1965.

Hall, C. S. The inheritance of emotionality. *Sigma Xi Quarterly,* 1938, **26,** 17–27.

Harlow, H. F. The formation of learning sets. *Psychological Reivew,* 1949, **56,** 51–65.

Heron, W. T. The inheritance of maze learning ability in rats. *Journal of Comparative Psychology,* 1935, **19,** 77–89.

Hirsch, J. Individual differences in behavior and their genetic basis. In E. L. Bliss (Ed.), *Roots of behavior: Genetics, instinct, and socialization in animal behavior.* New York: Paul B. Hoeber, Inc., medical book department of Harper and Row, 1962. Pp. 3–23.

Hirsch, J. Behavior-genetic, or "experimental," analysis: The challenge of science versus the lure of technology. *American Psychologist,* 1967, **22,** 118–130.

Hirsch, J., & Boudreau, J. C. Studies in experimental behavior genetics: I. The heritability of phototaxis in a population of *Drosophila melanogaster.* *Journal of Comparative and Physiological Psychology,* 1958, **56,** 647–651.

Hirsch, J., & Erlenmeyer-Kimling, L. Sign of taxis as a property of the genotype. *Science,* 1961, **134,** 835–836.

Hirsch, J., & Erlenmeyer-Kimling, L. Studies in experimental behavior genetics: IV. Chromosome analyses for geotaxis. *Journal of Comparative and Physiological Psychology,* 1962, **55,** 732–739.

Hoch, P. The etiology and epidemiology of schizophrenia. *American Journal of Public Health,* 1957, **47,** 1071–1076.

Hollingshead, A. B., & Redlich, F. C. *Social class and mental illness.* New York: John Wiley & Sons, 1958.

Hunt, W. A., Wittson, C. L., & Hunt, E. B. A theoretical and practical analysis of the diagnostic process. In P. Hoch and J. Zubin (Eds.), *Current problems in psychiatric diagnosis.* New York: Grune and Stratton, 1953.

Jackson, D. D. A critique of the literature on the genetics of schizophrenia. In D. D. Jackson (Ed.), *The etiology of schizophrenia.* New York: Basic Books, 1960.

Jones, H. E. Perceived differences among twins. *Eugenics Quarterly,* 1955, **2,** 98–102.

Kaij, L. Drinking habits in twins. *Acta Genetica et Statistica Medica,* 1957, **7,** 437–441.

Kallman, F. J. *The genetics of schizophrenia.* New York: Augustin, 1938.

Kallman, F. J. The genetic theory of schizophrenia: An analysis of 691 schizophrenic twin index families. *American Journal of Psychiatry*, 1946, **103**, 309–322.

Kallman, F. J. The genetics of psychoses: An analysis of 1,232 twin index families. *Congress of International Psychiatric Rapports*, 1950, **6**, 1–27.

Kallman, F. J. *Heredity in health and mental disorder.* New York: W. W. Norton, 1953.

Kallman, F. J. Psychogenetic studies of twins. In S. Koch (Ed.), *Psychology: A study of a science.* Vol. 3. New York: McGraw-Hill 1959.

King, H. E. *Psychomotor aspects of mental disease.* Cambridge, Mass.: Harvard University Press, 1954.

Klineberg, O. *Social psychology.* New York: Holt, Rinehart and Winston, 1954.

Lidz, T., Wild, C., Schafer, S., Rosman, B., & Fleck, S. Thought disorders in the parents of schizophrenic patients: A study utilizing the object sorting test. *Psychiatric Research*, 1963, **1**, 193–200.

Luxenburger, H. Vorläufiger Bericht über psychiatrische Serienuntersuchungen an Zwillingen. *Zeitschrift für die gesante Neurologie und Psychiatrie*, 1928, **116**, 297–326.

Mayr, E. Behavior and systematics. In A. Roe & G. G. Simpson (Eds.), *Behavior and evolution.* New Haven: Yale University Press, 1958.

McGonaghy, N. The use of an object sorting test in elucidating the hereditary factor in schizophrenia. *Journal of Neurology, Neurosurgery, and Psychiatry*, 1959, **22**, 243–246.

Moroni, A. Sources, reliability, and usefulness of consanguinity data with special reference to Catholic records. In *The use of vital and health statistics for genetic and radiation studies.* New York: United Nations, 1962.

Newcombe, H. B. Intelligence and genetic trends. *Science*, 1963, **141**, 1104–1109.

Newcombe, H. B., Kennedy, J. M., Axford, S. J., & James, A. P. Automatic record linkage of vital records. *Science*, 1959, **130**, 954–959.

Newcombe, H. B., & Rhynas, P. O. W. Family linkage of population records. In *The use of vital and health statistics for genetic and radiation studies.* New York: United Nations, 1962.

Pastore, N. The genetics of schizophrenia. *Psychological bulletin*, 1949, **46**, 285–302.

Payne, R. W. Cognitive abnormalities. In H. J. Eysenck (Ed.), *Handbook of abnormal psychology.* New York: Basic Books, 1961.

Pollock, H. M., & Malzberg, B. Hereditary and environmental factors in the causation of manic-depressive psychoses and dementia praecox. *American Journal of Psychiatry*, 1940, **96**, 1227–1247.

Powell, N. Vital and population registration. In *The use of vital and health records for genetic and radiation studies.* New York: United Nations, 1962.

Price, B. Primary biases in twin studies: A review of prenatal and natal difference producing factors in monozygotic twins. *American Journal of Human Genetics*, 1950, **2**, 293–352.

Raush, H. L. Perceptual size constancy in schizophrenia: I. Size constancy. *Journal of Personality*, 1952, **21**, 176–187.

Richter, C. P. The effects of domestication and selection on the behavior of the Norway rat. *Journal of the National Cancer Institute*, 1954, 15, 727–738.

Rosanoff, A. J., Handy, L. M., & Plesset, I. R. The etiology of manic-depressive syndromes with special reference to their occurrence in twins. *American Journal of Psychiatry*, 1935, 91, 225–362.

Rosanoff, A. J., Handy, L. M., Plesset, I. R., & Brush, S. The etiology of so-called schizophrenic psychoses. *American Journal of Psychiatry*, 1934, 91, 247–286.

Rosenthal, D. Some factors associated with concordance and discordance with respect to schizophrenia in monozygotic twins. *Journal of Nervous Mental Disorders*, 1959, 129, 1–10.

Rosenthal, D. Confusion of identity and the frequency of schizophrenia in twins. *Archives of General Psychiatry*, 1960, 3, 297–304.

Rosenthal, D. Problems of sampling and diagnosis in the major twin studies of schizophrenia. *Psychiatric Research*, 1963, 1, 116–134.

Rudin, E. *Zur Vererbung und Neuenstehung der Dementia Praecox*. Berlin: Springer, 1916.

Rundquist, E. A. The inheritance of spontaneous activity in rats. *Journal of Comparative Psychology*, 1933, 16, 415–438.

Scottish Council for Research in Education. *The trend of Scottish intelligence*. London: University of London Press, 1949.

Shields, J., & Slater, E. Heredity and psychological abnormality. In H. J. Eysenck (Ed.), *Handbook of Abnormal Psychology*. New York: Basic Books, 1961.

Slater, E. The inheritance of manic-depressive insanity and its relation to mental defect. *Journal of Mental Science*, 1936, 82, 626–633.

Slater, E. Psychotic and neurotic illnesses in twins. *Medical Research Council, Special Report No. 278*. London: Her Majesty's Stationery Office, 1953.

Smith, R. T. A comparison of socio-environmental factors in monozygotic and dizygotic twins, testing an assumption. In S. G. Vandenberg (Ed.), *Methods and Goals in Human Behavior Genetics*. New York: Academic Press, 1965.

Spuhler, J. N. On the number of genes in man. *Science*, 1948, 108, 279–280.

Stern, C. *Principles of human genetics*. San Francisco: Freeman, 1960.

Stumpfl, F. Untersuchungen an psychopathischen Zwillingen. *Zeitschrift für die gesante Neurologie und Psychiatrie*, 1937, 158, 480–482.

Taylor, J. A., & Spence, K. W. Conditioning level in the behavior disorders. *Journal of Abnormal and Social Psychology*, 1954, 49, 497–503.

Thompson, W. R. The significance of personality and intelligence tests in evaluation of population characteristics. In *The nature and transmission of the genetic and cultural characteristics of human populations*. New York: Milbank Foundation, 1957.

Tolman, E. C. The inheritance of maze-learning ability in rats. *Journal of Comparative Psychology*, 1924, 4, 1–18.

Tryon, R. C. Genetic differences in maze-learning ability in rats. In *39th Yearbook of the National Society for the Study of Education*. Bloomington, Ill.: Public School Publishing Co., 1940.

Watson, J. B. *Behaviorism*. New York: W. W. Norton, 1930.

Watson, J. D., & Crick, F. H. C. The structure of DNA. *Cold Spring Harbor Symposium on Quantitative Biology,* 1953, **18,** 123–131.

Williams, R. J. *Biochemical Individuality.* New York: John Wiley & Sons, 1956.

Yates, A. J. Abnormalities of psychomotor functions. In H. J. Eysenck (Ed.), *Handbook of Abnormal Psychology.* New York: Basic Books, 1961.

5.3   *Orientation*

Research on animal behavior has contributed much to our current understanding of human behavior. It is through such research that we are able to separate more clearly those aspects of behavior that appear to be inherited, those that are the result of social learning, and those that are modifiable through re-education, even if they are dependent upon genetic factors.

This article by Richard E. Whalen offers us a better understanding of human sexual behavior through his investigations on mating behavior in rats. He immediately points out that such behavior is exceedingly complex and cannot fully be covered by the term *innate.* His investigations clarify the various effects of heredity, hormonal balance, learning, and social development (peer contact). To explain the range of variations in mating behavior, he offers a "variance" formula which accounts for the interactive effects of these variables. Systematically, and with conceptual clarity, we are led to the point of discussion of sexual deviance in animals and the relevance of this research to deviance in humans.

5.3   The Determinants of Sexuality in Animals

Richard E. Whalen

Sex is a chameleon. It changes color to fit the background upon which it rests. When sex is seen in the context of Freudian psychoanalytic theory, sex is libido, a motive force which shapes perception and behavior. When seen in the context of sociological theory, sex is gender and all those characteristics that distingush male from female. When seen in the context of animal behavior, sex is the display of those observable responses that comprise the total reproductive pattern of the species. In the present article sex is seen in this last context. This article will attempt to make explicit the ways in which genetic, hormonal, and experiential influences control and modify the frequency and timing of animal sexual responses.

THE GENETIC DETERMINANTS OF SEXUAL BEHAVIOR

It has often been said that the sexual behavior of animals is innate and determined by the genetic constitution of the animal. Michael (1961a) expressed this belief in the following way: ". . . the pattern of sexual activity shown by the female domestic cat. It is an instinctual response, it is unlearned, and, presumably, is genetically coded into the activity of the central nervous system." This somewhat traditional concept of instinct may be characterized by the following simple equation:

$$R_{\text{instinct}} = f(\text{genotype})$$

Both Beach (1955) and Lehrman (1952) have cogently argued against the use of this model of instinct. On the one hand, Beach noted that the model requires proof of the null hypothesis in each case under investigation, namely proof that the behavior is not learned. On the other hand, Lehrman pointed out that no phenotype reaches expression independent of the environment. It must be the case, according to Lehrman, that

$$R_{\text{instinct}} = f(\text{genotype}) + (\text{environment})$$

This second model provides a more realistic representation of instinct, yet it itself suffers. This model is inadequate because it does not allow one to distinguish between the contribution of genotype and the contribution of environment to the performance of a given instinctive response in a given individual. *For the individual,* genotype cannot be distinguished from environment.

A useful concept of instinct must provide a means by which genetic and environmental influences on behavior can be separated. A variance model provides for such an analysis. For example,

$$\sigma^2{}_p = \sigma^2{}_g + \sigma^2{}_e$$

where

$\sigma^2{}_p$ = variation in phenotype
$\sigma^2{}_g$ = variation in genotype
$\sigma^2{}_e$ = variation in environment

In terms of this variance model, we expect individual differences in behavior (phenotypye) to be the result of individual differences in genotype and individual differences in environment. From this model we can estimate *heritability, h^2:*

$$h^2 = \sigma^2_g/\sigma^2_p$$

Heritability is a measure of the relative contribution which genotype makes to phenotype. Heritability is, therefore, a measure of the influence one generation can have upon the next generation through genetic transmission. Is this not what we really mean by "innate"?

The major point to be made here is that discussion of the genetic basis of behavior must focus upon individual differences in phenotype and individual differences in genotype. Only within such a context does instinct become a useful concept. With this proviso in mind, we may ask what is known of the genetic determinants of sexuality. Unfortunately, for the general reader, the answer to this question will be unsatisfying. We know very little about the genetic basis of sexual behavior. Since the research in this field does not yet form a cohesive body, only selected studies that illustrate major theoretical points will be discussed.

Strain Differences

The lowest level of genetic analysis involves the comparison of genetically different strains within a single species. Such studies do not lead to conclusions about the heritability of a behavior, but they do provide information about which components of a behavior are influenced by genetic variability. For example, Whalen (1961b) compared the mating performance of males from the S1, S3, RDL, and RDH rat strains that are maintained at the University of California, Berkeley. The S1 and S3 strains had been selectively bred for high and low performance, respectively, on problem solving tasks. The RDL and RDH strains had been selectively bred for low and high brain cholinesterase levels (Rosenzweig, Krech and Bennett, 1960). It was found that the S1 males achieved intromission with a shorter latency, and achieved intromission on a higher proportion of mounts than did the S3 males. The most striking difference between these strains, however, was in the amount of stimulation needed to produce ejaculation. The S1 males ejaculated after 14.6 intromissions while the S3 males ejaculated after only 7.1 intromissions.

The RDL and RDH males did not differ from each other on any measure of sexual performance. Both of these strains did resemble the S3 males in the amount of stimulation needed for ejaculation.

In a study of the same type, McGill (1962) examined the mating performance of three strains of mice. These strains were found to differ from each other on twelve of the sixteen behavioral measures taken. The C57BL males exhibited shorter intromission and ejaculation latencies than did the males from the other two strains. The DBA/2 males were characterized by few intromissions prior to ejaculation, and the BALB males were noted for the relative slowness with which they achieved ejaculation.

Using the guinea pig, Valenstein, Riss and Young (1954) also found strain differences in mating performance. These investigators examined the behavior of two highly inbred strains and one genetically heterogeneous strain of guinea pig. Using a complex "sex drive score" to describe the mating of these animals, they found that the inbred animals possessed a lower sex drive than the heterogeneous males. When the discrete components of the mating were compared, they found that the inbred family #2 males differed from the inbred family #13 males on some components (nuzzling, mounting, and ejaculation) and not on other components (sniffing and intromission).

Each of these studies of strain differences in mating demonstrates clear differences in mating performance in strains known to differ genetically. In each case, however, the strains were found to *not* differ from each other on some of the many facets of sexuality which were measured. These studies make it clear that sex is not a unitary dimension which is controlled in some simple way by genetic constitution. Since all facets of the behavior do not vary in the same way and to the same degree with variations in genetic structure, it would be meaningless to say that the sexual behavior of the male rat (or mouse, or guinea pig) is innate. One is forced to say, rather, that particular components of a complex mating pattern are relatively strongly (or weakly) influenced by gene action. These studies make it eminently clear, furthermore, that an adequate genetic analysis of a behavior requires precedent detailed analysis of the components of the behavior.

Selective Breeding

A more sophisticated genetic analysis of sexual behavior employs selective breeding techniques. In the simplest experiments of this type the sexual performance of two strains is measured. The males and females of these two strains are then interbred and their offspring studied. Finally, these F1 animals are bred back to their parent strains (backcrosses) and the offspring again examined. These procedures allow one to make reasonably accurate estimates of the genetic determinants of a behavior pattern.

Using this paradigm, Jakway (1959) and Goy and Jakway (1959) studied the sexual performance of male and female guinea pigs. These analyses indicated differential genetic controls over different components of the mating patterns. With respect to the males, it was shown that the circling, nuzzling, and mounting scores that are characteristic of the strain #13 males are inherited in a dominant fashion and that the intromission rate and ejaculation frequency characteristic of the strain #2 males exhibit genetic dominance. These data indicate that at least two different genetically controlled mechanisms contribute to the mating performance of male guinea pigs.

It was further found that three distinct genetically determined mechanisms modulate the mating performance of female guinea pigs. Measures of the latency of heat (in response to estrogen and progesterone injections), the duration of heat, and the percentage coming into heat were found to be consistently correlated and presumably controlled by the same mechanism. The duration of the lordosis response, the concave arching of the back which signals receptivity, was found to be inherited in a manner that is independent of the other measures of receptivity. Also found to be genetically independent was the control of the frequency of male-like mounting responses.

Using these same genetic crossing techniques, McGill and Blight (1963a; 1963b) studied the inheritance of sexual performance in male mice. Their results suggested the presence of three different types of inheritance of the different components of the total mating pattern, namely, "dominance of the behaviour pattern of one parent or the other, additive effects, and heterotic effects." This finding, which is similar to that of Goy and Jakway, further indicates that sexual behavior is extremely complex and cannot be covered by the term "innate."

The interbreeding technique described above is extremely useful to investigators because it can lead to conclusions about how phenotypic characteristics redistribute when the genes of two highly inbred strains are intermingled. In such studies, active selection pressure is not applied by the investigator. Randomly selected individuals are taken from the inbred strains to be the parents of the F1 generation. In studies of a slightly different type, the investigator does apply selection pressure. In these "artificial selection" studies the investigator selects for interbreeding only those individuals that score highest (or lowest) on some particular behavioral phenotype. Highest here may mean those animals scoring within the highest 25 percent (or 10 or 5 percent) of the population on some chosen phenotype *in each generation*. Genetically heterogeneous animals are usually used for the parent population in these studies so that the effects of artificial selection can be maximized. Studies of this type are particularly useful because they can lead to conclusions about the genetic lability of a characteristic and because they can yield reasonable estimates of the heritability of the behavioral phenotype.

Artificial selection studies differ from simple interbreeding studies in one important characteristic. Prior to the study, the investigator must select one component of the complex pattern to which selection pressure will be applied. In the simple interbreeding study, each component of the total pattern may be measured in the parents, in the F1 offspring, and in the backcross offspring. In the selective breeding experiment, one must focus on one single facet of the pattern.

Manning (1961) made an interesting and appropriate use of the artificial selection technique in his analysis of mating speed in the fruit fly *Drosophila melanogaster*. Manning measured the mating speed or copulation latency in two genetically diverse parent populations of fifty pairs each. From these populations the ten fastest and ten slowest pairs to mate were selected as parents for the F1 generation. In each succeeding generation, the ten fastest pairs to mate were used as parents for the "fast" line and the ten slowest pairs were used as parents for the "slow" line; the others were discarded. In this manner selection pressure was applied for twenty-five generations. Manning found a progressive increase over generations in the mean copulation latency in the lines artificially selected as slow maters, and a progressive decline in the copulation latency of the lines selected as fast maters. Control animals which were randomly interbred at each generation showed fluctuations in mating speed from generation to generation, but showed no consistent trend toward increased or decreased copulation latency. At Generation 17, some fast and slow maters were interbred. Their offspring when tested fell between the purebred fast and the purebred slow flies as would be predicted.

From his data, Manning was able to calculate the heritability of mating speed. h^2 was found to be approximately .30, indicating that about 30 percent of the variability between individuals on this behavioral phenotype may be accounted for in terms of genetic variability. It must be emphasized here that this heritability measure characterizes the *population* and not the separate individuals involved. According to our variance model of instinct, genetic studies deal with individual differences in behavior and not with individual behavior. For each individual, the genetic and environmental determinants of the behavior are inextricably confounded.

The data that we have summarized here show that sexuality in a wide variety of species is influenced by genetic factors. No mention has been made, however, of the mechanisms that translate genetic variability into behavioral variability. We know nothing of the proximal activity of the genes in these cases. We can make no statements about enzyme reactions or biochemical pathways. No work has yet carried us that far. We can, however, suggest that in the cases studied, the genes act at some level to alter the thresholds for the responses. For example, Manning was led to conclude that the effects of artificial selection in his study were to "raise the reaction thresholds of sexual behaviour in the S- (slow) lines and of general activity in the F- (fast) lines." Yet, we do not know where these thresholds are altered, at the receptor level, at the muscle effector level, centrally in the brain, or peripherally in the endocrine glands. The acquisition of these data will greatly advance our understanding of the genetic determinants of sexual behavior.

THE HORMONAL BASIS OF SEXUALITY

While it seems likely that genes control sexual behavior at least partly through their determination of hormone levels and through their determination of the reactivity of the substrate that responds to hormones, we cannot yet relate gene action to the effects of hormones on behavior. We can, however, examine questions of how hormones control sexuality.

Young (1961) emphasized the fact that we cannot discuss the problem of hormones and sexual behavior solely in terms of the action of hormones on the arousal or elicitation of behavior. Gonadal hormones seem to have two major types of effects, one activational and one organizational or differentiating. Here Young is distinguishing between effects of hormones upon the character of the substrate that responds to hormones (an organizational effect) and the simple stimulation of organized substrate by hormones (an activational effect). This distinction between organization and activation is most clearly made by comparing the effects of two types of hormonal manipulation. In the first experimental situation, a female (rat) is castrated shortly after birth and allowed to mature without endogenous hormonal stimulation. When mature, this animal is treated with exogenous female hormones and is tested with a sexually active male. If the animal displays the behavior characteristic of the normal female, that is, lordosis, the hormones are said to have a simple activational effect in that they stimulate substrate of normal character to activate normal behavior.

In the second experimental situation, the female (guinea pig) is treated with the male hormone prior to birth and allowed to mature. This female is again stimulated with male hormone when adult, and is tested with another, but normal, female. If the female treated with male hormone in infancy displays more male-like behavior under these conditions than a female not so treated during early development, the hormone is said to have an organizational effect in infancy since the behavior displayed is more congruent with the hormone administered in infancy than with the genetic sex of the individual. Both of these hypothetical experiments have been performed and the results indicate the existence of both organizational and activational hormone effects.

Activation

Two now-classical reviews exist on the relationships between hormones and behavior. The review by Beach (1948) contains much of the relevant literature up to the mid-1940s, and the review by Young (1961) contains both traditional material and the more contemporary studies of hormone-behavior relationships. Both of these sources are recommended to the reader who is interested in detailed information about the activation of sexual behavior by hormones. Since the activation of behavior has been so well reviewed, the present article will only point out a few well-established generalizations.

It seems quite clear today that gonadectomy, at least in nonprimate animals, ultimately results in the complete cessation of mating activity. It is also clear, however, that for male mammals the display of mating continues for some time past the point that significant amounts of testicular hormones are present in the circulatory system following castration. Since it seems unlikely that the post-castrational behavior in these cases is maintained by adrenal androgens (Cooper & Aronson, 1958), one must assume that the organism has some mating potential even in the absence of hormones.

For primate species, including man, castration also leads to a decline in sexual performance (Bremer, 1959; Money, 1961), but the degree of decline is less profound than that evident in lower animals.

In nonprimate female mammals, the presence of estrogen or estrogen and progesterone seems necessary for the display of mating. Following removal of ovaries in rat, cat, guinea pig, and so on, there is an almost immediate disappearance of all signs of receptivity. In primates, including man, ovarian hormones are not a sine qua non for the display of sexual responses. Rhesus monkeys, for example, are known to show sexual presentation responses at all times during the estrous cycle, although actual copulation is usually restricted to the period of estrus (Carpenter, 1942). In women, the ovaries seem to contribute even less to sexual behavior than they do in nonhuman primates. The complete removal of ovarian hormones has only a slight effect on the sexual desire or capacity of women (Bremer, 1959; Fuller & Drezner, 1944; Schon and Sutherland, 1963). This does not mean that sexuality in women is completely independent of hormones. It has been suggested that adrenal androgens are the primary libido hormone in women (Money, 1961; Waxenberg, Drellich, & Sutherland, 1959).

It is certainly reasonable to conclude from these data that gonadal hormones do underlie the display of sexual behavior in both sexes in a broad sample of mammalian species. Since this is so, we can ask how these hormones function to modulate sexuality. For many years we have assumed that the gonadal hormones induce sexual behavior primarily by their action on central nervous system structures. The first convincing evidence that this might be the case was provided by Fisher (1956). Fisher found that the application of sodium testosterone sulfate to the brain of rats could induce some components of the male mating pattern. Even more reliable evidence that hormones caused behavior by their action on the nervous system was provided by Harris, Michael and Scott (1958). These investigators reported that the implantation of estrogen directly into the brain of ovariectomized cats successfully induced behavioral receptivity. For their studies Harris et al. melted estrogen crystals and fused them to the tip of stainless steel needles. These needles were then permanently implanted into various regions of the cat's brain. The implanted females were regularly tested for receptivity by being placed with a vigorous male. At the same time, vaginal smears were taken to test for the presence of peripheral effects of the estrogen. Only those cats that mated and at the same time showed no evidence of peripheral hormonal effects were considered successful cases. The researchers found that estrogen implanted in the posterior hypothalamus of the brain was successful by their criteria. In some cases mating persisted for two months or more. Intracerebral implants in nonhypothalamic areas were not successful. In follow-up reports, Harris and Michael (1964) stated that eight of seventeen cats implanted with stilbestrol-di-n-butyrate in the mammillary region of the hypothalamus became receptive, while only one of twenty-three control animals with implants at other sites came to accept the male. Michael (1965) has more recently reported that similar effects could be induced by implants all along the base of the brain at the midline from the posterior hypothalamus to the preoptic region.

The hormone implantation technique has since been used in studies of the rat, rabbit, and chicken. Davidson and Sawyer (1961) implanted estradiol benzoate into the brains of rabbits and induced mating. Positive implants were found to reside in the posterior median eminence, the mammillary area, and the anterior hypothalamus. More recent work on the rabbit by Palka and Sawyer (1964) also found that the effective loci were quite widespread, but only in those cases where peripheral hormonal stimulation was noted as well. In the rabbits that exhibited receptivity, but no peripheral stimulation, the effective locus was found to be only in the posterior and central medial basal hypothalamic regions.

Using the female rat, Lisk (1962) found that estrogen implants led to receptivity only when placed in a relatively circumscribed region near the preoptic area of the hypothalamus. Implants in the posterior hypothalamus, in the arcuate and mammillary nuclei, induced ovarian atrophy but not sexual receptivity. Current research in our own laboratory, (Whalen & Hardy, unpublished), however, indicates that the areas that respond to estrogen to induce receptivity may be even more extensive than was suggested by Lisk.

Similar studies in male animals have been sketchy to date. Davidson (1966) has been successful in inducing copulatory behavior in castrated male rats with anterior hypothalamic implants of testosterone. Barfield (1964) studying capons also has been successful. He has found in ten cases that testosterone placed in the basal medial preoptic region of the hypothalamus induced capons to exhibit copulatory behavior. Copulatory behavior was not exhibited by another forty-one capons in which the hormone resided at other loci. Barfield also found that comb growth, a sensitive index of androgen in the general circulation, was uncorrelated with the presence or absence of mating in these animals.

These studies make it clear that particular localized neurons exist in the hypothalamus which respond to hormones to produce sexual behavior. Certainly we cannot think that the primary effect that hormones have on behavior is indirect, being mediated by changes in the peripheral genitals. It is also clear that the relevant neurons are located primarily in the hypothalamic region. The particular area within the hypothalamus that responds to the hormones is a function of the species. How the hormones work at these loci is still unknown.

On the basis of the findings reported here, one might be led to the conclusion that androgens are specific for masculine behavior and estrogens are specific for feminine behavior. This conclusion would be untrue. Although all of the studies using hormones applied directly to the brain have used nonhormone implants in control animals, only one of these studies (Palka & Sawyer, 1966) has reported on the effects of estrogen implants in the male or androgen implants in the female. Based on studies employing systemically administered hormones, we would predict that males implanted with estrogen would exhibit some masculine behavior, and that androgen implanted in the brain of females would induce both masculine and feminine behavior. Of the eight possible genetic-hormonal-behavior combinations, these seem the most likely to occur (Young, 1961). Androgens and estrogens are not entirely specific for masculine and feminine behavior respectively, although it does seem to be true that androgens are more likely to predispose the animal to display male behavior and estrogens are more likely to predispose the animal to display female behavior than vice versa. Some hormone-behavior specificity does exist, but the degree of specificity seems to be determined not by the genetic constitution of the animal, but rather by the hormonal stimulation that exists prenatally or during early infancy. Hormones not only stimulate neurons to induce behavior, they also stimulate neurons to determine their hormonal responsivity. Hormones are organizational as well as activational.

The Organization of Sexuality by Hormones

Two techniques have been used to study the organizational effects of hormones on the development of sexuality. First, exogenous hormones have been administered to the developing fetus via the circulatory system of the mother, or to the neonate directly. Using this technique, Phoenix, Goy, Gerall and Young (1959) found that the administration of testosterone to the pregnant guinea pig resulted in the birth of genitally pseudo-hermaphroditic female offspring. When tested for sexual behavior at maturity, following gonadectomy and estrogen and progesterone replacement, these females failed to mate normally. However, when the pseudo-hermaphroditic females were administered the male hormone, testosterone, they displayed more frequent male-like mounting responses than did control females.

In a similar study, Harris and Levine (1962) administered testosterone to neonatal female rats. These females never developed the 4–5 day ovarian and vaginal cycles typical of the female rat and did not mate when given exogenous estrogen and progesterone. When administered testosterone as adults, these females, like the pseudohermaphroditic guinea pigs, exhibited a higher frequency of male-like mounting responses than did control females.

Subsequent work (Goy, Bridson, & Young, 1964) has shown that these "masculinizing" effects of testosterone are restricted to a critical phase during the development of the organism. For the guinea pig, the hormone must be administered prenatally, preferably between 35–60 days post-conception. For the rat, the hormone may be administered up to about ten days post-natally and still be effective in producing virilization. In fact, it seems to be the case that the organization of the mating control system in the rat occurs only after birth. Female rats administered one of the artificial progestins, 17 α ethynyl–19 nor testosterone on days 15–19 of pregnancy give birth to female offspring which are highly virilized. Following high doses of this progestin, the females never develop an external vagina. When these females mature, however, they do behave in a feminine fashion, unlike female rats given androgen after birth. These prenatally virilized females show lordosis, the index of receptivity, when mounted by males both spontaneously and when primed with estrogen and progesterone. Of course, intromission does not occur, since these females have no vagina (Whalen, King, & LoPiccolo, 1966). These data show that genital and behavioral virilization need not be correlated and that only the former is induced by androgenic stimulation prior to birth in the rat. A similar contrast between the effects of pre- and post-natally administered androgen has been noted by Swanson and van der Werff ten Bosch (1964) with respect to the genital and ovarian systems.

The second technique that has been used to analyze the hormonal organization of sexuality involves castration of the neonate. Grady, Phoenix, and Young (1965) used this technique and found that male rats castrated at 1 or 5 days of age responded to estrogen and progesterone treatment in adulthood with the display of feminine responses. Males castrated at 10 days of age or later failed to behave as females in adulthood when given the same estrogen and progesterone treatment.

A similar study was performed by Feder and Whalen (1965). This study had the added feature of combined castration and hormone treatment. Male rats were castrated at birth, or castrated and administered estrogen to see if feminization was simply the result of the absence of androgen during infancy, or whether total feminization occurred only with the presence of the female hormone during the critical period. The results of this study are summarized in Table 1. The results showed that male rats castrated on the day of birth or five days after birth would behave as females in adulthood when given estrogen and progesterone, but only if they had not been treated with estrogen in infancy. Clearly, the feminization of the male rat results only from the absence of male hormones after birth and does not result from some positive feminizing action of estrogen.

TABLE 1. Feminine Behavior of Neonatally Treated Male Rats following Estrogen and Progesterone in Adulthood

Neonatal treatment[a]	N	Lordoses/Mounts (in percentages)
1A Castration only	8	40.0
2A Castration + estrogen	9	6.4
3A Estrogen only	9	14.0
4A No treatment	8	6.6
1B Castration only	6	19.5
2B Castration + estrogen	5	0.0
3B Estrogen only	9	0.0
4B No treatment	8	6.5

[a] "A" groups, if castrated, were castrated 16–32 hours after birth. "B" groups, if castrated, were castrated 96 hours after birth.

The experiments described above have led Young and his co-workers to the hypothesis that the presence of testicular hormones in the male, and the absence of such hormones in the female controls the development of the potential for male and female behavior respectively (Young, Goy, & Phoenix, 1964). Some findings, however, argue against this hypothesis. For example, Levine and Mullins (1964) found that female rats administered estrogen in infancy and testosterone in adulthood exhibit more frequent male-like responses than control females not given estrogen in infancy. (Such estrogenized females also do not behave normally as females either spontaneously or when ovariectomized and given estrogen and progesterone. Levine & Mullins, 1964; Whalen & Nadler, 1963, 1965.)

A second finding that argues against the hypothesis that masculinization occurs only in the presence of androgens and feminization only in the absence of androgens comes from studies in which males are castrated in infancy and administered testosterone in adulthood. Presumably such animals should exhibit only feminine responses, but this is not the case. In our own laboratory we castrated male rats on the day of birth (Whalen & Edwards, 1966). In adulthood these animals were divided into two groups. Group I males were given testosterone and tested with receptive females. Group II males were given estrogen and progesterone and were tested with sexually vigorous males. The results of this experiment are summarized in Table 2. The results show that the neonatally castrated male will behave as a male or as a female depending upon whether he

TABLE 2. MATING PERFORMANCE OF ADULT NEONATALLY CASTRATED MALE RATS FOLLOWING SUCCESSIVE TREATMENTS WITH TESTOSTERONE AND ESTROGEN AND PROGESTERONE

Group	Testosterone		Estrogen-progesterone	
	% Mounting	Mount frequency of mounting Ss	% Showing lordosis	% Lordosis/ mounts for positive Ss
Male then female	70.0	17.9	100.0	70.0

Group	Estrogen-progesterone		Testosterone	
	% Showing lordosis	% Lordosis/ mounts for positive Ss	% Mounting	Mount frequency of mounting Ss
Female then male	100.0	50.0	66.7	10.3

receives testosterone or estrogen in adulthood. Similar observations that the neonatally castrated male rat will show mounting behavior when given testosterone in adulthood have been reported by Beach and Holz (1946) and by Grady, Phoenix and Young (1965). Our study makes it evident also that, once the male reaches adulthood with the potential to display both male and female behavior, he maintains that potential permanently. An initial treatment with testosterone or estrogen does not prevent the neonatally castrated male from responding in the opposite fashion when the hormone treatments are reversed.

Our experiments to date have led us to believe that animals castrated prior to the end of a critical developmental period develop the capacity to display both male and female type responses. The female responses of the neonatally castrated animals are quite complete and differ very little from the responses shown by normal females. The male responses of these animals, however, are not always complete. When administered testosterone, the neonatally castrated males exhibit mounting and thrusting responses which appear normal, but intromission and ejaculation rarely occur. Following the hypotheses of Beach and Holz (1946), we believe that the absence of intromission and ejaculation represents not a failure in neural organization but rather a failure of the penis to develop fully. Male rats castrated in infancy exhibit markedly reduced penile growth (Beach and Holz, 1946; Grady, Phoenix, and Young, 1965), and reduced penile growth would reduce the probability of intromission and ejaculation. We feel that sexual performance should be distinguished from sexual motivation (Whalen, 1966) and that the neonatal castration does not interfere with the development of sexual motivation, but interferes only with the potential for complete sexual display. Our most recent experiments are consistent with this interpretation of the effects of hormones on the organization of sexuality (Whalen & Edwards, 1967).

The active experimentation in the area of the hormonal control of the organization of behavior is rapidly expanding our understanding of sexual behavior. A more complete understanding, however, must await a similar burst of activity on problems of the role of experience on sexuality, and studies that integrate hormonal control and the effects of experience. This latter problem, the experiential control of sexuality, has been studied only superficially to date.

THE EXPERIENTIAL DETERMINANTS OF SEXUALITY

Female monkeys deprived of normal mothering in infancy never themselves develop into successful, or even satisfactory, mates and mothers. Castrated male cats will continue to attempt to mate for months and years following gonadectomy, but only if they had successfully mated before castration. Both of these observations are appropriately classified as observations on the effects of experience on sexuality, although they represent quite distinct classes of experience. This section will review a few studies within each class of experience, since each contributes to our understanding of the experiential determinants of sexuality.

Variations in Early Experience

Since mating is a social activity, investigators have often asked whether the display of mating behavior requires precedent social experience, particularly social experience during maturation. Typically, investigators attempting to evaluate the role of early social experience on the development of sexuality separate the organism from the parent at the time of weaning or earlier, if possible, and allow the animal to mature in isolation from, or together with, species mates. In the studies done to date, isolation rearing means only isolation from species contact; interindividual visual, auditory, and olfactory contact has been permitted.

One of the earliest "isolation" studies of this type was done by Stone in 1923. Stone found that the isolation of male rats from 40 days of age until maturity had no detrimental effects on adult mating performance. This finding was not surprising, of course, since the rats were isolated quite late in development. Isolation at earlier ages, however, has yielded the same results. Beach (1942b, 1958) found that male rats isolated from conspecifics at 21 or 14 days of age were not inhibited in their adult sexual performance. In fact, isolation-reared males mated slightly more frequently than did males reared with other males. Kagan and Beach (1953) replicated this apparent facilitation effect when they showed that semi-isolated male rats (caged with a receptive female or another male 10 minutes each week for the 9 weeks preceding the mating tests) were less likely to ejaculate than were males which had been reared in complete isolation from 36 days of age until maturity. It appeared as though the weekly interactions with conspecifics during maturation led to the development of reponses that were incompatible with successful adult mating.

A similar absence of detrimental effects of isolation rearing on adult mating has been reported for female rats. Stone (1926) for example, reported that nineteen of twenty female rats showed receptivity and allowed intromission after having been reared in isolation from 20 days of age until maturity.

Valenstein, Riss, and Young (1955) used the same approach to this problem as Beach and reared three strains of guinea pigs in isolation from 25 days of age until maturity. For the males of each strain, nuzzling, sniffing, and abortive mounting occurred more frequently in those males that had been isolated than in those males not isolated during development. However, for each strain, intromission and ejaculation occurred more frequently in those males that had been reared in social groups. In this study, the detrimental effects of isolation rearing were striking for the two highly inbred strains and not for the genetically heterogenous strain. Thus, genotype may interact with experience to determine the development of sexuality. This gene-environment interaction appeared to be partially determined by the rate of development shown by each strain. When the rapidly maturing genetically heterogeneous males were isolated in a second experiment from 10 days of age instead of from 25 days of age they also exhibited a clear reduction in mating performance in comparison with males reared socially from 10 days of age.

The sexual behavior of the female guinea pig is also detrimentally affected by isolation rearing. Goy and Young (1956) noted that in each of three strains of female guinea pigs, prepuberal isolation was correlated with a reduced duration of heat and of mean maximum lordosis time. In addition, the absence of species contact during the first few weeks postpartum greatly inhibited the male-like mounting responses which were shown by socially reared females.

While isolation rearing may alter the probability, frequency, latency and duration of the component sexual responses of the guinea pig and rat, this treatment would not prevent the animals from reproducing. The appropriate mating responses necessary for insemination were displayed by both isolation-reared and social-reared males and females, although with different frequencies and timing. Such is not the case with monkeys. These primates show a very profound alteration in the development of sexual behavior as a result of isolation in infancy.

Mason (1960) separated three male and three female rhesus monkeys from their mothers one month after birth. Until these animals were tested at two and one-half years of age, their social contacts were restricted almost exclusively to the human caretakers. When mature, these animals were tested with each other and with control Feral monkeys that had been born and initially reared by their mothers in the wild. Mason tested "isolated-isolated," "feral-feral," and "isolated-feral" pairs and found that on measures of mounting frequency, duration of mounting, frequency of thrusts, and proportion mounting and thrusting, the feral monkeys greatly surpassed the monkeys that had been socially isolated in infancy. The sexual behavior of the isolated monkeys was grossly disorganized— they never mounted the female appropriately and often assumed inappropriate postures and body orientations.

Among the females, sexual presentation responses occurred more frequently with the feral animals than the isolates, but this difference was not statistically significant. The presentation postures that were assumed were more stereotyped among the feral animals.

When the isolated males were tested with the feral females, Mason observed a sharp increase in the frequency and appropriateness of mounting and in the frequency of thrusting, in comparison to the behavior of the "isolate-isolate" pairs. Presumably, the sexual experience of the feral females served to induce relatively appropriate behavior in the isolated males. This finding illustrates an important point with respect to studies of this nature. Sexual behavior is a social activity and the behavior of both individuals contributes to the totality of the mating observed.

The limited evidence that we have from these too-few studies would indicate that peer contacts during maturation do contribute to the development of organized sexual behavior, at least in the guinea pig and monkey. Individuals from these species that are isolated during development either fail to develop those postural adjustments and manual dexterities that are necessary for successful mating, or they develop extra responses that are incompatible with mating. Only in the rat is it the socially reared animal that develops responses that are partly incompatible with efficient mating. These studies do not indicate that species contacts are necessary for the development of sexual motivation, assuming, of course, that motivation and performance are partially independent characteristics of the organism, as we have suggested elsewhere (Whalen, 1966). Isolated male and female rats, guinea pigs, and monkeys do show approach responses to the appropriate partner and do attempt to initiate mating, which would indicate that the animals are motivated to perform the sexual responses, even though they do not have the appropriate responses in their repertoire to insure efficient mating performance.

Variation in Post-pubertal Experience

In some species the complete typical mating pattern is shown at the time of first contact with an appropriate partner. This is more likely to be the case for females than for males, and for rodents than for primates. However, this does not mean that once the behavior appears, it remains invariant. Although all of the components of the pattern may appear at the first contact, changes that may be attributed to experience do occur, particularly in the integration, frequency, and timing of the sexual responses.

With respect to studies of sexual experience, special care must be taken to distinguish between maturational effects and true experience effects. For example, McGill (1962b) noted a progressive reduction in the frequency of head-mounts (inappropriate mounting of the head of the female) by male mice as function of ejaculatory experience. Since in this study no animals were tested for the first time at the point when the experienced animals were exhibiting very few head-mounts, one cannot be certain that the reduction in head-mount frequency was a function of the ejaculatory experience obtained by the mice. The same problem exists for the interpretation of the data of Macirone and Walton (1938), which indicated that sexually experienced male rabbits mount the estrous doe in an "abnormal" fashion less frequently than do young males.

That the confounding of experience and maturation can pose real problems was clearly demonstrated by Larsson (1959). Larsson studied the copulatory behavior of male rats in four tests which occurred when the animals were between 105–138 days of age. He found that the frequency of ejaculations per hour increased, the frequency of intromissions per ejaculation decreased, and that ejaculation latency declined with age and experience. However, males tested for the first time at 138 days of age did not differ from the sexually experienced 138-day-old males on any of these measures of mating performance. The changes observed here were the result of maturational changes and were not a function of sexual experience. The only measure on which the sexually experienced and naive males did differ at 138 days of age was the duration of the post-ejaculatory interval, the time from ejaculation until the next intromission. The experienced males resumed mating after ejaculation sooner than the naive males.

In addition to the important methodological point made by Larsson, his study indicates that copulatory experience contributes very little to the organization of sexual behavior in the male rat. Rabedeau and Whalen (1959) and Whalen (1961a) came to the same conclusion with respect to male rats that are initially sexually vigorous, that is, very likely to copulate when placed with a female. Male rats that tend not to mate spontaneously, however, did seem to be positively influenced by mating experience (Rabedeau & Whalen, 1959).

In some respects, carnivores are more profoundly affected by sexual experience than are rodents. Male dogs, like male mice, become less likely to mount the head or side of the female as they achieve sexual experience (Beach, 1950).

For the female cat, sexual experience is quite important in facilitating receptivity (Whalen, 1963). Sexually naive female cats that are ovariectomized and administered large doses of estrogen give signs of receptivity, such as lordosis and treading, when stroked by the investigator. However, when placed with a male, these females display aggression rather than receptivity. Only after the male achieves an intromission does the female become receptive. As shown in Figure 1, the latency to intromission pro-

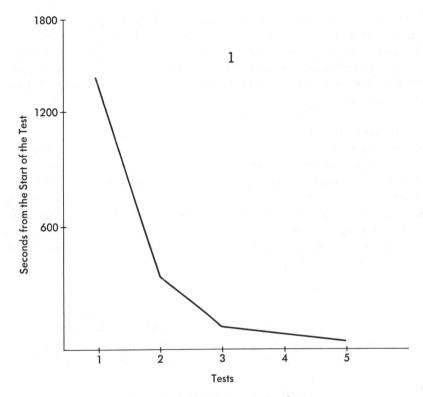

FIGURE 1. Mean intromission latency.

gressively declines in each test after the first test with intromission until it reaches the minimum characteristic of the experienced female. In this case, experience altered the receptivity (motivation?) of the female, but did not alter the motor components of the pattern. Adequate lordosis and treading were displayed before the time that the queen became truly receptive.

It is important to remember that the genetic, hormonal and experiential determinants of mating always act in concert. Hormonal and experiential determinants interact to control mating, just as genetic and hormonal, and genetic and experiential determinants interact to modulate mating performance. Hormone-experience interactions are particularly clear in the sexual behavior of the carnivores. Both sexually experienced male dogs and male cats respond quite differently to castration than do naive males of these species. Males of both species may continue to mate for up to two years after castration if they had mating experience before castration (Ford & Beach, 1951; Rosenblatt & Aronson, 1958). In the most complete study of this effect, Rosenblatt and Aronson (1959) castrated male cats at four months of age. When mature, these males were treated with testosterone, but only some of them were permitted sexual experience during the period of hormone treatment. All the males were tested with receptive females after the hormone treatment had been stopped, but only those males that had mated during the hormone therapy showed significant amounts of sexual activity in the absence of the testosterone. Even 15 weeks after the hormone withdrawal, the experienced males were showing more mating behavior than were the hormone-treated, but sexually inexperienced, males. Again in this case, it would seem that sexual experience can organize and facilitate sexual motivation.

Unfortunately, there have been no systematic investigations of the effects of sexual experience in primate species. From what we do know about sexuality in monkey and man we would certainly expect to find that experience and learning are the major determinants of sexual performance and sexual motivation in the primates.

IMPLICATIONS FOR HUMAN SEXUALITY

It must be admitted that studies of animal behavior have contributed little to a general theory of human sexuality. Some might argue that this must be the case because of vast differences in the nature of ontogeny of animal and human sexuality. This notion is difficult to accept. The similarities between humans and lower animals are striking—not the differences. The difficulties in generalization seem to arise from the fact that students of human and animal sexuality view sexuality with vastly different data languages and concept structures. Students of animal behavior describe copulation frequency, stimulus preference, and lordosis, while students of human behavior discuss libido and gender role. Rarely have attempts been made to define and establish the equivalences that must exist between animal and human sexual behavior, and, as a result, we have two worlds of thought.

Only in the past few years has research been done at both animal and human levels that can open the door for interactions between these two subdisciplines. The outstanding example at the human level is the work of Masters and Johnson (1966) on the nature of the human sexual response. This careful study has defined the cycle of human sexual responsiveness and provides a baseline for future research on the genetic, hormonal, and experiential determinants of human sexual arousability. The nature of the data collected by Masters and Johnson allows for ready comparison with already existing data from animal studies.

That interesting and useful comparisons between animals and man can be made has been demonstrated recently by Beach, Westbrook, and Clemens (1966) with respect to the ejaculatory response. These workers point out the great similarities that exist across species, including man, in the process and effects of ejaculation (or orgasm). Specifically, they note that erection and seminal emission are controlled by spinal mechanisms that are usually, but not always, activated by genital stimulation. Spontaneous emission is observed in the male of many species. Further, they report that simple activation of these spinal mechanisms does not result in the reduction in sexual arousability which characterizes ejaculation produced by coitus or masturbation. This post-ejaculatory refractory period (or resolution phase of Masters and Johnson) is a common feature of male but not female sexuality, and has important implications for theories of sexual motivation.

Recently this author prepared a detailed discussion of sexual motivation which incorporated data on the post-ejaculatory refractory period (Whalen, 1966). In this discussion sexual motivation was divided into two components, a transient component termed *sexual arousal,* and a more persistent component termed *sexual arousability.* In this framework, *arousal* represents the current level of sexual excitement and ranges from no excitement to maximal excitement (orgasm). *Arousability* is defined as the rate at which an individual approaches maximal sexual arousal. Orgasm was considered to produce an immediate inhibition of arousability such that no sexual stimulus, no matter how intense, could rearouse the individual. Arousability then recovered with time. Abundant data from animal and human studies were found to be consistent with this hypothesis.

Animal and human studies are also approaching each other with respect to another dimension of sexuality, namely gender-related behavior. One of the most obvious and interesting aspects of human sexuality is gender, all those facets of behavior that characterize an individual as male or female. At the human level, the determinants of gender have been under intensive study for the past several years (Hampson & Hampson, 1961; Money, Hampson & Hampson, 1957; Sears, 1965). At the animal level, this has not been the case; with animals the focus has been on primary sexual activity. Recently, however, attempts have been made to detect sex differences in nonsexual behavior in animals. Research at Harlow's laboratory has demonstrated, for example, clear differences between male and female rhesus monkeys in sex-related behaviors. These studies (Harlow, 1965) have shown that males exhibit more frequent threat responses than females, and engage in rough and tumble play more often than females. Females show more grooming and more frequent passive responses than males. The similarities between these male-female differences, and those observed in children (Sears, 1965) are indeed striking.

Furthermore, some of these male-female differences in behavior may be hormonally determined. Young, Goy, and Phoenix (1964) have shown that artificial pseudohermaphroditic female monkeys exhibit threat and play behaviors which more closely resemble those of males than females in frequency and intensity. This finding suggests that the predisposition toward masculine or feminine behavior may be hormonally determined, rather than environmentally determined as we are usually led to believe. A continuation of these studies of the ontogeny of the gender is likely to lead to a greater integration of data and theories of sexuality in animals and man.

SEXUAL DEVIANCE

Any concept of behavioral deviance, sexual or otherwise, may take one of two forms. The deviance concept may be either functional or statistical. With the functional concept, one assumes that a particular behavior has some major function in maintaining the status or integrity of the individual or of the species. The function of sexual behaviors, for example, may be assumed to be the reproduction of the species, and sexual behaviors that do not lead to reproduction may be termed deviant. With the statistical concept of deviance, the modal behavior of the species may be considered "normal," and behaviors that are exhibited by only a small proportion of the population may be termed deviant. By both functional and statistical criteria, homosexuality would be considered deviant, since it is reproductively ineffective and since it occurs only in a small proportion of the population. Masturbation, on the other hand, would be deviant only by the functional criterion of deviance, since it does occur in a high proportion of the human population and yet is reproductively ineffective.

It would not be wise to argue that either the functional or the statistical criterion provides a better definition of deviance. Both may be useful. Neither concept gives us insight into the causes of behavior because deviance is a descriptive and not an interpretative concept.

Functionally deviant behavior is common among animals. Homosexual, bisexual, and autosexual behaviors have been seen (Beach, 1942a; Ford & Beach, 1951; Michael, 1961b). Probably the most frequently reported functionally deviant behavior displayed by lower animals is the male-like mounting responses of females. These have been observed in several species. "Pseudo-female behavior," feminine responses by males, are also not uncommon (Young, 1961). These latter behaviors include presentation responses, lordosis, and so forth, depending upon the species. Finally, autosexual stimulation, and male-female oral stimulation have been observed, but these behaviors occur less frequently than male-like mounting by females and pseudo-female behavior by males (Ford & Beach, 1951).

Since the functionally deviant sexual behaviors of animals have been observed only in isolated individuals or in limited populations, it is difficult to assess the statistical deviance of these responses. That deviant responses have been observed by several investigators may indicate that these behaviors are characteristic of animals, but these observations still cannot tell us of their relative frequencies.

Do these observations have implications for our understanding of human sexual deviance? The answer to this question must be "yes," but only in a limited sense. That functionally deviant sexual behaviors do occur in lower animals of several species should lead us to expect to find similar behaviors in humans. These observations should not lead us to support any particular theory of sexual deviance. The data tell us nothing of the causes or controls of deviant sexual behavior. For an understanding of the causes and controls of sexual deviance we should look rather to our data on the genetic, hormonal, and experiential determinants of sexual behavior.

REFERENCES

Barfield, R. J. Induction of copulatory behavior by intracranial placement of androgen in capons. *American Zoologist,* 1964, 4, 113.

Beach, F. A. Execution of the complete masculine copulatory pattern by sexually receptive female rats. *Journal of Genetic Psychology,* 1942, 60, 137–142. (a)

Beach, F. A. Comparison of copulatory behavior of male rats raised in isolation, cohabitation, and segregation. *Journal of Genetic Psychology,* 1942, 60, 121–136. (b)

Beach, F. A. *Hormones and behavior,* New York: Hoeber, 1948.

Beach, F. A. Sexual behavior in animals and man. *Harvey Society of New York,* Series 42, Springfield, Illinois: Charles C Thomas, 1950.

Beach, F. A. The de-scent of instinct. *Psychological Review,* 1955, 62, 401–410.

Beach, F. A. Normal sexual behavior in male rats isolated at fourteen days of age. *Journal of Comparative and Physiological Psychology,* 1958, 51, 37–38.

Beach, F. A., & Holz, A. M. Mating behavior in male rats castrated at various ages and injected with androgen. *Journal of Experimental Zoology,* 1946, 101, 91–142.

Beach, F. A., Westbrook, W. H., & Clemens, L. G. Comparisons of the ejaculatory response in men and animals. *Psychosomatic Medicine,* 1966, 28, 749–763.

Bremer, J. *Asexualization.* New York: Macmillan, 1959.

Carpenter, C. R. Sexual behavior of free-ranging rhesus monkeys. I. Specimens, procedures, and behavioral characteristics of estrus. *Journal of Comparative Psychology,* 1942, 33, 113–142.

Cooper, M., & Aronson, L. The effect of adrenalectomy on the sexual behavior of castrated male cats. *Anatomical Record,* 1958, 131, 544.

Davidson, J. M. Activation of the male rat's sexual behavior by intracerebral implantation of androgen. *Endocrinology*, 1966, **79**, 783–794.

Davidson, J., & Sawyer, C. H. Effects of localized intracerebral implantation of estrogen on reproductive function in the female rabbit. *Acta Endocrinologica*, 1961, **37**, 385–393.

Feder, H. H., & Whalen, R. E. Feminine behavior in neonatally castrated and estrogen-treated male rats. *Science*, 1965, **147**, 306–307.

Fisher, A. Maternal and sexual behavior induced by intracranial chemical stimulation. *Science*, 1956, **124**, 228–229.

Ford, C. S., & Beach, F. A. *Patterns of sexual behavior.* New York: Harper and Bros., 1951.

Fuller, W., & Drezner, N. The results of surgical castration in women under forty. *American Journal of Obstetrics and Gynecology*, 1944, **47**, 122–124.

Goy, R. W., Bridson, W. E., & Young, W. C. The period of maximal susceptibility of the prenatal female guinea pig to masculinizing actions of testosterone propionate. *Journal of Comparative and Physiological Psychology*, 1964, **57**, 166–174.

Goy, R. W., & Jakway, J. The inheritance of patterns of sexual behavior in female guinea pigs. *Animal Behavior*, 1959, **7**, 142–149.

Goy, R. W., & Phoenix, C. H. A critical period for the suppression of behavioral receptivity in adult female rats by early treatment with androgen. *Anatomical Record*, 1962, **142**, 307.

Goy, R. W., & Young, W. C. The importance of genetic and experiential factors for the organization of sexual behavior patterns in the female guinea pig. *Anatomical Record*, 1956, **124**, 296.

Grady, K. L., Phoenix, C. H., & Young, W. C. Role of the developing rat testis in differentiation of the neural tissues mediating mating behavior. *Journal of Comparative and Physiological Psychology*, 1965, **59**, 176–182.

Hampson, J. L., & Hampson, J. G. The ontogenesis of sexual behavior in man. In W. C. Young (Ed.), *Sex and internal secretions.* (3rd ed.) Baltimore: Williams and Wilkins, 1961. Pp. 1401–1432.

Harlow, H. F. Sexual behavior in the rhesus monkey. In F. A. Beach (Ed.), *Sex and behavior,* New York: John Wiley & Sons, 1965. Pp. 234–265.

Harris, G. W., & Levine, S. Sexual differentiation of the brain and its experimental control. *Journal of Physiology*, 1962, **163**, 42–43P.

Harris, G. W., & Michael, R. P. The activation of sexual behaviour by hypothalamic implants of oestrogen. *Journal of Physiology*, 1964, **171**, 275–301.

Harris, G. W., Michael, R. P., & Scott, P. P. Neurological site of action of stilboestrol in eliciting sexual behaviour. In G. E. W. Wolstenholme & C. M. O'Conner (Eds.), *Neurological basis of behaviour.* Boston: Little, Brown and Co., 1958. Pp. 236–251.

Jakway, J. Inheritance of patterns of mating behaviour in the male guinea pig. *Animal Behavior*, 1959, **7**, 150–162.

Kagan, J., & Beach, F. A. Effects of early experience on mating behavior in male rats. *Journal of Comparative and Physiological Psychology*, 1953, **46**, 204–208.

Larsson, K. Experience and maturation in the development of sexual behaviour in male puberty rat. *Behaviour*, 1959, **14**, 101–107.

Lehrman, D. S. A critique of Konrad Lorenz's theory of instinctive behavior. *Quarterly Review of Biology*, 1953, **28**, 337–363.

Levine, S., & Mullins, R., Jr. Estrogen administered neonatally affects adult sexual behavior in male and female rats. *Science*, 1964, **144**, 185–187.

Lisk, R. D. Diencephalic placement of estradiol and sexual receptivity in the female rat. *American Journal of Physiology*, 1962, **203**, 493–496.

Macirone, C., & Walton, A. Fecundity of male rabbits as determined by "dummy matings." *Journal of Agricultural Science*, 1938, **28**, 122–134.

Manning, A. The effects of artificial selection for mating speed in *Drosophila melanogaster. Animal Behavior*, 1961, **9**, 82–92.

Mason, W. A. The effects of social restriction on the behavior of rhesus monkeys. I. Free social behavior. *Journal of Comparative and Physiological Psychology*, 1960, **53**, 582–589.

Masters, W. H., & Johnson, V. E. *Human sexual response*. Boston: Little Brown and Co., 1966.

McGill, T. E. Sexual behaviour in three inbred strains of mice. *Behaviour*, 1962, **19**, 341–350. (a)

McGill, T. E. Reduction in "head-mounts" in the sexual behavior of the mouse as a function of experience. *Psychological Reports*, 1962, **10**, 284. (b)

McGill, T. E., & Blight, W. C. Effects of genotype on the recovery of sex drive in the male mouse. *Journal of Comparative and Physiological Psychology*, 1963, **56**, 887–888. (a)

McGill, T. E., & Blight, W. C. The sexual behaviour of hybrid male mice compared with the sexual behaviour of males of the inbred parent strains. *Animal Behavior*, 1963, **11**, 480–483. (b)

Michael, R. P. An investigation of the sensitivity of circumscribed neurological areas to hormonal stimulation by means of the application of oestrogens directly to the brain of the cat. In S. S. Kety & J. Elkes (Eds.), *Regional neurochemistry: International neurological symposium*. New York: Pergamon Press, 1961. Pp. 465–479. (a)

Michael, R. P. "Hypersexuality" in male cats without brain damage. *Science*, 1961, **134**, 553–554. (b)

Michael, R. P. Oestrogens in the central nervous system. *British Medical Bulletin*, 1965, **21**, 87–90.

Money, J. Components of eroticism in man: I. The hormones in relation to sexual morphology and sexual desire. *Journal of Nervous and Mental Disease*, 1961, **132**, 239–248.

Money, J., Hampson, J. G., & Hampson, J. L. Imprinting and the establishment of gender role. *A.M.A. Archives of Neurology and Psychiatry*, 1957, **77**, 333–336.

Palka, Y., & Sawyer, C. H. Induction of estrous behavior in the ovariectomized rabbit by estrogen implants in the hypothalamus. *American Zoologist*, 1964, **4**, 289.

Palka, Y. & Sawyer, C. H. Induction of estrous behavior in rabbits by hypothalamic implants of testosterone. *American Journal of Physiology*, 1966, **211**, 225–228.

Phoenix, C. H., Goy, R. W., Gerall, A. A., & Young, W. C. Organizing action of prenatally administered testosterone propionate on the tissues mediating mating behavior in the female guinea pig. *Endocrinology*, 1959, **65**, 369–382.

Rabedeau, R. G., & Whalen, R. E. Effects of copulatory experience on mating behavior in the male rat. *Journal of Comparative and Physiological Psychology*, 1959, **52**, 482–484.

Rosenblatt, J. S., & Aronson, L. R. The decline in sexual behavior in male cats after castration with special reference to the role of prior sexual experience. *Behaviour*, 1958, **12**, 285–338.

Rosenblatt, J. S., & Aronson, L. R. The influence of experience on the behavioural effects of androgen in prepuberally castrated male cats. *Animal Behavior*, 1959, **6**, 171–182.

Rosenzweig, M. R., Krech, D., & Bennett, E. L. A search for relations between brain chemistry and behavior. *Psychological Bulletin*, 1960, **57**, 476–492.

Schon, M., & Sutherland, A. M. The relationship of pituitary hormones to sexual behavior in women. In *Advances in sex research*. Harper and Row, 1963. Pp. 33–47.

Sears, R. R. Development of gender role. In F. A. Beach (Ed.), *Sex and behavior*. New York: John Wiley & Sons, 1965. Pp. 133–163.

Stone, C. P. Further study of sensory functions in the activation of sexual behavior in the young male albino rat. *Journal of Comparative Psychology*, 1923, **3**, 469–473.

Stone, C. P. The initial copulatory response of female rats reared in isolation from 20 days of age to age of puberty. *Journal of Comparative Psychology*, 1926, **6**, 78–83.

Swanson, H. E., & van der Werff ten Bosch, J. J. The "early-androgen" syndrome; differences in response to pre-natal and post-natal administration of various doses of testosterone propionate in female and male rats. *Acta Endocrinologica*, 1964, **47**, 37–50.

Valenstein, E. S., Riss, W., & Young, W. C. Sex drive in genetically heterogeneous and highly inbred strains of male guinea pigs. *Journal of Comparative and Physiological Psychology*, 1954, **47**, 162–165.

Valenstein, E. S., Riss, W., & Young, W. C. Experiential and genetic factors in the organization of sexual behavior in male guinea pigs. *Journal of Comparative and Physiological Psychology*, 1955, **48**, 397–403.

Waxenberg, S. E., Drellich, M. G., & Sutherland, A. M. The role of hormones in human behavior. I. Changes in female sexuality after adrenalectomy. *Journal of Clinical Endocrinology and Metabolism*, 1959, **19**, 193–202.

Whalen, R. E. Effects of mounting without intromission and intromission without ejaculation on sexual behavior and maze learning. *Journal of Comparative and Physiological Psychology*, 1961, **54**, 409–415. (a)

Whalen, R. E. Strain differences in sexual behavior of the male rat. *Behaviour*, 1961, **18**, 199–204. (b)

Whalen, R. E. The initiation of mating in naive female cats. *Animal Behavior,* 1963, **11,** 461–463.

Whalen, R. E. Sexual motivation. *Psychological Review,* 1966, **73,** 151–163.

Whalen, R. E., & Edwards, D. A. Sexual reversability in neonatally castrated male rats. *Journal of Comparative and Physiological Psychology,* 1966, **62,** 307–310.

Whalen, R. E., & Edwards, D. A. Hormonal determinants of the development of masculine and feminine behavior in male and female rats. *Anatomical Record,* 1967, **157,** 173–180.

Whalen, R. E., & Hardy, D. F. Induction of estrus in female rats by intracerebral implants of estrogen. In Preparation.

Whalen, R. E., King, C. A., & LoPiccolo, J. Virilization of female rats by prenatally administered progestin. *Endocrinology,* 1966, **78,** 965–970.

Whalen, R. E., & Nadler, R. D. Suppression of the development of female mating behavior by estrogen administered in infancy. *Science,* 1963, **141,** 273–274.

Whalen, R. E., & Nadler, R. D. Modification of spontaneous and hormone-induced sexual behavior by estrogen administered to neonatal female rats. *Journal of Comparative and Physiological Psychology,* 1965, **60,** 150–152.

Young, W. C. The hormones and mating behavior. In W. C. Young (Ed.), *Sex and internal secretions.* Baltimore: Williams and Wilkins Co., 1961. Pp. 1173–1239.

Young, W. C., Goy, R. W., & Phoenix, C. H. Hormones and sexual behavior. *Science,* 1964, **143,** 212–218.

5.4 Orientation

Nothing is so basic to our own personalities as our biological sex— or so it would seem. Such a statement is seriously challenged by the remarkable case illustrations presented in the following article by Alexander C. Rosen.

For those of us who are not conscious of having questioned our basic sexual identity during our formative and adult years, it may come as a surprise to recognize that surgical transformations of adult "men" into "women" and adult "women" into "men" is not as uncommon an operation as we had thought. The basic questions that develop when we hear of such transformations center around "What went wrong?" Was the person biologically unsuited for his or her sex role? Was he psychologically unstable, leading to an uncertainty about appropriate gender role behavior? Were the conditions of early childhood such that only one kind of sex-typed behavior was acceptable? Do these persons go through severe psychological conflict subsequent to surgery?

Building on the previous article on mating behavior and sexual deviance in animals, Rosen presents information on the questions above and points to the relevance for theory and research on psychopathology. He does not offer final conclusions, but he does point to the combination of "biologic, genetic, social and psychological influences that [shape] the terminal adult gender identity."

5.4   The Inter-Sex: Gender Identity, Genetics, and Mental Health

Alexander C. Rosen

An individual who denies his own identity, that is, who denies his own person and assumes the identity of another, is generally suspect of psychosis, or has other deviant motives impugned to him by those who observe his behavior. The patient in the hospital who presents himself as a major historical figure or identifies himself with the deity is accepted both by mental health professionals and in common-sense discourse as psychotic.

Quite similarly, the individual who contends that there are serious lacks in his body, that is, that a portion of his innards have been stolen, strayed, or been removed, and therefore modifies his behavior because of this departure of a part of his body, may also be treated by society as deviant or described as psychotic, insane, or mentally deranged. It would then follow that a person who claims a gender identity in conflict with his history, his anatomy, and his genetic structure should be similarly viewed.

These persons in Goffman's terms (Goffman, 1963) display a marked discrepancy between "virtual social identity" (imputed character) and "actual social identity" (character and attributes actually possessed). They are people whose stigma (the gender identity discrepancy) places them in marked and significant danger of becoming a "discredited person." Once having become discredited, they lose the privileges associated with the prior social and personal identity.

Society expects that each person acknowledge his identity and so accords him the relevant rewards and taboos derived from the status associated with the social roles defined by that identity. The pressure for conformity to a determined status, whether derived by accident of birth (ascribed status), or from positive conscious effort (achieved status), is constant and pervasive. Any self-proclaimed shift in the socially recognized or established identity by the individual places him in direct jeopardy of controls or punishment by the social system. Such a person may well be assigned to a deviant group, defined as criminal or mentally ill, or may be considered deficient in some essential mental quality. The capacity to change identity and role vary in society's capacity to tolerate shift in specific social dimensions. Changes in vocational role as a consequence of personal achievement or education are clearly tolerated, as are shifts in nationality following geographical changes in residence. Even these nominally sanctioned shifts may involve an identity crisis for the individual and visible psychological effort in the transition to the newly achieved status and identity. However, it is relevant to note here that such shifts are differentially permitted and may well depend on the ethnic and religious background and the socioeconomic status of the individual attempting the change. Limited shifts in socioeconomic class levels are acknowledged, but the extent of change is very frequently circumscribed or may be limited to the dominant majority political, ethnic, or religious group. Changes in gender, ethnic affiliation, or subcultural affiliation, or movement into aristocracy and changes in personal identity are attended by greater resistance by society. The special instance of the person who assumes a name and personality different from his own is frequently rewarded with immediate social controls and limits. The tasks involved in these shifts are considered in detail in the literature on "passing" (Goffman, 1963; Stoller, Garfinkel, & Rosen, 1960), which includes such examples as the individual of Negro background who attempts to pass as caucasian, or the person involved in espionage who attempts to present himself in the spied-upon country as a native of that land. Passing involves careful control of information regarding identity to avoid the risk of disclosure and potential personal disaster. It would appear that persons who attempt to account for their present psychological character by a reconstruction of their life or by the denial of their own personal history may be assigned to a deviant group by both professionals and members of the laity.

THE RELATIONSHIP BETWEEN GENDER AND PSYCHOSIS

Let us consider, then, several individuals, each of whom engages in identifiable parological reasoning or who may exhibit disturbances in ego functioning or who may show disturbances in reality testing and demonstrate openly an alteration in their own identity as well as reveal an invasion of unconscious motivation into conscious behavior and thought processes. These qualities are commonly considered to be necessary and sufficient conditions to assign a person to the deviant category labeled "psychotic." Let us determine if these cases might not provide exceptions to this principle. These patients represent pardigmatic instances of a great number of persons seen in The Gender Identity Research Clinic by the author and others over the past nine years. They are, in this sense, not unusual instances but are persons who, in our experience, illustrate well the issues being discussed here.

CASE EXAMPLES OF VARIOUS GENDER ANOMOLIES

The first of these individuals was born apparently a normal genetic and biological male following an uneventful pregnancy. He was raised in a medium-size metropolitan community in the United States and was accorded all the privileges and restrictions generally directed toward boy children. He was always dressed in boy's clothing, treated as a boy, and from all reports lived as a boy and was equipped with male external genitalia. At puberty he began to become increasingly less involved with male contemporaries and peers and became more obviously socially isolated. He also began to develop perceptible growth of the breasts. He became increasingly less comfortable in public school and finally withdrew to be taught by a visiting teacher. At seventeen he visited members of his family living in a distant city and during the trip purchased women's clothing and discarded all of his male garb, commencing then the full act of "passing." From that day forward he lived as a woman and continues to do so with resounding success. "His" breast enlargement continued and he developed a characteristic female body structure, becoming an attractive and shapely young woman. He presented himself to physicians as a woman and requested that the deviant member, his male genitalia, be removed and a vagina be constructed through cosmetic plastic surgery. In recounting his history, he insisted that he had never been adequate or successful as a male, that he had never been happy in his role as a male and insisted that as early as he could remember, he preferred to play with dolls and with other girls rather than with boys or with baseballs and masculine toys.

This individual, although possessing visible male genitalia, managed to live successfully as a woman, to persuade the attending physicians of his deep and intense feminine identity, and to induce responsible, prudent, and competent doctors to perform surgery, removing the penis and testes and constructing surgically a sexually adequate vagina. Since that time "she" has married and lived quite adequately as a woman with a full and complete female heterosexual life. "She" claims sexual gratification, female sexual response, and orgasm. "She" states that no one, even those in intimate contact with her, suspects that "her" early history is at variance with "her" presenting gender. "She" has shown great skill in managing the shift to the new gender identity and has demonstrated persistent application to the tasks of learning the essentials of the female role and status.

This case illustrates the management of biography and history as well as the control of social information in conventional social intercourse. This individual demonstrates active, presistent, and continued application to essential learning tasks to avoid being discredited. This history is ample testimony to the manner in which strong motivation can carry the individual through the successful sex transformation and can provide the ego strength to tolerate the most urgent social and personal stress.

AN EXAMPLE OF A LATE SHIFT IN GENDER

The second patient was identified at birth as a female and raised as a female. Although possessed of a large, rubbery organ which appeared to be a clitoris, the family in general treated her as a female, and she had few doubts as a child that she was a girl. However, the large, rubbery organ (actually a small bound-down hypospadic penis) was a source of some embarrassment, and the phallic-like appendage was surgically removed when she reached the age of 18. Subsequent efforts to make an adequate female heterosexual adjustment failed. Despite family pressure, she found it more and more difficult to play the role of the woman and finally fell into a series of seeming homosexual relationships with other women. She then perceived herself as a homosexual female and played that role as the aggressive member of a homosexual couple. She is, in appearance, a large, raw-boned person with heavy coarse fingers and broad shoulders and husky build. The apparent homosexual adjustment continued until other medical difficulties led her to a medical center where careful evaluation could be made of her medical status. At that time it was determined that she was, in fact, a biological male who had been erroneously assigned to the female gender because of the anomalous genitals. Having been informed of this fact she then completed the psychological transformation into full masculine role behavior and indeed managed to transfer legal as well as psychological identity to that of male. Following this shift, "he" became more relaxed, less anxious and certainly more at ease with "himself" and with "his" functioning in society.

In this individual, the persistent function of biological influence may well be seen, with the resolution of genetic and role conflict resulting from gender role shift, as yielding a decrease in anxiety and more adequate adjustment. This reflects essentially a lessening of the necessity to manage the social identity and lowering of general energy involved in this passing when there was coherence between social identity, personal identity, and ego identity.

THE BIOLOGICAL MALE

A third case is of a normal biological male exposed to normal patterns of child rearing who as an adult became increasingly interested in dressing like a female. As he became less and less identified with his identity as a male, he became more anxious and more "psychotic." After some considerable difficulty and negotiation, a castrating operation was performed outside of the United States and a cosmetic vagina constructed. Competent mental health professionals evaluating this individual before and after the sex transformation operation reported that there was a marked and significant diminution of psychotic-like personality content and a reduction of anxiety level following the sex transformation operation. In effect, therefore, the operation resolved conflicts leading to the psychotic ideation and restored some measure of balance to the personality. The resolution of role conflict by the sex transformation operation has been observed by several investigators as generating a more stable and less anxious adjustment in other individuals as well.

Clearly for this patient the gender change moved him from a state of gender ambiguity and confusion to a state in which bodily structure was consistent with psychological and self-ascribed gender identity.

SHIFTING IN A BIOLOGICAL FEMALE

Consider the fourth case, an only child born and raised as a normal genetic female, who, while attending school as a female, secretly dressed as a male and so successfully masqueraded as to be able to interact socially, without detection, with those individuals who knew her as a female. Despite their familiarity with her as a girl, they did not recognize her in her male garb. Her insistence on transformation into a male became increasingly more manifest as this individual passed through puberty, until finally at the age of 18, she was consistently presenting herself as a male in dress and manner with such eloquence that her mother and father accepted the transformation although surgical intervention was impossible. Henceforth, this individual, despite the contrary evidence of prior rearing, prior identity, legal identity, genetic constitution, and the physical evidence of the body itself, proceeded to live entirely as a male. She dates with women and finds ways to attempt a successful sexual adjustment. Although at times disturbed and angry, this person struggles hard to deal with the reality of her decision and to find a successful way to live as a male despite the demanding contrary evidence of anatomy and ascribed gender. Despite transient turmoil caused by society's resistance to this change, "he" manages to make a reasonable adjustment to life.

Here one can see clearly the overwhelming dominance of biological, genetic, and physiological influences by psychological and motivational factors. Despite the powerful forces acting against such a move, the strong wish to alter gender became dominant.

SHIFTING WHERE BIOLOGY AND ENVIRONMENT CLASH

The fifth case was a child born following normal delivery and identified at birth from an inspection of the external genitalia as a girl. The child was reared as a girl with no apparent difficulties in early childhood. As puberty approached, her behavior became more extroverted and aggressive, and difficulty began to become overtly manifest with increasing huskiness of body structure and apparent change in the quality and character of the voice. The parents reported a school phobia with increasing behavior problems. Careful physical examination by the family physician led to medical studies in greater detail including studies of the chromosome distribution. This yielded, following buccal smears, the discovery of a typical male XY chromosome distribution and possession of internal male gonads. With psychiatric and medical assistance, a shift was made from female to male gender, personal identity, and social role with accompanying corrective and cosmetic surgery. The shift was swift and easy, occurring literally overnight. The surgery made possible the external appearance of the genitalia which was more nearly consistent with the youngster's masculine sex and male gender identity. He moved very quickly and very easily into a male role and has been successfully living in that role subsequent to that time. In fact, the parents report the disappearance of all previously reported problems in adjustment. To all intents and purposes, the change was made, although with great effort, at least without the production of major psychological pathology. In this case, biological forces might be seen as providing powerful undercurrents in the personality producing the successful gender role shift.

This young man illustrates the futility of hasty generalization from such cases as described above. In contrast with case number four, we find the genetic and physiological influences thrusting to the fore despite the host of social and psychological forces acting to hold the youngster in the gender of ascription at birth. The disappearance of behavioral difficulties following the shift again demonstrates the anxiety- and psychopathology-reducing effects of reducing ambiguity or resolving conflicts in the totality of gender role identity.

THE PERSISTENT EFFECTS OF ENVIRONMENT

For the sixth case, let us consider a 19-year-old woman who presents herself for medical care complaining of never having experienced the menses. Extended medical examination determined her to be a young woman of relatively nonfeminine physical build with small, poorly developed genitals, and an extremely small, blind-pocketed vagina. Chromatin staining studies and other evidence indicated that she suffered from a form of Turner's Syndrome, with XO chromosomal pattern. She had been raised, as well as identified at birth, as female, and after a most careful psychological examination was found to be normally identified with the female gender. This person is notable since in this instance, although biologic determinants were in the masculine direction, the gender of rearing clearly established the gender identity rather than the genetic determinants.

FAMILIAL GENESIS OF TRANSVESTISM

The seventh case is that of a boy born biologically and genetically male and identified at birth as a male. From birth he was raised in intimate association with his mother and treated almost as an extension of the mother both physically and psychologically. In a sense, the youngster was an appendage of this mother with a visible merging of identity between the mother and child. The father was psychologically or physically absent a major portion of the time, and interviews indicated that the father was an indifferent and uncommitted part of the family. The father was visibly uninvolved in the rearing of the child and expressed indifference to the nature of that rearing. He provided neither control, affection, nor personal example to the growing boy. The focal responsibility for all physical and psychological care rested with the mother. As an infant, the boy was dressed in "fussy" clothing. As the child began to walk, he insisted on wearing feminine clothes which he obtained either from an older sister or from his mother. His first step was reported by the mother to be taken while wearing his mother's high-heeled shoes. He continued to wear feminine clothes and to insist on cross-dressing without great concern to the parents until he was approximately 4 years old. The family came for psychiatric consultation following strong criticism and ridicule of the boy's cross-dressing by family and friends and confusion regarding the sex of the child by passers-by in the street. After extended contact, it was revealed that the mother had recollections of her own tomboy childhood and recounted her own reluctance to assume the feminine stance. It would seem that the confusions in the boy's gender identity and the cross-dressing behavior seemed related to the above described phenomena. It might be inferred that the mother could not or would not permit her son to become a masculine male and so unconsciously fostered the transvestite behavior. This was reinforced by the father's absence and the lack of an adequate identification model.

This case shows a sharp difference from case number five, since in this instance the complex developmental factors in psychological growth could be so distorted as to generate grave confusions in gender relevant behavior. Nurture rather than nature proved to be the more powerful force.

NUMBER AND TYPICALITY OF CASES

It cannot be sufficiently emphasized that the selection of the individuals cited are typical of those seen by the author and his colleagues in a setting concerned with problems of gender and sex (The UCLA Gender Identity Clinic). One can perceive in the clinic any combination of biologic, genetic, social, and psychological influences that might bear upon the terminal adult gender identity of the individuals portrayed. In the human, it is difficult indeed to see clearly, as it may be in lower animals, the consistently overpowering influences of either genetic or environmental determinants (Whalen, 1963, 1960). In most cases one can palpate a delicate and subtle blending of these influences on gender-relevant behavior, but the specific, precise, and exact accounting for behavior by a single dominant influence cannot reasonably be assumed.

Parenthetically, it is interesting to note that each of the persons described above did not appear either on careful psychological testing or on psychiatric examination to be psychotic in the usual meaning following the successful resolution of the crisis in gender identity. These persons did, however, display a visible denial of physical reality by denying the substance of the evidence presented to them by their own bodies of their anatomic gender. They had as well, as a result of insistent and intense desire, shifted from one gender identity to another which was contrary to the presenting evidence. In the first cited case, this intense desire for sex transformation and the skillful manipulation of the environment was achieved by invoking the active cooperation of an ethical and sincere group of professionals. The management of the shift in gender identity for all of these individuals represented careful and intense thought, organized planning, and a meticulous concern for the details that must be attended to in order to pass successfully from one significant identity to another. The common-sense concerns that most of us may be aware of in our own behavior as adequate members of our own gender and sex are more than considerably excelled by these individuals who must literally learn bit by bit those things that reflect gender and which most people very much take for granted in their own behavior. These individuals must consciously model themselves after persons of the sex toward which they are changing and whom they can perceive about them. The intense effort in the change and the severe threat attendant to public discovery require remarkable control, notable skill, and sensitive acuity in dealing with the environment.

In terms of the usual criterion for psychosis, these individuals show a defect in ego, that is, they deny the reality of their own bodies but yet they also show extraordinary strength of ego in the vigor and enthusiastic concern they direct toward the active and successful alteration of their environment and in the pursuit of their warmly desired change in identity. These persons deny their own history, and frequently they retreat from those individuals for whom they may have deep and intense emotional relationships in some prior portions of their life in order that they might reconstruct their image of themselves and their life history with an intent to support the reality of the newly adopted gender identity.

Most persons take presenting gender as given and irrevocable. Most of society takes the presenting data of the visible anatomic sex as beyond the possibility of change and consider it an intrinsic part of identity. Change in gender appears on the surface to represent a major departure from reason, as gender is frequently seen as intensely tied to biological qualities and to be invulnerable to change. The denial of identity, that is to say, the denial of one's own sexual and biological history, is behavior apparently as psychotic as that of the person who presents himself as J. Edgar Hoover or God and therefore violates his established identity, his name, his history, and his associated experiences.

For most people, the qualities ascribed to men and women are generally seen as unique, separate, and peculiar to each gender. The stereotyped models of male and female behavior are generally described in a nonoverlapping and present in a logically distinct fashion. There is great agreement between men and women about the models of gender-relevant behavior, and these similar descriptions of the two sexes as they are, and as they ought to be, overlap but little (Bennett & Cohen, 1959). This is true despite the fact that empirically observed traits, qualities, values, and beliefs are visibly overlapping and found to be so in all investigations of masculinity-femininity (Aaronson, 1959; Aaronson & Grumpelt, 1961; Barrows & Zuckerman, 1960; Dahlstrom & Welsh, 1960; Engel, 1962; Panton, 1960; Butler & Marcuse, 1959; Grugier, 1957; Lynn, 1959; McHugh, 1963; Sappanfield, 1959; Wheeler, 1949; Yamshiro & Griffith, 1960). Very few qualities visible in one gender cannot also be found in representative members of the opposite gender, but despite this, most persons on a common-sense basis consider that masculine and feminine behavior are separate and unique (Bennett & Cohen, 1959). It is significant that the experimentally demonstrated low correlation between masculinity and femininity tests and the shaky character of these tests runs quite contrary to common-sense beliefs (Barrows & Zuckerman, 1960; Engel, 1962).

In effect though, any person who violates normal expectancies about the differences between the male and female gender by assuming alterations in gender or by professing the elective character of gender runs counter to the culture and violates many of its taboos and reward systems. Generally, gender and gender identity is not considered elective and is not vulnerable to the same change as one's religion, one's occupation, or one's geographic place of residence. It is most usually perceived as having the same meaning for most social observers as ethnic background, which is largely part of one's genetic history or of the same immutability as other physical and anthropological characteristics such as head size, head shape, or bone length.

It is generally postulated by most investigators that gender identity is established by the age of 2½ and clearly set by 5 (Brown, 1958, 1959, 1960; Money, 1955, 1957; Stoller, 1965; Hartup, 1963; Hooker, 1958, 1959). This early fixing of gender reflects the close relationship between the developing image of oneself as a person and the maturing concept of oneself in a gender-status role. It would appear that the sense of gender identity is woven closely into the basic fabric of the psychological mechanism and parallels the formation of other basic elements of the personality. It is true that in many respects gender is intrinsic to the structure of one's identity, and the early development of this psychological quality appears to be a part of the development of the self, personal identity, and ego identity. The denial of gender may well parallel the denial of self and therefore the loss of a fundamental and relevant bench mark which defines the person as a psychological entity. In theory, therefore, such a denial of gender surely should not be vulnerable to the kind of easy and comfortable shift as would be a change in jobs or a move to another city, and it should involve violent psychological disruption.

There is ample evidence in animals that the administration of steroids at crucial moments in development can lead to sex-related structural change and to gender- and sex-linked behavioral changes (Whalen, 1963, 1966). By inference from these excellent and convincing studies, the sheer possession of XX and XY chromosomes is not the sole information of the necessary and sufficient condition to make an assignment to a particular sex and gender. It appears necessary that other kinds of supporting phenomena be present before the individual can be assigned to the appropriate gender and sex. There are many other biological and physiological structures that contribute to sex, such as the genital organs, the secondary sex characteristics, the internal and external genital structures, the gonads, the hormonal titres in the bloodstream, and certain as yet undefined brain systems which generate sex-specific and gender-specific behaviors.

The learned phenomenon of gender is influenced by and reflects many psychological, societal, and experimental factors. The models presented to the child by the family and by society may be influenced by biological sex, but in the larger sense gender and gender-relevant behavior is largely learned, although perhaps influenced by significant biological states.

GENDER AND SEX A MANY TEXTURED THING

The variety of possible combinations in the cases cited illustrates clearly the multidetermined nature of gender. It is all of these which play a determining role in the assignment to the male sex and female sex, and the emergent behaviors subsequent to that. At birth however, the possessions of organs that appear characteristic of the genitals of either sex are generally the major significant basis on which sex assignment is made. It is only later that other features may influence sex typing and gender assignment. In rare instances medical intervention can alter physical structure and the assigned sex, either in order that it be made consistent with gender identity, or in order to achieve other resolutions of inconsistencies in assigned sex gender identity and gender role.

Therefore, it is presumed that basic and fundamental gender identity and gender-relevant behavior is biological in two senses. There are first of all the direct effects of biological determinants on behavior. Behavior is influenced by brain mechanisms, as is inferred from the various studies of influence of hormonal states on both structural and psychological development. There are differences in activity levels in neonates and differences in other types of gender relevant behaviors that support this. The second sense in which gender is influenced by biological qualities in a more direct fashion is by the reaction of the surrounding social environment to the physical structure possessed by the individual at birth. The physician perceiving normal male genitalia on a newborn infant assigns that child to the male sex, which in turn leads to the reinforcement by parents and others of behavior compatible to the socio-cultural stereotype of masculine-gender behavior. In this fashion, therefore, gender-relevant behavior and fundamental gender identity is a learned phenomena, with the selective character of the learning influenced by biological factors.

As indicated, then, environmental factors manifest themselves on gender identity through the agencies of emotional conditioning, behavioral shaping, imitation of like-sexed parent, modeling, and other influences that direct behavior and mold it to a significant extent. The amount to which any individual achieves the characteristic behavioral role of a given gender is part of a complex relationship among his given biological structure, the nature of the learning circumstances, the affect associated with learning activities, a variety of unconscious phenomena, and the nature of the relationship to the parents or other major models for such learning.

AMBIGUITY OF GENDER YIELDS AMBIGUITY OF TESTING

There is, as a consequence of these factors, differential learning of the psychological components of gender, that is, the behavior, the attitudes, the characteristics, the response modes, the personality traits, and the other related phenomena that distinguish men and women. These may yield for an appropriately gendered person a broad variety of possible combinations of psychological states and behaviors that are gender consistent. This may account for the low correlations between various so-called M-F tests and suggest that no one test can adequately measure M-F since no one test can adequately sample all domains of human functioning that contribute to gender and gender identity (Engel, 1962).

Powerful influences occurring as a consequence of social learning and learned phenomena can be assessed from the examination of the cases cited above in which the experiences and environmental influences were able to overpower the biological influences and lead to cross-gender identifications. Case number six is an eloquent testimonial to the power of environmental shaping in overwhelming genetic influence. As noted in the clinical examples cited above, several of the individuals described presented clearly consistent biological pictures of gender and sex, which under most visible circumstances should have led to a psychological identity, whose gender was consistent with that of the physical and biological determinants. In point of fact, however, despite the apparent influence of these biological determinants, the impact of the immediate environment, the influence of the parents and the social milieu were indeed more relevant, more important, and more effective in determining the gender identity of the individual.

The pervasive quality of gender-relevant phenomena provides further affirmation of the heroic dimensions of the efforts made by the transexual in shifting from one gender assignment to that of the opposite achieved gender. It is relevant that only rare instances can be cited of persons who appear to remain poised on dead center between the two gender identities and gender roles, although such *intersexed* individuals are by no means unknown. Most individuals tend to fall, at least in sum total of qualities, more in one gender direction or another. In many instances of gender change, it is assumed that the shift in gender serves to resolve a prior state of identity ambiguity with an accompanying state of psychological distress and anxiety. There is for many such persons a history of unsureness and doubt which is thrust aside by the final resolution. In those cases where individuals tend to be poised in the intersexed position, that is, without significant balance in one direction or another, there seems to be greater propensity for emotional disturbance and psychological upheaval and distress.

It is suggested that persons who make the shift in gender identity cannot be considered to have normal or conventional developmental histories. For those persons who shift after early childhood, that is to say, in the ages following 6–7 years, there are data indicating the presence of a failure in the assumption of appropriate gender identity or anomalies in biological determinants or in other subtle psychological influences that serve to press the individual away from that gender and sex assigned to him at birth (Money, Hampson, & Hampson, 1955, 1956, 1957). This difficulty may be a function of parental influences, both subtle and overt, as well as other causes leading to failures in identifying with the like-sex parent. Most frequently the shift appears to be from the state of gender ambiguity, gender conflict, or gender confusion toward a resolution of the confusion or distress by the assumption of a new given gender identity. This certainly is reflected in a seeming reduction in psychiatric symptoms and allaying of evidences of emotional distress in the individuals which had existed prior to the gender shift and the quieting or perhaps even the disappearance of the symptoms following the successful transmutation.

Assigned sex, biological sex, and gender identity in the normal individual in all respects are coincident and affixed early in life. Where discrepancies are present, that is, where there are conscious or unconscious uncertainties and where gender identity is incompatible with assigned sex or where identity is disturbed or ambiguous and there is no clear gender identity, then this unstable equilibrium is resolved by a seeming shift in the appropriate direction toward a more stable resolution. The direction of the shift, and the nature of the eventual gender is a function of the complex weighting of a number of factors, none of which is the single necessary and sufficient condition for the establishment of gender.

SHIFT IN GENDER AS MOVEMENT TOWARD STABILITY

What in fact appears in the patients described in the cases cited above to be an apparent denial of reality may in fact be an attempt to restore equilibrium and balance by movement in the direction of greater stability. The fact of the shift, the fact that the individual has been troubled with this psychological issue, is not evidence in itself of either a retreat from reality or a departure from reason.

For those persons who are unable to make the shift successfully, one can see increases in psychological symptoms, increases in distress and confusion, and clearly what one sees in the unsuccessful shift became visible because the change did not resolve the ambiguity of gender identity arising out of environmental and biological factors. This might well occur where the individual could not successfully deny or psychologically evade the evidence of his body and the fact that his achieved gender, that is, the gender identity toward which he wished to move, was in sharp and dramatic conflict with that gender assigned to him by virtue of biology and birth. In effect, then, the shift in gender leads not to a state of greater equilibrium or harmonious balance in the psychological forces involved, but to a state of greater conflict and greater imbalance. By extension, the psychological determinants such as the strength of motivation and the power and force of the cross-gender identification, must be carefully evaluated before surgical intervention is initiated.

This is best illustrated in the conventional transvestite where the cross-dressing behavior does not ever represent to him the strong desire to *become* a woman, but, quite to the contrary, the wish to mock or simulate a woman while still remaining a man. With the transvestite, the central and most important issue is that he is accorded the rights and privileges of a woman by cross-dressing and that he can as well maintain his awareness of his possession of normal male genitalia while engaged in the masquerade. For this person the complete shift in gender identity, and most certainly the surgical intervention and subsequent cosmetic surgery which would make him become structurally female, would not lead to the resolution of the psychological conflict; it might well produce greater distress and the evocation of more malignant psychological disorder. The subtle difference between a seeming male who feels himself to be a woman and the male who wishes to appear to be a woman is a crucial and significant one in separating the individuals who can successfully change their gender identity and those for whom this gender identity change might well lead to disaster.

At times it appears as if gender identity and the qualities of personality concerned with the transformation of gender represents a carefully circumscribed area isolated from other features of personality functioning. These individuals are frequently otherwise supremely able to deal with their environment, and in several instances, far better able than most. They can manage the most overwhelming tasks of reorganization of life patterns, reorganization of interpersonal patterns, and organization of personal history in a fashion that might well be impossible for many otherwise normal individuals.

Although these individuals show apparent evidence of psychological defects which may be perceived as grave and profound disturbances in ego, there are clear evidences of more adequate ego functions than in many people. One might say that these individuals are psychotic because they deny themselves, because they deny physical reality, and because they deny a part of their basic identity intrinsic to the whole warp and weft of personality. But because of their supreme ability to manage the environment, they must be seen in another light, as perhaps possessing defects in ego functioning but certainly not in reality testing mechanisms. These individuals are not like the average person in the community, but they are well able to function in society, they clearly demonstrate their capacity to hold jobs, to make lasting personal relationships, and to relate themselves to the community as a whole. In this instance, these persons are supremely able to handle the world and show the gender shift to be not a denial of reality but a personal resolution in the direction of a greater and more powerful contact with reality. As a consequence, the dilemma concerning the apparent psychotic state is no longer evident and some underlying consistency is manifest.

The observation of individuals who have engaged in this massive task of gender switch has significant implications for an understanding of mental illness and psychosis. This massive reorganization of personality, and the assumption of a major behavioral repertoire markedly different from those previously possessed, as well as a major disruption of significant dimensions of personality generally considered to be structural to the ego, suggests that there are conditions under which "ego" reorganization can occur, and indeed quite massive disruption of ego mechanisms can take place, without attendant psychosis. Under ordinary circumstances it is assumed that disruption of the ego and the denial of reality are necessary and sufficient conditions to describe psychosis. For persons who have successfully attained a gender apart from that in which they were originally assigned and seemingly reared, grave reorganization of the ego has occurred without subsequent disruption. It is thus possible to assume that many significant reorganizations of the substrata of personality can occur that can lead to a resolution yielding a more adequate adjustment. In some circumstances, as cited above, denial of reality, that is to say, denial of one aspect of the reality of the structure of one's body, can aid in achieving psychological balance rather than leading to destruction of the fabric of personality. These cases can therefore bring a new frame of reference, or at least a new attitude, to bear on considerations of the context as well as the necessary and sufficient conditions for the identification of psychosis. It might well be assumed that other varieties of ego dissolution and reorganization under conditions of control and with a clearly defined goal can yield a more effectively functioning personality rather than necessarily yielding psychosis.

REFERENCES

Aaronson, B. S. A comparison of two MMPI measures of masculinity-femininity. *Journal of Clinical Psychology*, 1959, **15**, 48–50.

Aaronson, B. S., & Grumpelt, H. R. Homosexuality and some MMPI measures of masculinity-femininity. *Journal of Clinical Psychology*, 1961, **17**, 245–247.

Barrows, G. A., & Zuckerman, M. Construct validity of three masculinity-femininity tests. *Journal of Consulting Psychology*, 1960, **24–25**, 441–445.

Baughman, E. E., & Guskin, S. Sex differences on the Rorschach. *Journal of Consulting Psychology*, 1958, **22**, 100 401.

Bennett, E. M., & Cohen, L. Men and women: Personality patterns and contrasts. *Genetic Psychology Monographs*, 1959, **59**, 101–105.

Bieliauskas, V. J. Sexual identification in children's drawings of the human figure, *Journal of Clinical Psychology*, 1960, **16**, 42–44.

Brown, D. G. Inversion and homosexuality. *American Journal of Orthopsychiatry*, 1958, **28**, 424–429. (a)

Brown, D. G. Masculinity-femininity development in children. *Journal of Consulting Psychology*, 1958, **55**, 232–242. (b)

Brown, D. G. Sex-role development in a changing culture. *Psychological Bulletin*, 1958, **55**, 232–242. (c)

Brown, D. G. Psychosexual disturbances: Transvestism and sex-role inversion. *Marriage and Family Living*, 1960, **22**, 218–227.

Butler, R., & Marcuse, F. L. Sex identification at different ages using the draw-a-person test. *Journal of Projective Techniques*, 1959, **23**, 299–302.

Dahlstrom, W. G., & Welsh, G. S. An MMPI handbook. Minneapolis: University of Minnesota Press, 1960.

Diamond, M. A critical evaluation of the ontogeny of human sexual behavior. *Quarterly Review of Biology*, 1965, **40**, 147–175.

Engel, I. M. A factor analytic study of items from five masculinity-femininity tests. Unpublished doctoral dissertation, University of Michigan, 1962.

Goffman, E. *Stigma. Notes on the management of spoiled identity*. Englewood Cliffs, N.J.: Prentice-Hall, 1963.

Grygier, T. G. Psychometric aspects of homosexuality. *Journal of Mental Science*, 1957, **103**, 514–526.

Hart, D. B. On some points in regard to the conditions of the human male and female termed hermaphroditism and pseudohermaphroditism. *Internal. Clinics*, 25th Series, 1915, **4**, 135.

Hartup, W., & Zook, E. Sex-role preferences in three- and four-year-old children. *Journal of Consulting Psychology*, 1960, **24**, 420–426.

Hartup, W. W. Some correlates of parental imitation in young children. *Child Development*, 1962, 85–96.

Hartup, W., & Moore, S. G. Avoidance of inappropriate sex-typing by young children. *Journal of Consulting Psychology*, 1963, **27**, 467–473.

Haworth, M. R., & Normington, C. J. A sexual differentiation scale for the D-A-P Test (for use with children). *Journal of Protective Techniques*, 1961, **25**, 441–449.

Hooker, E. Male homosexuality in the Rorschach. *Journal of Projective Techniques*, 1958, **22**, 33–53.

Hooker, E. What is a criterion? *Journal of Protective Techniques*, 1959, **23**, 278–281.

Lindzey, G., Tejessy, C., & Zamansky, H. S. Tat Test: An empirical examination of some indices of homosexuality. *Journal of Abnormal and Social Psychology*, 1958, **57**, 67–75.

Lynn, D. B. Sex differences in masculine and feminine identification. *Psychological Review*, 1959, **66**, 126–135.

McCully, R. S. A projective study of a true hermaphrodite during a period of radical surgical procedures. *Psychiatric Quarterly Supplement*, 1958, **32**, 1–35.

McHugh, A. F. Sexual identification, size, and associations in children's figure drawings. *Journal of Clinical Psychology*, 1963, **19**, 380–381.

Meketon, B. W., Griffith, R. M., Taylor, V. H., & Wiedeman, J. S. Rorschach homosexual signs in paranoid schizophrenics. *Journal of Abnormal and Social Psychology*, 1962, **65**, 280–284.

Money, J., & Hampson, J. G., Hampson, J. L. An examination of some basic sexual concepts: The evidence of human hermaphroditism. *Johns Hopkins Hospital Bulletin*, 1955, **97**, 301–319. (a)

Money, J., Hampson, Joan G., & Hampson, J. L. Hermaphroditism: Recommendations concerning assignment of sex, change of sex, and psychologic management. *Johns Hopkins Hospital Bulletin*, 1955, **97**, 284–300. (b)

Money, J. Hampson, J.G., & Hampson, J. L. Sexual incongruities and psychopathology: The evidence of human hermaphroditism. *Johns Hopkins Hospital Bulletin*, 1956, **98**, 43–57.

Money, J., Hampson, J. G., & Hampson, J. L. Imprinting and the establishment of gender role. *AMA Archives of Neurology and Psychiatry*, 1957, **77**, 333–336.

Nelson, M. O., Wolfson, W., & LoCascio, R. Sexual identification in responses to Rorschach, card III. *Journal of Protective Techniques*, 1959, **23**, 354–356.

Panton, J. H. A new MMPI scale for the identification of homosexuality. *Journal Clinical Psychology*, 1960, **16**, 17–20.

Rabban, M. Sex-role identification in young children in two diverse social groups. *Genetic Psychology Monographs*, 1950, **42**, 81–158.

Pascal, G. R., & Herzberg, F. I. The detection of deviant sexual practice from performance on the Rorschach test. *Journal of Protective Techniques*, 1952, **16**, 366–373.

Rado, S. A critical examination of the concept of bisexuality. *Psychosomatic Medicine*, 1940, **2**, 459.

Sappenfield, B. R. Perception of masculinity-femininity in Rorschach blots and responses. *Journal of Clinical Psychology*, 1961, **17**, 373–375.

Silverstein, A. B. Identification with same-sex and opposite-sex figures in Thematic Apperception. *Journal of Projective Techniques*, 1959, **23**, 73–75.

Stoller, R. J. A contribution to the study of gender identity. *International Journal of Psycho-Analysis*, 1964, **45**, Parts 2–3, 220–226.

Stoller, R. J. The Hermaphroditic identity of hermaphrodites. *Journal of Nervous and Mental Disease*, 1964, **139**, 453–457.

Stoller, R. J. Gender-role change in intersexed patients. *Journal of the American Medical Association*, 1964, **188**, 684–685.

Stoller, R. J. Passing and the continuum of gender identity. *Sexual Inversion*. New York: Basic Books, 1965. Pp. 190–210.

Stoller, R. J. The sense of maleness. *The Psychoanalytic Quarterly*, 1965, **34**, 207–218.

Stoller, R. J., Garfinkel, H., & Rosen, A. C. Passing and the maintenance of sexual identification in an intersexed patient. *A.M.A. Archives of General Psychiatry*, 1960, **2**, 379–384.

Stoller, R. J., Garfinkel, H., & Rosen, A. C. Psychiatric management of intersexed patients. *California Medicine*, 1962, **96**, 30–34.

Stoller, R. J., & Rosen, A. C. The intersexed patient. *California Medicine*, 1959, **91**, 261–265.

Whalen, R. E., & Nadler, R. D. Suppression of the development of female mating behavior by estrogen administered in infancy. *Science*, 1963, **141**, 273–274.

Whalen, R. E. Sexual motivation. *Psychological Review*, 1966, **73**, 151–163.

Wheeler, W. M. An analysis of Rorschach indices of male homosexuality. *Journal of Projective Techniques*, 1949, **13**, 97–126.

Whitaker, L., Jr. The use of an extended draw-a-person test to identify homosexual and effeminate men. *Journal of Consulting Psychology*, 1961, **25–26**, 482–485.

Worden, F. G., & Marsh, J. T. Psychological factors in men seeking sex transformation: A preliminary report. *Journal of the American Medical Association*, 1955, **157**, 1292–1298.

Yamshiro, R. S., & Griffith, R. M. Validity of two indices of sexual deviancy. *Journal of Clinical Psychology*, 1960, **16**, 21–24.

5.5   Orientation

In recent years, a major controversy in mental illness research has centered around whether schizophrenia can be explained as a result of social or chemical causation. The leader of the group that holds firmly to the view that it is socially determined is the author of this article. His arguments have been powerful and compelling, and as such they have served to clarify the basic illness and concepts involved.

In this article, John R. Weakland points out many of the difficulties inherent in previous research on the sociocultural determinants of schizophrenia, and disordered behavior in general, and suggests what steps need to be taken to improve the quality of the research. He offers his own model for interpreting and explaining schizophrenic behavior and its underlying causes. An analytic viewpoint is taken from the study of the family as an ongoing interaction system with communication as the prime means of interaction. Schizophrenia is seen as a mixed resultant of psychological and social influences and is dependent upon incongruent messages in familial situations. As such, the research emphasis is less on what constitutes pathology and more on the underlying nature of primary communications and social influence.

5.5   Schizophrenia: Basic Problems in Sociocultural Investigation

John H. Weakland

This article represents an attempt to develop and convey a fresh picture of the significant general problems presently inherent in investigating various aspects of schizophrenia (for example, its nature, etiology, prevalence) in relation to its sociocultural environment, and to outline some approaches to effective handling of these problems. This is to be done by bringing into view the general aims, premises, and problems exemplified but not made explicit in much of the existing work in this area, and contrasting these with a different viewpoint developed in the course of first-hand studies of schizophrenia in the family context—a kind of sociocultural environment in miniature.

Accordingly, there is here no comprehensive review of past work in this area, nor critique of specific aspects of such work within its own frame of reference. Instead, I shall only sketch certain main outlines of such work, neglecting details to clarify the broad fundamental picture, and emphasizing what is amiss more than acknowledging accomplishments. A more inclusive and balanced view of this already sizable field, for other purposes, is readily obtainable by reference to various bibliographies (Baldwin et al., 1962; Clausen, 1956; Driver, 1965) and conventional reviews (Clausen, 1959; Benedict, 1958; Benedict & Jacks, 1954; Dunham, 1961; Hunt, 1959; Leacock, 1957; Lemkau & Crocetti, 1958). Particular mention should be made of Mishler and Scotch (1965) who review the field at length, citing original work, other reviews, and methodological discussions, and themselves consider from another viewpoint some of the main issues raised here.

SCHIZOPHRENIA IN SOCIETY: TRADITIONAL APPROACHES

Some selective examination of existing work on sociocultural factors and schizophrenia (including some related material on society and mental illness more generally) is necessary here to provide a concrete basis for discussion. For this purpose, I shall rely on two articles that already report on large areas of the field in brief and orderly fashion. These will be used to formulate a description of typical studies, largely in their own terms, and a summary characterization of them. Then, by further examination based on the family viewpoint to be described, it will be shown: (1) that these studies involve a common, but largely implicit, structure of aims and premises as well as procedures; (2) that this structure fits poorly with the inherent nature of the subject matter; and (3) that these studies themselves indicate some awareness of this discrepancy but fail to meet it directly and take it seriously.

The two sample articles are, in the main, representative of two closely related yet significantly different groups of studies. One group deals with schizophrenia within a given society—most commonly the United States. The other is concerned with schizophrenia in other kinds of societies; these studies are therefore at least implicitly cross-cultural. Aims and approaches correspondingly differ somewhat between these groups.

Intrasocietal Studies

Hunt's (1959) review provides a well-organized descriptive sample of studies of the first type, and some pertinent discussion. Hunt first mentions demographic studies as the oldest and crudest type of investigation in this field. These studies relate rates of incidence of mental disorder to such variables as age, sex, marital status, and race. It is noted from more extensive reviews by Felix and Kramer (1953) and Rose and Stub (1955) that schizophrenia in males is more frequent among foreign-born and Negro groups than native whites, and its onset is concentrated in the 20–35 age range.

Ecological studies are characterized as explorations of relationships between mental disorders and a variety of environmental factors such as high population density, poverty, and high delinquency rates, in defined urban districts. These studies are correctly noted as having been a very influential type since the pioneer study by Faris and Dunham (1939); they have been reviewed extensively by Queen (1940) and Dunham (1955). Workers in this area have, interestingly, exhibited a clear concern about possible *causal* relationships between the factors studied and schizophrenia, but at the same time have maintained a certain caution and distance from this question. That is, none of the factors studied were necessarily presumed to be causally significant, and the possible causal means or connections were largely left undiscussed. The findings have indicated higher rates for schizophrenia in geographical districts characterized by the factors mentioned.

Social stratification studies, examining relationships between mental disorders and various indices of socioeconomic status, appear as a development and refinement of the prior ecological studies. Chief among these, and typical of problems and methods, is the extensive study headed by Hollingshead and Redlich (1958) at Yale. These investigators devised a scheme for assigning individuals studied to one of five social class strata, defined in terms of occupation, education, and area of residence. They were careful to use a normal control sample and to control for population distribution of class membership. Perhaps even more carefully, "The investigators take pains to point out that their results have reference only to diagnosed or treated and not 'true' rates [Hunt, 1959, p. 98]." They found that, on this basis, schizophrenia is more common among lower status groups (Hollingshead & Redlich, 1954a, 1954b, 1958). Similar findings are cited from the work of Tietze, Lemkau, and Cooper (1942a), Frumkin (1955), and Clark (1949). Hunt (1959) himself already points toward the need for a critical overview of such findings: "It may be that whether a given patient is classified as . . . schizophrenic when diagnosis is uncertain, will be in some measure a function of his social status. If this is true the studies reviewed . . . would, at least in part, refer only to status factors in the *diagnosis* of mental disorder [p. 99–100]."

A number of studies attempting to relate rates of mental disorder to social mobility also are largely a development from earlier ecological studies. Work of this kind is found in Tietze, Lemkau, and Cooper

(1942b), in parts of Hollingshead and Redlich (1954a, 1954b), and in Hollingshead, Ellis, and Kirby (1954). A study by Ellis (1952) is of special interest, since in attempting to test the hypothesis that mobility is often partly inspired by emotional drives resulting from unsatisfactory primary group relations, but then leads to further deteriorations of these relations with accompanying neurotic symptoms, she took a step beyond the usual studies by suggesting a possible mechanism—disturbances in primary group relations—as relating mobility and mental disorder. In general, these studies showed no clear results concerning spatial mobility, but indicated that patient groups, especially schizophrenics, tend to be more mobile in status than nonpatients—but mobile *upward,* contrary to certain expectations.

A final group of studies is concerned with relations between social variables and treatment of mental disorders; that is, how much therapy of what sort (for example, psychoanalysis, other psychotherapy, organic therapy, custodial care), and by whom (for example, psychiatrists, psychiatric residents, social workers) is received by patients of various classes. The work of Hollingshead and Redlich (1954a, 1954b, 1958) was important in this area also, along with work by Robinson, Redlich, and Myers (1954), Myers and Schaffer (1954), Auld and Myers (1954), Winder and Hersko (1955), and Hunt, Gursslin, and Roach (1958). These studies suggest that the likelihood of treatment, its extent and intensity, and the status both of the form of therapy and of its practitioner all increase wih higher class status.

Hunt also points out (1959, p. 103) that differential treatment according to class status could influence the interpretation of studies relating social class and incidence rates of schizophrenia, since observed incidence may, in complex ways, depend also on the treatment situation—the two may be measured separately without being independent.

Finally, Hunt discusses explicitly the strong yet largely implicit interest of these studies in causal or etiological connections between the social factors and related mental disorders. Three main kinds of hypotheses have been put forth. The first is the "drift" hypothesis, which argues that schizophrenics, especially, will be unable to function effectively in a society because of their disorder, and will "drift" downward in status and residential area. The second is the "social isolation" hypothesis of Jaco (1954). This proposed that social isolation, "the cutting off or minimizing of contact and communication with others" (measured by such variables as number of acquaintances, membership in fraternal organizations, visits with friends) is an etiological "precipitating variable" specific for schizophrenia, and that "those communities having high rates of schizophrenia will have a concomitantly high degree of social isolation." The third hypothesis is that of "culture contact," that experiencing sociocultural conflict or disorganization from immigration, assimilation of new cultural influences, or cultural complexity would provoke mental illness. Various studies already cited bear on this, as does the work of Goldhamer and Marshall (1953) on social change over a period of time and mental illness, by studying rates of first admissions to hospital for psychosis in Massachusetts over 100 years. In Hunt's judgment, none of these hypotheses has been confirmed. Yet whether such hypotheses result from the studies in question or merely underlie them, they help to fill out our view of their general nature.

"Cross-cultural" Studies

We may now consider the group of studies concerned with mental illness in other societies. This group differs from the first, not only in studying various foreign or primitive societies different from our own, but also in their concern with a wider range of "cultural" problems; for example, the possible variation in nature or manifestation of mental illness, or in rates of incidence, in relation to specific or general characteristics of a given culture. Such studies especially tend to give more consideration to various theoretical and methodological problems, including some that also inhere in studies of the first group but receive little explicit attention there.

The valuable article by Lin (1953), which combines a report of an empirical study, a review of much related work, and significant consideration of a number of issues general to such research, is mainly drawn upon here to illustrate the nature of such studies. Lin first notes some prior general predictions about the probable incidence of various types of mental illness in China, based on deductions from conceptions of the nature of Chinese culture and character, and a few very limited or unclear surveys. He then discusses various possible methods for measuring incidence of mental disorders of the population of a given geographical unit. The more common general method is based on hospital admission statistics, which may miss many cases, particularly where hospital facilities are not well developed. The other general method is investigation of a sample taken to represent the total population. Of several possible kinds of samples, all have evident serious flaws, except the census method, based on examination of all inhabitants of one area taken as a sample of a larger geographical unit.

This method was used by Lin, since hospital facilities were minimal in Formosa, the site of his study, and tolerance of Chinese families in regard to abnormal behavior is rather high, and a large proportion of mental cases would therefore remain in the community even if hospital facilities were sufficient (1953, pp. 315–316). Also the method gave an opportunity to collect demographic and ecological data along with that on mental disorders. First, inquiries were made, using local census records and official personnel, to gather information about all inhabitants and suspected mental cases. Next, the investigators questioned family members or neighbors to get detailed accounts of these cases, and interviewed these persons where feasible. Finally, a confirmation visit was made, by teams which visited every house, checked the information from local records, briefly interviewed each family member, and interviewed in detail all reported cases plus anyone showing any sign of abnormal conduct.

Lin reports the incidence of schizophrenia and other mental disorders thus found, tabulated against the areas studied, and against his demographic and ecological data on age, occupation, and socioeconomic status. Lin also surveyed studies of the incidence of mental disorder in a dozen other societies, and compares them with his own findings. The Formosa rates for the major psychoses and epilepsy did not differ appreciably from those of other countries, but reliable comparison could not be made for nonpsychotic mental disorders, as the problems related to differences in sampling, intensity of study, criteria of mental illnesses, and data handling were too great. Lin also indicates awareness of other important empirical and theoretical complexities in such studies. "It must be re-emphasized that contemporary psychiatry lacks adequate data regarding incidence of types of mental disorders in different cultures. . . . Most European authors on this subject have emphasized hereditary and constitutional factors, and have made little of the cultural and environmental side of mental illness. But modern anthropologists . . . are making contributions to the study of relationships between psychological and cultural patterns frequently at the cost of oversimplification and generalization of hypotheses obtained through observation of primitive societies [1953, p. 335]." Even if these opposing difficulties about data are met, there are basic problems in interpretation, and therefore in the development of a theoretical framework for effective organization of data. For example, Lin's study indicated an absence of obsessive-compulsive neurosis, and this is consistent with other observations. However, "LaBarre (1946) noted the low incidence of obsessive-compulsive neuroses, and thought that the poorly developed 'sphincter-morality' in Chinese character might account for it; thus this lack in Chinese character structure might be related to the lack of strictness in the early training of children. Carothers (1947), on the other hand, attributed the absence of obsessional neurosis in Kenya Negroes to the fact that their culture itself was essentially obsessive-compulsive. In Chinese culture, the rituals connected with ancestor worship may provide an outlet for compulsive tendencies" (Lin, 1953, p. 334).

Hunt's limited consideration of "cross-cultural studies" has little factual to report. He does suggest, on the basis of the reports of Carothers (1953), Stainbrook (1952), and Linton (1956), that the fundamental types of psychosis recognized by Western medicine all appear in other societies, although rates and symptoms may vary considerably, and that specific localized types of psychosis seem very rare, but the situation is more variable for neuroses. Also he reports the assertion by Weinberg (1952) and others that schizophrenia is less frequent in cultures that are homogeneous and have intimate contacts than in cultures which are heterogeneous and have impersonal and hostile contacts, but concludes that, as with Jaco's similar isolation theory, there is as yet no adequate proof or disproof of this sweeping proposition. Hunt's review puts more emphasis on the severity of methodological and interpretative problems in cross-cultural studies, including conflicting tendencies that are likely to exist. The lack of hospitals interferes with usual survey methods, but census methods may also be biased; in one way by the difficulties of survival in primitive societies for anyone seriously psychotic, or in the opposite by acceptance of less serious cases merely as part of the society, not as "mental cases." Diagnoses are also apt to be vague or arbitrary in such studies.

Summary

In summarizing the foregoing, we may say that the intersocietal studies in form are rather simple and repetitive typical sociological investigations except for their specific focus on mental illness. They are fundamentally concerned with collecting data on the incidence of schizophrenia, based on hospital admission records for cases diagnosed as schizophrenia, or less often based on some sort of census survey of a selected population sample, all the members of which are examined psychiatrically, although perhaps quite briefly, to see if this diagnosis could be applied. The resulting raw figures on numbers of cases are converted into rates by relating them to the total population of whatever social or geographical unit is presumed to have been sampled. Such overall rates are then often broken down by tabulation of incidence of various stock sociological categories, differentiated according to simple demographic variables. Data on the handling of schizophrenia or other mental illness may be gathered and utilized similarly; such work especially has included studies of the kind of treatment given various classes of patients. Rather separately, there has also been some concern with outcomes of mental illness, although such studies have mainly been clinically and individually aimed except for work concerned with the "therapeutic community," and with social attitudes toward the mentally ill (see reference in Baldwin et al., 1962, Ch. 18; and Driver, 1965, Chs. 7–8).

It is striking that although most of this work is only empirical or parametric, an interest in causal connections or wider theoretical problems is repeatedly evidenced; but such questions are very seldom brought into the center of the stage for explicit and careful examination. Instead, there is usually only some rather vague postulation of mechanisms connecting mental illness and social factors, or of similarities which interrelate them—as in suggesting "isolation" as common to the individual and social aspects of schizophrenia without much critical scrutiny of either the concept or the phenomena it is so freely used to characterize.

Two significant points characterize the cross-cultural studies. First, they bring up a number of important wider issues. They are concerned with the possibility of different manifestations of mental illness in different cultures, and different handling of it. There is more concern with methodological problems—for example, it is noted more that to determine the incidence of schizophrenia is itself no simple task. And there is more direct attention to issues about theory or about connecting mechanisms between cultural factors and mental illness. This is not to say that care is always exercised in these matters, however. An example to the contrary is the rather casual pronouncement of sweeping and conflicting statements about *the* nature of "primitive" society. When actually observed, primitive society is more like the stock market as characterized by J. P. Morgan. That is, it is hard to make any general statement with certainty, except "It fluctuates"; different cultures are remarkably different. Nevertheless, and perhaps largely because of this fact (it is hard to proceed with scientific "business as usual" in other cultures, as the evident differences in social facilities, practices, and attitudes force one to stop and consider, in research as in other areas of life, ideas and procedures taken for granted in our culture), the cross-cultural studies do tend to exhibit somewhat greater scientific sophistication, if they less readily produce neat quantitative tabulations. But, second, it is generally evident that these studies still want to produce these tabulations; they are basically concerned with the same kind of questions and aims as the intrasocietal studies. The methodological and theoretical problems they notice (are perhaps forced to notice) are seen as obstacles to these aims, not as suggestive of reorientation to a different, broader, and more connected viewing of culture and mental illness.

SCHIZOPHRENIA IN THE FAMILY:
AN INTERACTIONAL APPROACH

In contrast to this persistent orientation, under rather similar influences the research work of my colleagues and myself on schizophrenia and family interaction (Bateson, Jackson, Haley, & Weakland, 1956, 1963; Haley, 1959a, 1959b; Jackson, 1957a, 1957b; Jackson & Weakland, 1959, 1961; Weakland, 1960, 1962; Weakland & Fry, 1962; Weakland & Jackson, 1958) became increasingly oriented toward investigating the nature of schizophrenia, its social contexts, and their interrelation, all viewed similarly in terms of communication.[1] This work itself in important senses was a study of "cultural factors in schizophrenia." That is, although our research group included people trained in psychiatry and communications analysis as well as anthropology, and dealt with schizophrenia and families in our own society, it considered these matters as if they were new and foreign, and as if the family were a small society, so that this work could be viewed largely as an anthropological study of the culture of schizophrenic families. Thus, certain fundamental features of our theoretical or even epistemological orientation and research procedure also seem pertinent for extrapolation to the examination of schizophrenia in larger social contexts, and the basic scientific viewpoint they embody appears useful as an analytic tool for obtaining a new view of the usual work on schizophrenia and culture, by comparison and contrast.

It is significant that our present focus of study and our accompanying set of basic orientations largely developed, or became clearer and more explicit, jointly during the course of our research. Our interest in schizophrenia was at first only an outcome of Bateson's prior interest in the general nature of communication, especially the paradoxes and conflicting messages that may arise because human communication does not involve single, isolated messages, but always proceeds via multiple messages on different levels and different channels. Our research on these matters was being carried on in a mental hospital, and, urged on by Haley, we became interested in interrelations between the obviously disturbed communication of schizophrenics and our wider theoretical interests. The schizophrenic's "inappropriate affect," for example, in communicational terms stands out as an extreme case of conflict or incongruence between two messages, often one verbal and the other via facial expression, about one situation. The general value of examining the ex-

---

[1] The account of our work and its bases presented here is my own formulation; although it often depends on observations and ideas from my colleagues, they might view and describe our joint work differently in various respects.

treme or pathological to illuminate the usual or normal is well known—
and quite different from a focus on the "abnormal" alone in the studies
considered above.

Therefore we began to study the communicative behavior of schizophrenics. Since we conceived of communication as interaction, and there
was then almost no verbatim interview material available even in tran-
script, let alone the tape or film records required to give nonverbal messages, we became involved in conducting our own interviews with the
patients and recording them for detailed study. We were less interested
in content than in the *formal* aspects of communication; study of our
interview records at this level led us to see the presence of certain confusions in discriminating the logical types of messages as characteristic of
the schizophrenics we studied. We then considered how such a failure of
discrimination might have been learned; that is, what sort of formal
pattern of communication directed to the child would produce this
pattern in return? From this arose our concept of the double bind—a
communication involving two conflicting, incongruent messages, at different levels—as a message pattern that should have such an effect. We
therefore began to observe and record schizophrenics and their parents
communicating in joint interviews. At this point in our alternations
between theorizing and observation, we were into "family anthropology"; the only remaining development was partially to enter "applied
anthropology," that is, to explore ways and means of family therapy
with such families. This final state is relevant here not because of its
practical significance, but because some aspects of a family or other social
system become clear only when changes in functioning are attempted.

Family Studies of Schizophrenia:
The Basic Framework

From the summary above, our work might seem not just varied, but
diffuse. Yet one body of interrelated fundamental principles and premises can be discerned as underlying all this work and defining our general
approach. These may be stated, proceeding from the general toward the
more specific, as follows:

1. Our viewpoint was fundamentally interactional rather than atomistic. In particular, we aimed to understand and explain any selected
item of behavior by viewing it in relation to its wider context of social
interaction, as part of a related larger whole, rather than attempting to
correlate two "separate" items.

2. We were especially concerned with ongoing systems of interaction,
in which the system is more than and different from the sum of individ-

ual parts that may be distinguished within it. The family was viewed as a social system in this sense.

3. Systems are both characterized and maintained by the existence of recurrent patterns of interaction—for example, typical styles of relationships among the members in a family, or cultural patterns in a given society. Such patterns, and their significance, can only be found by close observation; they may not be foreknown or obvious.

4. Homeostasis—the ways interaction of elements within the system contribute to the correction of deviations, so as to maintain its ongoing existence—is a fundamental aspect of system functioning.

5. Emphasis on systems and interaction implies a primary interest in "contemporary causality"; that is, how existing behaviors are reciprocally stimulating and reinforcing, and contribute to the total pattern. This contrasts with a more linear-temporal view which seeks root causes of present behavior in the past, and also with a noncausal focus on empirically observed association alone.

6. *Communication* is seen as the key means of interaction. In human social systems, communication in this sense must be understood, and examined, as involving various kinds of messages—verbal and nonverbal, overt and covert, congruent and incongruent, at various levels—and as involving both report and command aspects—that is, influence as well as information. The concept of communication also provides a single framework for viewing both individual and group behavior.

7. The schizophrenic is viewed primarily as a member of his family —part of this social system, not primarily as isolated or outside of it.

8. "Schizophrenia," correspondingly, is taken as the behavior of that family member labeled as the patient or the crazy one (although other members may by certain standards seem equally "sick"). This behavior, like the behavior of family members generally, is examined first and foremost in terms of its observable nature as communication, and the significance of such communication in the overall family patterns and the maintenance of this functioning system.

9. This view also requires consideration of the patient's "saner" behavior together with his "crazy" behavior, rather than separating these elements of his overall individual pattern of communication—and equally, consideration of any "crazy" aspects of the behavior of other family members.

In work along such lines, it can be rather difficult to discriminate neatly between theoretical or epistemological orientations and general considerations of methodological approach; they are too closely interconnected. However, four other interrelated points from our work may be mentioned as being closer to the empirical pole:

1. Our research was based, not on a thorough grounding in past work on schizophrenia, but rather on the existence or assumption of a relatively naïve observational stance, as if we knew little of schizophrenia and of families, or as if members of families of schizophrenics were the natives of some newly discovered tribe. The purpose of this is to maximize prospects of seeing something new and significant. In any area where major problems remain in spite of a history of extensive and intensive study, it is only reasonable to suspect that traditional observations and conceptions are inadequate or inappropriate in important respects, so that reliance on them prejudices research at its very foundations.

2. Therefore, apart from our very broad theoretical orientations, our basic work was heavily concentrated on close observation and description of raw data—the actual behavior of schizophrenics and their families, or at least on comprehensive recordings of such behavior on tape or film—carried on by our senior research personnel.

3. Fresh observation must be accompanied by *positive* description and definition. We aimed, at all levels of behavioral observation, to state what something is or is like, rather than what it differs from or is not. This is, in fact, a correlate of our general emphasis on studying interaction and systems, which focuses on inclusion rather than exclusion. The opposite position is all too prevalent, especially in fields concerned with deviant behavior; witness the common use of such terms as "illogical," "disorganized," or "word-salad," which characterize something negatively by contrast, by exclusion, or by labeling as a "mish-mash"—that is, there is heavy use of residual categories and labels for the very matters of central interest. Such characterizations may express well a negative evaluation or a sense of frustration, but are of little scientific use; even a rough or partial characterization in positive terms is much more informative, although harder to make.

4. In dealing with interaction and systems, from primary observation and description right through building up concepts and theories, to get too simple makes matters more complex. True simplicity, to whatever extent it is possible, can only be achieved by taking all the essential interrelated elements in a system into consideration *together*. If C is a resultant of A and B interacting, then we may find much by studying these factors all together, but despite the apparent simplicity of minimizing the factors to be handled, we may find *nothing at all* by studying A and C, or B and C. If Occam's razor is used too forcefully, it will only cut up units. This principle seems plain, but it is so readily neglected in practice that two more concrete examples will be given. (a) Communication always involves a multiplicity of messages; if a communication

includes the message "Do that" and also the message "Don't do that," observation and analysis of the behavioral effects of the communication based on half of the communication—either half—will only be confusing, and averaging the two messages will be even worse. (b) If schizophrenia has to do with family interaction, it may be simpler—more informative and efficient—to study the schizophrenic even in the apparent chaos of his family than in "simple" isolation (if that were really possible—there is always interaction with the researcher to consider).

REVIEWING THE TRADITIONAL APPROACH

In now utilizing this point of view to reexamine the traditional kind of sociocultural studies of schizophrenia (and other mental illness), there is no intention to criticize the ability, care, time, and effort expended in them in terms of their own premises and orientations. This is rather a viewing from a different angle of the kinds of problems they selected for study, the observations made, the concepts involved, and the interrelations between these. Any body of work, including our own research, could similarly be examined from some outside viewpoint; the results would probably always be both painful and profitable.

This examination will first show how these traditional studies, although manifestly only concerned with empirical correlations, implicitly involve a coherent epistemological position which we here point out and criticize. Next, certain further comments will be made concerning these studies' handling of their inherent major foci. Finally, an explanation of the occurrence and nature of many of these features will be proffered.

In this examination, it is naturally postulated from the very existence and labeling of these studies that they assume (1) that mental illness has some relationship with social life, and (2) that significant aspects of these factors or their relationships are unknown and problematic. Nevertheless, to begin with, these studies appear to take too much as known, or at least as simply and easily knowable, in several respects. They proceed as if schizophrenia were clearly recognizable and comprehensible, and as if there were a good list of the social factors that might be significant for it, so that the only problem is to tabulate a variety of these factors against rates of schizophrenia, in order to pick out the proper ones from the existing list. In our view, it is highly doubtful if such knowledge existed, or even exists yet. And as Mark Twain said, "It's not so much what people don't know that makes trouble; it's what they know that isn't so." Despite this danger, the usual studies do not appear to observe their subject matter sufficiently, meaning sufficiently in terms of quality, intensity, and openness. They do include a sizable *quantity* of observations, but these observations largely are based on existing records, and cannot excel these in quality or scope; even where census surveys have been made, the time devoted to direct observation of any one situation or person, normal or schizophrenic, is quite brief. Related considerations hold for description or labeling in these studies. Standard sociological and psychiatric terms and categories are applied extensively and rather routinely; their relevance and adequacy are not questioned, although various terms used appear to be overly simplistic or to involve constructs quite remote from directly observed data. Such use of standard variables facilitates data collection and recording by assistants; but from another standpoint, this means facilitation of *nonobservation* of basic raw data by the presumably most competent research personnel.

A different aspect of the same overall orientation is manifested in these studies' strong antitheoretical, and even antirelational, stance. These studies say little about either a general or a specific theoretical orientation. Although their basic aim is to investigate relationships between social and psychosocial variables, this investigation is highly restricted by almost exclusive reliance on empirical correlation. There is little consideration given to the *nature* of possible relationships between these spheres, in either theory or observation, so that even when there is some empirical evidence of association there is no basis for meaningful or logical connections, causal or otherwise. As an example, we may again consider the concept of "isolation." This is, in fact, fundamentally a relational concept. It might be used heuristically to promote further observation and exploration of what kinds of social interaction schizophrenics do engage in, and this might be useful in clarifying and connecting individual and social aspects of schizophrenia. But in the rush to use it quantitatively—that is, to move at once to a more abstract and narrow level of relationship—these possibilities are largely neglected. Also, even when various social factors are recognized (especially in crosscultural studies) as being of interest and as necessarily interrelated—such as varying manifestations of mental illness, social recognition and attitudes, and treatment or other handling—the fact of significant relationship is not followed up. It is noted in a cautionary way ("This must be considered") and quickly set aside to get on with more specific and delimited tasks. If such an antirelational approach worked well, criticism might be inappropriate. But the studies themselves indicate an inadequacy in this respect; considerations of theory, causal connections, and other relationships keep cropping up, late in the game and in *ad hoc* fashion. The picture, overall, is one of determination and effort to cast out any theorizing, and its recurrent reappearance, rather surreptitiously. The whole matter resembles struggling with sin and temptation, and the proscribed relational thinking, correspondingly, enters these studies only through the back door and in varying disguises. This hardly seems as good as open and direct consideration of such important matters.

Furthermore, this antirelational, atomistic framework appears to operate strongly not only at this general level, but also at more specific levels, where its isolating effects are invidiously reinforced by marked tendencies to approach "mental illness" in negative or residual-category terms. The outstanding example of this is so common as ordinarily to be taken completely for granted. Again and again these studies, in their titles and in their texts, refer to "mental disorders." That this is a stock term means only that its use is prevalent and habitual, not that it is necessarily appropriate. Like any other "disorder" or "disorganization" reference (including both explicit and implicit references to "social disorganization" in these studies) it characterizes, isolates, and stigmatizes by negation and exclusion. Its use thus obstructs needed inquiry into what kinds of positive characteristics and organization the "disorder" exhibits, as it necessarily must if it identifiably exists at all, and how it is related to anything else. It is also quite consonant with such an emphasis that in these studies there is almost no positive functional view of mental illness either at a general social level (although the cross-cultural studies at least should recognize that deviant behavior, including behavior resembling that of our mental patients, is often clearly important for overall social functioning—for example, the role of the shaman) or at an individual level. The patient is seen as isolated, if he is seen at all, and not as actively involved in any social functioning. Even in relation to a diagnostician, he tends to disappear behind his symptoms, as if these had independent existence.

Indeed, a great deal of the foregoing is exemplified in condensed form in the concept of schizophrenia as a "syndrome" or "disease entity," which is basic to these studies. A syndrome is not behavior; it is an isolable (and isolating) fixed, distinct, and separate existent; it tends somehow to be more real than the patient himself. Perhaps this is because it apears simpler to deal with. Yet even in medical work on schizophrenia, this "reality" appears to exist mainly as an ideal; particular cases, or even cases generally, have a distressing tendency to conflict with the neat textbook picture of a fixed entity—even when any more normal behavior by patients is quietly ignored.

These studies are necessarily concerned with three main foci, namely *relationships* between certain *social variables* and *mental illness*—primarily its incidence, and secondarily its handling. Yet the social variables or categories in these studies are hardly ever social in the senses that seem crucially important. The groupings constructed by the investigators, presumably because they should be environmentally influential in producing schizophrenia, have little or no relevance to actual social interaction systems, which might be significant in the etiology of such a condition. (In some instances they have some relevance to this negatively, to situations conceived as lacking social interaction.) At best, they may imply some concern for groupings that might have certain common social attitudes or definitions of life situations, but what these may be or their supposed significance for schizophrenia is little considered. The categories, in short, appear to reflect a "fishing expedition" approach, but at the same time they are such stock categories of social research that their relevance as bait for hooking the elusive determinants of mental illness is already suspect.

Also, as mentioned above, these studies in many significant respects turn their attention and efforts away from rather than toward considering possible interrelations among the factors with which they are concerned. It might only be added here that although they pronounce their identity as social studies, the approach to interrelating variables that is used—that is, establishing empirically correlations between factors that are partially on a social level, partially on a psychological level, and even partially on a biological level (for example, the factors of age and sex)—does nothing toward providing some common framework relevant to social interaction, within which the various factors of interest can be viewed together. It is perhaps no wonder that investigators in this area seem impelled repeatedly to step out of the framework they have themselves originally set up and seek for some kind of connective concepts. But this is better done earlier and more deliberately.

Then there is the matter central to all this work, concern with determining the incidence of mental illness, especially schizophrenia. There have been specific misgivings on this score (for example, awareness of certain kinds of diagnostic difficulties), but quite regularly these have been noted in passing, as it were, only to be overridden in the need to get on with the research. Moreover, they have not only not been taken seriously enough, but critical consideration of the whole question of incidence has not been sufficiently wide and deep. In the first place, when schizophrenia is taken as an isolable syndrome (the studies allow that there may be certain problems of diagnosis because of different standards of psychiatric training and so on, but these are seen as only unfortunate but specific practical difficulties, beyond which lies a definite knowable entity), then these studies, although they are seeking significant connections between schizophrenia and social factors, begin with an attempt to radically separate schizophrenic behavior from its social context, and even to separate schizophrenic behavior from any other behavior of the same individual.

Two more specific problems are promoted by such a conception of schizophrenia. First, different indexes are used to identify cases without adequate consideration of what is being done differently. As noted earlier, the cases on which incidence figures are based are selected in two main ways—by making a diagnostic census, or by collecting records of hospital admissions. These methods may differ not only in completeness, which is often recognized, but, at least in part, in *what* they measure. A census, whatever the nature or reliability of its criteria and procedures, is based on judgment of symptoms in an interview situation within the general context of daily life. Thus, inclusion in a count of cases by this method is based on what are at least seen as purely psychological criteria (since the social relationship with the diagnostician, although necessarily present, is ignored), and ordinarily leads to no practical social consequences. Hospitalization, however, even where a similar diagnosis is made, is always subsequent to and partially dependent upon some kind of gross disturbance in the relationships of the patient-to-be with other people; an individual may have symptoms and not be hospitalized so long as he does not bother other people too much with them (see Goffman, 1959). There are therefore "cases" of schizophrenia in hospitals less "sick" in terms of psychological or psychiatric diagnostic criteria than some "noncases" in the outer society; all this requires is that they be less disturbed but more disturbing. In short, in addition to its other vagueness and complexities, the category "schizophrenic" in practice always involves an element of social judgment of behavior in relation to others, and an element of psychological judgment of "symptoms," conceived as purely individual in nature. This problem can be seen as another consequence of an atomistic rather than an interactive viewpoint, as the latter would view symptoms as just one part of individual behavior, and individual behavior generally as something to be considered in relation to its environing social system. But even disregarding this more general view, it is evident that in the usual studies, data on incidence rest on two conflicting bases.

Second, the tendency to consider schizophrenia as if it were a known phenomenon also has unfortunate influences in attempts to relate its incidence to other variables. It is true enough that the present state of diagnosis and nosology is adequate to achieve consensus on the identification and even description of many or even most cases, by the psychiatrically trained and indoctrinated. But identification is not equivalent to scientific characterization; to know a case is X is not necessarily to know what X is, in any basic sense—not even if there are stock labels for bits of symptomatic behavior. And it is the essential, basic elements of any phenomenon that need knowing more than ever when the aim is to investigate its significant relationships with other phenomena of a different sort. Viewing "isolation" or "withdrawal from reality" as characterizing schizophrenia may be of some descriptive or communicative value in a context of hospital administration but still be of little value in any attempt to relate schizophrenia to social factors; in fact, assuming such characterization as sufficient blocks further examination and understanding.

Many of the points of criticism mentioned above have been made before, but they have not been seen as interrelated and pervasive aspects of a general approach common to these studies, nor has the extent of their implications been recognized. In sum, it appears that the traditional sociocultural studies of schizophrenia recurrently rely upon existing, standard psychiatric labels and methods of observation, standard sociological categories, numerical procedures and measures of association as if all these are both appropriate and sufficient to the objects of investigation, and consonant among themselves—even in the face of repeated evidence to the contrary in these studies themselves.

There are, as usual, rather compelling if not really good reasons for the recurrent appearance of such difficulties, and for the recurrent tendency of the studies to ignore or override them. Quite simply, the nature of studies of schizophrenia, like their object, is very much enmeshed in and influenced by practical rather than scientific considerations. People acting in crazy ways, and methods of labeling and dealing with them (that is, conceptions of mental disease, diagnosis, hospitals and record keeping, and so on) are urgent practical matters of social life, for individuals and for the social system. Correspondingly, these are deeply entwined with systems that are highly ordered but not scientifically ordered; that is, with the administrative, legal, and medical systems in our society, or their analogues in customary behavior elsewhere. Such systems, quite expectably, are normative; they are geared and ordered toward handling certain selected problems within established social frameworks and limits, not toward the clarification and understanding of basic general relationships among social phenomena. There is a natural tendency in research work toward utilizing the ordering represented in these established categories and procedures—but it is done at a scientific price, which rises rapidly if the nature and inherent limitations of this approach are ignored.

Moreover, although science itself is not a practical matter in basic principle, even science is a social activity, and it seems that the general scientific approach used in these studies also has probably been affected by similar practical biases and limitations. Given the social prestige of science (it knows all, or is just about to) and the prestige of atomistic discriminations, hard data, and quantitative methods in its enterprises at present, there are natural difficulties in recognizing openly that we really know little about schizophrenia and related social factors, and that a more deeply and frankly exploratory approach, based on observation and thinking, guided by a broad interest in interaction, may be more appropriate now and for some time yet than the piling up of empirical correlations of this with that, in hope of finding some important relationship.

Our own studies, however, in contrast to the traditional ones, did proceed along such lines, and this approach can be defended as scientific in the most fundamental sense, and as ultimately more productive. Some of the premises and principles described earlier were fairly clear and definite early in our research. Others became so only as we looked at schizophrenics from a communicational view and in a family context, first in idea and later in actuality. And in particular, our work began, largely, without initial specific definition or assumption of what is essential in schizophrenia, in families, or in their systematic study. These matters were left to become progressively clearer, within the framework of our most general orientations, during and in relation to the course of our research. This was realistic because it constituted an acknowledgement and acceptance of a basic general ignorance about these matters. This was possible because practical, official, or traditional criteria can suffice initially to identify and select objects for observation and description while still being quite inadequate to characterize them well. And, moreover, this was positively desirable, since the looseness and flexibility of this approach, in combination with a general framework and much empirical observation, promoted the gradual development of a new but unified and interrelated set of observations, methods, and concepts, all adapted to the objects of study and to each other. Such mutual adaptation of its various aspects, although seldom discussed, seems essential for penetrating and productive research.

This is, obviously, a procedure based on successive approximation, with repeated revision and increasing refinement of all aspects of the research. Research necessarily always involves such successive approximation, since we can never know adequately in advance what is relevant, and how, for a problematic situation. The more problematic the situation (and schizophrenia is an excellent example), the more this approach is fundamentally appropriate to all aspects of a study, yet the more difficult it may be to accept and use. To begin with so little definition may, very understandably, seem uncertain or threatening, yet it does offer a fundamental promise of gradually discovering research means appropriate to a largely unknown situation, which will progressively bring order out of chaos—or more accurately, will allow us to perceive and describe inherent order not seen before.

FUTURE DIRECTIONS

After all the foregoing criticism, what constructive views can be offered? As just indicated, our approach is not one that promises too much in the way of quick results (although our family studies have rapidly become useful both in understanding and in treating schizophrenia), but it seems possible at least to outline positively some significant factors for the sociocultural study of schizophrenia and make suggestions toward their investigation from our standpoint.

Factors for Study

In fact, the very studies criticized have a quite positive contribution to make in this respect. As a group they have demonstrated that social factors are significant, and shown the basic elements that must remain central to this area: studies in this field are and will be concerned generally with *interrelating* information about the *occurrence* (or possibly absence) of schizophrenia, as behavior necessarily manifested by an individual or a number of individuals, with information about the *social contexts* of such behavior.

More particularly, as to occurrence, information must be gathered on the observable manifestations for each individual case, or set of cases, in a social group. In a framework that bears in mind that schizophrenic behavior is a mixed resultant of psychological and social organization and influence, and may be a different mixture in different societies, we should then look at relevant examples to see their general nature and any special characteristics, variations in such behavior, its severity or intensity, and (although perhaps finally rather than initially) its prevalence in the society or social group. That is, the question of rate of incidence should not be abandoned, but also it should not be put first in such investigations either in time or emphasis. Such overall incidence rates, although apparently a simple variable because of the high level of abstraction, may actually be more complex and less rewarding to study than examination of other aspects of schizophrenic behavior. Indeed, rough indications or estimates of incidence might for many purposes be preferable to concentration of effort on achieving precision that may be misleading, or even inherently impossible to obtain.

As to the social contexts of schizophrenia, to facilitate linking this broad concept with factors that in past work have been noted on a more separate basis, we may broadly discriminate between social factors concerning the *circumstances* of schizophrenic behavior and those concerning its *handling*. Among the circumstances that need investigation would be the general cultural patterns of the social group, charactcristic styles of social interaction, and family and child reading patterns. More specific factors would include social conceptions of the nature and etiology of mental illness, and related evaluations. For example, is schizophrenic behavior socially classified or labeled as an entity, and if so, as a disease, as spirit possession, as bad behavior, as a special personality type, or what? Such labels can be most important for the manifestation and outcome of schizophrenic behavior, since they strongly influence social judgments as to the existence and nature of certain behavioral phenomena, and also influence responsibility for and social reaction to them (witness the extent of efforts in our own society in recent years to label certain "delinquent" behavior, or alcoholism, as diseases and thus as involuntary). Such social conceptualization must be inquired about, as its nature can never be safely assumed or guessed. For example, it is reported that in Timbuctu syphilis, which is ubiquitous in the population, is considered a minor disease to be caught and got over with as soon as possible—about the way we view measles (Miner, 1965).

With regard to the social handling of schizophrenia much more may need investigation than the matter of psychiatric treatment, although this is an example within this category, and is of major importance in our society. In other social groups there may be other forms of treatment, or handling that is not conceived as treatment—for example, the person whose behavior would here put him in the role of patient may elsewhere move into a quite different role—a high status as a shaman, a feared one as a witch, or perhaps some tolerated but menial role. The roles that persons behaving in schizophrenic ways are apt to assume may vary not only in status, but also in the extent and nature of their integration with the rest of the social system. Changes of role with onset of schizophrenia, and then subsequent changes—whether toward "cure" and thus reversion to the former social role, or toward further development in a new role, and general social expectations about the temporal course of behavior and eventual outcome of schizophrenia, all need careful inquiry. The social fate of persons whose behavior we would call "schizophrenic" may be very different in different societies.

Such conceptions and expectations about social handling and outcomes of schizophrenia evidently may also be significant for its development and characteristics. Thus, in fact, sharp discrimination of circumstances and handling as if one were simply antecedent and the other consequent is fundamentally inappropriate. The two must ultimately be considered together, keeping in mind that in a social system, because of interaction and feedback, all factors must be seen as having both these aspects. The usual social consequences of any behavior are also a part of the circumstances of its occurrence.

An Approach to These Factors

It is perhaps evident already from the discussion above that the main positive suggestion here is that some basic aspects of our family studies' viewpoint be tried out on a larger social scale, with a focus on the particular kinds of factors cited. In broad terms, it is proposed that the behavior patterns of schizophrenic individuals, including both normal and "crazy" aspects, be closely examined within and in relation to their particular sociocultural settings. The criteria for and definition of schizophrenia could be rather loose initially, so long as actual behavior was observed and described carefully in each case. Such observation and description should explicitly focus on schizophrenia as communicative behavior, and within this frame, on its general features, especially at a formal level (that is, such aspects as the recurrent combination of incongruent messages). Limited attention might be given to the content of schizophrenic communication as related to cultural themes. This has been a topic of interest in previous cross-cultural studies, but, while finding such connections provides evidence for social influence on the manifestations of schizophrenic behavior, it also may draw attention away from the more important general features of structure and relationship, as has occurred before in the psychological study of symbolic and personal-history aspects of schizophrenic productions.

The use of such loose initial criteria is allowable because such studies would assume that in any event this category "schizophrenia" is unclear and needs investigation, and also because the research emphasis would be more on viewing clearly social contexts and associated behaviors than on these behaviors as such. The main emphasis throughout, in fact, would be on investigating the social system from an interactional viewpoint, and schizophrenic behavior as a sector within this—that is, less on "pathology" and more on social science. Such investigation and interrelation is facilitated by focusing on communication, which refers to observable behavior, is directly concerned with interaction (since communication is the main vehicle for the transmission of influence as well as information among human beings), and is a concept applicable to descriptions of behavioral phenomena at the level of the social system, the family system, and the individual, so that these may all be examined within one common framework.

At the societal and family levels, attention would again be focused first on recurrent general patterns. On both anthropological and psychiatric grounds it appears that such general and formal patterns are of much more fundamental significance for determining the nature of individual behavior of members of a social system than are specific and unusual events. Although these may be more dramatic, and in some instances quite influential, even such influences can only be predicted or understood if the more pervasive context has first been seen (see Jackson, 1957b). This holds whether causality is considered with a historical emphasis, in which case general contexts are crucial to more specific learning and change, or with a more contemporary, circular view emphasizing reciprocal reinforcements of behavior patterns within an interactive system. The latter is the primary viewpoint proposed here; attention in theorizing, observation, and description (which themselves are highly interconnected) would be concentrated on any society or social group as an ongoing system, on its homeostatic nature, and on seeing the interactive and homeostatic functioning of behavior. This needs stressing especially for deviant behavior such as schizophrenia, since just these functional relations are apt to be overlooked or overshadowed by the factors of difference and distance apparent in such behavior, which have led to views emphasizing "isolation," "broken homes," "deterioration of primary group relations," and the like, which emphasize the overt and neglect covert organization and functioning. In our family studies, an emphasis on function and interaction has been revealing and rewarding; it leads to a picture of tightly intermingled contact *and* isolation of the schizophrenic and other members of the family system, which serves importantly in the maintenance of the typical behaviors of other members and the nature of the system as a whole. Not only is this visible on observing the interaction of family groups where the patient is present; even if a patient has long been hospitalized and his family far away it is often easy to see that they still affect each other strongly—perhaps by correspondence (Weakland & Fry, 1962), or in its absence (itself a message), by their recollection of unfinished business with each other. It seems probable that a similar approach to schizophrenia and a wider social system would also be valuable, and there is evidence of this in anthropological studies, which often show how the deviant individual and his behavior fill social roles that are of importance as part of the total cultural system.

Consistent with the foregoing emphasis on interaction within a social system, it may be suggested that work in this area should for some time focus on case studies, at a social level, using comparative information only as an aid to clearer observation of the main target. General cross-cultural comparison is a more complex task which should be deferred for some time.

Schizophrenia and Culture: Some Broad Problems

The suggestions above obviously are quite general; they certainly do not provide any specific research design. This is appropriate to our view of the field as one that most needs exploration, so that guidance must be based on stating general principles to be used in connection with careful and intensive examination of relevant data. To be more specific would limit and bias study more than assist it. However, it is possible in conclusion also to consider certain particular problems related to any such studies as proposed.

These problems are chiefly concerned with broad aspects of the relationship of schizophrenia and culture. A relatively simple one, for a starter, is embodied in speculations as to the possible existence of a "schizophrenic society." From the standpoint taken here, the answer is "yes and no, but mostly no." Its basis may be seen by considering, first, whether a pattern of individual psychological organization identifiable as schizophrenic might independently exist. This is very dubious, because the organization of individual behavior is so highly interrelated with social organization and interaction. But even if this were possible, there are only two possibilities at the social level. Either no functioning society could exist based only on such individuals, or some kind of cultural patterns involving such individual organization, such that an ongoing social system would result, could exist. But in this case, the term schizophrenic, without serious qualification, would really not be applicable for either the individuals or the society, because, as noted earlier, our usual concept of schizophrenia fundamentally involves certain elements of social deviance and malfunctioning, which by definition are absent in this case.

In other words, our "schizophrenic society" or more general "sick society" ideas are rough and mixed concepts usually used, for some given society, to point toward the presumed existence either of a predominance of individuals with schizoid (or other "pathological") personality organization, or of a social organization we see as undesirable and somehow analogous to schizoid patterns. Although these terms are poor, there is some evidence of reference to significant social realities. According to Fortune (1932), the people of Dobu were generally paranoid in personality make-up, yet they had a society which, although to our eyes it was riddled with hostility, suspicion, and black magic, nevertheless functioned. And the character structure of the Balinese, as described by Bateson and Mead (1942), appears highly schizoid in terms of our psychological standards, yet, in connection with cultural patterns and social mechanisms which they describe, an extensive and considerable culture flourished.

Indeed, many features of the Balinese patterns of culture and personality organization seem to have parallels in several important Oriental societies, and it is worth considering how social and personal levels of organization seem to be geared together in such instances. Speaking broadly (as a basis for further investigation rather than as a definite account) sociocultural systems that strongly involve schizoid personality types appear correspondingly to involve distant rather than intimate social relationships. Such distance may not be obvious, as it is with many schizophrenics. On the contrary, the dominant impression, as in Bali, or in China or India, may be of a great deal of social activity and interaction, at close quarters. These two apparently opposed views are not really incompatible, but complementary. In such cultures there is much social interaction in large groups and in close physical proximity, but much less in terms of one-to-one relationships and emotional intimacy. And social relationships are largely carried on, not in terms of interaction whose nature is worked out between participant individuals, but in terms of extensive impersonal rules and standards of behavior and interaction that are given, known in advance. Such a system obviously can best exist in a traditional society, although the necessary rules could conceivably come into play otherwise—for example, as part of a social movement joined by true believers; it is certainly adequate to serve as a basis for even large and complex societies.

The implications of such a system for psychological functioning or malfunctioning (it seems almost impossible yet to avoid negative or residual categorizations) are interesting here, especially in their dualistic functioning. It is likely that individuals of schizoid character ordinarily would function well in such a social system, since its patterns are congruent with their relationship tendencies; indeed, these tendencies might well be rewarded and promoted more than other possible types of psychological organization. Thus, if surveys are possible, one might expect in such a society to find considerable schizophrenia or near-schizophrenia with a test delineating deep psychological patterns, but little schizophrenia if evaluation were based more on social functioning (as with hospitalization). As a further complication, however, it seems likely that the few cases that would thus be found (those that somehow exceeded such a social system's functional limits) might be very severe ones.[2] These considerations, taken together with the possible existence of positive social roles even for quite deviant schizophrenics, give some view of the relational complexities that may lie behind the deceptively

[2] For the development of this line of thinking I am indebted to discussions with John W. Gittinger.

simple concept of the "rate of incidence" of schizophrenia, and how little such rates may indicate directly about the "mental healthiness" of either the social system or of the population involved.

Culture-contact may also be considered in a related light, as another important situation that has suffered from over-simplified viewing, largely in relation to ideas about conflict and "disorganization." There has been little real study of culture contact—what changes, restructurings and developments occur and how, which must vary with the nature of the two cultures in each instance; it has only been noted in a few studies that schizophrenia does not appear to be associated with immigration. If one has a more positive conception of schizophrenia, as embodying a characteristic organization of its own, it is not so surprising that it should not regularly arise out of the many different ways in which customary behaviors might be rather randomly blocked or frustrated in various kinds of cultural contacts.

But if schizophrenia is both positively organized behavior and largely a matter of social interaction and influence, how can one conceivably explain the apparent fact of its occurrence in a vast variety of cultures? (This may not be established for all cultures, but the evidence still is considerable, and our experience with several quite different cultures also indicates a widespread core of similar behavior.) Certainly no definite answer to this problem is at hand, but a conceivable answer is. We view schizophrenia—both in nature and in etiology—as based essentially on certain formal patterns of communication involving incongruence between related messages of different levels, and the behavioral influence of such communication (Bateston et al., 1956). To illustrate these matters with examples requires bringing in some content, but the essence of schizophrenia depends on the structuring of certain universal factors of human communication and social interaction into patterns that, although distinctive, are of such high abstraction and generality as to be relatively independent of any lower-level cultural phenomena; thus schizophrenia can be supra-cultural to a considerable extent without being an organic illness. Furthermore, this view still allows room for the possible existence of partial interrelation of schizophrenia with factors within a given culture: (1) The content of a culture, being at a relatively specific level, may be reflected in the content of schizophrenia. (2) At a somewhat higher level, it is possible at least to imagine a society (one version of the psychiatric utopia often sought) in which cultural patterns would somehow encourage a minimal production of incongruent messages, with resulting influences on schizophrenia in the society. (3) And, at a yet higher level of cultural learning and patterning of interaction, societies may well vary in the extent to which congruence, as against incongruence, in communications is normal or expected; this should affect responses to otherwise schizophrenogenic communications in complex and fascinating ways.

Finally, what can be said of the most central problem in the study of schizophrenia when approached as suggested here—the interrelations of the individual, family, and social system? Perhaps not too much, beyond pointing out how badly this topic needs investigation, in a variety of societies (for example, would the family seem of equal importance for schizophrenia if our own work were repeated in a different society, or even in this society with more attention given to the wider social system?), and that the concept of communication provides a common framework for such investigation. Yet two further observations may suggest the kind of relationships that need looking into. On one hand, it has been suggested earlier that schizoid character structure, here seen tentatively as primarily a resultant of the family interaction system, could be the basis of a viable society (rather than the basis of deviance and pathology), given interaction patterns in the culture generally that would fit such character organization without undue strain, and thus simultaneously reinforce it. This in fact implies that the family and the social system are apt to have patterns that are parallel or similar to a large extent. On the other hand, in our own family work and related work by others, there is evidence suggesting that individuals may be very schizoid, yet be functioning and not labeled as sick, in their own family settings, which presumably foster such behavior but are also adapted to contain it. Such families also are often marked by the limited extent their members interact outside the family—they are closed systems to an unusual degree —but as children grow older, even in such families opportunities and pressures for extrafamilial contacts increase markedly (for example, school, work, military service, sexual relationships). And a schizophrenic break—the rapid appearance of overt psychosis—often seems to be related to such an individual's developing increased contact with some world of social interaction outside the family, although this outer world appears much "healthier" than that in the family. That is, there is here some indication of overt schizophrenic behavior as being related to certain incongruences between the *systems* of interaction at the family level and a wider social level, contrasting with the previous example of viable functioning where there is congruence between these systems of interaction. Such considerations may provide that sort of beginning for fruitful inquiry which in science traditionally is at least supposed to be as significant as specific findings.

REFERENCES

Auld, F., Jr., & Myers, J. K. Contributions to a theory for selecting psychotherapy patients. *Journal of Clinical Psychology*, 1954, **10**, 50–60.

Baldwin, J. A., Gelfand, S., Kelly, J. G., Lange, H., Newbrough, J. R., & Simmons, A. J. *Community mental health and social psychiatry: A reference guide*. Cambridge, Mass.: Harvard University Press, 1962.

Bateson, G., Jackson, D. D., Haley, J., & Weakland, J. H. Toward a theory of schizophrenia, *Behavioral Science*, 1956, **1**, 251–264.

Bateson, G., Jackson, D. D., Haley, J., & Weakland, J. H. A note on the double bind—1962. *Family Process*, 1963, **2**, 154–161. (Includes extensive bibliography of the group's work.)

Bateson, G., & Mead, M. *Balinese character: A photographic analysis*. New York: Special Publications of the New York Academy of Sciences, II, 1942.

Benedict, P. K. Sociocultural factors in schizophrenia. In L. Bellak (Ed.), *Schizophrenia, a review of the syndrome*. New York: Logos Press, 1958. Pp. 694–729.

Bendict, P. K., & Jacks, I. Mental illness in primitive societies. *Psychiatry*, 1954, **17**, 377–389.

Carothers, J. C. A study of mental derangement in Africans, and an attempt to explain its peculiarities, more especially in relation to the African attitude of life. *Journal of Mental Science*, 1947, **93**, 549–597.

Carothers, J. C. The African mind in health and disease. *World Health Organization Monograph 17*. Geneva: World Health Organization, 1953.

Clark, R. E. Psychoses, income, and occupational prestige. *American Journal of Sociology*, 1949, **54**, 433–440.

Clausen, J. A. *Sociology and the field of mental health*. New York: Russell Sage Foundation, 1956.

Clausen, J. A. The sociology of mental illness. In R. K. Merton, L. Broom, & L. S. Catrell (Eds.), *Sociology today*. New York: Basic Books, 1959. Pp. 485–508.

Driver, E. D. *The sociology and anthropology of mental illness: A reference guide*. Amherst, Mass.: University of Massachusetts Press, 1965.

Dunham, H. W. Current status of ecological research in mental disorder. In A. Rose (Ed.), *Mental health and mental disorder*. New York: W. W. Norton, 1955. Pp. 168–179.

Dunham, H. W. Social structures and mental disorders. In *Causes of mental disorders: A review of epidemiological knowledge, 1959*. New York: Milbank Memorial Fund, 1961. Pp. 227–265.

Ellis, E. Social psychological correlates of upward social mobility among unmarried career women. *American Sociological Review*, 1952, **17**, 558–563.

Faris, R. E. L., & Dunham, H. W. *Mental disorders in urban areas*. Chicago; University of Chicago Press, 1939.

Felix, R. H., & Kramer, M. Extent of the problem of mental disorder. *Annals of the American Academy of Political and Social Science*, 1953, **286**, 5–14.

Fortune, R. F. *The sorcerers of Dobu*. New York: Dutton, 1932.

Frumkin, R. M. Occupation and major mental disorders. In A. Rose (Ed.), *Mental health and mental disorder*. New York: W. W. Norton, 1955. Pp. 136–160.

Goffman, E. The moral career of the mental patient. *Psychiatry*, 1959, **22**, 123–142.

Goldhamer, H., & Marshall, A. *Psychosis and civilization*. Glencoe, Ill.: The Free Press, 1953.

Haley, J. An interactional description of schizophrenia. *Psychiatry*, 1959, **22**, 321–332. (a)

Haley, J. The family of the schizophrenic: A model system. *Journal of Nervous and Mental Diseases*, 1959, **129**, 357–374. (b)

Hollingshead, A. B., Ellis, R., & Kirby, E. Social mobility and mental illness. *American Sociological Review*, 1954, **19**, 577–583.

Hollingshead, A. B., & Redlich, F. C. Social stratification and schizophrenia. *American Sociological Review*, 1954, **19**, 302–306. (a)

Hollingshead, A. B., & Redlich, F. C. Schizophrenia and social structure. *American Journal of Psychiatry*, 1954, **110**, 695–701. (b)

Hollingshead, A. B., & Redlich, F. C. *Social class and mental illness*. New York: John Wiley & Sons, 1958.

Hunt, R. G. Socio-cultural factors in mental disorder. *Behavioral Science*, 1959, **4**, 96–107.

Hunt, R. G., Gursslin, O., & Roach, J. Social status and psychiatric service in a child guidance clinic. *American Sociological Review*, 1958, **23**, 81–83.

Jackson, D. D. The question of family homeostasis. *Psychiatic Quarterly Supplement*, 1957, **31**, 79–90. (a)

Jackson, D. D. A note on the importance of trauma in the genesis of schizophrenia, *Psychiatry*, 1957, **20**, 181–184. (b)

Jackson, D. D., & Weakland, J. H. Schizophrenic symptoms and family interaction, *Archives of General Psychiatry*, 1957, **1**, 618–621.

Jackson, D. D., & Weakland, J. H. Conjoint family therapy; some considerations on theory, technique, and results. *Psychiatry*, 1961, **24** (Supplement to No. 2), 30–45.

Jaco, E. G. The social isolation hypothesis and schizophrenia. *American Sociological Review*, 1954, **19**, 567–577.

LaBarre, W. Some observations on character structure in the Orient: II. The Chinese, Parts One and Two. *Psychiatry*, 1946, **9**, 215–237, 375–395.

Leacock, E. Three social variables and the occurrence of mental disorder. In A. H. Leighton, J. A. Clausen, & R. N. Wilson (Eds.), *Explorations in social psychiatry*. New York: Basic Books, 1957. Pp. 308–337.

Lemkau, P. Y., & Crocetti, G. M. Vital statistics of schizophrenia. In L. Bellak (Ed.), *Schizophrenia: A review of the syndrome*. New York: Logos Press, 1958. Pp. 64–81.

Lin, Tsung-yi. A study of the incidence of mental disorder in Chinese and other cultures. *Psychiatry*, 1953, **16**, 313–336.

Linton, R. *Culture and mental disorders*. Springfield, Ill.: Charles C Thomas, 1956.

Miner, H. *The primitive city of Timbuctoo.* (Rev. ed.) Garden City, N.Y.: Doubleday Anchor Books, 1965.

Mishler, E. G., & Scotch, N. A. Sociocultural factors in the epidemiology of schizophrenia. *International Journal of Psychiatry*, 1965, **1**, 258–305.

Myers, J. K., & Schaffer, L. Social stratification and psychiatric practice: A study of an outpatient clinic. *American Sociological Review*, 1954, **19**, 307–310.

Queen, S. A. The ecological study of mental disorders. *American Sociological Review*, 1940, **5**, 201–209.

Robinson, H. A., Redlich, F. C., & Myers, J. K. Social structure and psychiatric treatment. *American Journal of Orthopsychiatry*, 1954, **24**, 307–316.

Rose, A., & Stub, H. R. Summary of studies on the incidence of mental disorders. In A. Rose (Ed.), *Mental health and mental disorder.* New York: W. W. Norton, 1955. Pp. 87–116.

Stainbrook, E. Some characteristics of the psychopathology of schizophrenic behavior in Bahian society. *American Journal of Psychiatry*, 1952, **109**, 330–335.

Tietze, C., Lemkau, P., & Cooper, M. Schizophrenia, manic-depressive psychoses, and social-economic status. *American Journal of Sociology*, 1942, **47**, 167–175. (a)

Tietze, C., Lemkau, P., & Cooper, M. Personality disorder and spatial mobility. *American Journal of Sociology*, 1942, **48**, 29–39. (b)

Weakland, J. H. The double-bind hypothesis of schizophrenia and three party interaction. In Jackson, D. D. (Ed.), *The etiology of schizophrenia.* New York: Basic Books, 1960. Pp. 373–388.

Weakland, J. H. Family therapy as a research arena. *Family Process*, 1962, **1**, 63–68.

Weakland, J. H., & Fry, W. F. Letters of mothers of schizophrenics. *American Journal of Orthopsychiatry*, **32**, 604–623 (1962).

Weakland, J. H., & Jackson, D. D. Patient and therapist observations on circumstances of a schizophrenic episode. *A.M.A., Archives of Neurology and Psychiatry*, 1958, **79**, 554–574.

Weinberg, S. K. *Society and personality disorders.* New York: Prentice-Hall, 1952.

Winder, A. E., & Hersko, M. The effect of social class on the length and type of psychotherapy in a Veterans Administration mental hygiene clinic. *Journal of Clinical Psychology*, 1955, **11**, 77–79.

5.6 Orientation

"A voice out of the past which speaks of the future" is perhaps an appropriate description of the paper by Bernard Rimland.

The assumption that all psychopathological behavior is based on constitutional-genetic determinants was considered a tenable hypothesis in the nineteenth and early twentieth centuries. Since the rise to prominence of Freudian concepts, however, functional explanations of pathology have tended to put organic-oriented explanations into disrepute. Thus, to speak out publicly about such hypotheses has usually meant relegation to research oblivion.

Dr. Rimland's ideas are bold and controversial. He assumes that all personality disorders are organically based and that psychosocial influences are minor in the development of these disorders. He presents the arguments for both sides clearly and objectively before marshalling an impressive array of evidence against functionally based theories. The sacred cows of current beliefs about mental illness are systematically destroyed by his arguments and his manner of presentation.

Not content simply to criticize existing functional theories, the author offers strong evidence of biogenic causation in mental illness. If "environmental upheaval" is far more serious than "social upheaval," as Rimland concludes, he is becoming the voice of the future in pointing to the coming directions of research.

5.6   Psychogenesis versus Biogenesis: The Issues and the Evidence

Bernard Rimland

Millions of people throughout the world are so disturbed in thought and behavior that we call them "mentally ill." We know the cause of the disorder in many of these people: infections of the brain, tumors, toxic effects of chemicals or drugs, vitamin deficiencies, head injuries, and metabolic disorders are among the recognized causes of mental illness. In the case of millions of other affected persons, however, no specific cause can be ascribed. To these latter cases many psychiatrists and psychologists attach the label "functional" or "psychogenic" mental illness, indicating their belief that no physical or chemical impairment accounts for the disordered behavior. Rather, they claim that the disorder is a

This paper is a highly condensed version of material which will appear in a forthcoming book, *The Psychogenic Hypothesis*. Because references to the literature will be available in the book, and would be unduly space-consuming here, I have limited the number of works cited. Some of the documentation not included here may be found in my book *Infantile Autism*, especially in Chapter 3.

consequence of faulty relations with other people, especially in early childhood.

In using the terms "functional" and "psychogenic" the professionals explicitly assume that the patient has no biological defect to which his disorder might be traced, and they implicitly assume that there is in actuality a general class of disorders correctly called "psychogenic." That is, they assume that mental illness *can* be caused by faulty interpersonal experiences.

It is the purpose of this essay to question that assumption; to ask, "Why do psychiatrists and psychologists believe there are people whose mental disorder is functional rather than organic? Why do they reject the plausible premise that the 'functional' cases differ from the organic cases only in that our knowledge is at present too limited to identify the 'organic' defect in the 'functional' cases?"

The concept of psychogenic mental illness is so widely accepted today that most readers may regard these questions as too naive to deserve consideration. Yet, I maintain, they are not. These are extremely important questions which must be asked—often and insistently. Though the questions need asking, I think it is not yet possible for us to provide more than a fairly good guess (or should I say prediction?) at the ultimate answer to the question, "Is there a sound basis for the widespread belief in 'functional' mental illness?"

Let me emphasize, before we enter into any very detailed examination of the matter, that our task, at this stage, is more like that of a bettor at a race track than that of a juror in a court of law. That is, our task is not to reach a *conclusion*—any conclusion would be premature—but to make a *prediction,* albeit a prediction based on the available evidence. We know so little about mental illness, how to define it, what causes it —and for that matter, about how the normal brain functions—that to try to solve this problem may appear as futile as to try to describe a rainbow to a man born blind. Yet the problem of determining causation of mental illness is obviously an important one. Not only do our ideas about causation bear directly on how vast expenditures will be made in research and treatment, but they also have important implications for such every-day human affairs as child rearing, the management of criminals and delinquents, and even our attitudes toward ourselves and others.

What will the textbooks say 50 or 100 years from now about the causes of what we now term "functional" psychoses? Will they refer to the psychogenecists of the 1960s in the same half-amused, half-pitying way our current texts refer to the nineteenth century physicians who considered paresis a "moral disease"? Or will those who insist on the primacy of biological factors be seen in the wisdom of restrospect to have been foolishly misguided? How will the eclectics fare in retrospect—those who say it takes *both* a faulty constitution *and* a history of adverse social relationships to cause the disorder? Is it logically inescapable, as some seem to believe, that the eclectics *must* be right?

The outcome of the search will not be a function of how popular each choice is with the current experts, nor of how confident each authority feels in asserting that he is right. The history of science is replete with instances of respected authorities who turned out to be very wrong.

I have stressed the tentativeness of the present picture to encourage the reader to consider my own prediction with an open mind. I predict that research will ultimately show psychosocial influences to have minor —if any—relevance in causing the limited disorders called "neuroses," and even less relevance in causing the severe disorders known as psychoses. This view is today an exceedingly unpopular one, unpopular both in the statistical sense of being relatively rare or uncommon, and in the affective sense—to doubt any long-held belief, perhaps particularly the belief in psychogenesis, makes people angry. Nevertheless, a number of years of close consideration of the available evidence has caused me to doubt that faulty interpersonal relations will appear in the textbooks a century hence as a significant factor in the cause of mental disorder. At the very least, I predict that it will be seen to have been grossly over-rated as a causal factor.

My own professional training was similar to that of most psychologists. I was led to believe that psychosocial causation of mental illness was a fact established beyond doubt. I also learned (and many present textbooks continue to give this impression) that the few die-hards who questioned the psychogenicity of much mental illness were not only biased, old-fashioned, and irrational, but motivated by evil, antihumanistic intentions as well. This being so, I was later distressed to find occasional statements in the literature which suggested that my beliefs might be incorrect, and that what I was then teaching the next generation of students might be no more than myth. For example:

If the experiences of childhood importantly influence the later personality, we should expect to find some correlation between such experiences and the later occurrence of mental disorders. In fact, no such correlations have ever been shown [Stevenson, 1957, p. 153].

There are no data to prove that . . . there is a class of "functional" mental illness that is produced by emotional disturbance alone [Hebb, 1949, p. 271].

There seems to be no clearly demonstrated instance of either a cultural or social factor being known to be a predisposing factor in mental illness. . . . The absence of clear-cut evidence does not show that the hypothesis is incorrect

ſ

but only that it has not been demonstrated even once [Milbank Memorial Fund, 1961, p. 379].

Psychologists have reasoned that the experiences the individual has in his early life at home . . . are major determinants in . . . the development of psychopathology. A review of the research of the past 40 yrs. failed to support this assumption. No factors were found in the parent-child interaction of schizophrenics, neurotics or those with behavior disorders which could be identified as unique to them or which could distinguish one group from the other, or any of the groups from the families of the controls [Frank, 1965, p. 191].

Statements such as these surprised me. If they do not surprise you, read them again. If you remain unsurprised you are either an unusually sophisticated psychologist, or you are reading this chapter some years after it was written.

Upon finding assertions so discordant with my beliefs, and with the beliefs of the vast majority of other psychologists (including virtually all textbook authors), I decided to take a long, hard look at the research evidence myself.

My prediction that psychogenicity of mental illness will eventually be abandoned as a tenable hypothesis results from the negative outcome of my search for unambiguous or even strongly suggestive evidence favoring the hypothesis, and from my discovery that the belief is psychogenesis is founded on some rather amazing misinterpretations of the negative evidence. On the other hand, I found what I consider to be a good deal of solid evidence favoring biological causation even in those cases called "functional."

I don't imagine I can change the minds of many readers in the few pages allotted to me here. Nor do I pretend personally to have a very thorough understanding of this very complex matter. But I do want the reader to share my doubt of what is usually presented as fact. I feel strongly that if we accept as true anything that purports to be based on science rather than on faith we should be able to say why—to state the basis and cite the evidence for our belief. And I feel that the current high level of belief in psychogenesis has resulted from an unfortunate suspension of critical judgment—amounting almost to ideology—among people who regard themselves as scientists.

As an offshoot of the original problem, the problem of the belief system itself has intrigued me. Why is it that so many psychologists, psychiatrists, and other professional workers are convinced that there is such a thing as functional mental illness? Is it possible (Heaven forbid!) that *I* am wrong, and they have good reason for arriving at a view much different than mine? Self-deception should never be ruled out lightly.

On the following pages I have tried to present, as clearly and succinctly as I can, the major issues and assumptions that I feel underlie belief in the psychogenesis of mental illness. In conjunction with the discussion of these issues, I will present a sampling of the research evidence which bears on the problem.

Because of space limitations, most of the discussion will be confined to *severe* mental disorder—the psychoses. By limiting our concern primarily to severe disorder we can avoid becoming enmeshed in what I refer to further on as "the continuum fallacy." However, after having considered in detail some of the errors entailed in attributing psychological cause to the severe behavior disorders, we will be in a better position to discuss causation of the less severe disorders. The reader will find, I believe, that much of our discussion has implications relating to the causes not only of mental illness, but of individual variation within the normal personality range as well.

THE ISSUES

Much of the confusion regarding psychogenesis stems from fuzzy thinking. Let us start by defining terms as explicitly as we can, and by recognizing the fact when we cannot be completely explicit.

The Concept of Biogenesis

A biogenic mental disorder is a severe behavior disorder that results solely from the effects of biological factors, including both gene action and the effects of the physical-chemical environment. Biological factors may exert their effects prenatally, during labor and birth, and at any subsequent time. There are many examples: paresis, a consequence of syphilitic infection; pellagric psychosis, which results from a lack of certain vitamins; and various permanent and transient effects of such substances as alcohol, LSD, and amphetamine. An important point here is that we *know* that such biological factors can cause severe behavior disorders. We may not be able to say of a certain specific individual whether or not his disorder is biogenic, but we know that the *class* of biogenic disorders is a real one.

The Concept of Psychogenesis

Psychogenesis is harder to define, partly because very few writers have been very explicit in articulating what the word means. Psychogenic or functional mental illness refers here to severe behavior disorder *purportedly* caused by adverse experience in the psychosocial environment, that is, by *socially meaningful stimuli* whose point of entry is the *sense organs* of the individual. In practice, the definition is usually tacitly limited to refer only to adverse interpersonal interactions. The distinction that psychogenic variables must input through the sense organs has not been made before, so far as I know, but it is important and I wish to make it explicit. The individual is assumed to be organically intact, or organic problems are assumed not to be the direct cause of the behavior disorder. The body is regarded as normal, and the abnormal behavior stems from consciously, or more often, unconsciously, remembered experience.

The age at which the supposedly pathogenic events took place varies somewhat from one psychogenic theorist to another, though physical or psychological mishandling of the infant by the mother, usually in a vague and undefined way, is a commonly held view. Other psychogenic theories focus upon the developmental years, and refer to loss of a parent, or inconsistent or self-contradictory communication patterns within the family as creating confusion. Somewhat more plausible, though still very weak from the evidential view, are the theories which focus upon the circumstances immediately preceding the breakdown. Even here, the fact that some persons break down readily under stress, while others endure far greater stress without breaking down, is often attributed to differences in child-rearing practices.

There is a rather trivial sense of the words "biogenic" and "organic" in which the distinction between biogenic and psychogenic disappears: since all learning and memory take place in biological organisms, even "functional" disorders can be reduced to a biological basis. Let me make it clear that my objection to the validity of the concept "psychogenic" is *not* based on this rather sophistic argument. It is instead based on the empirical position that there is little or no scientific *evidence* that one's social experiences do in fact cause or predispose one to become mentally ill. Stated somewhat differently, what I object to is acceptance of the assumption that the critical *difference* between mentally ill and non-ill persons resides totally or partially in differences in their social (largely familial) experiences, that the illness of affected persons could have been averted had they been raised in a "better" social environment, and that people who are not mentally ill would be ill if their social (largely familial) experiences had been sufficiently adverse. I contend that the bulk and perhaps even the entirety of presently available evidence contradicts the view that one's social experience has any important causative effect on whether or not he will become mentally ill.

An important distinction between the biogenic and the psychogenic concepts is that the latter can only be tentative in any given case. We can only be inferring when we say a patient has psychogenic or functional mental illness. This is so for two reasons: In the first place, one may question the *assumption* that there is, in reality, a class of disorders legitimately called functional, in contrast to the biogenic class, which demonstrably does exist. Throughout the history of science and medicine, firmly accepted immaterial causes of phenomena have been discarded when physical causes were discovered. To label an illness functional is obviously tenuous if tomorrow a virus, a vitamin deficiency, or some other biological factor may be discovered as the true cause.

If the reality of class of functional disorders may be questioned, use of the terms "functional" or "psychogenic" becomes even less defensible at the individual case level. Aside from not being sure there is such a category as "functional," one faces the additional hazard that the patient may later turn out to have an identifiable organic defect sufficient to account for his odd behavior. The literature of psychiatry is replete with cases of patients called psychogenic and given psychotherapy, only to succumb to an undetected brain tumor or degenerative CNS disease. Ross (1959) gives an example of this. A young girl had been given intensive physical examinations at three large medical centers. All findings were negative. Intensive psychotherapy was given to remedy her mother's "intellectualized" affection, which supposedly caused her strange behavior. When the girl suddenly died, a postmortem examination of her brain revealed massive degeneration which the neurological examinations had failed to discover. Malamud (1959) gives several similar examples.

Considering that present neurological and EEG methods often fail to discover even *gross* brain pathology which is clearly visible upon postmortem examination, and considering our virtually complete ignorance of how the normal brain operates (a famous neurophysiologist was quoted recently as saying, "We know *zero* about how the brain really works"), it would seem presumptuous to label any given case "psychogenic"—even if we were sure that some cases were psychogenic. Each of the ten billion neurons in the human brain is far more complex than any transistor or vacuum tube. We don't know how a neuron works, and we certainly have no instrument for determining the adequacy of even one of these neurons. To proclaim a behavior disorder "functional" under these circumstances seems as unreasonable as applying the same label to a malfunctioning television set when one lacks a tube tester, voltmeter, wiring diagram, and an understanding of electronics.

The terms "functional" and "psychogenic," if used at all, should be applied very tentatively, and then only *after* it has been shown that the category is not an imaginary one. Our present task is to try to predict whether the category will in time prove to be real or imaginary.

The Concept "Environment"

In discussing the concepts "biogenic" and "psychogenic," I distinguished between the physical-chemical and the psychosocial environments as the inferred sources of adverse effects. Many writers fail to make this discrimination and erroneously ascribe all adverse environmental (nongenetic) effects to the psychosocial environment. This failure represents an important source of the belief in psychogenesis. Examples are numerous. A striking one is Bettelheim's (1959) case of a psychotic girl whose illness he regarded as functional. In attributing her problem to the *presumed* effects of lack of mother love, Bettelheim ingnored four *known* causes of behavior disorder. The girl had been conceived and raised by her Jewish parents in a tiny, dark, cramped hole beneath a farm building in Poland in World War II. German soldiers were nearby (they sometimes fired shots into the building), and the mother had to smother the child's cries. Bettelheim emphasized such psychological factors as the mother's dislike of the father and the child's being unplanned, not deigning to mention such established adverse influences on the child as (1) prenatal development in an unbalanced endocrinal environment due to maternal stress; (2) extremely poor pre- and postnatal sanitary and (3) nutritional factors; and (4) extreme postnatal sensory deprivation. Each of these factors is known to have *demonstrable* effects on the young. One would think biological factors such as these at least warrant mention.

The relative potency of the physical and social environments may be compared by considering the "sensory deprivation" studies. When one's sensory input is sharply curtailed, such as by submersion in a water tank (with a breathing tube, of course!) in a silent and dark room, he is unable to tolerate the experience longer than 8 hours at most. By contrast, if a person is isolated only from *social,* as opposed to *physical,* stimuli, he can endure indefinitely, although he may become lonely. Hermits, forest rangers, marooned sailors, prisoners, and life-raft survivors are among those who have undergone lengthy *social* deprivation with no evident harm.

At times even biologically sophisticated people make the error of equating "environment" with "psychosocial environment." The cases of identical twins of which only one is schizophrenic are sometimes incorrectly cited by those who commit this error. They conclude that while inheritance may be relevant, the normality of the co-twin somehow proves that social factors play a role in causing the disorder. Actually, of course, one of the twins might have suffered adverse biological effects in the uterus, at birth, by postnatal infection, and so on, and the schizophrenia might have nothing to do with his psychosocial experiences.

A recent review of the literature in fact showed that of 26 pairs of identical twins of which only one twin was schizophrenic, in 19 cases the schizophrenic twin had been the lighter of the two in birth weight—a statistically significant difference (Pollin, Stabenau, & Tupin, 1965). (This, incidentally, is similar to the finding on IQ scores of identical twins: the greater the birth weight difference, the lower the IQ score of the lighter twin.) However, Pollin, Stabenau, and Tupin show the usual preference for a psychogenic explanation: they suggest that the mother's special solicitude for the weaker child led to his schizophrenia. This type of explanation troubles me. If the heavier twin had turned out to be the more prone to schizophrenia, it could be said that his mother's solicitude for the weaker sib caused him to feel rejected and to withdraw. Either or both of these explanations would be more convincing if there were some independent evidence showing that a mother's attitude has *any* causal relevance in the development of schizophrenia in her children.

When a psychogenecist cites evidence that a mental disorder is "environmental," in most instances he has ruled out the physical-chemical environment merely by ignoring it.

The "Moderate" Approach—Biogenic and Psychogenic Causation

The proposition that *both* an individual's biological makeup *and* his psychosocial history are important in determining whether or not he will become psychotic is so widely accepted that it has earned "sacred cow" status. One hardly dares question it. It may even be true, but I doubt that it is. As in the case of many other self-evident "truths"—"The sun revolves around the earth," "A heavy object falls faster than a light one," "A heavier-than-air machine cannot fly," "The atom is indivisible"— neither plausibility nor wide acceptance, even by the scientifically trained, confers validity. Nor is validity conferred by stating the reasons why such propositions *must* be true: "If the earth were round, people would fall off it." "The atom cannot be divided because it is already the smallest particle of matter." These matters are empirical ones that can be evaluated only on the basis of scientifically valid evidence. The scientist's job is to question and test assumptions, not merely to accept those that are plausible or widely believed.

The "it takes both" position has no better claim to acceptance on faith than the alternate purely psychogenic or biogenic positions. It is quite conceivable that schizophrenia is as purely organic (nonfunctional) as paresis. I will accept the idea that social interactions contribute to the causation of schizophrenia, just as I will accept the idea that a cosmic ray striking one's navel is a contributing cause of schizophrenia, when I see good evidence that it is so—not before.

Let us look at the "it takes both" position more closely. It is of course true that genetic mental disorders, such as those associated with hypothyroidism and phenylketonuria, are dependent upon certain kinds of environments. These two disorders can be corrected by altering the environment with regard to the amount of thyroid and phenylalanine the patient ingests. It thus cannot be denied that these problems reside not only in heredity but also in the environment, providing you mean the physical-chemical environment. The misconception that psychosocial factors *must* play a role in the cause of mental illness can be traced in part to the confusion concerning to what the word "environment" refers, that is, to the tendency to ascribe the same potentialities to the psychosocial as to the physical-chemical environment. The well-known geneticist, Dobzhansky, in his book *Heredity and the Nature of Man* (1964), makes a statement that many would misconstrue so as to cause the kind of confusion I describe: He explains (p. 18) that the frequent dichotomization of human traits into hereditary and environmental is "false and misleading." Using skin color to illustrate the point that heredity cannot be separated from environment in its effects, he says that one could be strongly tanned by outdoor life or bleached by living indoors, "yet nobody doubts that the skin pigmentation is influenced by heredity." Exactly the same holds true for mental illness: many will claim that "You must have bad heredity and bad environment." But note again that it is the physical-chemical environment which is important in Dobzhansky's example, except for such brief and transient changes as blushing and blanching. If one asserts that the psychosocial environment has much effect on long-term and significant changes in skin color, I will willingly listen, but it will be his burden to prove the point. Similarly in the case of behavior disorders, I want to see evidence that the social environment is influential in causing the disorder; don't just assert it *must* be so. (I might add, on the subject of skin color, that freckles make perhaps a good analogy to schizophrenia. Only a small fraction of the population is genetically predisposed to become freckled, but whether they do or not depends on the environment—the physical-chemical environment, to be sure.)

The analogy with skin color (and freckles) serves to illustrate the point I had in mind, but I hasten to admit that it may be misleading. After all, behavior disorders involve nervous system functioning, and unlike skin coloration, the nervous system is responsive to the social environment. True enough. Even a child who is organically intact will not learn to speak unless he is exposed to speech. Thus, within the *normal* range of behaviors, the social environment can be said to have a demonstrable effect on the emergence of certain behaviors. Our basic question is: Does the same hold true for *abnormal* behavior, such as mental illness? My position is that I doubt that it does, but the question is one that must be answered empirically, and not, as my illustration was intended to show, one that can be answered by uncritically saying, "It takes both." The distinction between normal and abnormal is obviously crucial to this point, and it is not being taken lightly. It will be discussed in detail a little further on.

The "both" position has certain dangers which warrant special mention. (1) It is seductively attractive. Many people seem to derive notable satisfaction from proclaiming, "Mental illness cannot be entirely biological nor entirely psychological. We must reject both extremes. It must be both." Attractiveness notwithstanding, "both" may be an entirely wrong answer. (2) The "both" position often pays lip service to biogenic possibilities, then slides too quickly to what is in essence a wholly psychogenic position. "It takes both, but since we can't do anything at present about the biological part, let's concentrate on the other." Thus society is led to massive expenditures on completely unproven remedies and preventatives such as psychotherapy (which we will discuss shortly) and ultrapermissive child rearing.

In summary, the "both" answer is neither harmless nor *ipso facto* correct. Like the purely biogenic and psychogenic positions with which it competes, it must be judged on evidence.

The Concept of Causation

There are various ways of conceiving of causation, as evidenced by such adjectives as "precipitating," "predisposing," "necessary," and "sufficient." Despite the variety of ways in which psychosocial influences *might* be causative of mental disorder, I know of no reason to believe that they are *in fact* causative. Most studies which purport to demonstrate a causative relationship merely demonstrate a correlation. A surprisingly large number of writers on mental illness have apparently never heard of, or do not understand, the admonition, "Correlation does not imply causation." The studies on maternal deprivation, on so-called schizophrenic mothers, and on social class differences in mental illness, for instance, have all been criticized severely and justifiably because their authors accepted simple correlation as evidence for psychosocial causation, when competing hypotheses, such as the biogenic one, could equally well or better account for the findings. For example, many writers, knowing that schizophrenics are found disproportionately often in slum areas (that is, schizophrenia correlates with socioeconomic status), conclude that poor social conditions must *cause* schizophrenia. Several recent studies, however, such as Dunham's *Community and Schizophrenia* (1965), show clearly that most schizophrenics have *migrated* to the poorer parts of cities, quite possibly as a *result* of their disability.

In addition to these rather commonplace points, the problem of psychogenesis versus biogenesis presents some rather unique and interesting features regarding causation. One of these concerns use of the concept for the individual as against the group. For instance, if we consider the hypothesis that biogenic and psychogenic factors *are* equally involved in causing schizophrenia, the following possibilities are still open:

1. In half the population the disorder is entirely psychogenic, in the other half, entirely biogenic.

2. In each individual in the population, psycho- and biogenesis contribute equally.

3. The relative contribution of psycho- and biogenesis within individuals varies between rather wide limits, and the average contribution of the two factors is equal for the total group.

Positive results in the studies of psychogenesis would require us to try to untangle this complex problem. The strongly negative findings we actually have spare us this task.

Another problem stems from the difficulty attached to proving a negative proposition. When one hears or reads of a case of functional or psychogenic disorder, the label "psychogenic" is intended to indicate that some special features of the individual's psychosocial environment are considered to have caused the disorder. The burden of demonstrating the systematic exclusion of organic causation would seem to lie with the one who attached the functional label. This, as we have seen, is not possible, since neither do we understand how the brain works in general nor do we have instruments adequate to determine whether any individual brain is functioning properly. Thus, the assumed pathogenic features in the environment are pointed to. But for each person who develops a behavior disorder in an adverse environment, there are easily dozens in similar or more adverse environments who do *not* manifest the disorder. At this point, it seems to me, the psychogenecist is forced into postulating an organic or constitutional weakness in the patient. Once this concession is made, it would seem much more economical, scientific, and straightforward to attribute the *entire* disorder to the constitutional weakness, rather than to postulate nebulous, undemonstrated, and quite possibly purely imaginary factors in the psychosocial environment, as having caused or contributed to the disorder.

The Fallacy of Confusing Content and Cause

The answer to the question just raised—Why postulate psychogenic causes if organic cause cannot validly be ruled out?—resides, I think, in an erroneous equating of the conceptual content of a disorder with its cause. If a person raised in a French home becomes psychotic, his bizarre speech is ordinarily in French. If he is raised in a deeply religious home, his hallucinations and concerns may well relate to religious matters. Raised in a home stressing wealth and power instead, the same person might dwell on these matters in his rambling. This is quite understandable, even if one is willing to regard the case as purely biogenic. Yet who has not read or heard of cases where the *content* of the disordered person's concern was used as evidence that the disorder was psychogenic?

Inferring cause from content is a particularly important source of the widespread belief in the psychogenesis of mental illness, because this type of reasoning is often presented in an apparently scientifically approved way in the public press.

The case of Marilyn Monroe is a good example. I have read many popular accounts of her repeated episodes of mental disorganization and depression, long-term psychoanalysis, and eventual suicide. Most of these accounts stress her unhappy early marriage and her concern with her fading beauty. Little heed has been paid to possible biogenic causes, although her own hospitalization for "breakdowns" and the fact that her mother had been institutionalized for many years suggest possible genetic causation. Has the "fading love goddess" aspect any real relevance? No matter. The public finds the psychogenic material more interesting, and thus the belief in psychogenic factors is reinforced.

Charles Whitman, the young man who in 1966 shot 14 persons from the University of Texas tower, presents a similar case. Massive publicity was given to his dislike for his father, which was regarded as the psychogenic cause, but very little publicity was given to his malignant brain tumor, to the remarkable change in his personality which took place before the shooting, nor to the large quantities of psychoactive drugs he had been taking.

Much has been written about the man who piloted the airplane that dropped the atom bomb on Hiroshima. His subsequent mental illness is widely believed to be the consequence of guilt. Little mention is made of his long-term record of mental instability, nor of the failure of the remainder of the men on the several atom-bombing missions to become mentally ill. Was his Hiroshima experience at all relevant?

The fact that a mentally ill person was or was not a "love goddess," had too much or too little affection for his father, or felt deeply guilty because he killed in wartime or because he evaded the draft—all these and many more things may be part of the *content* of the patient's consciousness if he does or does not become mentally ill. To claim, as is commonly done, that these things somehow *cause* the illness involves, I think, quite an unwarranted assumption.

The Post Hoc *Explanation Fallacy*

Closely related to the last point is the ease with which plausible psychogenic explanations can be concocted—and accepted—after the fact. Students are readily convinced by textbook case histories which make it appear logical that the sophomore should be found running naked in the snow claiming he is the reincarnation of Joan of Arc. After all, he *was* an only child whose parents insisted on his getting good grades and becoming a doctor and . . . Hah!

Quite often, in lecturing on the supposed psychogenicity of mental illness, I have illustrated the fatuousness of *post hoc* psychodynamic explanations by singling out in turn several members of the audience at random and asking:

> You, yes, you in the third row, with the red shirt. Suppose you were to suddenly become psychotic tomorrow morning at 10 o'clock, because I picked you out at random and shot you with my imaginary mind-disintegrator ray gun. And suppose someone investigated your case to find a plausible psychological explanation for your cracking up. Could they do it? For instance, your fiancee may have told you she is leaving you to marry a fat short-order cook, or maybe your wealthy granduncle died and is leaving all his money to found a monastery, or the dean's office may have said you are about to be expelled, or your mother used to say she loved your baby brother more than you, or. . .

After only a moment's reflection, everyone I've ever asked this question agrees: "Yes, if I become psychotic, there would be no trouble in ascribing a logical environmental (psychosocial environmental) cause." (If you doubt this, ask yourself the question.) This being so, how much credence should one give the textbook examples, the TV shows, the newspaper accounts, and the other sources of the prevailing belief in psychogenesis?

Looking back at my own training, which like that of most psychologists, instilled in me the belief that psychosocial causation of mental illness had been scientifically established, it seems to me that I was very much influenced by those fascinating case histories which appear in small print in the textbooks. The author used them with assurance to *illustrate* the operation of psychological factors in a given case. We students never questioned the author's designation of the case as "functional." The possibility that there might be an undetected organic disorder, such as a metabolic dysfunction, was never even mentioned, nor did I appreciate the now obvious point that plausible after-the-fact psychodynamic explanations of any behavior—either normal or abnormal—can be devised by any person with even modest imagination.

As part of a research study on normal males, Renaud and Estess (1961) conducted intensive clinical interviews with 100 "above average" young men. Renaud and Estess reported that they were quite surprised to find just as much supposedly "pathogenic" personal history material in this superior group as they were accustomed to finding in clinically abnormal persons. Needless to say, I was not a bit surprised.

Psychologists aren't the only experts in concocting after-the-fact explanations. Following an election, or football game, or a squiggle on the stock market curve, the experts come out in full force to explain why what happened was inevitable and should have been anticipated. This is part of human nature, I suppose, and it is not very surprising. It is not science, however. Science requires that one demonstrate understanding of a phenomenon by predicting it; postdiction is quite insufficient. That *post hoc* explanations are so easily devised does not mean they are invariably invalid, of course. It does mean that we should look beyond them for evidence of validity.

The Continuum Fallacy

Most textbooks in psychology, psychiatry, and sociology present the psychogenic viewpoint, or the combined psychogenic and biogenic viewpoint, as though psychogenicity was of established rather than hypothetical relevance in mental disorder. An argument often used to advance this position is that the continuity of troublesome behaviors—the fact that behavior forms a spectrum ranging from a mildly offensive habit to the widely assaultive behavior of a schizophrenic—somehow demonstrates that these kinds of behavior merely represent differences in degree and not in kind. This is an unusually appealing type of argument, and it is, in my opinion, at the root of a large proportion of the fuzzy thinking that characterizes what are called the social sciences. It is demonstrably specious. It embarrasses me to admit that as a student I accepted this reasoning uncritically, and as a teacher I espoused it enthusiastically. In general, the idea is that if it is difficult to make a distinction between two neighboring points on a hypothetical continuum, no valid distinctions can thereafter be made even at the extremes of the continuum. There are thus persons who would argue that the existence of several variations of gray precludes a distinction between black and white. Hokum. While I will agree that some patients in mental hospitals are saner than some nonpatients, and that it is sometimes hard to distinguish between deep unhappiness and psychotic depression, I do *not* agree that the difficulty sometimes encountered in making the distinction between normal and abnormal necessarily invalidates all such distinctions.

Many books and articles are devoted to asserting that mental illness is merely a myth, and that we are faced with only a distribution of normal personalities having more or fewer quirks, or having habits which conform to others' expectations in varying degrees. Yet even the most psychodynamically inclined psychologist who believes this will seldom be found driving his auto without lights at 11 P.M., however imperceptible may have been the change from the bright daylight of 3 P.M. to the complete darkness of 10 P.M. Similarly, we may guess that no "mental-illness-is-a-myth" psychologist swelters in his long underwear in July, even though the change of temperature from winter cold to summer heat is not only mere matter of degree(s), but an uncertain and overlapping one at that, since some days in May are colder than some days in February.

If the continuum fallacy had misled investigators of overtly physical illness as it apparently has misled investigators of "mental" illness, modern medicine would not exist. Instead, we would be advised that since such measures as temperature, blood pressure, and white cell counts all fall along continua having no natural dividing points, there are really no such things as fevers, hypertension, or infections. These are merely gradations or variations from average, and they thus have no special significance. ("Besides, where are you going to draw the line?")

It should be evident that the distribution of phenomena along smooth gradients can lead the unwary to erroneous conclusions. The fact is that there *are* people who are mentally ill, many millions of them, and they exist in every land on earth, the continuum notion notwithstanding.

The Parallel Planes Concept

Since the continuum fallacy obviously may lead to some rather absurd conclusions, it needs to be viewed with skepticism. (One can use this pseudologic to demonstrate that the nose is the same as the ear: after all, each blends smoothly into the skin of the cheek, and surely no one wants to draw the line arbitrarily!) However, my criticism of the continuum concept should not lead us to reject it prematurely. I demonstrated that it was not necessarily a valid view; I did not demonstrate that it is invariably an invalid one.

Despite my criticism, I find that it *is* helpful to conceive of a population as falling along a continuum in terms of the psychological normality of its members. The distribution along the continuum may or may not be a "normal" curve in the mathematical sense; for our purpose it doesn't matter. At one end of this distribution are people whose behavior is so peculiar that protective custody is required for their own sake and for the welfare of others. A little closer to the main body of the population are individuals who are less disordered in their behavior and for whom custody is problematical, and so forth. At the other end of the distribution are people who are so completely rational and in control of themselves that there is not the slightest doubt about their stability. Since there are no gaps in this distribution, it *is* hard to draw the line. Who is to say that the most deviantly behaving people are not just a little different in *degree* from the others?

But suppose we now learn that 10 percent of the population had taken a few cocktails. This subgroup would tend to be concentrated toward the deviant-behavior end of the scale, though of course, the behavior of the silliest of the people who had not been drinking might be more peculiar than the behavior of the most serious and alcohol resistant of those who had. A better way of depicting the distribution of deviancy values, now that we know about the alcohol, would be to draw two separate but overlapping curves, so that the one for the drinking population is displaced to a different plane parallel to and a little in front of or in back of the plane of the first curve.

From our original vantage point, we felt sure there was but one single continuum. From our new vantage point, a somewhat different angle (now that we know about the cocktails), we can appreciate that there were always two separate curves that had overlapped along their base lines and that we were originally in error in not seeing the data in proper perspective. Suppose now that we learned that a second small subgroup of the population had taken a minute dose of LSD. These people—most of them—had appeared near the tip of our original continuum, acting more bizarrely than almost anyone else in our population. Again project this group to another parallel plane, since they represent a different (though ostensibly overlapping) population. It was only our original inability to perceive these subgroups that led us to believe there was but a single continuum ranging from the solidly rational to the wildly deviant.

Now suppose there is a subgroup of people who are unable to metabolize adrenaline properly, as has been proposed in the schizophrenia theory of Osmond and Smythies (1952; see also Hoffer, Osmond, Callbeck, & Kahan, 1957), and whose bodies thus become loaded with the hallucinogenic substance, adrenolutin? We know that an analogous process operates in the metabolic disorder phenylketonuria (PKU), and that if the population we started our hypothetical study with was large enough, it would include several very bizarrely acting people who, if examined, would turn out to be victims of PKU. In fact, Benda has pointed out that some children with PKU are routinely classed as schizophrenics, until the diagnosing psychiatrist is told about the positive PKU test (1959).

The foregoing presentation of the "parallel planes" concept does not, of course, show that any or all mental illness is biogenic rather than psychogenic. It does show, I think, that writers such as Adams, Jackson, Menninger, and Szasz, who call mental illness a myth, do not necessarily have a valid point in the apparent lack of other than arbitrary lines separating people called "normal" from those called "ill." The problem is that we do not yet have laboratory tests for such disorders and are thus forced to rely on behavioral symptoms. There are good reasons, to be presented shortly, to believe that these writers are quite mistaken.

Perhaps at this point I should note the argument, advanced by some, that since bizarre behavior of certain kinds is accepted as normal by certain primitive peoples, especially in their shaman (witch doctor), we Westerners are being provincial in thinking of such behavior among our own people as a sign of sickness. As Leighton and Hughes (1961), among others, have pointed out, behavior appearing psychotic or hysterical to Westerners may be the result of deliberate learning and practice on the part of the shaman, and thus is only superficially similar to the acutely psychotic behavior it resembles. And as Edgerton (1966) has noted, even very primitive African societies have, and recognize as abnormal, severe behavior disorders coinciding in detail with what we call schizophrenia.

The Matter of Diagnosis

It is indeed true, as many proponents of the psychogenic view have argued, that there are hardly two informed people who agree on what schizophrenia is in general, or on whether or not a given patient is schizophrenic. They assert that schizophrenia does not exist and that "schizophrenics" are people who have failed to adjust to their social environment. Menninger, for example, in his book *The Vital Balance*, lists the many conflicting classificatory schemes for mental illness which men have devised over the centuries to support his contention that the patients so classified are not ill but have merely lost their mental balance.

It takes but little thought to dispose of this specious conclusion, though the perspective of history should spare us the exercise. A century ago one might have similarly pointed to the hodgepodge of physical disorders known as "consumption." Noting that there were just a few symptoms in common among the patients, and that chances for recovery varied markedly from case to case, one might have erroneously concluded that such chaotic information could be due only to human diversity (or perversity!) and that no physical cause for consumption could possibly be found. Today we understand our ancestors' confusion, since the "disease" they called consumption included diabetes, tuberculosis, and other now identifiable disorders. Kanner (1958) has pointed out that the same problem existed not very long ago with "the fevers," which included malaria, cholera, and diphtheria. So it may be with a "mental" illness such as schizophrenia, which is very probably a conglomerate of separate diseases, each having disorientation of the higher functions of the brain as one of its most prominent symptoms. Obviously, until we know the exact cause of a disease, it is often difficult, if not impossible, to distinguish it from other diseases on the basis of symptoms alone—particularly if the other "diseases" are also a mixture of conditions of unknown cause. How can it be concluded that "mental illness," or "schizophrenia," must be of psychosocial origin because at the present time we are unable to label and classify it accurately? Of course, when the necessary laboratory tests are developed, the biogenic versus psychogenic dispute will be essentially over, though no doubt some will argue that the social environment *caused* the observed physical changes. Judging from the history of science and medicine, however, those who would argue for mystical, dynamic, intangible functional forces will probably lose out.

That we don't *now* have a test for, say, schizophrenia is clearly no argument for psychogenesis. As Curt Stern has pointed out, we also have no way of detecting Huntington's chorea until the victim reaches middle age and his brain begins to deteriorate, and Huntington's is clearly a Mendelian dominant genetic disorder. Considering the unimaginably small quantity of a substance, such as LSD, that can affect the working of the brain, it is not surprising that there should be a number of biogenic disorders difficult to detect biochemically.

Biogenesis and the Pessimism Problem

I have talked with many people in an attempt to discover why they believe in the psychogenesis of mental disorder. Those who are most frank sometimes espouse a position which logically should have no bearing on the matter: "If you think mental illness is organic, you are giving it up as hopeless. I prefer a more optimistic approach."

One need only cite cretinism, PKU, galactosemia, epilepsy, and diabetes among the many organic diseases with clear mental or behavioral involvement which are readily amenable to medical control. Those who believe that psychological problems are necessarily more hopeful than physical ones seem oblivious to history, which shows that centuries of lawmaking, teaching, preaching, threatening, punishing, explaining, persuading, and cajoling have not resulted in a notably more exemplary Man. Preventive and remedial medicine, on the other hand, have made remarkable strides, even in many disorders that defied solution while they were called "functional."

Is Mental Illness Unhappiness Magnified?

It is widely believed that if a person becomes unhappy enough, he will "reject reality" and become severely ill mentally. This assumption seems to underlie a great deal of the belief in psychogenesis. It is a seriously held belief, though one often hears it expressed in a half-joking way: "It's enough to drive you crazy." (I have even caught myself saying that!) A great deal of thought on this matter leads me to doubt that unhappiness is of consequence in bringing about mental illness, though there is no doubt that mental illness is one of the prime causes of unhappiness.

In addition to this problem, there is the interesting associated problem of people who are unhappy but not disordered being *called* mentally ill. This latter problem is well illustrated in the book *Mental Health in the Metropolis* (Srole, Langner, Michael, Opler, & Rennie, 1962). Based on interviews with nearly 2000 persons in Manhattan, the study reported only 18.5 percent of the population to be mentally "well"!

Inherent in the unhappiness-leads-to-mental-illness concept is the idea that all humans are vulnerable to psychosis and will succumb if conditions become sufficiently grim. An interesting refutation of the "everyone has his breaking point" hypothesis is seen in the studies of World War II pilots who flew many missions despite high casualty rates among their companions. After the weakest broke down early in their assignment, the others seemed able to continue almost indefinitely, despite severe loss of weight and other signs of stress (Milbank Memorial Fund, 1961).

More interesting data on this matter come from a study of U.S. soldiers who were formerly prisoners of war in Korea (Strassman, Thaler, & Schein, 1956). Conditions were so intolerable—hunger, beatings, filth, cold, uncertainty—that some prisoners simply stopped eating, curled up into a ball, and died. For them, life was not worth living. Their surviving companions, who reported these cases, said emphatically that those who died in this way were sane and lucid until the end.

Considering the tragic plight of some humans whose sanity never falters, and the enviably favorable life circumstances of many who become psychotic, I find the hypothesis that unhappiness causes or contributes to mental illness patently inadequate. A more plausible hypothesis is that people who are becoming psychotic mismanage their affairs so badly as a *result* of their mental impairment that quarrels, loss of jobs, and other unhappiness-provoking events become common.

Psychotherapy

I am sometimes asked, "If you don't think the psychosocial environment contributes to mental illness, how do you account for the effectiveness of psychotherapy (or psychoanalysis) in helping victims?" This question, as probably most readers know by now, has a very obvious answer: there is no scientific evidence whatever that psychotherapy helps the mentally ill (psychotics or neurotics), despite the numerous studies which have attempted to show its beneficial effects.

In 1949, in his celebrated book *The Organization of Behavior*, D. O. Hebb briefly reviewed the evidence on the effectiveness of psychotherapy and psychoanalysis and concluded flatly: "There is no body of fact to show that psychotherapy is valuable" (p. 271). A few years later H. J. Eysenck made a more intensive review and came to the same conclusion (see Eysenck, 1964, for a more recent review). The literature on the effectiveness of child psychotherapy has been separately reviewed by several authors (Levitt, 1963; Lewis, 1965) with similar findings. Levitt, basing his conclusion on more than 50 studies involving thousands of children, said the conclusion was "inescapable" that psychotherapy could not be claimed to be effective.

The studies which claim that benefits are derived from psychotherapy seem to be only those in which no control group is used, and in which anecdotal and testimonial evidence make the findings scientifically useless. These are the kinds of studies that medicine (except for psychiatry) wisely learned to ignore long ago.

Space limitations prevent our reviewing the massive research literature on the efficacy of psychotherapy. It is possible only to note briefly that the proponents (usually practictioners) of psychotherapy have fought back vigorously, but their claims are peculiarly small. Pointing to what they regard as technical shortcomings in the research, they say, for the most part, "Psychotherapy has not been proven useless—it simply has not been proven useful" (Astin, 1961). They have also, as Astin has noted, deemphasized the "cure" aspects and have instead suggested rather nebulous general benefits, such as self-actualization or, perhaps, happiness, but again proof of efficacy is lacking. The burden of proof of usefulness traditionally rests on the advocates of any treatment. Be that as it may, the failure of psychotherapy (and I do think it is a failure, to put the matter bluntly) to ameliorate mental disorder in children and adults, while it does not prove biogenesis, is precisely what one would expect if the "insight" which psychotherapy is intended to provide had no bearing whatever on the genesis of the disorder.

Contrary to what most psychodynamic doctrine indicates, research shows that a substantial proportion of the mentally ill recover spontaneously, as do many people with the majority of illnesses that *are* widely recognized as physical in origin (Wolpe, 1961).

Since anyone questioning the claims of the psychotherapists is probably considered even more antihumanitarian than one who questions psychogenesis, let me attempt to redeem myself by adding, as an aside, that I am in general agreement with the position of William Schofield in his book *Psychotherapy: The Purchase of Friendship*. Most people feel a desire to talk to a sympathetic person about their problems, and they should be given an opportunity to do so. To pretend, however, in the face of existing evidence, that such conversation has curative powers, or that the listener needs to be highly sophisticated in psychology or psychiatry, is quite unjustified. In any event, it is clear that the proponents of the psychogenic view cannot turn to psychotherapy research for support of their position.

Behavior Therapy

This discussion has been concerned with "insight therapy," as contrasted with a newer and apparently much more helpful treatment for behavior disorders—behavior therapy. Behavior therapy is based on a learning theory approach to the modification of behavior. In certain forms of neurosis, the symptoms are attacked directly, the old fear of symptom substitution being discarded as a superstition. Based on just a few years' evidence, the results of behavior therapy seem surprisingly good—good enough to have converted me from strong skepticism to rather enthusiastic endorsement.

Certain behaviors of psychotics, like the fears of neurotics, have proven amenable to a behavior therapy approach. The usual method of dealing with psychotics is operant conditioning, but in the case of psychoses, unlike neuroses, behavior therapists seldom if ever claim to have actually cured a patient.

The efficacy of operant conditioning in modifying pathological behavior is thought by many behavior therapists, including some leaders in the field, to indicate psychogenesis of the behavior problem. I doubt, however, that behavior therapy tells us anything about the *cause* of the problem. One can use conditioning successfully on a mongoloid child, a schizophrenic adult, or a decorticate dog. Does this imply in each case that the nervous system is sound and intact?

Does the demonstrated effectiveness of operant conditioning in improving the behavior of a child with, say, infantile autism mean that the autism must have been *caused* by selective reinforcement by the child's parents, of behaviors of an autistic sort, as some writers have suggested? No more than the usefulness of aspirin in relieving a headache means the headache was *caused* by a lack of aspirin.

While I have learned to respect the conditioning techniques of behavior modification as unexpectedly powerful devices for improving the behavior of both mentally ill and retarded children and adults, I have no sympathy for the naive belief of the many "behaviorists" or "Skinnerians" who have leaped to the untenable conclusion that because a mentally ill person can sometimes be taught to discontinue some of his "crazy" actions, he must be a normal person who has merely learned maladaptive habits.

Similarly, I cannot agree with the enthusiasts of the behaviorist approach who argue that because in laboratory-type studies you may be able to manipulate a normal person into temporarily acquiring a very specific behavior of a bizarre sort, *all* bizarre behavior must have been similarly produced. This is as logical as asserting that because you have discovered that natural blondness can be simulated with peroxide, *all* blondes must use peroxide on their hair. Further, this mode of thought ignores the basic question of *why* some persons acquire bizarre behavior in the real world and others do not: the essential problem of biogenesis or psychogenesis. The answer, "Their reinforcement histories differ," is merely an assumption, not a fact. As indicated in the quotations cited earlier, the available evidence contradicts the assumption. To focus on the behavior alone is to commit the error of confusing content and cause. Are the behaviorists willing to face the question: Does anything resembling their carefully contrived laboratory procedures actually occur in real life, and if it does, can it produce enduring changes in personality?

It seems to me that the Skinnerians should have learned from the horrible example of the Freudians that there are real dangers in making extravagant generalizations from scanty, albeit interesting, data. Perhaps I should suggest to Professor Skinner that when his classic book *The Behavior of Organisms* is revised, he ought to give it a more seemly title, like *Some Behavior of Some Organisms.*

The Problem of Neurosis

Neuroses present a more difficult problem than the more severe disorders because they are harder to define and harder to discriminate, clinically and conceptually, from mood changes, anxiety, unhappiness, and other psychological variations among normal (nonsick) individuals. It is of more than passing interest to our main concern with possible functionality of psychotic illness that statistics show that neurosis is not simply a way station on the path to psychosis; psychotics, contrary in particular to the views of the psychoanalysts, are *not* ordinarily recruited from the ranks of the neurotics.

I have not devoted nearly as much study to the etiology of the neuroses as to that of the psychoses; nevertheless, since I am frequently asked my views on the topic, I will briefly state my present position, which is fundamentally a behavioristic one.

Those called neurotics fall into three categories: (1) Some are temporarily anxious or unhappy because they have a right to be—life has been or threatens to be unkind. If one wishes to call them neurotics (I would not), these *would* be functional neurotics. (2) Some have temperaments or dispositions that lead to what appears to be chronic unhappiness. A good deal of research suggests a genetic element here. I know of no scientific research that shows child-rearing practices to have the causal influence on this condition that the popular and professional literature implies. (3) Some have a severe and specific problem, such as enuresis or a phobia. Behavior therapists have taken the view that in these cases the symptoms *are* the disease; the idea of an underlying emotional problem is rejected as a myth. As noted above, the danger of symptom substitution is scoffed at by the behavior therapists as merely a deduction from psychoanalytic theory, bolstered by a few anecdotal instances. "Therapy" consists of training designed to eradicate the undesired habits or to teach new ones. Grossberg (1964) has provided an excellent review of this approach and Paul (1966), in his book *Insight vs. Desensitization in Psychotherapy,* has described an impressive experiment in which the behaviorist approach is shown to be superior to the traditional one.

Insofar as such specific behaviors as phobias are learned and usually present a rather circumscribed problem, I might accede to their being called "functional." However, (1) these problems are perhaps better described as bad habits than as mental illness, (2) there is no reason to believe that their occurrence is in any way influenced by the patient's early family life or social relationships, and (3) since so few people are afflicted, the problem, despite its being amenable to psychological modification (which I would term "educational" and not "therapeutic"), would appear to be at its roots a biogenic one. Despite these reservations, I feel that learning theorists have made a substantial contribution in this area.

Weak Inference, or "Don't Confuse Me with the Facts"

In a paper in *Science* that attracted a good deal of attention, John Platt (1964) attributed the very rapid progress made in the fields of high energy physics and molecular biology to the use of a systematic research strategy which he named "strong inference." The strategy consists in carefully spelling out various alternative hypotheses for phenomena of interest, devising and performing studies capable of rejecting the incorrect hypotheses, then employing the confirmed hypothesis in a repetition of the cycle at the next point of uncertainty. The process is akin to finding the shortest path through a maze by carefully planning the steps to take at each point of choice.

It is no secret that psychology is not a pacesetter among the sciences. Psychology's sluggish progress is often attributed to the complexity of its subject matter. While this is no doubt a valid explanation, I think another important factor in the failure of psychology and the other social sciences to move ahead is their rejection of the strong inference model in favor of what I will call, by analogy, the "weak inference" approach.

Rather than being guided by their data, psychologists seem determined to cling to certain favored hypotheses regardless of the outcome of the research they may do. It will come as no surprise to the reader that I regard the psychogenic hypothesis as the prime example of this backwardness.

Biochemist Roger J. Williams (1956), among others, has also observed this phenomenon and has seen the need to protest it:

> We therefore make a plea for an unprejudiced facing of the facts of heredity. We urge that such facts be accepted with as great readiness as any others. This plea seems necessary in view of the attitude which we have repeatedly noted, namely, that of willingness to arrive at "environmentalistic" conclusions on the basis of slender evidence while rejecting points of view which would emphasize the role of heredity, even though the weight of the evidence, viewed without prejudice, appears overwhelming [p. 16].

My own plea for "an unprejudiced facing of the facts" includes not only hereditary explanations but those implicating the nonsocial environment. A few illustrations of weak inference will have to suffice, out of the dozens of examples which could be cited.

Osterkamp and Sands (1962) studied the birth and pregnancy problems, and the incidence of breast feeding, in mothers of schizophrenic children as contrasted with the mothers of less disturbed neurotic children. The more severely afflicted children were found to have more often been the product of a troubled pregnancy and delivery. Breast feeding was found to have taken place *more* often in the severely disturbed group of children. Despite these findings, "the results were interpreted in terms of the mothers' unconscious negative feelings toward the infants" (p. 366).

Psychoanalyst René Spitz has won fame for his studies supposedly showing that when an infant is deprived of "affective interchange" with his mother, for example, when the infant is hospitalized, he experiences a major deterioration of his personality. Pinneau (1955), on analyzing Spitz's published data, made the interesting observation that of the 59-point drop in the average Development Quotient of the children, which Spitz reported as resulting from the mothers' departure, 43 points were lost *before* most of the mothers were separated from their infants.

Spitz's findings, however, were supported in a later study by Fischer (1952). Or were they? Fischer reported that her sample of "maternally deprived" institutionalized infants performed very poorly on the tests she used, and asserted the children's deficiencies were "environmentally fostered." However, as Pinneau (1955) pointed out, Fischer had chosen for her study the lowest scoring 62 infants out of a group of 189—a group whose mean IQ on the Cattell test was 76.1! Again the data appear to have been collected only as a formality, as a means of "proving" what the researcher knew to be true.

Beisser, Glasser, and Grant (1966), basing their conclusions on structured interviews with parents, reached the not surprising conclusion that "children of schizophrenic and psychoneurotic mothers are seen to have a greater rate of behavioral deviations than children of 'normal' mothers, as judged by the mothers themselves" (p. 114). A number of possible explanations are evident, including (1) "sick" mothers may be poor judges of their children, (2) some children may have inherited the mother's tendency toward having behavior problems, (3) the interviewers may have been biased (the report does not indicate safeguards against this possibility). Despite the unmentioned and apparently unconsidered alternate explanations (especially the second one), it is concluded that the results "provide support for the proposition that the family milieu and the nature and quality of its interactions has a significant contribution to the mental health or lack of it of its members" (p. 114).

Still another example of weak inference is found in the report of a large five-year comparison of psychotherapy with three drugs in a group of 299 women (Brill, 1966). The psychotherapy group was seen at least once a week for an hour, while the drug groups were seen for only 10 or 15 minutes weekly, biweekly, or monthly, over a shorter total period of time. To summarize the rather complex report of findings, in this study, as in scores of others, the psychotherapy group showed no improvement over the other groups (and appeared to be somewhat less improved than the meprobromate group). The author says, "These findings were unexpected. They suggest that the widespread preference for the traditional out patient psychotherapy is based as much on the physician's bias as on its *proven* greater effectiveness" (italics mine). But are these findings accepted, and the simpler, less expensive, more convenient methods recommended? No. "The findings do not justify any departure from the principle of providing treatment which is based on an understanding of psychodynamics and unconscious factors in emotional illness" (p. 253).

I will not lengthen this depressing list with further examples. It should be evident by now that psychologists and psychiatrists believe what they want to believe. Perhaps when the reader sees the additional examples of this sort of "science" that abound in the research literature, he will be reminded, as I am, of the small printed sign that one often sees posted on office walls as an intended joke: "Don't confuse me with the facts. My mind is made up." Or perhaps he may prefer Norman Maier's (1960) way of saying it. "Maier's Law" is "If the facts don't conform to the theory, they must be disposed of."

A BRIEF LOOK AT BIOGENIC FACTORS

I have said that I believe that psychogenic factors will ultimately be shown to have little, if any, relevance in mental illness, that the bulk of the available research evidence strongly counterindicates the psychogenic theory of mental illness, and that the present high level of belief in psychogenesis is based largely on a series of irrelevant arguments, unwarranted assumptions, and misinterpreted evidence. This is essentially what I set out to do—to point to the large and alarming gap between what is believed and taught about psychogenesis and what research has actually shown. Many with whom I've discussed this matter have tried to excuse this deplorable state of affairs by saying, in effect, "So what if the evidence for psychogenesis doesn't hold up very well? The evidence for biogenesis is just as weak."

Obviously there is no biogenic evidence for any disorder called psychogenic that will convince the psychogenicists. If there were, the disorder would immediately be reclassified "organic" (as has happened so often in the past) without challenging the belief system. But despite the lack of conclusive biogenic evidence for disorders (like schizophrenia) called psychogenic, it is simply not true that the scoreboard for biogenesis is as vacant as the scoreboard for psychogenesis.

The space remaining does not permit more than brief mention of some of the reasons for believing that biological factors are operative in the causation of mental illness. Let us look briefly at some of the evidence for biogenesis of schizophrenia.

Schizophrenia resembles physical illness in a number of ways. For one, untreated schizophrenia comes and goes, as do many chronic physical illnesses in which remissions and relapses for unknown causes are the rule. For a long time we failed to appreciate this because of our preoccupation with the psychogenic model, which did not lead us to anticipate relatively symptom-free periods. This error has proven disastrous to un-counted thousands of schizophrenics who have been "put away" in the past. Only lately have we begun to realize that schizophrenics, like other ill and incapacitated persons, must be motivated toward constructive activity to avoid the lassitude and deterioration which severely impedes recovery.

The extraordinary success of biochemical methods in treating schizo-phrenia, while not proof of biogenicity, certainly provides a strong impetus toward that conclusion, especially when it is contrasted with the utterly dismal record of psychotherapeutic methods. It is well known by now that after increasing at the rate of about 10,000 cases per year for many years, the number of mental patients in state and local public hospitals reached a peak of 559,000 in 1955, when the introduction of the new antipsychotic drugs began decreasing the number of hospitalized patients until at the end of 1965 there were 83,000 fewer patients than in 1955. This decrease occurred despite a sizable increase in the total U.S. population.

It is sometimes explained, in apparent seriousness, that all the drugs do is make the patients amenable to psychotherapy. I am reminded at this point of the article which appeared in the April 5, 1966, issue of *Look* magazine, under the title *Breakthrough in Psychiatry*. The "break-through," which, judging from my mail following publication of the article, excited many readers, consisted essentially of the "direct analysis" method of psychotherapy for schizophrenia, wherein the therapist exerts his total effort and personality in the task of therapy. Previous employ-ment of psychotherapy with schizophrenics was assumed to be not inten-sive enough to do the job. Photographs of this remarkably effective new approach were shown, and several dramatic cases illustrating its curative power were provided. Unfortunately, when a 5-year follow-up of direct analysis of schizophrenia was published later that year in the *American Journal of Psychiatry*, *Look* magazine didn't report it. Unlike the 15,000 or so subscribers to the *American Journal of Psychiatry*, the 7,200,000 subscribers of *Look* were not told that the schizophrenics in the untreated control group did just as well as the "direct analysis" group, and perhaps even a little better.

Also adding weight to the biogenic position is the experimental pro-duction of psychotic behavior in normal persons through biochemical means. One often hears the assertion that drug psychoses are not really very much like real-life psychoses. This is not so. While LSD may not realistically simulate schizophrenia, reserpine produces depression in some persons, according to Kety (1966), that is practically indistinguishable from endogenous depression. Lemere (1966) observes that amphetamine may mimic schizophrenia, especially paranoid schizophrenia, so closely as to be indistinguishable except for the presence of amphetamine in the urine. As indicated previously in this paper, there is no evidence that any psychogenic factors can produce such aberrant behavior, and still less evidence that they do.

Additional evidence on the biogenic side comes from the stability of the incidence and symptoms of schizophrenia from one century to the next, from one part of the world to the others, and from times of peace to times of war and turmoil. Despite common belief, statistics show the proportion of psychotics to be no greater in 1965 than in 1865, no greater in rushing, bustling competitive countries than in slow-moving underdeveloped lands, no greater in England during the nightly bombings of World War II than in the years before (Milbank Memorial Fund, Reid, 1961).

The least refutable and most consistent evidence for biogenesis, however, is probably that compiled by the geneticists. To briefly summarize the data from a number of studies (Buss, 1966, p. 319), the likelihood that a person will be a schizophrenic is a function of the presence of schizophrenia in his blood relatives, according to the following table:

No schizophrenic relatives	1%
Grandparents, cousins, nephews, and nieces	3–4%
One schizophrenic parent	16%
Both parents schizophrenic	39–68%
Half-siblings	7%
Sibling	5–14%
Fraternal twin	3–17%
Identical twin	67–86%

Various objections have been raised to the above data, none of which to me seem very compelling. A common objection is that the percentage differences between studies cast doubt on the validity of the research. Yet all but one of the twelve studies which have included identical and fraternal twins show the concordance rate for identicals to be four to six times as great as for fraternals, even though the actual rates themselves vary from one country to another as a result of diagnostic differences and other problems. The kinds of objections raised might explain away concordant rate differences of, say, 10 percent, or even 20 percent, but to assert that errors in the diagnosis of schizophrenia, or in the determination of zygosity in twins could account for the differences of 400 to 600 percent which have been found seems rather far fetched.

I have already discussed another objection: the fact that there are identical twins who are discordant for schizophrenia. Discordance in identical twins shows merely that schizophrenia is not *entirely* genetic. It is not evidence for psychogenesis, since pre- or postnatal differences in physical environment have not by any means been ruled out. The study referring to the significantly lighter birth weight of the schizophrenic member of discordant identical twins has already been mentioned as specifically consistent with the prediction based on biogenic theory. Actually, genetic familial data on *known* physical disorders, such as tuberculosis and diabetes, give results very similar to those reported above for schizophrenia. The question of a psychogenic element in diabetes is seldom raised.

Some critics claim the above data do not show genetic causation. By this they mean that the percentages do not follow the simple Mendelian model for dominant and recessive genes. Genetic disorders do not necessarily follow the Mendelian model.

Among the many embarrassments these data hold for psychogenicists is the difficulty of explaining why a fraternal twin of a schizophrenic is no more likely to become schizophrenic than is an ordinary sibling—about 10 to 15 percent in each case. The family and social environment is certainly more similar for twins, even fraternal twins, than for siblings, who may be much younger or older than the one who becomes schizophrenic.

Another embarrassment to psychogenesis, as Lewis Hurst and Curt Stein have both pointed out, is that a schizophrenic father is as likely to have a schizophrenic child (about 15 percent likelihood) as is a schizophrenic mother. Since the mother tends to have much more contact with the child, this is hard to explain on psychogenic grounds, but it is entirely consistent with biogenic causation.

Two studies have been published during the last year which cast new light on the causation of schizophrenia. Both studies involved the use of children of schizophrenic mothers in a control group design. Higgins (1966) compared 25 Danish children reared by their own schizophrenic mothers with a matched group of 25 similar children who were raised apart from their schizophrenic mothers. "It was predicted that the mother-reared children would display greater maladjustment on the various measures than would the reared-apart children. The results failed to support the hypothesis" (p. 166). While Higgins' study is a valuable one, the subjects were children, and we do not know which, if any, will actually become schizophrenic in adulthood.

A landmark study, for a number of reasons, is Heston's (1966) follow-up of children born between 1915 and 1945 to schizophrenic mothers confined in an Oregon psychiatric hospital. Heston was able to obtain follow-up data into adulthood for 47 such children who had been adopted as infants into foster homes in which there was no suspicion of schizophrenia. By comparing this group with a carefully matched control group of children born of nonschizophrenic mothers who had also been adopted in the first few days of life by a matched group of foster parents, he was able to determine what effect, if any, the genetic element might play in the later development of schizophrenia. The results were strongly in accord with genetic expectation. Five (16.6 percent) of the adopted children of schizophrenic mothers and none of the matched adopted children of normal mothers were found at follow-up to have been schizophrenic. Other psychiatric problems were also found more often in the former group. For example, 8 out of 21 of the adopted children of schizophrenic mothers had later records of psychiatric or behavioral discharge from the armed forces, while only one of 17 of the adopted children of normal mothers had such a discharge record.

The design and procedures Heston used appear to be airtight. Unlike the majority of studies which have concluded in favor of psychogenic causation, Heston's study ruled out competing hypotheses through the use of a control group and through refinements in the experimental procedures, rather than by simply ignoring them.

Further support for the biogenic causation of schizophrenia—by far the most important of the "functional" disorders—is now emerging from a variety of other sources, and some of these carry implications as to the nature of the possible biochemical defect which may be involved in schizophrenia. A good deal of interest has been aroused by a study by Dohan (1966), in which the per capita wheat consumption of five countries during World War II was compared to the number of hospital admissions for schizophrenia during the same period. In the three countries (Finland, Norway, and Sweden) whose wheat consumption was reduced by about 50 percent because of shipping shortages during the war, the number of admissions for schizophrenia was also cut nearly in half. In the U.S. and Canada, where wheat consumption did not change, neither did the incidence of schizophrenia. Although it is indirect, this study is of special interest because there are several studies linking schizophrenia with celiac disease, a metabolic disorder involving an unusual sensitivity to wheat and certain other grains. (On Formosa, natives eating very little of these grains are reported to have a schizophrenia rate one-third that of Northern Europe.) In a very recent study, Dohan was able to manipulate schizophrenics' behavior by secretly controlling the gluten in their diet (Dohan, 1968).

Further evidence linking schizophrenia and its possible treatment to a metabolic error comes from the adrenolutin theory of schizophrenia of Osmond and Smythies and Hoffer et al. referred to earlier. This theory has met great controversy since it was introduced some 15 years ago. It is of interest that biochemist Seymour Kety, who had earlier been highly critical of this work, wrote recently (1966) that he had found "new and compelling evidence" favoring the hypothesis. Hoffer and his colleagues have reported favorable results in treating many schizophrenics with massive quantities of niacin, one of the B vitamins, in what Kety has described as an ingenious application of the theory (Hoffer & Osmond, 1966).

I find the niacin approach to the treatment of schizophrenia intriguing in view of a study by Kaufman (cited by Williams, 1962), in which massive doses of niacin were found to be remarkably beneficial in providing objectively measured improvement in joint movement in arthritics. Since several studies of large populations of schizophrenics have shown a much lower rate of arthritis than would be expected, some interesting possibilities seem apparent. Could the niacin that normal persons use in CNS metabolism be lost into the bloodstream of certain predisposed individuals, thus producing the cognitive and emotional disturbances of schizophrenia, while protecting the victim from arthritis?

I have described but a few of many studies favoring biogenesis. My primary task, however, is not to support biogenesis, but to expose the tenuousness of the widespread belief in psychogenesis. I trust the reader now appreciates why I predict that the term "functional mental illness" will disappear from use as science progresses.

I am quite in accord with the thinking of Dalbir Bindra (1959), who said, "The available research . . . suggests that the psychodynamic approach, like so many other ideas in the history of science has turned out to be a wrong 'lead' " (p. 138). Like Bindra, I urge that psychologists give serious consideration to abandoning this dead end of research and practice, and turn their talents to endeavors based on logic and evidence rather than on wishful and muddied thinking.

REFERENCES

Adams, H. B. "Mental illness" or interpersonal behavior? *American Psychologist,* 1964, **19**, 191–197.

Astin, A. The functional automony of psychotherapy. *American psychologist,* 1961, **16**, 75–78.

Beisser, A. R., Glasser, N., & Grant, M. Level of psychosocial adjustment in children of identified schizophrenic mothers. *California Mental Health Research Digest,* 1966, **4**, 113–114.

Benda, C. E., & Melchior, J. C. Childhood schizophrenia, childhood autism, and Heller's disease. *International Record of Medicine,* 1959, **172**, 137–154.

Bettelheim, B. Feral children and autistic children. *American Journal of Sociology,* 1959, **64**, 455–467.

734   Nature-Nurture and Perspectives on Pathology

Bindra, D. Experimental psychology and the problem of behavior disorders. *Canadian Journal of Psychology,* 1959, **13,** 135–150.
Bookhammer, R. S., Meyers, R. W., Schober, C. C., & Piotrowski, Z. A. A five year clinical follow-up study of schizophrenics treated by Rosen's "direct analysis" compared with controls. *American Journal of Psychiatry,* 1966, **123,** 602–604.
Brossard, C. Breakthrough in psychiatry. *Look,* April 5, 1966.
Brill, N. Q. Results of psychotherapy. *California Medicine,* 1966, **104,** 249–253.
Buss, A. H. *Psychopathology.* New York: Wiley, 1966.
Dohan, F. C. Wheat "consumption" and hospital admissions for schizophrenia during World War II. A preliminary report. *American Journal of Clinical Nutrition,* 1966, **18,** 7–10.
Dunham, H. W. *Community and schizophrenia.* Detroit: Wayne State University Press, 1965.
Edgerton, R. B. Conceptions of psychosis in four East African societies. *American Anthropologist,* 1966, **68,** 408–425.
Eysenck, H. J. The effects of psychotherapy. *International Journal of Psychiatry,* 1964, **1,** 97–142.
Fischer, L. K. Hospitalism in six-month-old infants. *American Journal of Orthopsychiatry,* 1952, **22,** 522–533.
Frank, G. H. The role of the family in the development of psychopathology. *Psychological Bulletin,* 1965, **64,** 191–205.
Grossberg, J. Behavior therapy: A review. *Psychological Bulletin,* 1964, **62,** 73–88.
Hebb, D. O. *Organization of behavior.* New York: Wiley, 1949.
Heston, L. L. Psychiatric disorders in foster home reared children of schizophrenic mothers. *British Journal of Psychiatry,* 1966, **112,** 819–825.
Higgins, J. Effects of child rearing by schizophrenic mothers. *Journal of Psychiatric Research,* 1966, **4,** 153–167.
Hoffer, A., & Osmond, H. *How to live with schizophrenia.* Hyde Park: University Press, 1966.
Hoffer, A., Osmond, H., Callbeck, M. J., & Kahan. Treatment of schizophrenia with nicotinic acid and nicotinamide. *Journal of Clinical and Experimental Psychopathology,* 1957, **18,** 131–158.
Jackson, D. D. *Myths of madness.* New York: Macmillan, 1964.
Kanner, L. The specificity of early infantile autism. *Zeitschrift f. Kinderpsychiatrie,* 1958, **53,** 379–383.
Kety, S. S. Research programs in the major mental illnesses: I. *Hospital and Community Psychiatry* (Aug.) 1966, 12–18.
Leighton, A. H., & Hughes, J. M. Cultures in the causes of mental disorder. New York: Milbank Memorial Fund, 1961. Pp. 341–365.
Lemere, F. The danger of amphetamine dependency. *American Journal of Psychiatry,* 1966, **123,** 569–572.
Levitt, E. E. Psychotherapy with children: A further evaluation. *Behavior Research and Therapy,* 1963, **1,** 45–51.

Lewis, W. W. Continuity and intervention in emotional disturbance: A review. *Exceptional Children*, 1965, **31**, 465–475.

Maier, N. R. F. Maier's law. *American Psychologist*, 1960, **15**, 208–212.

Malamud, N. Heller's disease and childhood schizophrenia. *American Journal of Psychiatry*, 1959, **116**, 215–220.

Menninger, K. *The vital balance*. New York: Viking, 1964.

Milbank Memorial Fund. *The causes of mental disorder*. New York: Milbank Memorial Fund, 1961.

Osmond, H., & Smythies, J. Schizophrenia: A new approach. *Journal of Mental Science*, 1952, **98**, 309–315.

Osterkamp, A. & Sands, D. J. Early feeding and birth difficulties in childhood schizophrenia: A brief study. *Journal of Genetic Psychology*, 1962, **101**, 363–366.

Paul, G. L. *Insight versus desensitization in psychotherapy*. Palo Alto: Stanford, 1966.

Pinneau, S. R. The infantile disorders of hospitalism and anaclitic depression. *Psychological Bulletin*, 1955, **52**, 429–452.

Platt, J. R. Strong inference. *Science*, 1964, **146**, 347–353.

Pollin, W., Stabenau, J. R., & Tupin, J. Family studies with identical twins discordant for schizophrenia. *Psychiatry*, 1965, **28**, 119–132.

Reid, G. D. Precipitating proximal factors in the occurrence of mental disorders: Epidemiological evidence. In *Causes of mental disorders*. New York: Milbank Memorial Fund, 1961. Pp. 197–216.

Renaud, H., & Estess, F. Life history interviews with one hundred normal American males: "Pathogenicity" of childhood. *American Journal of Orthopsychiatry*, 1961, **31**, 786–802.

Rimland, B. *Infantile autism: The syndrome and its implications for a neural theory of behavior*. New York: Appleton-Century-Crofts, 1962.

Rodale, J. I. Do gluten and milk cause mental illness? *Prevention*, July, 1968, 18–19.

Ross, I. S. An autistic child. *Pediatric Conferences*. Babies Hospital Unit, United Hospitals of Newark, N.J., 1959, **2** (2), 1–13.

Stevenson, I. Is the human personality more plastic in infancy and childhood? *American Journal of Psychiatry*, 1957, **114**, 152–161.

Strassman, H. D., Thaler, M. B., & Schein, E. H. A prisoner of war syndrome: Apathy as a reaction to severe stress. *American Journal of Psychiatry*, 1956, **112**, 998–1003.

Szasz, T. S. The myth of mental illness. *American Psychologist*, 1960, **15**, 113–118.

Williams, R. J. *Biochemical individuality*. New York: John Wiley, 1956.

Williams, R. J. *Nutrition in a nutshell*. New York: Doubleday, 1962.

Wolpe, J. The prognosis in unpsychoanalysed recovery from neurosis. *American Journal of Psychiatry*, 1961, **117**, 35–39.

Name Index

Ash, P., 68
Astin, A., 722

Bacon, M. K., 159–175 *passim*
Barry, Herbert, III, 155–176
Bateson, G., 86
Beach, F. A., 628, 634, 640, 641, 646–647
Beaglehole, Ernest, 199–217
Becker, Howard S., 508–509, 559
Beers, Clifford, 48
Beisser, A. R., 727
Benda, C. E., 719
Bendix, R., 459
Benedict, Ruth, 81, 95, 97–98, 230–232
Bettelheim, Bruno, 709
Bindra, Dalbir, 733
Blackwell, G. W., 366

Blau, P. M., 459
Blumer, G. A., 293
Boas, Franz, 95
Böök, J. A., 608, 613–614
Bowman, Karl, 510–511
Brill, N. Q., 727–728
Brown, J. K., 163–164
Bryan, James H., 556–577
Burchinal, L. G., 383
Burton, R. V., 163, 164

Cannon, Walter B., 99
Caplow, Theodore, 544
Cattel, R. B., 68
Cavalli-Sforza, L. L., 621
Cayton, H., 621
Chapman, T. A., 296
Chein, L., 506–507, 512, 519–520

Child, I. L., 158–176 *passim*
Clausen, J. A., 351, 377, 505, 507, 510
Cohen, Y. A., 160, 165, 169, 173, 174
Corbet, W. J., 291
Crawford, Fred R., 241–256
Cuber, J. F., 319

Davidson, J., 635, 636
Dawson, W. R., 296
Demming, J. S., 385
De Motte, Marshall, 268
Devereux, G., 52–53, 113, 120, 121
Dohan, F. C., 732
Dohrenwend, B. P., 331
Downie, N. M., 384–385
Drake, St. C., 328
Dunham, H. Warren, 336–363, 374, 458, 713
Durkheim, Emile, 135, 138, 463–465, 475–477
Duster, Troy, 522–538

Eaton, J. W., 614
Edgerton, Robert B., 49–72
Ellis, E., 460, 675
Enright, J. B., 211
Erikson, E. H., 91, 175
Eysenck, H., 722

Fantini, A. E., 224, 232, 234, 237, 238
Faris, R. E. L., 374
Feder, H. H., 638
Fenechel, O., 368, 504
Finestone, Harold, 513
Finney, J. C., 101–102
Fischer, L. K., 727
Fisher, A., 635
Flügel, J. C., 163
Forster, E. B., 73
Foster, F. H., 206

Frank, G. H., 705
Freedman, R., 374–375
Freud, Sigmund, 27, 80, 90–91, 98, 163, 170, 175, 289, 305–306
Fried, M., 387
Fuller, V., 384
Funkenstein, D., 434

Gens, H. J., 322
Garfinkel, Harold, 484, 525
Geertsma, R. H., 68
Gerard, D. L., 351, 376, 498
Gibbs, J. P., 328
Gilliland, C. H., 384
Glasser, William, 44
Goffman, E., 654
Goldhamer, H., 84, 294, 676
Goodman, Paul, 581
Gorer, G., 91–92
Gorwitz, Kurt, 249–250, 251
Gottesman, I. I., 614
Goy, R. W., 630, 637, 642
Grady, K. L., 638, 640
Gray, J. P., 293
Greenwald, Harold, 559, 574
Greenwood, M., 397
Grossack, Martin, 248
Grossberg, J., 725
Gurin, G., 342

Haggard, H. W., 494
Hallowell, A. Irving, 96
Harlow, H. F., 158, 647
Harris, G. W., 635, 637
Hart, H. L. A., 490
Hayden, C. D., 292, 294, 297
Hayner, N. S., 257
Hebb, D. O., 704, 722
Higgins, J., 731
Hillery, G. A., Jr., 366
Hirsch, Jerry, 596–627
Hoffer, A., 732–733

Hollingshead, A. B., 319, 322, 328, 331, 332, 366, 377, 459, 460, 674
Honigmann, J. J., 232
Hooker, E., 559
Horney, Karen, 329
Houston, L. A., 351–376
Howard, Jan, 251
Hughes, H. M., 518
Hughes, J. M., 719
Hsu, Francis L. K., 230, 231
Hunt, R. G., 673–676, 678
Hurst, Lewis, 731

Jackson, D. D., 611, 612–613, 614
Jackson, E. F., 328
Jaco, E. G., 218–220, 221, 230–239, 246, 373, 376, 459, 675–676
Jaeckle, W. R., 211
Jakway, J., 630
Jamieson, Dr., 290–291
Jarvis, E., 298
Jefferson, Thomas, 288
Jones, R., 291

Kaelbling, R., 109
Kagan, J., 641
Kallman, F. J., 607–609, 611, 613, 614
Kanner, L., 720
Kantor, Mildred, 364–394
Kardiner, A., 92
Keller, Mark, 496–497
Kenkel, W. F., 319
Kety, Seymour, 729, 732–733
Kidd, C. B., 450–451
Kiev, Ari, 106–127
King, H. E., 122
King, R., 511
King, S. H., 434
Kitano, Harry H. L., 256–284
Klein, Melanie, 86
Kleiner, Robert J., 326, 327, 328, 331, 372–373, 457–479

Knutson, A. L., 223
Kohn, M. L., 351, 377
Kreg, C. L., 451
Kramer, Morton, 247, 250

Lambert, W. W., 159, 168
Lambo, T. A., 114–115
Langner, Thomas S., 422–440, 460
Lapouse, R., 377
Larsson, K., 644
Lazarus, J., 371
Lee, E. S., 84, 370–371
Lehrman, D. S., 628
Leighton, Alexander H., 115, 179–199, 719
Leighton, D., 351
Lemere, F., 729–730
Lemert, E. M., 509
Lenski, Gerhard, 327
Le Vine, R. A., 162
Levine, S., 632
Levitt, E. E., 722
Lewis, Oscar, 321
Leybourne, G., 381
Liddle, G. P., 384–385, 386
Lin, Tsung-Yi, 676–677
Lindesmith, Alfred, 505, 508–510
Linton, Ralph, 24, 92
Lipset, S. M., 459
Lisk, R. D., 635–636
Locke, B. Z., 371
Loftus, T. A., 69
London, Perry, 31–48
Lystad, M. H., 376, 459

MacAndrew, Craig, 438–501
McClatchy, V., 268
McClosky, H., 458
McGee, R., 580
McGill, T. E., 629, 631, 643–644
McGonaghy, N., 617
McHugh, Peter, 538–555

Macirone, C., 644
McLean, Helen, 248, 251
Madsen, William, 217–241
Major, H. C., 291
Malzberg, Benjamin, 84, 370–371, 394–421
Manning, A., 632
Marshal, A. W., 294
Marshall, A., 84, 676
Martin, W. T., 328
Marx, Karl, 317–318
Mason, W. A., 642–643
Masters, W. H., 646
Mayr, Ernst, 618–619
Mead, Margaret, 204
Meer, B., 451
Mehlman, B., 68
Menninger, Karl, 136, 719
Mensh, Ivan N., 440–456
Merton, R. K., 463–464, 533
Michael, R. P., 628, 635
Monroe, Marilyn, 714
Moroni, A., 621
Mowrer, O. H., 557
Murdock, G. P., 170
Murphy, Raymond J., 312–336
Murray, Harry G., 596–627
Myerson, A., 351

Nagi, S. Z., 327–328
Naroll, Raoul, 127–155, 174
Newcombe, H. B., 620–621
Nisbet, R. A., 319

Omari, T. P., 382
Opler, Marvin, 77, 87–105, 219–220
Osmond, H., 718, 732–773
Osterkamp, A., 726

Palka, Y., 635
Parker, S., 112, 326, 327, 328, 331, 372–373, 457–479

Pasamanick, Benjamin, 248
Paul, G. L., 725
Payne, R. W., 616
Pedersen, F. A., 387–388
Peters, R. S., 489
Phelan, Joseph D., 268–269
Phillips, E. L., 386
Phillips, L., 68
Phoenix, C. H., 637
Pinneau, S. R., 727
Pitt-Rivers, J. A., 231
Platt, John, 725–726
Plog, Stanley C., 287–312
Prothro, E. T., 170

Rabedeau, R. G., 644
Ramos, Samuel, 226
Ranney, M. H., 295
Ray, M., 517
Rayner, H., 294
Redlich, F. C., 377, 674
Renaud, H., 716
Revitz, P., 386
Riesman, D., 232
Rigney, F., 579
Rimland, Bernard, 701–736
Ritchie, J. E., 209–210
Rogler, L. H., 332
Roheim, G., 91
Romano, O., 223, 225–226
Rose, A. M., 381–382
Rosen, Alexander C., 653–671
Rosenblatt, J. S., 646
Rosenthal, D., 609, 611, 613, 623
Rosenzweig, N., 68
Ross, I. S., 708
Rubel, A. J., 108, 225, 228

Sanseigne, A., 109
Sapir, Edward, 92, 95
Sarbin, Theodore R., 9–31
Sawyer, C. H., 635

Schneider, P. B., 138
Schofield, William, 723
Schroeder, C. W., 338
Schur, Edwin M., 501–522
Schutz, Alfred, 484
Shenker, S., 386
Shields, J., 614
Shryock, H. S., 365
Simpson, G., 136
Singer, J. L., 77
Skinner, B. F., 174
Slater, E., 614
Smith, Bradford, 271–272
Smith, L. Douglas, 577–593
Smith, W. D., 385
Snipes, W. T., 384
Spiro, Melford E., 96
Spitz, René A., 158, 726–727
Srole, Leo, 89, 92, 93, 99, 219–220, 341, 422–440, 459, 460, 721
Stearns, H. P., 291, 295
Stein, Curt, 731
Stephens, W. N., 162, 163
Stern, Curt, 720
Stevenson, I., 704
Stoller, R. J., 68
Stone, C. P., 641
Sullivan, E. J., 387–388
Sutherland, E. H., 528
Swanson, H. E., 638
Szaz, Thomas, 11, 21, 43, 51, 67

Terashima, S., 281
Teresa of Avila, 12–13
Tetresu, E. D., 384
Thompson, W. R., 622
Tietze, C., 382
Tilly, C., 382
Tooth, G., 79
Tuke, E. H., 294

Uchimura, Y. Imu, 107

Valenstein, E. S., 630, 641
Venables, P. H., 122

Waldstein, E., 138
Wallace, Anthony F. C., 74–87, 114
Warner, W. L., 319, 320, 331, 459
Warshay, L., 381–382
Weakland, John R., 672–701
Weber, Max, 318, 319
Wegrocki, H. J., 220
Weil, R. J., 614
Weinberg, S. K., 678
Weiss, J. M. A., 452
Whalen, Richard E., 627–653
White, William A., 291–292, 295, 296
Whitehead, A. N., 484, 486
Whiting, Beatrice, 165
Whitman, Charles, 714
Williams, J. S., 702
Williams, Roger J., 619, 726
Wilson, G. S. D., 213–214
Wisse, Jakob, 133
Wittgenstein, L., 484, 486, 496
Woodward, J. L., 342
Wright, G. O., 161

Yap, P. M., 107, 115
Youmans, E. G., 447–448
Young, F. W., 165, 173
Young, W. C., 633, 634, 638, 639
Yule, G., 397

Zigler, E., 68
Zubin, J., 122, 123

Subject Index

Actors (professional), 538–555
  audience, one-way communication with, 546–548
  career prospects, 543–544
  celebrity, 544–545
  collegial social organization, 551–552
    uncertainty and, 552–555
  competence, indeterminate standards of, 545–546
  downward mobility, 543–544
  group practices and sentiments, 548–552
  identification with occupation, 548, 549
  income, 543–544
  interaction, 550–552
    competition for work, 551
    personal dislike, actors' view of, 551
  prestige and, 551
  occupational conditions of, 541–548
  procedure of study, 540–541
  public behavior of, 539–555
  readings, 541–543
  self-criticism, 549–550
  socioeconomic uncertainty, 541–545
  technical conditions, 545–548
  typecast, public behavior toward, 545
  unemployment, 543
Adjustment, in psychiatry, 43–46
Africa
  East, 53–66
  Nigeria, psychiatric disorder in, 179–199
  Nigerian folk psychiatry, 99–100
  West, 79–80
Aggression socialization anxiety, 160–162

Aging, 440–456
Agrinado, 235
Alcoholism, 483–501
oral stage experience, 159, 167–168, 170
Anglo-Americans, mental illness among, 217–241
See also Texas
Animal research, *see* Sexual behavior, animal
Anomie, 457–479
Anthropology, psychiatry and, 76, 88–105
cultural anthropology, role of, 90–91
epidemiology of illness, 88–92
etiology of illness, 88–92
fields of crucial importance for, 94
Nigerian folk psychiatry, 99–100
research, types of, 99–104
transcultural studies, 92–99
See also Culture-bound disorders

"Beats," 577–593
attitudes toward, 579–580
characteristics of, 581–582
drug use, 591
females
mildly disturbed, 589–590
severely disturbed, 585–586
males
mildly disturbed, 586–588, 590
severely disturbed, 582–584, 586
mild psychological disturbance, examples of, 586–590
money-making, role of, 591
pacifism, 591
racial tolerance, 591
sense of direction, 592
severe psychological disturbance, examples of, 582–586
sexual license, 591–592
social values, attitude toward, 580–581
study method, 579

Behavior, causal explanations of, 9–10
Behavior-genetic analysis, 597, 615
See also Heredity
Behavior therapy, 723–724, 725
Biochemical approach to mental illness, 75–77
Biogenesis *vs.* psychogenesis, 702–736
behavior therapy, 723–724, 725
biogenesis
case for, 728–733
concept of, 706
as pessimistic outlook, 720–721
"both" factors causative approach, 710–712
causation
concept of, 712–713
content confused with, 714–715
continuum fallacy, 716–717
diagnosis, 719
environment, concept of, 709–710
neurosis, 724–725
pain of mental illness, degree of, 721–722
parallel planes concept, 717–719
post hoc explanations, fallacy of, 715–716
psychogenesis, concept of, 706–708
psychotherapy, effectiveness of, 722–723
"strong inference" research, 725–728
Body functions, conflict about, 169–171
Bohemia
nature of, 578–579
role of, 593
Bohemians, *see* "Beats"
Bouffée delirante aigue (Haitian), 109–111

Call girls, *see* Prostitutes
Canada, psychiatric disorders in, 179–199
Catholics, *see* Protestants
Chicanos, *see* Mexican-Americans

China, 676–678
Choice, role of, 27–28, 35–36
Cities, mental illness distribution patterns in, 336–363
changing attitudes toward mental illness, 342–343
changing rate patterns, 338–350
evidence of, 344–350
definition of mental illness, widening, 340–342
differential rates, significance of, 350–361
psychiatric facilities, increase in, 343–344
social change, role of, 338–340
Class, mental illness and, 477
among immigrants, 406–407
See also Stratification
Collegial social organization, 551–555
Conformity, psychiatry and, 43–45
Conservatism, in psychiatry, 43–45
Conversion hysterias, 101–102
Crime, 35–37, 175, 522–538
drug addiction and, 512–514
law and, 523–524
Criminal
as immoral, 524–525
mental illness theory and, 536–538
as psychically inadequate, 525–527
social context of crime and, 534–536
social theory, 536–539
societal ambivalence and, 531–533
treatment of, 529–533
as victim of external forces, 527–530
Cross-cultural studies, 115–116
cultural differences and, 196–199
epidemiological studies, 88–89, 246–248, 458–461
incidence, new approaches to, 245–248
prevalence, new approaches to, 245–248
of schizophrenia, 676–678, 679
shortcomings of, 244–245
Cultural anthropology, social psychiatry and, 90–91

Culture, role of, 73–176
"bad mother" theory, 85–86
change, 92–93
in Polynesia, 199–217
role of, 83–84
clinical diagnosis, 120–123
comparative study with consistent data, 179–199
conflict, role of, 83–84
as content of neurosis, 81–82
cross-cultural study
of traditional disorders, 115–116
of disability caused by disorders, 117–118
value of, 123
cultural differences, 179–186
cross-cultural studies and, 196–199
cultural epidemiology, 77–78
culturally enjoined disorders, 82
current conceptions of, 77–86
Europe and New Zealand compared, 205–210
Fiji, 213–214
Hawaii, 210–212
heterogeneity, 92–94, 97
New Zealand and Europe compared, 205–210
Nigeria, 179–199
as pathogenic influence, 78–79
direct, 80–86
indirect, 79–80
as per se cause of neurosis, 80–81
role conflicts, 84–85
in rural North America, 179–199
schizophrenia and, 695–698
and sick society concept, 127–155
stress, 203–205
symptoms defined by, 82–83
syndromes, identification of, 118–120
value conflicts, 84–85
"zonal theories" of, 91
See also Anthropology; Early experience; Japanese-Americans; Negroes; Polynesia; Suicide; Texas

Culture-bound disorders
anthropological study of, 109–111
concept of, 106–107
factors contributing to, 107–109
follow-up studies of, 115
and identification of syndromes, 118–120
intensive clinical studies of, 114–115
psychodynamic study of, 111–113
research approaches to, 113–123
recommended, 124–125

Dependence, early experience and, 167–169
Detroit, schizophrenia in, 351–361
Deviant behavior
ideology among groups, 559–560
as labeling process, 508–510
positive, 577–593
stigmatization, role of, 557–558
successful, 557–558
See also specific entries
Distal ecology, the, 16–17, 21
Drug addiction, 501–522
area studies of, 506–508
compulsory therapy, 518–519
crime and, 512–514
in Great Britain, 514–516
laws and enforcement policies, 510–511, 517–519
legal prescription of drugs, 518, 519–520
as physiological pathology, 502–503
processual approach to, 508–510
deviance as labeling process, 508–510
psychiatric theories, 503–505
criticisms of, 505–506
relapse, 516–519
secondary deviation produced by, 512–514
societal reaction and addict behavior, 510–516
subcultures produced by, 512–514

Synanon House, 516–517
treatment, 516–519

Early experience, cross-cultural study of, 155–176
advantages of, 172
body functions, conflicts about, 169–171
conclusions of study, 174–176
cultural universals and variations, 156–171
disadvantages of, 171, 172–173
evaluation of research methods, 171–174
household type and sex role, 162–165
independence and dependence, conflict between, 167–169
love and hate, conflict between, 160–167
materials available for, 172
multivariate analyses in, 173
need for, 155–156
sex role and household type, 162–165
social organization features, 165–167
trust and fear, conflict between, 158–160
Epidemiological studies, 246–248
of social mobility, 458–461
Epidemiology, etiology interdependent with, 88–89
Ethnic origin, mental illness and, 408–409
Etiology, epidemiology interdependent with, 88–89
Europe, mental illness in, Maori tribe (New Zealand) compared with, 205–210

Fear, and trust, conflict between, 158–160

Fiji Islands, pathology in, 213–214
Folk psychiatry, 99–101

Galenic medicine, 13–16, 23, 27, 29
Gender identity, shifting, 653–671
  biological female, 658–659
  biological male, 658
  when biology and environment
    clash, 659
  case examples of, 656–661
    number and typicality of, 661–
      664
    environment, effects of, 664
    persistent, 660
    testing ambiguity produced by,
      665–666
  late shift, 657–658
  as stabilizing movement, 666–669
  transvestitism, 660–661
Genetics
  alleles, 598
  assortative mating, 605
  behavior-genetic analysis, 597
  chromosomes, 598
  defined, 597
  DNA, 598
  dominant alleles, 599
  gametes, 599
  gene pool, 604
  genes and gene action, 598
  genotype, defined, 597
  Hardy-Weinberg law, 605
  inbreeding, 605
  independent assortment, law of, 601
  meiosis, 599
  Mendelian populations, 604
  mutation, 605
  nature-nurture controversy in, 603–
    604
  phenotype, defined, 597
  polygenic inheritance, 602–603
  population genetics, 604–607
  recessive alleles, 599
  RNA, 598

segregation, law of, 601
selection, 605
and sexual behavior, animal, 628–
  633
transmission of genes, 598–602
zygote, 599

Hate, and love, conflict between, 160–
  167
Hawaii, pathology in, 210–212
Heredity
  historical review, 291
  and individual differences, 597–607,
    618–622
  and psychopathology, 607–623
    dimensional-polygenic model, 615–
      618
    family studies, 607–609
    population studies, 613–615, 618–
      622
    twin studies, 610–613
  See also Genetics; Sexual behavior,
    animal
Homosexuality, 41–42
  See also Gender identity, shifting;
    Sexual deviation
Hospital facilities, increase in, 343–
  344
Hospitalization rates, historical, trends
  in, 299–300

Identity, see Social identity
Immigrants, 394–421
  first admissions data, 395–409
  schizophrenia among, 409–418
  See also Migration
Individual differences, see Heredity
Internal migration, see Migration

Japanese-Americans, 256–284
  anti-Japanese attitudes, 268–269
  attitudes toward mental illness, 278–
    279

classification of mental illness, 266–267
community organization, 269–272
crime rates, 257–258
diagnosis difficulties, 277, 281
epidemiology, 258–266
ethnic identity, 273–274
expectations, 275–278
family, 272–278
future predictions, 282–283
hospitalization data, 263–266
individual-group orientation, 274–275
masculinity, 274
means *vs.* ends values, 274
nontheoretical hypotheses, 267–268
and other forms of deviant behavior, 279–282
passivity, 275
responsibility, 274
scientific interest in, 257–258
social agencies caseload, 261–262
stereotypes of, 256–257, 268–269
theoretical hypotheses, 267–268
therapeutic need and use, 259–260
Jews, *see* Protestants

Liberalism, in psychiatry, 45, 46
Love, and hate, conflict between, 160–167

Machismo, 225–229
Maori tribe (New Zealand), 205–210
Mental Health Association of America, 46–48
Mental hospitals, 21
Mental illness
changing attitudes toward, 342–343
choice and, 27–28, 35–36
concept of, 368–370
heuristic implications of, 21
history, 11–19
illness concept, history of, 11–16
implications of, 19–22
internal causal locus of, 20–21
mind concept, history of, 16–19
misconduct as illness, 12–13
model, inadequacy of, 10
pejorative nature of, 20–21
semantic analyses of, 11
stigmatizing nature of, 20
definitions of, 50–51
widening, 340–342
diagnosis of, 49–72, 719–720
in aging patients, 450–455
external causal factors, reflection of, 20–21
germ theory model and causes of, 21
hereditary factors, historical review of research, 291
hospitalization rates, historical trends in, 299–305
metaphor, scientific status of, 9–31
morals and, 32–48
pain, degree of, in, 721–722
physicians, role of, 21
recognition process, 49–72
action, 50
of cases not both severe and chronic, 57–65
cross-cultural evidence, 52–53
defined, 49–50
in East Africa, 53–66
labeling of, 50–51
negotiation, role of, 58, 69–70
perception, 49–50
process defined, 49–50
of psychotics, chronic, 53–57, 65
self-recognition, 51
thesis of, delineated, 511
in United States, 66–69
social causes of, 22–29
term, origins of, 11
See also specific entries
Mexican-Americans, *see* Texas
Midtown Manhattan Mental Health Research Study, 89, 92, 93, 99, 219–220, 248, 341, 422–440, 459, 460, 721

Migration, 364–394, 477
adjustment data, 380–390
characteristics of migrants, 383–386
circumstances surrounding, 386–388
concept of, 365–368
interstate, effects of, 378
local moving distinguished from, 365–368
mental illness, concept of, 368–370
mobility characteristics and, 379–380
patient status data and, 370–380
receiving communities, 381–383
sending communities, 381–383
See also Immigrants
Mobility, *see* Migration; Social mobility
Mother
"bad mother" theory, 85–86
and sex role development, 162–165

Negroes, 235, 316, 327, 328, 331, 339–340, 370–372, 513, 535
care, quality of, 251–252
expectations, 252–253
history of research on, 296–298
incidence, new approaches to, 245–248
incidence rates, variations in, 248–251
prevalence, new approaches to, 245–248
prevalence rates, variations in, 248–251
social mobility and, 465–476
values, 252–253
whites compared with, 241–256
Neurosis, 724–725
New Zealand, pathology in, 205–210
Nigeria
folk psychiatry in, 99–100
mental illness in, 179–199

Oedipus conflict, 162–165
Oral stage, cross-cultural study of, 158–160

Polynesia, 199–217
cultural stress in, 203–205
Fiji Islands, 213–214
genetic basis of culture in, 200–203
Hawaii, 210–214
New Zealand, 205–210
Poverty and mental illness, 380
in historical theory, 295–298
Professionals, moral problems of, 38–46
criteria of disorder, problem of, 40–41
the law and, 39
restricted numbers of, 39
sexual morality and role of, 41–42
social biases of, 42–46
social engineering by, 41–42
Prostitutes, high class, 556–577
counter-morality, 565–567
entrance phase, 561–562
ideology, 565–567, 570–571
teaching of, 563–564
individual attitudes of, 567–569
interaction, 567–569, 571
sample, described, 560–561
social system of, 561–569
stigmatization and, 571–572
strain, sources of, 572–575
suicide among, 573–574
traditional psychological orientations toward, 558–559
training period, 562–565
Protestants, Catholics and Jews compared with, 422–440
impaired mental health category, 436–439
parental religiosity and, 427–435
patient-history factor, 436–439
professional orientation, 436–439
religious mobility and, 435–436

Psychiatry
  anthropological contributions to, 88–
    105
  classification of disorders, 98–99
  conformity and, 43–45
  conservative bias in, 43–45
  effectiveness of, 722–723
  folk, 99–101
  Galenic medicine and, 29
  ideology of practitioners, 41–46
  liberal bias in, 45, 46
  recognition of mental illness, 67–69
  social biases in, 42–46
  transcultural, 106–127
  See also Anthropology; Biogenesis vs.
    psychogenesis;   Culture-bound
    disorders; Social psychiatry
Psychosis
  biochemical approach to, 75–77
  chronic, recognition of, 53–57, 65
  psycho-social approach to, 75–77
  specific, cities and, 336–363
Psycho-social approach to mental ill-
    ness, 75–77

Radicalism, in psychiatry, 45–46
Religion, see Protestants
Role-relationship, social identity and,
    23–24
Rural areas, immigrant mental dis-
    order in, 404–406

Schizophrenia
  "bad mother" theory and, 85–86
  biogenetic approach to, 728–733
  cities and, 336–363
  culture and, 695–698
  diagnosis of, 718–720
  gluten intake and, 732
  heredity and
    dimensional-polygenic model, 615–
      618
    family studies, 607–609

  population studies, 613–615, 618–
    22
  in twins, 610–613
  among immigrants, 409–418
  niacin and, 733
Schizophrenia, problems in sociocul-
    tural study of, 672–701
  communicative behavior, study of,
    680–684
  cross-cultural studies, 676–678, 679
  in family, international approach to,
    680–684
  future directions, 691–698
    culture and schizophrenia, 695–
      698
    factors for study, 691–694
  intrasocietal studies, 673–676, 678–
    679
  traditional approaches, 673–679
    review of, 684–691
  twins, 709–710, 730–731
Sex changes, see Gender identity, shift-
    ing
Sexual behavior, animal, 627–653
  deviance, 648–649
  experiential determinants of, 640–
    646
    early experience, variations in,
      641–643
    post-puberal experience, variations
      in, 643–646
  genetic determinants of, 628–633
    selective breeding, 630–632
    strain differences, 629–630
  hormonal basis of, 633–640
    activation, 634–637
    organization, 637–640
  human sexuality, implications for,
    646–649
Sexual behavior, human, 646–649
  See also Gender identity, shifting
Sexual deviation, 37–38
  See also Homosexuality
Sexual role development
  household type and, 162–165
  status-envy theory of, 163–164

Sick society, cultural determinants and concept of, 127–155
Social change
and cities, mental illness in, 338–340
See also Culture
Social class, *see* Class
Social deviance, *see* Deviant behavior; specific entries
Social engineering, morals of, 41–42
Social identity transformation, 22–30
choice, role of, 27–28
degraded identity, 26–29
involvement dimension, 27–28
nonperformance of roles, 26–27
status dimension, 24–25
value dimension, 25–27
Social mobility, 457–479
definitions of, 460
Negro, 465–476
procedure of study, 465–468
race perceived as barrier, 471–472
racial identification, 469–471
research design, 461–465
self-esteem, 474–475
status aspirations, 472–474
research on, 459–460
status, measurement of, 460–461
Social organization, early development and, 165–167
Social psychiatry
anthropological contributions to, 88–105
and classification of disorders, 98–99
control factors, complexity of, 306–308
cultural anthropology and, 90–91
and drug addiction, 519
Freudian psychiatry, historical influence of, 289, 305–306
future of, 308–309
historical data, comparability of, 299–305
historical review of research, 287–312

Jefferson, Thomas, and, 288
past and present comparisons, 308–309
See also related entries
Social role theory, 22–30
role conflicts, 84–85
Social stratification, *see* Stratification
Society, 33–38
deviance, tolerance of, 33–34
wealth and, 34
economic threat, 33
moral issue in, 37
psychological threat, 33
sick, concept of, 127–155
See also Culture; Professionals
Sociocultural disintegration, 198
Status, 24–25
measurement of, 460–461
Stirling County Study, 186–199
Stratification, United States, 312–336
class concept and, 317–322
mental health research implications, 329–331
as continuum, 317–322
mental health research and, 329–330
mental health research and, 325–333
subculture, class as, 320–322
mental health research and, 330–331
subjective perceptions, significance of, 322–324
mental health research and, 331–333
values, 320–322
mental health research and, 330–333
variation, high degree of, in 314–317
mental health research and, 326–329
"Strong inference" research (Platt), 725–728
Subculture, class as, 320–322, 330–331

Suicide, 37–38
  divorce and, 131
  among high-class prostitutes, 573–
    574
  as measure of societal sickness, 128–
    135
  mental illness linked with, 138–139
  psychiatric factors, relevance of, 135–
    137
  rarity of, 130–131
  social disorientation and, 135–136
  source wordage ratio, 133–134
  statistics, validity of, 131
  thwarting disorientation hypothesis
    of, 135–139
    cross-cultural survey of, 139–153
  See also Anomie
Synanon House, 516–517
Syndromes, identification of, 118–120

Taboo
  sex, 163, 166, 171
  violation, 99, 108
Texas, Mexican-Americans and Anglo-
    Americans compared, 217–241
  the agrinado, 235
  anglicization, 234–235
  background of study, 220–222
  children, 229–235
  death, 232–234
  difficulty of accurate measurement,
    238–239
  family, 224–225
  female roles, 225–229
  guilt and shame, 230–232
  individual, role of, 224–225
  male roles, 225–229
  mental illness, 236–241
  Midtown Manhattan study and, 219–
    220
  parents, 229–232
  sex, 226, 227–230

  sickness, 232–234
  society, 224–225
  world views, 222–224
Toilet training, early experience and,
    169–171
Totem and Taboo (Freud), 90–91
Transvestites, see Gender identity,
    shifting
Trust and fear, conflict between, 158–
    160
Tryps, 79–80
Twins
  heredity and pathology study of, 610–
    613
  schizophrenia, 709–710, 730–731

United States
  attitudes toward mental illness in,
    34
  ethnic groups, study of, 104
  recognition of mental illness in, 66–
    69
  See also Japanese-Americans; Strati-
    fication; Texas
Urbanization and mental illness
  control factors, complexity of, 306–
    308
  historical review of research, 287–
    312
  among immigrants, 402–404
  Jefferson, Thomas, on, 288
  population shifts, historical theory,
  See also Cities; Poverty; Social psy-
    chiatry

Voodoo, 99

Yoruba tribe (Nigeria), psychiatric disorder among, 179–199